Lecture Notes in Medical Informatics

Lecture Notes in Medical Informatics

Edited by P. L. Reichertz and D. A. B. Lindberg

25

Medical Informatics Europe 85

Proceedings, Helsinki, Finland
August 25–29, 1985

Edited by F. H. Roger, P. Grönroos,
R. Tervo-Pellikka and R. O'Moore

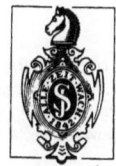

Springer-Verlag
Berlin Heidelberg New York Tokyo

CR Subject Classifications (1985):

ISBN-13:978-3-540-15676-5   e-ISBN-13:978-3-642-93295-3
DOI: 10.1007/978-3-642-93295-3

2145/3140-543210

INTRODUCTION

The European Federation for Medical Informatics (EFMI) is a regional
coordinating body for the National Informatics Societies of Europe.
EFMI has organized a number of congresses. The Congresses in Cambridge
1978, Berlin 1979, Toulouse 1981, Dublin 1982 and Brussels 1984 were
all successful in providing the wide variety of people in the caring
and specialists in the computing profession with up-to-date information from the expanding multidisciplinary field of medical informatics.

We hope that the sixth European Congress on Medical Informatics,
MIE-85 in Helsinki will be equally successful.

You have in your hand the pre-publication of papers to be presented
at MIE-85 as well as the short abstracts of the posters. The proceedings enable the participants to follow work presented at sessions
that they are unable to attend. It also provides a permanent record
with relevant bibliography for workers in the field of medical computing. All the papers have been refereed and the referees' suggestions incorporated in the final text. Rapid publication, using camera-
ready paper, reduces the time required for editing and indexing.
The editorial board has worked hard to improve the standard of the
communications and to reduce the number of errors. Very few papers
did not arrive in time to be included in the proceedings; these are
marked with * in the table of contents.

The papers for MIE-85 Helsinki present a broad range of topics in
Medical Informatics with a trend towards papers that particularly
present the use of computers in clinical practice and in the handling
of data collected from the care of patients. This is a sign of the
increasingly important role of the computers in the delivery of
health care. The rational progress in the use of computers in this
field could significantly increase the efficiency of the health care
system. This is very important today when the rising cost of health
care is of major concern to all the European countries.

We would like to thank the Programme Committee for their hard work
in selecting papers for the Congress and the authors for their contributions.

We hope that this book, that gives an overview of the current status of medical computing, will be valuable to individuals responsible for the development of better health care computing systems.

Francis Roger   Paul Grönroos

Rory O´Moore   Raija Tervo-Pellikka

TABLE OF CONTENTS

* Paper not available

Session A1:   Hospital Information Systems
Chairmen: P. Reichertz (Fed. Rep. Germany) and
R. Tervo-Pellikka (Finland)

Session B5:   General Practice Office Systems
Chairmen: G. Gell (Austria) and
M. Kataja (Finland)

* Paper not available

Session C3: Clinical Laboratory and Intensive Care Systems
Chairmen: S. Bengtsson (Sweden) and
E. Karjalainen (Finland)

* Paper not available

Keynote Speech

Posters

* Paper not available

* Paper not available

NEW TRENDS IN MEDICAL INFORMATICS IN EUROPE

Francis H. ROGER

President of the European Federation for Medical Informatics

University of Louvain, Faculty of Medicine, 1200 Brussels, Belgium.

Computer technology as well as medicine are moving rapidly. It appears therefore difficult to determine where we will be in five or ten years from now.
However, lessons might be learned from the past and the present extension of similar new trends in different countries might be a good sign to take into account for the future.

Fears of computers coupled with excessive expectations.

Twenty years ago, when physicians became aware of the increased availability of digital computers, there was already a large debate about many potential adverse effects of this new technology in medicine. Wouldn't the patient-physician relationship be dehumanized ? Wasn't there a serious risk of dependency from a centralized bureaucracy that could control health care personnel ? How could patients right to privacy be protected ? Wouldn't the medical way of thinking be colonized by programs developed in foreign countries ?

Although all these concerns are still present in our mind, the development of health information systems made progress in most instances without destroying the human relationship between the patient and the physician, as well as between health care personnel and the society. Doctors have not been replaced by machines. Coupled with these excessive concerns were excessive expectations. It is often true that the less direct experience people have with a machine, the more they tend to react to it with both fear and unreasonable admiration (1). The electronic digital computer is indeed an awe-inspiring device. It allows to process large amounts of information with great speed and accuracy, and to communicate more rapidly. It is supposed to give a more precise knowledge of facts to hospital and department managers, to facilitate clinical and epidemiological research, and to help medical decision making as well as the teaching and documentation in health care.

This development of computer technology in medicine has been, however, slower than expected. The myth of total hospital information systems existed already in the sixties.
Comprehensive and integrated hospital information systems proved to be very hard to build. With few noticeable exceptions, most hospitals use at best partial information systems that contain often remarkably little medical information.
A great deal of money has sometimes been spent with little results in return, usually partially working billing systems, payement of employees and a lot of printed reports. Much of what is done in hospitals appears to be a linear extension of the experience gained with older generations of equipment and software.

Concerning the computer aid to medical diagnosis and decision making, most descriptions remain experimental and few programs are used routinely in the wards.

Medical imaging made considerable progress with the creation of computerized tomography and nuclear magnetic resonance but the replacement of XRay films by digitized video-disks takes more time than was predicted five years ago.

In summary, the advent of informatics in medicine has generated fears that did not have often enough grounds as well as great expectations that were frequently disappointing.

New trends in Europe

Spinoza, the great philosopher of the XVIIth century, stated that humanity would
be saved the day when it would find a tool harmonizing centralisation and decen-
tralisation. J. Basile (2) remembered this statement during MIE 84 as he believed
that networking between macro,mini and micro-computers might provide now this tool
expected by humanity.

In medicine, macro-computers were first introduced for administrative purposes.
Medical technology such as the clinical laboratory, XRay department, intensive
care monitoring and physiological measurements were soon thereafter developed
mainly on mini-computers. These machines allowed more real time oriented applications.
Today, the advent of the micro-computer invades all areas where people were prevented still to use computers.
With few exceptions programs used on mini- and micro-computers are, however, often
isolated from one another and unable to share information. Yet they pioneered the
introduction of computing into health care.

Several trends are now developing among European countries. We will try to identify
a few of them.
Some aim at the development of isolated new technologies. Others are more management oriented in order to obtain more integrated medical and administrative information systems. All are influenced by the economic crisis. European countries react
differently following historical and social constraints.
Let's see three main areas of influence.

1. Management imperativeness in health care.

If informatics can be defined as a way to process information rationally (with
all the techniques and instructions that can be used with computers), management is the art and the science to handle an organisation rationally.

Informatics and management cannot be separated. Computer technology requests
systems analysis. This process puts many organisations into question. Adjustments are therefore unavoidable. A better efficiency of health information handling follows generally a good organisation.

The management of health care systems appears, however, extremely complex, much
more complicated than in industrial enterprises (3). Objectives vary strongly
among the diverse partners. They might differ between patients, health care personnel, third party payers, corporate organisations and national authorities.
Even professions in health care are widely diversified. Hierarchy is complex
e.g. it is well known that a nurse is answerable vertically to her headnurse and
has to follow laterally orders from the patient's care team. Furthermore, the
nature of patients information is not only medical. It is also administrative as
decisions to admit or discharge a patient as well as the process of medical
techniques have financial consequences.

These differences in objectives of multiple partners have a particular strenght
in Europe because of the traditions gained by the diverse disciplines. Changes
in behaviour appear therefore harder to obtain than in the New World. Difficulties to obtain integrated hospital information systems seem to be much more linked to human factors than to technological problems. There are many "border con-
tests" between health professionals as soon as computers are introduced.
But two factors, cost containment and new technologies, might induce a profound
change in the next future.

2. The challenge of cost-containment measures.

The first factor is the influence of society in a period of economic crisis.

The growth of health care expenditures has been more rapid than the one of the Gross National Product (GNP). These expenses account for 7 to 10 % of the GNP in European countries (4). Governments are worried about this situation that they all observe. They take cost-containment measures almost everywhere, especially in the hospital sector considered to be the source of the largest expenses.

Given this shortage in financial means, only one solution appears reasonable in order to continue to deliver better care : it is to improve the efficiency of care in order to maintain its quality.

Most governments have oriented their policy toward prospective budgeting and fixed budgets (5). The base line, in the beginning, is retrospective, based on the last year budget. New indicators are necessary thereafter to adjust hospital financing to population needs. Information should be incentive rather than coercitive.
There is a strong tendency to adopt systems like the Diagnosis related groups (DRGs) (6) but many health professionals are expecting results from the United States before implementing such a system. Reforms come in a somewhat smoother fashion in Europe. Some European countries have already morbidity statistics, others not.

Nobody knows how far cost-containment measures will go but one thing is clear : we need comparable indicators about the efficiency and quality of health care. The European Minimum Basic Data Set recommended by the Commission of the Communities (7) should help to reach some uniformity in hospital morbidity statistics. Grouping of diagnoses and operations might be a further step as well as severity of disease indices and measurements of nursing care workload. International Classification and nomenclature problems remain a key issue.

Most physicians have been teached to practice medicine in an individual relationship with their patients. Time has come to consider also the management of groups of patients with similar characteristics.

In this perspective, the computer should play an increasingly important role. Budgeting in health care could rapidly modify situations that were earlier much more difficult to change. For the future, a top priority is ensuring the quality of medical records and the coding of medical diagnoses and procedures.
New trends to shift patients from inpatient care to ambulatory services, homecare and same day surgery will require appropriate indicators of activity.
The patient's degree of dependency on health personnel should also be taken into account as an important measure for management in the next decade.

3. Technological innovation.

The second factor that will shape the future is technological innovation.

Behaviours are changing following the availability of microcomputers, local area networks (LAN), and data base management systems (DBMS). Spreadsheet programs can be learned and applied quickly on microcomputers by physicians, nurses and health administrators. The cost of implementation is low. Ambulatory care, clinical research and hospital management should benefit from these developments. Use of optical disks and LAN technology may solve problems of communication that are still challenging in hospital information systems. For example, two people in different location could access a same record at the same time and modify it to reflect activity without creating inconsistencies between copies.

DBMS should help to solve maintenance problems and allow to devote more time to the development of applications.

In-house versus shared services approaches are the object of a new debate. Larger hospitals are more likely to develop in-house programs while smaller hospitals choose more and more shared services companies that provide a more generalized product. Both approaches have their limits as in-house development might take more time than expected and be confronted with integration difficulties, while turnkey systems might not meet the total needs of the hospitals. Standard software maintained by the industry but allowing for local developments in health care systems appears to be the combination to be promoted.

A few years ago, the objective of medical informatics was often to try to computerize informations generated by the health care system. Now, a more fundamental question is asked : given the present development of technology, the new availability of industrialized software products and cost-containment measures, who should get what information, when and why ?

<u>Each country has experiences to share : the example of Finland.</u>

In this process, each country has made its own experiences, with failures and successes. It is one of the richnesses of Europe to allow experiments in different social and historical structures. For the future, a lot can be learned from our neighbours.

As MIE 85 is held in Finland, allow me to quote three remarkable developments that very few other countries could claim :

(1) FINN STAR, an adaptation from Costar, has become here a standard in medical software. Too many of us try to reinvent what we could obtain from others. This congress provides a good opportunity to estimate the efficiency of this shared system.

(2) The organisation of the medical record in Finland is impressive. It is a hierarchical information system that reflects most probably the high organisational level of the society. Shouldn't we visit Finish hospitals to understand how it works ?

(3) Some computerized information systems such as clinical laboratories have been developed in one center and then implemented by others. I have been told that this lack of redundancy was due to a shortage in public funds. Why doesn't it happen elsewhere ?

There are, of course, many other lessons to learn from Finland especially concerning public health indicators and child care, but I could not quote all of them. The exchange of experiences is one of the main purposes of an international conference.

<u>In conclusion</u>, management becomes more and more involved in medical informatics, mainly because of the economic crisis. New solutions might be at hand with the development of new technologies and we can learn from the experience of others.

The good manager is not the one who undergoes change. Isn't he the leader who can predict change and who can utilize it to innovate ?

REFERENCES

(1) BLEICH H.L., BECKLEY R.F., HOROWITZ G.I., et al.
Clinical computing in a teaching hospital.
N. Engl. J. Med. 1985 ; 312 : 756-64.

(2) BASILE J.
The impact of new technologies on the society and the medicine of tomorrow.
In "Lecture Notes in Medical Informatics", 24 (Lindberg D.A.B. and
Reichertz P.L., Ed.).
Medical Informatics Europe 84, Brussels, (F.H. Roger et al., Ed.).
Springer Verlag, Heidelberg, 1984 ; 4-8.

(3) SCHERRER J.R.
Management approach to selection, evaluation and implementation of HIS.
MEDINFO 83 Seminars (O. Fokkens et al., Ed.).
North Holland, Amsterdam, 1983 ; 84-89.

(4) Council of Europe.
Elements of a policy aiming at reducing the growth of hospital expenditures without prejudice to patients and without compromising progress in
medical sciences.
Special report, Strasbourg, 1983, 143 p.

(5) MAYNARD A.
Budgeting in Health Care.
Effective Health Care, 1984, 2, (2) : 41-49.

(6) FETTER R.B. et al.
Case-mix definition by diagnosis related groups.
Medical care (suppl.) 1980, 18, 52 p.

(7) LAMBERT P.M. and ROGER F.H.
Hospital statistics in Europe.
North Holland, Amsterdam, 1982, 200 p.

MEDICAL INFORMATION MANAGEMENT

IS A RETURN TO NATURAL LANGUAGE POSSIBLE ?

Roger A. Côté, M.D.
Faculty of Medicine
University of Sherbrooke
Sherbrooke (Québec) J1H 5N4
CANADA

INTRODUCTION

In September 1984, Working Group 6 of the International Medical Informatics Association (IMIA) held a working conference in Ottawa, Canada
on the " Role of Informatics in Health Data Coding and Classification
Systems ". Fifty experts from fifteen countries were invited to discuss the basic issues of medical nomenclature and classification in
this computer age. The organizers had expected the group to recommend
a completely new expanded nomenclature from which could be extracted
an equally novel and logical statistical classification. Following
all the discussions, the experts actually recommended a return to natural medical language. We quote from the Proceedings: " The outcome
of the two and a half days of deliberations was the recommendation that:

1. In future health care information systems, the user inter-
    face should be based upon natural language. The generation
    of numerical or alpha-numeric codes should occur within the
    computer.

2. Automatic encoding of natural language be used. This will
    simplify, at the conceptual level, the linkage between dif-
    ferent health care information systems such as: drug,
    hospital management, laboratory, medical records, occupa-
    tional health, primary care, etc.

3. There is need to enhance the involvement of physicians and
    other health care professionals in the original entry of
    medical and other relevant data to increase its accuracy
    and quality.

4.   Multiple health care information systems are required to
     meet the different needs in health care delivery and mana-
     gement, be they primary, secondary or tertiary care.
     Wherever possible these systems should be based on common
     underlying information representations.

5.   Future health care information systems must be able to
     adapt to changing requirements in health care delivery
     and management.

6.   Under the umbrella of Working Group 6, working parties
     should be formed to survey the existing health care in-
     formation systems related to hospital and ambulatory care,
     occupational and environmental health, accidents and in-
     juries, and disability and rehabilitation, with a view to
     recommending improvements.

7.   The morbidity and mortality statistical classification re-
     quirements of national and international groups should be
     the by-product of medically-based health care information
     systems.

8.   As a result of the historical difficulties in converting
     from one ICD version to another, no final decision on
     ICD-10 should be reached until the findings of this wor-
     king conference are explored and evaluated."

In examining these recommendations in their historical context, it
appears that we have gone full circle from natural language classified
back to natural medical language.

NATURAL LANGUAGE CLASSIFIED

The desire of the early statisticians to count cases of mortality, then
morbidity, according to the diseases or injuries led them to take natural medical language, classify it, and then give code numbers to the
different classes.

The International Classification of Diseases (ICD), a statistical classification, is used to compile disease data and to furnich quantitative
data that will answer questions about groups of cases. The classification of diseases and injuries maintained a class structure based on pre-

valence and importance. Although the number of classes expanded, the aim was always to obtain information about groups of diseases and not to manage the medical information of a specific case.

Classifying the natural medical language used for denoting diagnoses by the early and current statisticians was, and is done, to serve a very general statistical purpose. Therefore, once the medical information in a specific patient chart has been coded and analyzed, the case is classified in one ICD category and counted for statistical purposes at the national and international level, and the specific information can no longer be obtained.

At this point, this same case can be coded either in a Diagnosis-related Group (DRG) or in a case-mix group (CMG) for hospital re-imbursement for the care provided to the particular patient.

CLASSIFICATION TO NOMENCLATURE: A NATURAL EVOLUTION

As the need arose for obtaining more coded bits of medical information from patient charts to determine therapy, to associate signs and symptoms to specific diseases for clinical studies and to related all types of medical and surgical procedures to specific diagnoses, it was evident to almost everyone, that a well organized medical nomenclature had become a necessity to manage the detailed more specific medical information. The first such endeavour, was to take all the more common terms of the current natural medical language and to systematically organize and code this language according to various axes as was done in the Systematized Nomenclature of Medicine (SNOMED).

NOMENCLATURE IS ORGANIZED NATURAL LANGUAGE

SNOMED was the first systematized nomenclature for medicine. It is comprehensive, multiaxial, computer compatible and is open-ended allowing for the incorporation of additional axes in the future. Currently it is composed of seven axes.

Axis 1, is a hierarchical anatomic list called Topography and is used to anchor all diseases and injuries to body sites, organs, regions or entire systems.

Axis 2, Morphology, represents pathological anatomy. The included terms refer to abnormalities in the form or structure of the body or its parts.

Axis 3, Etiology, lists all causes as well as causal agents of diseases, dysfunctions and morphological alterations that occur in
the human body.

Axis 4, Function, contains all the normal and abnormal functions,
functional states and physiological units of the body, its glands
and its major body systems. In essence it is physiology and pa-
thophysiology.

Axis 5, is called Disease and consists of an organized list of diseases
and syndromes. Combinations of terms from the first four categories or
axes are equal to a diagnosis in the Disease category, which is actually
the classification axis of SNOMED, while the first four are the true nomenclature.

In addition, there is a Procedure axis as well as an Occupation axis,
the latter being the official classification of occupations of the International Labor Office (ILO).

The building of SNOMED served the purpose of collecting and systematically organizing medical terminology into a form that allows the coding
of specific medical diagnostic elements and the management of this information in a relational data base type system. Built into the system
are qualifiers of information, some syntactic links, a certain logic
and the potential for the development of medically significant algorithms.

NATURAL MEDICAL LANGUAGE INPUT

In the near future, natural medical language, somewhat standardized
with accepted qualifiers of information as well as a recognized useful
syntax, will be used to communicate with computer systems. The language will be coded within the machine using some type of built-in
nomenclature and logic. A nomenclature such as SNOMED or some future
more complex offspring will be embedded within the system.

For the last few decades the major fundamental impediment to widespread
adoption of computer-based information systems in medicine has been the
absence of a standardized nomenclature or even a standard vocabulary.
The creation of such a unified medical language now appears to be a
high priority research goal of the National Library of Medicine of
the United States.

CONCLUSION:

Natural medical language in the form of nouns and nouns accompanied
by qualifying adjectives has been classified to represent groups of
diseases and injuries. This grouping soon gave way to splitting so
that each entity would have its own code. Classification therefore
gave way to nomenclature as more and more specificity was sought.

With the advent of the computer to facilitate knowledge engineering
on a wide scale, a built-in medical nomenclature can be coupled to
a high level syntax to create a uniform medical language that would
allow natural medical language input by the health professional.

Within the next 10 years it will be possible to use a uniform somewhat standardized natural language, typed, written or oral to communicate to a computerized health care management system all the necessary detail from a medical record or a biomedical scientific article.

The generated by-products of such a system will be any classification,
whether for statistics, such as the ICD, or for re-imbursement, such
as that of diagnosis-related groups (DRGs). In fact, we will have
comme full circle.

THE INDIVIDUAL PORTABLE MEDICAL FILE ON MEMORY CARD (The smart card) ;

ACCESS TO NETWORKS

F. P. BEGON

(University Hospital - Poitiers - France)

INTRODUCTION

The idea of an individual portable medical file is an old one which recent technology in micro-processer on cards has made possible. The required features of such a card are :

- confidentiality,
- dependability,
- multiple usage.

Thanks to modern technology, the Portable Medical File is becoming a reality.

I - THE CARD

What holds the micro-circuit is a plastic rectangular card (85 x 54 mm) on which there is :

- a memory of 8 K bits (1,000 letters corresponding to 300-400 coded words),
- a micro-processer,
- an interface allowing information exchange.

a- The memory card looks like a credit card ;

b- 300-400 coded words can be recorded.

The micro-processer assures rapid access to coded information stored in the memory which can be entered by using a password known only to the card owner.

I.1. Confidentiality

When dealing with medical files, confidentiality must be strictly guaranteed.

Each card holder has a secret code.

The micro-processer makes the card completely inviolable because it is the card holder himself who enters the secret code into the memory at the moment when the card is used for the first time.

After the secret code is entered, the corresponding zone of the memory can no longer be read or changed externally.

With each new card the card holder can change the code, if desired.

Without using the secret code, certain people would have access to part of the information (in case of emergencies).

No information can be given without using the secret code. However, in special cases consultation of certain specific zones of the card can occur, bypassing the secret code.

The content of the recorded information cannot be erased, which implies replacing the cards regularly.

I.2. Dependability

The dependability of the stored information is guaranteed by the high retention level of the memory and by the checks activated by the micro-processer (checking the expiration date, the number of uses, etc ...).

I.3. Multiple uses

The memory card, at a cost of approximately 10 $ per card, will certainly become one of the most frequently used sources of confidential information in the future.

Low operating costs.

Its primary use will be in the banking area, as a means of payment and deposits, as well as a portable file of bank statements.

It is obvious that the smart card is a particularly rich growth area within the micro-processer field since it requires a high number of dependable facts, strict user identification, and a high guarantee of confidentiality.

The wide-spread use of this card is linked to the development of information networks, notably Telecom, and in particular to the installation of Teletel in France and Prestel in U.K.. In fact, the full benefits of the card will not be fully realized unless there are terminals that read the cards at the doctors' offices. This service must be inexpensive to use, the same price everywhere, and the rental of terminals should not exceed 7 $ per month.

The wide-spread use of the card depends on the development of information networks.

II - THE INDIVIDUAL PORTABLE MEDICAL FILE

This file has 2 parts - one administrative, the other medical.

II.1. The administrative section

Whatever health care system is concerned, be it private medecine, group medicine, public hospitals, prevention centers or private clinics, proper patient

identification and registration with Social Protection
Services are essential.

The card makes this easier and also paves
the way to facilitating medical care payment procedures,
especially by using a telepayment system.

*a- For Social Service
Organisations : sim-
plification of proce-
dures ;*

Correct and speedy patient identification
also improves admission procedures in Medical care
Institutions.

*b- For hospitals : less
paperwork.*

II.2. The medical section

The medical section of the smart card
includes :

*Portable Medical File
under 3 headings :
- emergency information,
- medical information,
- existing files (dates,
  locations).*

- an EMERGENCY file,
- references to previous files,
- a minimum medical file.

a) The EMERGENCY file

Its contains information necessary to protect
the life of the card holder in case of extreme emergency
(ie-automobile accident, heart attack, stroke, coma).
This information includes blood type, allergies, any known
reactions to medecines, if the patient is undergoing
treatment, wearing a pace maker.

*In case of emergency,
the patient may be
unable to furnish the
necessary information.*

It is hoped that emergency organisms be equipped
with specific readers capable of uncoding this particular
zone without recourse to the secret code.

b) References to previous files

A large part of the file should be devoted
to references to medical records. Each reference would
include the information necessary in order to find the
corresponding file in each medical care center.

*Everyone has several
medical files in va-
rious locations - there
must be access to this
information.*

c) The medical file

Taking into account the relatively small amount
of space left in the card's memory, only a limited medical
file can be recorded. It could include several diagnoses
and their corresponding treatments, coded under the OMS
list, and perhaps recent biological or other tests could
be included as well. Patients with chronic ailments
(diabetes, heart problems, thyroid...) would have several
cards. These specialized cards would greatly help patients
with their periodic check-ups and their treatment.

*a- Standardisation of
medical information
will make the card
universal ;*

*b- Patients will have
several cards ; some
cards will be specia-
lized : chronic ail-
ments, dental care ...*

The recording of this medical information
must be done extremely carefully, making sure that the
information entered is only that which is pertinent.

II.3. <u>The memory card : NETWORK ACCESS KEY</u>

Every patient within the medical care system will have a computerized medical file containing a resume of the patient's medical history, with the diagnoses and treatments prescribed. This will be kept in the medical center's mass storage. When the patient leaves, his card will be made and the file references will be entered into it.

a- Besides the information it contains, the card will act as an access key to an information network ;

In fact, the memory card can not, by itself, be the base of the entire medical file. Its primary utility will be to stock file references recorded in the mass storage of the medical care centers' computers.

b- The network gives access to mass storage memories and to complete files.

In the case of further treatment, analysis of previous recordings will allow identification of the corresponding medical care center. Then, using the secret code, there will be intercommunication between computers, in order to consult or transfer the complete file.

III - <u>OPERATION</u>

Every person entering into the preventative or medical care system will be issued a card.

Determining the organisms capable of controling and managing the cards.

The making of the card must be regulated. The following organisms qualify :

- Social Protection System,
- Public Hospitals,
- An organisation specialized in making cards, their regeneration, and in the technical problems posed by cards and the reading of cards.

Whichever organism is in charge, they will make up the first card (or its renewal), recording the card holder's identification criteria, and eventually putting his photograph on the card.

Every medical care or consultation center must be equipped to read the content of the card protected by the secret code, but only certain places are capable of completing the medical information.

Specify who can record information on the card.

These recording places should be closely linked to the departments of Medical Information or to the Archive Services.

Coordinating the medical words index is very important. The existence of the OMS nomenclature and for various other internation systems is a starting point.

The OMS classification is a starting point for the standardization of medical information.

All the members of the Medical Care System must participate in this organisation - doctors, pharmacists, prevention centers, social service organisations. The memory card will become more valuable when all the makers and users of the data are involved.

The cards efficiency depends on the generalisation of its use.

CONCLUSION

The card is light, safe, universal, and seems well adapted to the problems posed by medical information.

It can be used by medical care and Prevention Centers :

- as an information base, a way to identify patients, for emergency medecine and care,

- as an access key to a network of intercommunication between computers of medical care centers.

INTEGRATION BY DISTRIBUTION - A CONTRADICTION OR AN EVOLUTIONARY METHODOLOGY TO DEVELOP MULTI-FUNCTIONAL HEALTH INFORMATION SYSTEMS?

Karl Sauter
Department of Medical Informatics and
Statistics, University Hospital Kiel, F.R.G.

1. DISTRIBUTED HEALTH INFORMATION SYSTEMS

The overall objectives of computer-supported information systems (IS) in the health care field are to raise the quality and relevance of information, and to improve the flow of information within and between the respective organizations. Historically the application of electronic data processing (DP) tended first - for technical and economical reasons - towards a centralization of the computing resources yielding in centralized IS. During the last years essential progress in information technology, especially with regard to mini/micro-processors and data communications, allowed for a controlled decentralization of system components and functions by creating distributed information systems (DIS). Their global goal is to improve the organization's effectiveness and efficiency based on a better matching of information processing and organizational structures.

In the medical field an increasing trend to decentralization of DP has recently been stated by several authors (e.g. 06, 09). Some of the numerous objectives claimed for DIS are:
- increased DP autarchy of the users
- high data and system availability for the users
- good system performance, esp. short response times
- transparency to user location.
The notion of 'distribution' has sociological, methodological, technical and managerial aspects. Of all these issues the methodology will be considered in more detail.

2. METHODOLOGICAL ISSUES

Major elements of IS methodology comprise socio-technical approaches for the system environment, software engineering issues, data management and data communication. These various methods are strongly interrelated:

database and communication issues e.g. are relevant to all phases of system development, also data protection aspects which will, however, not be considered further (see e.g. 07).

In the context of DIS, the notion of <u>integration</u> has to be redefined in its various dimensions, the basic idea being a change of meaning replacing the centralization of all DP resources by a global or corporate system concept with centralized control functions based on global models for data and processes, at the same time distributing the DP resources. The major dimensions of "integration" to be considered here are:
- integration of data resp. <u>information</u>, oriented at global models and preserving the logical coherence of shared information
- integration of common or shared DP <u>functions</u>, especially by means of a tool-kit for data acquisition, storage, management, retrieval and evaluation tasks
- integration of <u>technical components</u>, with special regard to communication channels allowing for a balanced use of central and local DP resources.

One of the key problems to be solved is the appropriate <u>management of information</u>. Within a complex organization consisting of numerous functional units, e.g. a hospital, there exist local as well as global interests in information. Historically databases have been developed as centralized systems (see e.g. 03, 08), but there is an increasing trend to distribution, allowing for a physical replication, partition or (mixed) distribution of data (02) in preserving their logical coherence.

Another important methodological issue in the context of DIS is that of minimizing the interdependence of applications by developping loosely coupled systems. The notion of <u>loose coupling</u> has various aspects:
- With regard to the processed <u>information</u>, the set of common or global data has to be minimized (see e.g. 11),
- with regard to application <u>functions</u>, the degree of interdependence of the processes involved should be minimized. Considering communication processes, preference has to be given to queued message communication instead of closely coupled message/reply solutions,
- as to <u>system development</u>, this principle may allow for a prototype-oriented development of pilot systems on the base of powerful and flexible centralized resources, and a following realization of the routine system on a distributed base. This evolutionary procedure may

be substantially supported by appling an appropriate methodology for
IS modelling, e.g. as outlined in (10).

These considerations are of general interest for multi-functional hospital information systems (HIS, 09). At a specific site however, local conditions are important as well: organizational structures, priorities,
resource restrictions and, especially, the "data processing history"
which calls for an evolutionary system development, characterized by
stepwise transitions from historical structures to integrated components
and functions of the global target system. Between the extremes of fully
centralized and fully decentralized systems, a multitude of distributed
system configurations may exist, due to the fact that the DIS elements
can be distributed at a various degree (see e.g. 05).

3. THE MEDICAL INFORMATION SYSTEM KIEL

The general approach for a DIS, as outlined above is based on experiences gained in realizing, operating and developping further several disease registries and an integrated HIS (04), all components of the Medical
Information System Kiel (MEDIK). Major long-term projects with varied
tasks to support patient care, research, education, consultation and
organizational coordination are: a supra-regional lymph-node registry
with 72.000 specimen from 56.000 patients, a pediatric EEG registry
with 84.000 findings from 12.000 patients, a supra-regional pediatric
tumor registry with 7.500 findings from 6.500 patients and the after-
care registry of the tumor center Kiel, integrated with the HIS. The
patient-oriented part of the HIS is characterized by a central database
with basic medical and administrative information of 230.000 patients
with more than 380.000 hospital stays. Various departmental systems are
under development, among others a dedicated IS for blood-donors, the
prototype version being realized on the central computer system whereas
the final version will be implemented as a mainframe - microcomputer
interconnection with an appropriate distribution of data and functions.

The cope with the various degrees of integration for patient information,
the following 3-level shell-concept has been developped:

Level 1: This DBS-controlled IS-nucleus comprises data of high integration and communication value, particularly medical and administrative base data and references to distributed information

Level 2: This level comprises a number of dedicated documentation subsystems, managing additional medical data profiles for various
subgroups of the patient population

Level 3: This outer shell is built up by the various - more or less autonomous - peripheral computer systems coupled loosely to the IS
nucleus. With regard to the data structures involved, the minimal intersection consists of a defined set of identification
information allowing for specific aggregations of distributed
patient data, subject however to data protection rules.

The role of microcomputers within the University Hospital and their inclusion into the global strategy for a DIS is defined by guidelines based
on the general policy of the university aiming at a coordinated and
- where relevant - integrated application of DP resources. The major
features are:

a) Basic configurations:
- Exclusive use of the central computer system
- Use of an isolated microcomputer
- Use of a microcomputer connected to the mainframe.

All configurations have their specific advantages and disadvantages.
With regard to the specific application the decision for the most
appropriate solution is found according to the following catalogue
of criteria.

b) Catalogue of decision criteria for a graded integration resp. distribution:
1. Application area (research, routine patient care etc.)
2. Target functions (straightforward, specific)
3. Recource needs (cpu power, storage, languages, DBS etc.)
4. Specific requirements (process control, continous availability etc.)
5. Data protection requirements (data integrity, usage integrity)
6. Availability of trained staff (for system installation, operation
and maintenance)
7. Provision of application software (development by end user/medical
computer center; commercial software)
8. System usage (long-term/project-bound; sporadic/continuous)
9. Relationship with the central system (no relationship; conceptual,
technical and organizational interfaces).

4. SUMMARY AND CONCLUSIONS

First the various aspects of distributed information systems are considered. With regard to the underlying methodology key issues are a
differentiated understanding of the integration aspect and the concept
of a loose coupling of system components and functions. As to system
development the use of an adequate IS modelling concept is pointed out.
In the context of the operational Medical Information System Kiel, DP
policy aspects are addressed, in particular the need for an evolutionary
system development and guidelines for the inclusion of microcomputers
into the MEDIK concept. Concluding, an integration by distribution is
a promising principle to develop multi-functional health information
systems in a flexible way.

REFERENCES

(01) Bracchi, G., Lockemann, P.C. (eds.): Information Systems Methodology.
Lecture Notes in Computer Science 65 (Springer, Berlin-Heidelberg-
New York, 1978).
(02) Champine, G.A.: Distributed Computer Systems - Impact on Management,
Design and Analysis (North-Holland, Amsterdam, 1980).
(03) Collen, M.F. (eds.): Hospital Computer Systems (John Wiley, New
York, 1974).
(04) Griesser, G.: Das Klinik-Informationssystem des Klinikums der
Christian-Albrechts-Universität zu Kiel (Kiel KIS). (University
Press, Kiel, 1975).
(05) Peterson, H.E., Isaksson, A.I.: Communication Networks in Health
Care (North-Holland, Amsterdam, 1982).
(06) Reichertz, P.L.: The challenge of medical informatics - Delusions
or new perspectives? In: O'Moore, R.R., Barber, B., Reichertz, P.L.,
Roger, F. (eds.): Medical Informatics Europe 82 (Springer, Berlin-
Heidelberg-New York, 1982) 909-924.
(07) Sauter, K.: Information Systems Methodology related to Data Protection. In: Griesser, G., Jardel, J.P., Kenny, D., Sauter, K.
(eds.): Data Protection in Health Information Systems - Where do
we stand? (North-Holland, Amsterdam, 1983) 91-101.
(08) Sauter, K.: Databases in Medical Information Systems. In: Lindberg,
D.A.B., Kaihara, S. (eds.): MEDINFO 80 (North-Holland, Amsterdam,
1980) 44-452.
(09) Sauter, K.: Distributed Health Information Systems. In: van Bemmel,
J.H., Ball, M.J., Wigertz, O. (eds.): MEDINFO 83 (North-Holland,
Amsterdam, 1983) 1122-1126.
(10) Sauter, K., Hedderich, J.: Methodological Aspects of Information
Management with Special Regard to Disease Registries and Hospital
Care Statistics. In: van Eimeren, W., Engelbrecht, R., Flagle, Ch.D.
(eds.): Proc. 3. Int. Conf. on System Science in Health Care
(Springer, Berlin-Heidelberg, 1984) 743-746.
(11) Spector, M., Elgard, M.-C., Grémy, F.: Project Analysis of a
Hospital Information Network: Total or Partial Integration of
Existing Applications? In: van Bemmel, J., Ball, M.J., Wigertz, O.:
MEDINFO 83 (North-Holland, Amsterdam, 1983) 1147-1150.

PATIENTS FLOW THROUGH A UNIVERSITY HOSPITAL

R. BAUD, G. THURLER, A. ASSIMACOPOULOS and J.-R. SCHERRER
Hôpital Cantonal Universitaire de Genève et Faculté de Médecine
Division d'Informatique
1211 Genève 4 - Switzerland

ABSTRACT

This paper presents an exhaustive analysis of patients flow (admissions, transfers
and discharges) during one year at the University Hospital of Geneva. Specific
characteristics of different medical specialities are enlighted, such as : admission
mode, duration of stay, age of patients, rate of transfers, etc.

The impact of a fully automated graphical presentation of pertinent data issued from
a Total Hospital Information System is emphasized, as well as the benefits of an in-
depth understanding of the leading parameters governing the patient flow.

INTRODUCTION

The rising cost of health care in western countries has worried hospital managers
and decision makers for a long time. No simple answer is expected in a near future.
The complexity of the health care delivery process shared between private and public
pratices, from preventive health maintenance actions to non-for-profit oriented medical researches, is a reality which cannot be escaped.

In such a situation, any model of the patient population is of value when trying to
estimate trends. If in addition, the model is simple, easy to understand, and presents a strong connection to real facts, it becomes a basic prerequisite to any decision.

Models are often built from a sample of the observed population, and are subject to
biais : this well-known problematic limits the validity of the conclusions. But in
some particular situations, the model can be derived from the total population,
avoiding the aboved mentionned difficulty. This is the case in the present study
realized at the University Hospital of Geneva, where the Total Hospital Information

System DIOGENE [1, 2, 3] as completed at the end of 1984, six years of full production without discontinuation gathering exhaustive data about in-patient flow.

THE MODEL OF THE HOSPITAL

Presently, the model is limited to in-patients only. All medical specialities are present at the 1 700 beds University Hospital of Geneva, except psychiatry. In 1984, the number of patient days was about 487 000 for 35 000 patients. The average length of stay was less than 14 days.

The hospital is composed of a set of independant services according to usual medical specialities. Each patient when hospitalized belongs to one and only one medical service at a given time. A stay at the hospital is made of one or more periods in services. The movement of a patient from one service to another, i.e. changing the medical responsability, is called a transfer.

In addition, there is an emergency rooms center open seven days a week, 24 hours a day. This service is in charge of a first evaluation of the patient before choosing the most appropriate service for the stay. When it is possible, this center treats patient with ambulatory cares, escaping in such way the costly process of hospitalization.

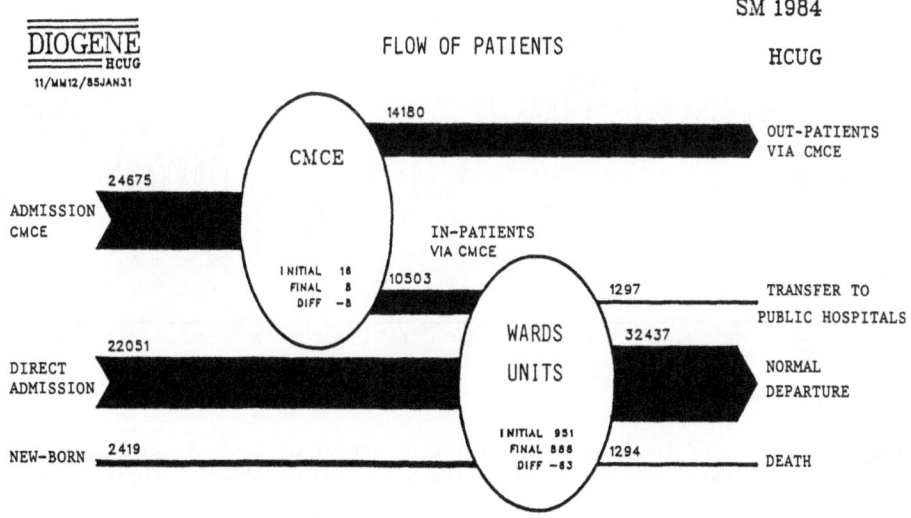

TOTAL NUMBER OF PATIENTS : 49145

Figure 1

Basic patients flow within 2 entities : the emergency rooms center (CMCE) and all wards grouped in a set of medical services.

When admission has been scheduled appropriately, the patient will go directly to the medical service where he has an appointment. Birth is a third way to enter the hospital.

Discharge of patients is possible from any service. In some cases, discharges are oriented to particular public hospital, such as geriatry, long-term recovery, psychiatry, etc. Death at hospital is another situation of discharge.

GENERAL DATA

The basic assessment of the model of the hospital is the patient flow within two boxes : emergency rooms center and the set of medical services. Figure 1 presents these data over a period of one year.

The number of patients present for each day of the year is an estimation of the patient load of the hospital. Figure 2 is the presentation of this charge related to elderly people only.

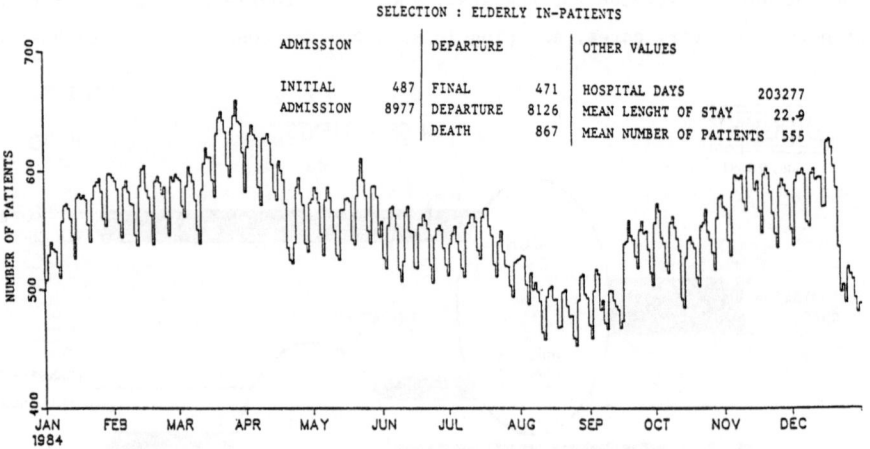

Figure 2 : Charge of the hospital in terms of number of patients present each day of the year. In this histogram, the selection of elderly people is set.

The distribution of the length of the stay at hospital is displayed on an histogram. From this data, the mean duration of a stay is calculated (13,9 days for the total population of patients).

The distribution of the age of the patients is another basic distribution. It is available under different situations, for example with the selection of female only,

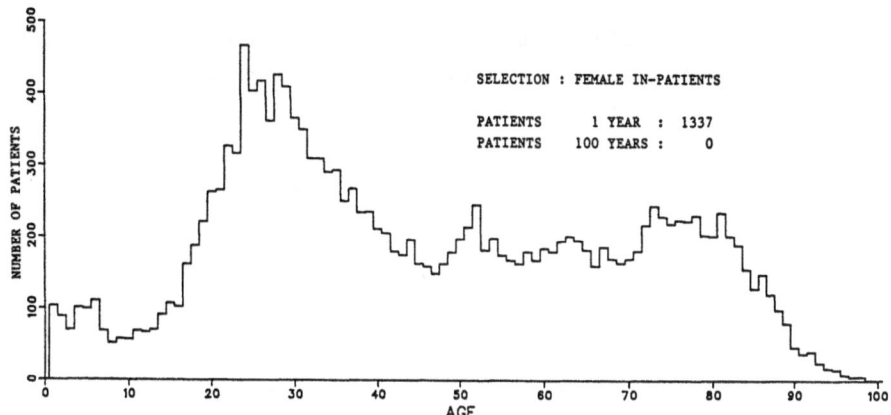

<u>Figure 3</u> : The distribution of the age of the total population of female during one
year. The large pic at age 26 is due to obstetric, as it can be shown
when selecting the same distribution for this medical service only.

Other presentations of data are possible, i.e. histograms, apple pie and tables.
Special selections for sex, age, period of time, admission mode, etc, are available
on request. Moreover data files of raw figures are prepared for further mathematical
analysis.

DATA FROM MEDICAL SERVICES

The histogram of the patient load for each service is presented on a similar way as
in Figure 2. Seasonal effects in some services are strongly evidenced.

The distributions of the length of stay show typical pattern for each service. The
shape is quite different from one medical speciality to another. Figure 4 is a good
example.

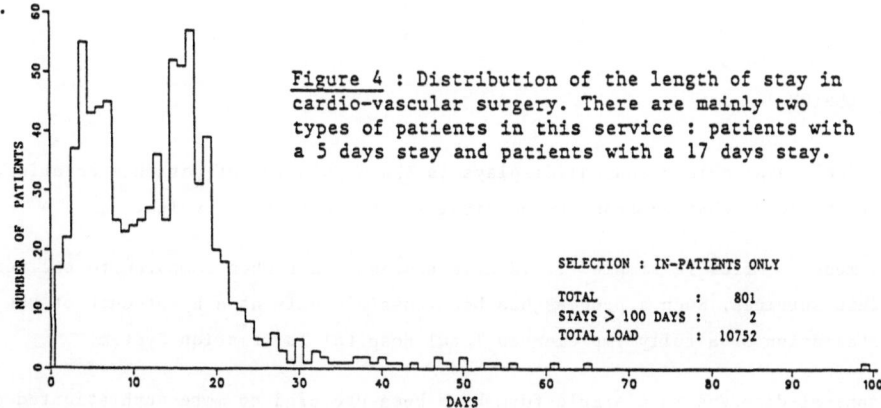

<u>Figure 4</u> : Distribution of the length of stay in
cardio-vascular surgery. There are mainly two
types of patients in this service : patients with
a 5 days stay and patients with a 17 days stay.

The repartition of the load between the different wards of the same medical service is shown with an apple pie. A table gives additional information about mode of entry and discharge for each ward.

Finally, a graphical view of entries and discharges is available for each medical service as on Figure 5.

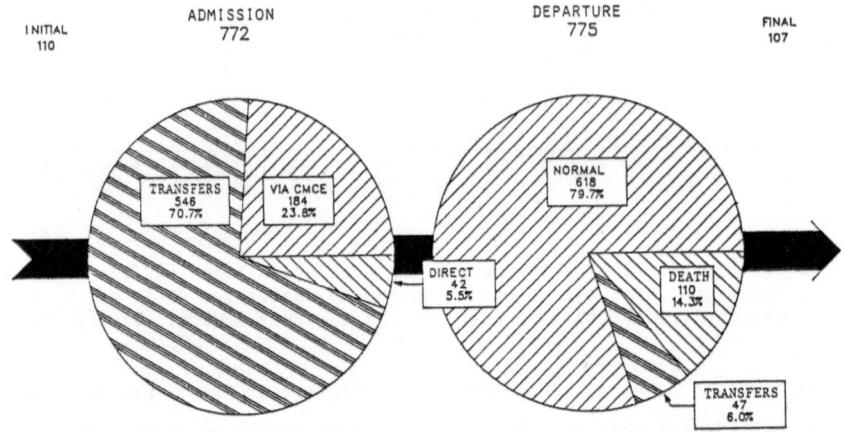

Figure 5 : How the patients enter a medical service and they leave it

IMPLEMENTATION

Every graphical presentation of data is available on request as a dedicated program, part of a general statistical application.

An atlas of all the medical services is edited once a year. In addition, special outputs with particular selections and options in the analized period of time are available as standard products.

CONCLUSION

Routinely available graphical displays on the population of patients entering, staying and discharged from the hospital is of considerable value.

The model of flow is simple. It is nevertheless exact when compared to the real life within services. Such a process has been possible only as a by-product of the installation of a fully implemented Total Hospital Information System.

Graphical displays in a simple form have been prefered to more sophisticated data manipulation. A large audience has been reached without any complex explanation.

Further analysis and developments will be necessary on the following topics : trend analysis, detection of patient load displacement, cross plotting of laboratory data and X-ray data with patient load for each medical service, etc. An analytical view of the consumption of hospital resources and costs, broken down by medical services, will thus be possible.

*
*   *

References

[1]   R. BAUD, E. MESSMER, A. ASSIMACOPOULOS and J.-R. SCHERRER : "The monitoring of a Hospital Information System" - MEDINFO 80, Lindberg/Kaihara Ed., North-Holland Publishing Co. - 1980, p. 1038-1042.

[2]   E. MESSMER, R. BAUD : "Functional decomposition of a Hospital Information System" - MEDINFO 83, van Bemmel/Ball/Wigertz Ed., North-Holland Publishing Co. 1983, p. 22-25.

[3]   A. ASSIMACOPOULOS, R. BAUD and J.-R. SCHERRER : "A ten years retrospective for the HIS DIOGENE, its learning for the next decade" - MEDINFO 83, van Bemmel/ Ball/Wigertz Ed., Nort-Holland Publishing Co. - 1983, p. 73-76.

DESIGN AND PROTOTYPING OF COMPONENTS OF A HOSPITAL INFORMATION SYSTEM

R. Sawinski, J.R. Möhr, J. Wiederspohn, A. Koch
Institute for Medical Documentation, Statistics & Data Processing
University of Heidelberg, Heidelberg, D6900, F.R.G.

Abstract: Many Hospital Information Systems for University Hospitals have to meet increased demands with severely restricted ressources. This situation is characterized and an approach to meet the resulting challenge is described. It consists of the design of a very general application system on the basis of a fourth generation software environment, compatible with the available mainframe alternatives. Selection and design process are described and the results evaluated put into perspective for future plans. The available evidence points to a more than five fold productivity increase in the production of a very general tool system which will enable coordinated but decentralized application system development and maintenance in a very heterogeneous environment.

1 Introduction

The challenges for hospital information system have changed considerably in the last two decades. The users of the information services place higher demands on availability, employment of predefined application components for increased and new applications, which satisfy user needs comprehensively on an integrated basis. Significantly increased expectations in ease of programming and maintenance, on the basis of in house or external services, distributed services and increased use of expert system approaches all require increased involvement of the end user and meet with an increased readiness of the end user to play a responsible part in shaping his application environment. These demands are based on decreasing hardware cost and increasing availability and entail a shift in investment from hardware to software and beyond to development and application suport. As a consequence the traditional approach to hospital information systems (2), (5), (6) has to be adapted. In the following some work is described which can be seen as an initial step in the direction to meet this challenge.

2 Local Conditions

The University of Heidelberg includes a large decentralized hospital complex with research & teaching facilities. Within the hospital numerous more or less autonomous EDP systems ranging from office systems to departmental information systems and realized with a wide array of technical alternatives have been put into operation. Also the fraction of use of the university computing center through medical staff is significant. Attempts to complement these diverse approaches with an integrating system date relatively far back but have so far led mainly to an admission discharge-transfer (ADT) system and consequent administrative applications on the basis of SIEMENS 75XX hardware, BS 2000 operating system (1). There are several small groups within different subdivisions of the hospital with considerable EDP expertise and operations and diverse system orientation and a small centralized group for development.

3 Goals

From this background arise the following goals:

- adoption a system architecture that allows to meet the diverse demands of the hospital with minimal total man power consumption and maximal voluntary involvement of the various EDP Groups irrespective of their current focus of EDP application and habitual environment.
- integration of existing and future applications, irrespective of their having a predominantly medical or administrative orientation hopefully by increasing the fraction of applications based on a common and compatible system architecture.
- maximal respectation of the various end user groups' responsibility for information processes, as well as their requirements of data protection acts.

4 Realization

4.1 Alternatives:

The alternatives for meeting the specified goals include
- (I)   resorting to existing application systems, perhaps with adaption to local requirements
- (II) employment of advanced ("4th generation") tool systems for construction of the system
- (III) conventional system development based on (third generation) languages
- (IV) combinations of the above

4.2 Chosen Approach

4.2.1 Project Evolution

In our case we decided to investigate realization possibilities on alternatives (I) and (II), observing the side conditions that the systems chosen would have to be put into operation on SIEMENS BS 2000 or IBM mainframe compatible systems.

The system alternatives taken into consideration initially included

code	System Designation	Vendor(s)
a	PCSK	IBM Deutschland, UPDATE GmbH
b	ACTION/RADIUS	SMS Deutschland GmbH
c	SESAM/SESAM DRIVE	SIEMENS DV
d	ADABAS/NATURAL	SOFTWARE AG
e	IDMS/R, ADS-online	ADV/ORGA, Cullinet

Based on vendor information (literature, presentations) system alternatives a) and b) were excluded early in the selection process.

Among the remaining was based on a one week training period for 12 participating senior programmers and analysts after installation of all three systems at the University of Heidelberg. This group based their selection on accepted standards for state of the art end user systems (2, 3).

The selection employed the technique of 'Nutzwertanalyse' NWA (4, 7, 11, 12). Execution of NWA resulted in system alternatives d, c and e reaching 74, 63 and 48% respectively of the maximum score. As a consequence it was decided to investigate system alternative c (ADABAS/NATURAL) thoroughly (rather than testing all three systems alternatives superficially).

This test application (DEMOSYS demonstration system) was thoroughly planned with respect to design considerations, selection of features to be realized, distribution of subtasks among project group members, and time schedule.

4.2.2: Features of DEMOSYS

The features realized include:

- all functions are realized in (procedural) NATURAL programs and masks.
- database structures are specified in third normal form.
- mask sequence is controlled by mode specification (e.g. input, look up, print etc.).
- system modules are used to realize menues, branches, command processing, data security, help and error messages.
- these modules are table driven.
- system tables may be adaptable through maintenance functions.
- user interface:
  - commands may be issued in a user defined command language
  - functions, menues and command language are always available as alternatives
  - help functions are available at all application levels
  - masks and menues are composed in a standardized fashion
  - features such as waste basket, transactions, set default etc. are included.
- data security/confidentiality:
  - functions may be activated by authorized users only
  - usermodes are user specifically controlled (e.g. read only)
  - tuples, fields and field values may be protected for defined users or user groups.

- applications:
  - administration of documentation entities (e.g. personnel, patients, investment goods)
  - documentation support (acquisition, plausibility checks, validation, storage, retrieval, presentation of data)
  - maintenance support, menue maintenance, user maintenance
  - production of manuals
  - user training.

4.2.3 Results

While the globally relevant features were planned to be realized as comprehensively as possible the applications were realized for rather rudimentary sample applications. In this way it was attempted to employ available man power ressources which were in the range of 15 man months while the scope of the function to be realized was estimated to be in the range 100 man months on the basis, of conventional third generation languages using the function point method (9).

The more than five fold productivity increase could be met subsequently, although termination of the project was delayed by four weeks beyond the estimated 20 weeks due to the reduced availability some team members which became occupied by different duties with higher priority.

For tests and demonstration purposes a test data base containing close to 30 000 "patients" and close to 100 000 treatment periods was synthetized. These case data are used for performance tests, demonstration purposes and end user training.

So far one application of modest complexity (information system for out patient department in dermatology) is scheduled to be realized on the basis of the demonstration system within 2 man months.

5 Conclusions, Critique

The selection process had to take some short cuts by not evaluating all system alternatives with equal thoroughness. Therefore we cannot be certain to have made an absolutely correct decision. The realization of the predictined goals within a predefined schedule supports us in the assumption that the selection decision was not entirely wrong.

The shift of emphasis away from programming to design was an essential prerequisite to meeting the specified goals. The features of the selected programming language (NATURAL) proved to be very elegant for simple programming tasks while the solution of complex tasks however made us appreciate the features of more stringent and coherent languages e.g. PASCAL. Some of our activities had to compensate for minor deficiencies in the available release of NATURAL (e.g. with respect to modularization). The increase in efficiency for application production (see above) and the reduction of redundancies and dependencies in subsequent application development and maintenance seem to us to make this effort worthwhile.

Similar results have cost benefit considerations concerning the selection process. Excluding the initial phase which resulted in the decision to test one of the three tool systems the effort was in the range of DM 50 000 (DM 30 000 for training, DM 20 000 for man power). If the choice is correct, this amount is easily compensated by the decision against system e which was the preferred system prior to this phase and had a purchase price more than 100 thousand DM above the selected system.

References:

(1) Alle, W., Eckert, U.:
Das Konzept eines kompatiblen Datenbanknetzes am Klinikum der Universität Heidelberg. In Haas, P. (Hrsg.):
Datenverarbeitung in der ambulanten und stationären Versorgung
Tagungsband, 5. Arbeitstagung für Medizinische Informatiker, 4./5. Mai 1984, Schloß Reisensburg (Darmstadt,1984) 96-119

(2) Bakker, A. R., Mol, J. L.:
Hospital Information Systems
Effective Health Care, Vol. 1, No. 4, (1984) 215-223

(3) van Bemmel, J. H., Duisterhout, J. S., Franken, B.:
Fourth-Generation Software for Medical Information Systems (AIDA)
In Cohen, S. (Ed.):
Proceedings of the Eigth Annual Symposium on Computer Applications in Medical Care, 4.-7.11.1984, (Washington, D.C., 1984) 818-821

(4) Daenzer, W. F.:
System Engineering
(Zürich: Verlag Industrielle Organisation, 1982/83)

(5) Ehlers, C. Th. et al.:
Data Processing in the Hospital of the Georg-August-University Göttingen
(Göttingen: Georg-August-Universität, Department of Medical Data Processing, 1980)

(6) Lordieck, W., Reichertz,P. L.:
Die EDV in den Krankenhäusern der Bundesrepublik Deutschland
Reihe Medizinische Informatik und Statistik, Band 45
(Berlin, Heidelberg, New York, Tokyo: Springer, 1983)

(7) Möhr, J. R. et al.:
On Selecting Commercial Information Systems
Medical Informatics Europe 84
(Berlin, Heidelberg, New York, Tokyo: Springer, 1984) 686-692

(8) Anonymous:
Hospital Computing: Prognosis
(Nolan, Norton & Co.: Cambridge, Mass., 1983)

(9) Noth, T., Kretzschmar, M.:
Aufwandschätzung von DV-Projekten
(Berlin, Heidelberg, New York, Tokyo: Springer, 1984)

(10) Reichertz, P. L. et al.:
Das "Patient Care System" in den USA
Institutsinterne Dokumentation
(Hannover, Medizinische Hochschule Hannover, Institut für Medizinische Informatik, 1984)

(11) Sawinski, R. et al.:
Methodische Unterstützung bei der Auswahl von EDV-Systemen
In Abt, K., Giere, W., Leiber, B. (Hrsg.):
Krankendaten, Krankheitsregister, Datenschutz
(29. Jahrestagung der GMDS, 10.-12. Okt. 84, Frankfurt)
(Tagungsband noch nicht erschienen)

(12) Zangemeister, C.:
Nutzwertanalyse von Projektalternativen.
(Scientific Control Systems Ltd. & Co. GmbH, 1970)

AN ICU COMPUTER SYSTEM COUPLED WITH A HIS

J.C. Helder, H. Verweij, H. Kamp
Central Computer Department and
Biochemical Laboratory, Department of Neurology
University Hospital, Utrecht, The Netherlands.

One of the intensive care units has been equipped with a data processing system. This system has been coupled with the Hospital Information System. Experiences with this system and with the use of this coupling for laboratory data are described.

Introduction

During the long-term decision process of building a new intensive care unit (ICU) for patients from the neurological, neurosurgical, otorhinolaryngological and dental surgery departments of the University Hospital in Utrecht, it was decided to computarize this unit. Reasons for this decision were expectations about improvement of patient care and some reduction of nursing manpower and the wish to get experience with this setup in view of the planned new building of the whole University Hospital.

Except in the field of automated patient monitoring, the hospital had a lot of computer experience. The presence of an extensive hospital information system, called (in Dutch) ZIS (1), implied that a coupling of the ICU-system and this ZIS should be considered.

The ZIS is a hospital information system, running on a large minicomputer (PDP 11/70), serving an extensive terminal network (now about 300 terminals) and a large patient data base. Its basic software and applications are developed and expanded in a cooperation of many Dutch hospitals, and covers nowadays more than 10,000 beds in Holland.

The ICU computersystem

For the ICU we decided to buy a commercially available system, which could be modified to cope with the requirements of this specialized Care and could be coupled with the ZIS. After a selection procedure the Kontron DPS 100 was chosen. Principal arguments for this choice were the system's fast response times and easiness of handling, the presence of sufficient and satisfactory functions, among them graphical review of patient data, structured alphanumerical information, an automated fluid balance and so on. Also a competitive price and above all, a fieldproven usefulness of the system were decisive criteria.

The DPS 100 system runs on a minicomputer (PDP 11/23), with three 5 Mbyte disk units (RL01), (2 for programs and online data, 1 for backup purposes and copying procedures), and supports alphanumerical displays with graphical extensions. Bedside equipment can be coupled in an analogous way or digitally.

The operating system, including the resident I/O drivers are dedicated to this application. It is designed for reliable operation and fast response. Application programs, all written in MACRO, are split up in modules of 1 K bytes and have 2 K bytes databuffers for disk I/O. The communication with the data base occurs via macros, which issue an EMT. Each terminal has its own partition.

The data base consists of a number of files for each patient, e.g., for monitored data, for medications, etc. Each file consists of a forward and backward linked chain in strict time order.

The modularity and the strict separation between application programs and the operating system warrant that modifications or additions at the application level will marginally interfere with other parts of the system or not at all. However, the use of MACRO and the small partition size are handicaps for fast program development.

On the application side we have programs for the monitored parameters (see Table 1) like heart rate, blood pressures and fluid output. Specific for this intensive care is the monitoring of the respiration by means of the digitally coupled Spirolog and the measuring of the intracranial pressure. All parameters are measured every 30 seconds and can generate an alarm. Storage intervals may run from 30" to 1 hr. A special pump program controls the digitally coupled IVAC infusion pumps and alarms for malfunctioning.

Table 1   Monitored parameters

Automatic parameters	Respiratory parameters
Heart rate	Tidal Volume
Arterial Systolic Pressure	Respiration Rate
Arterial Mean Pressure	Minute Volume
Arterial Diastolic Pressure	Peak Pressure
Central Venous Pressure	Mean Pressure
Intracranial Pressure	End Exp. Pressure
Pulmonary Systolic Pressure	Compliance
Pulmonary Mean Pressure	Resistance
Pulmonary Diastolic Pressure	Plateau Pressure
Temperature 1	FiO2
Temperature 2	
Respiration rate	Derived parameter
End exp. CO2 %	Fluid balance
Infusion 1	Cerebral Perfusion Pressure
Infusion 2	
Urine production	
Drain loss	

Other programs encompass the fluid balance, which uses the automatically measured input (pumps) and output combined with manual data, a prescription and medications program which warns the nurse when an order has to be done and records the actions, input or retrieval of laboratory and manual data, and structured and free text nurse notes. Reporting is fully parameterized and can be done periodically or on request.

The coupling with the HIS

The presence of a HIS and a computer in the ICU implies that patient data may be present in both systems. It is of paramount importance that these data are and remain equal. Error reduction and manpower considerations require that data are put in only once. From the user point of view it is important to avoid different terminals for the two systems.

Originally a very close coupling between the two systems was intended. In this setup also patient administrative data like name and birthdate would be derived from the HIS when a patient was registered at the intensive care. It appeared, however, that this setup would require too much programming.

Therefore, we simplified the coupling setup, and kept as possibilities
- the use of every terminal in the ICU as a ZIS terminal;
- the possibility that the ICU printer acts as a spooling terminal of the ZIS;
- the automatic storage of laboratory data;

- the possibility for the ZIS subsystems to obtain data from the ICU
system like medications, bills due to actions and data for research
purposes.
The first three possibilities are operational, the last one is in
preparation.
The first two possibilities could be met with an extra printer and VDU
directly coupled to the ZIS, but the required space was prohibitive. The
storage of lab data in the system was foreseen by the manufacturer by
means of the installation of an extra terminal in the laboratory. Since
in our hospital all laboratory data are already present in the ZIS, and
since laboratory analyses for the ICU are performed in different
laboratories, this solution was not feasible in our situation.
Log in on any terminal is started by depressing a function key, called
ZIS. All characters on the ZIS line, a normal terminal connection both
for ZIS and DPS100, are then transmitted to the VDU screen, all keyboard
data are transmitted to the ZIS, except the RELEASE command which
generates a log out sequence. The ZIS has provisions to prevent logging
in when it is spooling to the login terminal. Since a terminal user
might lock up another user who is willing to log in, each user is given
a maximum connect time. In most cases this link is used to interrogate
the ZIS about patient data that are not available in the DPS 100. The
ZIS has the option to give a written report which in this case will be
printed on the ICU printer.
In order not to interfere with the above described ZIS-terminal use,
spool reports and laboratory data are transmitted by another line.
Normally all characters on this line are transmitted to the ICU printer
(spooling). Since the ZIS has an acceptance dialogue after printing, the
DPS 100 generates this dialogue, asking for retransmission when the
system sees an irregularity. This spooling is used for printing of
reports prepared elsewhere in the hospital concerning ICU patients.
In the stat reporting laboratory program (RAP) of the ZIS a routine is
added which for patients of this ICU issues another output of the
laboratory data. These data, for the ZIS merely another spooling but
recognized by the DPS 100 by means of a special header, are sent over
and are stored by a DPS 100 program in the laboratory data file. The
patient is recognized by its patient number, the sample is identified by
its sample number. Different transmissions of results originating from
the same samples are combined internally and enable corrections made by
the laboratory. Transmission quality is checked by means of a checksum.
After transmission the DPS 100 generates a message which causes an alarm
saying laboratory data are ready. By means of one keystroke the terminal
operator can ask for these data. The RAP program still generates
spooling which appears on the printer, mainly for backup reasons.
This setup amounts to a connection (fig. 1) from the laboratory
equipment via the laboratory preprocessor and the ZIS to the ICU which,
after insertion of the patient material in the laboratory equipment,
requires only one human interaction, namely the preliminary validation
of the data and the request for spooling (RAP), and allowing for almost
immediate reporting of stat laboratory data. Reporting of laboratory
data on the DPS 100 screen is in a cumulative way.
In our organization the laboratory is responsible for the quality of the
data. Therefore, a few measures are taken to maintain this
responsability. First, all DPS 100 output is marked as preliminary,
since after the preliminary validation data may be changed and such an
update, although also transmitted to the system may not be observed. The
cumulative fully authorized report, which also can be spooled to the ICU
printer is considered to be the final document. ICU personnal is not
authorized nor able to change laboratory data. Extensive checks of the
system have proven that all data arrived correctly in the DPS 100 files,
and that these data are complete. This could never have been reached in
a human driven system in our situation where the same type of analysis
is done in a different laboratory for stat analysis at night.

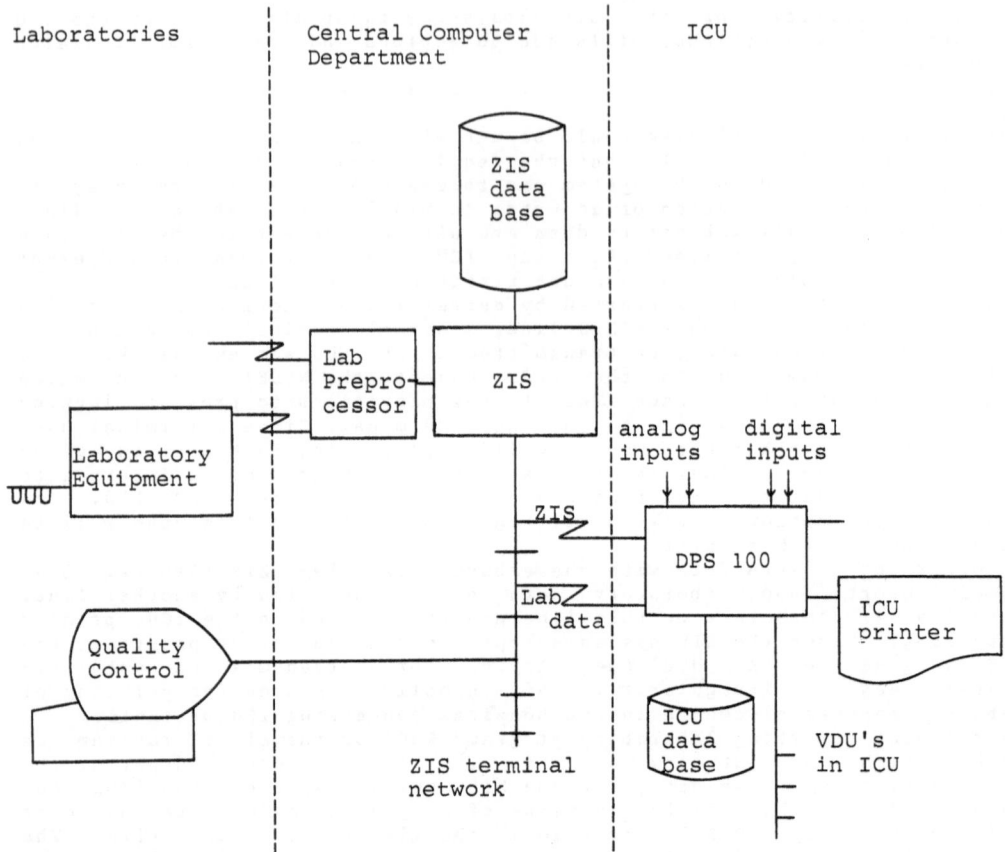

Fig. 1 : The hardware connection between laboratory equipment and ICU

After the DPS 100 system became operational in the middle of 1984, it was decided to obtain experience with the system and to implement more essential changes before using the other way, namely sending data to the ZIS. In the mean time written reports are used to sample data for medications and billing.

Experiences

Our first experience was very disappointing. At the opening of the ICU (March 1983), the computer system was not bug free. The manufacturer clearly underestimated the amount of work involved with adaptations of the hardware and software to our equipment and to the requirements of this type of ICU. He also appeared to have not sufficient support personnel available. For this reason we decided to take over the software debugging and development, supported in this decision by the manufacturer. We needed an extensive testing period, since all parties distrusted the system because of the preliminary experience. So, instead of a flying start, we had a gradual take off.
However, once operational, the system appeared to be easy to handle, requiring only minimal instructions to novice personnel. It received acceptance by the routine personnel very quickly. In practice, the nursing staff is almost completely responsible for entering data in the

system, the medical staff uses the system mainly for retrieval purposes. The use of a computer necessarily changes some of the procedures in the ICU. This might be welcomed by the routine personnel, but for temporarily workers who do not have computer experience, e.g. nurses from other intensive cares that give a helping hand during peak times, it is embarrassing.

A few parts of the system cause problems, sometimes unforeseen. The system is not able to handle the various ways in which a medication infusion is prescribed. The balances for the automatic fluid output function well for urine, but for the smaller amounts of drain leakage they lack accuracy. The free text notes are used very heavily, but for this heavy use the editing possibilities are too restricted.

One main experience looks like a trivial one. In most sites the system is used in a recovery room or in a cardiac surgery care, with a rather rapid patient turnover. A considerable amount of patients in our intensive care are patients that remain there for more than a few days, e.g. traumatological patients. The system has been designed to give a manageable review of data for at most a few days. Considering patient data belonging to a longer period requires different presentation methods, which were not present in the system. Therefore, we implemented a few review programs which present data for longer periods.

Procedures in an intensive care environment are changing more rapidly than a computerprogrammer can work. This implies that the reduction of paper work proceeds less fast than was hoped. It also forced us to adapt a few computer procedures. For medications we now no longer use only a fixed list of about 300 medications and orders, but give the terminal operator the possibility to phrase his own medication. A similar procedure is implemented for infusion fluids.

Legal and hospital requirements, too, require written and undersigned documentation.

Conclusion

In spite of the starting problems, the system functions well and is very well accepted by the staff. The reduction of paperwork already exists, and can be improved by implementing computer procedures better tuned to the organizational procedures in the unit.

A large amount of personnel reduction was not expected and is indeed not realized. Nursing care of the patients has been improved. A computerbased intensive care system, adapted to the specific needs and the specific procedures in this intensive care, making use of other computer procedures existing in the hospital, is a valuable and important tool in patient management, but certainly not the universal remedy for all problems.

Acknowledgements

The authors wish to thank Dr. Z. Kalenda, Dep. of Anaesthesiology, for his critical comments, and the medical and nursing staff of the ICU for their endurance.

References

(1) A.R. Bakker, W. Heijser, M. Mulder "A centralised system still the best network" Medinfo 1983, North Holland, Amsterdam, Augustus 1983 pp 243-247

IMAGIS : A RELATION BETWEEN PACS AND HIS.

Part 1 : Storage and simulation.

J.P.J. de Valk, K. Bijl, W. Heijser, R.C. van Rijnsoever and A.R. Bakker

BAZIS, Leiden University Hospital

Bld. 50, AZL, Rijnsburgerweg 10

2333 AA Leiden, Netherlands.

ABSTRACT

The IMAGIS (Image Information System) approach demonstrates that a PACS (Picture Archiving and Communication System) in a radiology department can take advantage of a relation with a HIS (Hospital Information System).

It is emphasized that use of HIS-data on patient and image data flow can assist in improving the management of images in a multilevel storage structure.

Moreover the presentation of HIS-data may increase the value of PACS multimodality medical image workstations.

In this paper particular attention is focused on the set-up of a digital mass data storage structure. In our opinion the division of the storage component of an IMAGIS prototype into multiple layers is absolutely necessary, if considering the properties of equipment as available nowadays.

Before actually installing any hard- and software, a computer simulation model can be of great assistance in dimensioning the configuration. We have been constructing such a model until now with respect to the storage structure and strategy, of which the first simulation results are discussed in this paper.

We conclude that our model, as far as we can judge thusfar, can yield useful data leading to a well-founded choice of storage equipment, although still a lot of simulation runs, using HIS-data as input, have to be carried out.

INTRODUCTION

The rapid developments in the field of information technology and the growing knowledge and experience about the human visual perception will finally result in the feasibility of an integrated system for storage and (re)presentation of radiographs (and other medical images) within hospitals [e.g. 1,2].

Seven fields of technological developments deserve special attention :

1. The development of storage systems for huge amounts of data (one image may contain several megabytes of data).

2. The development of very fast data communication facilities (with datarates of dozens of megabaud), organised within LANs (Local Area Networks).

3. The development of (very) fast central processing units (16-32 bits wide), sometimes incorporating the bit-slice principle.

4. The development of very fast array-processors, especially for image processing purposes.

5. The development of (colour) image displays with high resolution in space, large image refresh rate and a wide range of intensities.

6. The development of ergonomics, both in software and in hardware, especially with respect to image input and output manipulation (trackball, joystick, lightpen, graphic tablet, touch screen, sophisticated keyboard with programmable function keys, facilities for threedimensional display and time-series presentation etc.).

7. The development of complete systems for handling of graphics and image data, mostly called PACS, in the medical field.

In particular departments of radiology have traditionally tried to cope with large amounts of medical images, always applying photographical procedures. These procedures suffer from several drawbacks, such as :

1. The availability of images can be rather poor (sometimes images are even missing), resulting in problems with lending, management and image statistics.

2. The size of the archive can easily become a big problem because of the huge volume of space which all radiographs occupy together.

3. All images are basically unique, and only available on photographic hardcopy, which implies that image processing methods are hard to use.

4. The use of photographic procedures is quite expensive, if compared to digital procedures both with respect to personnel and to material costs.

Systems which are aiming to cope with the problems mentioned above are denoted in the literature [1,2,3] as PACS (Picture Archiving and Communication Systems).
In the Dutch project we use the terminology IMAGIS (Image Information System), referring to a PACS coupled to the existing HIS.
The Dutch Hospital Information System [4], as developed in the Leiden University Hospital (in fact called "ZIS" - Ziekenhuis Informatie Systeem) is presently in use in 20 Dutch hospitals. These major hospitals serve 11,500 acute beds out of the total amount of 65,000 in the Netherlands.
In 1984 the Central Development and Support Group BAZIS, situated in Leiden, has initiated a considerable research effort to realise a feasible IMAGIS within 10 years. Since then a close cooperation has grown within the project with the Departments of Radiology and Nuclear Medicine of the Utrecht University Hospital and also with the Department of Radiology of the Leiden University Hospital.

A change from the current practice of using a mixture of analogue and digital image acquisition devices to a situation where all the images are stored in a digital format in a central archive will undoubtedly be a very complicated process.
Eventually, however, the following effects should be achieved by the realisation of IMAGIS :

1. Image and patient data become highly accessible;

   The archive is fast, well-ordered, complete and approachable in a simple and flexible way (i.e. from multiple locations with possible use of multiple reference keys).

2. Images can be processed in many ways [5,6];

   The processing techniques may range from "simple" operations (such as panning and zooming) to complex filtering methods, use of colour, threedimensional representation and dynamic series presentation (thus making possible emphasis and quantification of desired details).

3. A positive balance of costs and benefits is realised [7,8];

   Reductions may be caused by saving of material, personnel and archival space, whereas benefits can also be immaterial, e.g. forthcoming from more ergonomic ways of working.

One of the most necessary prerequisites to realise a feasible IMAGIS is a satisfactory procedure for the archival and retrieval of digital medical images [9,10]. The next sections of this paper will deal with the retrieval process, our software simulation model and some of the results of the simulations thusfar.

In our simplified model of a radiological department we consider the room where patients are waiting to visit a medical specialist.

The specialist himself uses a workstation where he can retrieve all images desired concerning the entering patients.

In our current model one or two parallel workstations are included. No large waiting times are permitted for the (re)viewing process. The specialist must be able to dispose of every image within 5 seconds, with an average waiting time of 2 seconds at most. The only way to achieve such short waiting times is to prepare the retrieval of the images in advance belonging to the patients that (have) enter(ed) the specialist's waiting room. This requires at least intelligent scheduling.

Therefore we propose a basic configuration of three storage layers, organised as follows :

1. A central archive of infinite size, but rather slow;
2. A storage buffer of large size (gigabytes), and rather fast;
3. An active image storage layer of moderate size (hundreds of megabytes), and very fast.

(Of course the terminologies "slow", "moderate" etc. are relative).

Ad 1. This layer might be some type of jukebox containing a large number of digital optical disks [11] and at least one read/write unit for these disks,

Ad 2. This layer might consist of one or more large Winchester disks,

Ad 3. This layer could be either a real-time disk or a large semiconductor memory, with capabilities to store and retrieve (processed) images at videoframe rate at least.

From the HIS-data concerning patients and their images (tracking information) we have the possibilities to schedule images correctly, since daily (and sometimes even future) appointments of all patients concerned are registered there.

With respect to the storage strategy, the following remark must be made. If the examination results are stored per patient, the accesstime of his history, containing all examinations, is the same as the accesstime of any examination in his history. One should notice that an examination can contain one or more radiographs. If the "patient-oriented" strategy is applied, a significant additional amount of storage capacity is required, since storing per patient needs an organisation such that in general more images belonging to the same patient can be stored together. This strategy results in more empty space and overhead.

If, however, examination results are stored chronologically, of course longer accesstimes will accompany increasing numbers of examinations, although the total storage capacity can be smaller.

Although a (reversible) compression technique [12] might help to decrease the totally needed amount of storage space, one should seriously consider the loss of time caused by the decompression process, if an image is retrieved. Datacompression and -reduction techniques applied to digitised radiological images are subjects of our current research.

Finally, before describing an actual model, we want to mention the use of clinical (functional) parameters, such as the number of patients and visits, the time needed for image inspection and judgment, the time between visits etc.

Details concerning these parameters as well as details with respect to technical parameters, such as used by us until now, can be found in the following section.

THE SIMULATION MODEL AND ITS PARAMETERS

In cooperation with the Delft University of Technology we have implemented a computer simulation model, as referred to before.

Thusfar only archiving and retrieval of radiological examinations have been included in the model, however we also want to simulate the image data communication network and interfaces in the future. We applied a computer language that has especially been developed for simulation problems at the Delft University, named PROSIM.

We have successfully employed this language until now, but we will also try to use an other computer language for our aims, called SIMULA, which is more widely used.

In PROSIM so-called "components" are defined, each with its own process description.

The following shortlist shows the most important components in use :

Patient	Archive	& Queue
Examination	System	& Queue
Workstation User & Queue	Generator	
Workstation & Queue	Request	
Buffer & Queue		

In our current model two workstations at most are defined, each used by one medical specialist.

A short functional description of the model is given below, whereas the schematical architecture can be seen in Figure 1.

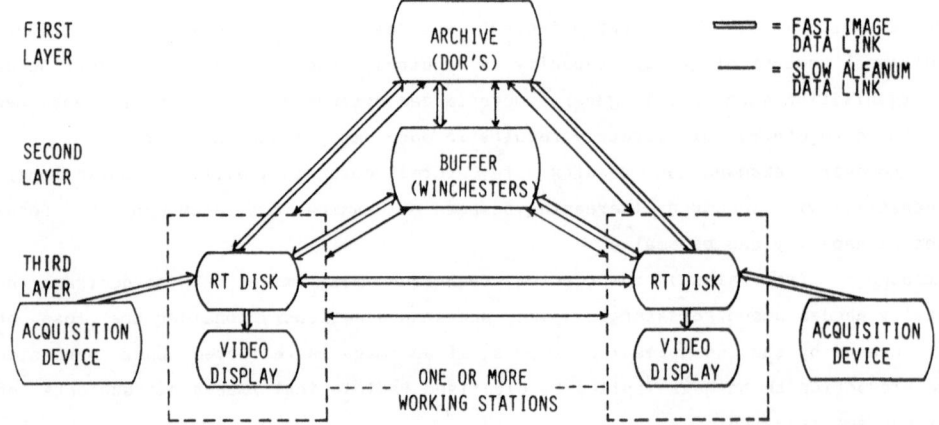

FIGURE 1. Configuration model (the system or control layer are not explicitly contained).

New patients are generated at regular time intervals (INTARRT).

If necessary, a request for the transfer of a patient's history is sent to the buffer if either the patient has been generated, or if he has entered the waiting room. The patient visits (a number of times) the specialist after a particular period of time (ACT_T and VISITS). After a treatment or consult the patient has to wait (INTVISITTIME) before the next specialist is visited. If a specialist admits a patient from the waiting room, a request is sent for the activation of the patient's (and the next patient's) history from the buffer to the real-time disk (belonging to the workstation). Each (set of) requested image(s) is inspected during some time (INSTIME) with a particular time delay at the end (INTPATTIME) between the inspection of the image and the serving of the next patient. Multiple requests can be made per patient (NROFREQ) for the complete history (or part of it). All requests are ranked according to their priority within one of the queues mentioned above.

Our model can be easily adapted by variation of its parameter values. The values of the clinical parameters have been determined thusfar from (pseudo)random distribution functions, with shapes approaching those of the distributions as described in the literature.

However, the choice of these shapes is not a trivial one and our initial choices will be changed in future simulation runs, according to statistical information we will extract from HIS-data.

PRELIMINARY RESULTS

The program output consists of histograms of waiting times for the medical specialist at a workstation, while he is requesting (already digitally acquired) images of restricted size (6 Mbyte per examination average). It is also possible to get data concerning the workload of the three components archive, buffer and workstation (disk), which can help to spot bottlenecks in the system.

Two simulation runs will be discussed here as an example, indicating the trends in the experiments.

In the first run one workstation and 6 generated patients per hour are modeled, in the second run two workstations and 12 generated patients per hour. The most important information desired by us in this primary stage of the simulation project is the peak load behaviour of the three-layered storage hierarchy.

The simulated time was 12 hours for both situations, of which the first 4 hours were meant to bring the system into a stationary state.

With the parameter values given before as input we found the average waiting time to be about one third of a second. Only 4 percent of the waiting times exceeded 2 seconds, whereas all waiting times remained less than 5 seconds.

The following figures give an indication of the amount of requests in an average simulation run: in the last four hours of the runs mentioned above in total about 150 visits to the specialists were recorded, resulting in nearly 1700 requests to the image database.

The load of the system remained rather low, whereas for the time being the archive seems the most likely component to become the bottleneck in the storage structure for increasing loads, due to its large accesstime of 20 seconds.

DISCUSSION

The outcomes of our model thusfar have not contra-indicated the possibility of a real system for storage such as simulated, with images of restricted size (see [9,10]).

However, the validation of the model and the reliability of its results are still subject of our attention.

The high number of parameters to be manipulated forces us to carry out a high number of simulation runs before the results can be completely overseen with respect to reliability.

We also intend to incorporate network properties within our model, thus bringing a complete IMAGIS one step closer.

At this very moment high priority is given to the extraction of parameter values from HIS-data, as available in the database of hospitals using the Dutch ZIS.

Parameter values, which cannot be derived from the HIS, must be determined by observation of the daily routine at the radiology department.

The IMAGIS project has still a long way to go.

ACKNOWLEDGEMENTS

It is a pleasure to thank Prof. G.L. Reijns for his support in the research work reported here.

The preparation of the manuscript has been carefully done by Mrs. A. Venema-v.d. Linden, for which the authors are grateful.

REFERENCES

[1] Proc. SPIE First Int. Conf. and Workshop on PACS for Med. Appl. (PACS I), A.J. Duerinckx (Ed.), Newport Beach, Jan. 1982, SPIE Vol. 318.
[2] Proc. SPIE Sec. Int. Conf. and Workshop on PACS for Med. Appl. (PACS II), S.J. Dwyer III (Ed.), Kansas City, May 1983, SPIE Vol. 418.
[3] Special Issue on Digital Picture Archiving and Communication Systems (PACS) in Medicine, Computer, Vol. 16, 8, Aug. 1983.
[4] Bakker, A.R. "Hospital Information Systems", in : Proc. NATO ASI on Pict. Inf. Syst. in Med., Springer, Berlin, Series F : Computer and Systems Sciences, 1985, in press.
[5] Wang, D.C.C., Vagnucci, A.H. et al "Digital Image Enhancement : A Survey", Computer Vision, Graphics and Image Processing, Vol. 24, 1983, pp. 42-66.
[6] Rosenfeld, A. "Picture Processing; 1983 : A Survey", Computer Vision, Graphics and Image Processing, Vol. 26, 1984, pp. 347-393.
[7] Dwyer III, S.J., Templeton, A.W. et al "The Cost of Managing Digital Diagnostic Images", Radiology, Vol. 144, 2, 1982, pp. 313-318.
[8] Nudelman, S., Capp, M.P. et al "A Study of Photoelectronic - Digital Radiology", Proc. of the IEEE, Vol. 70, 7, 1982, pp. 700-726.
[9] Van Rijnsoever, R.C., de Valk, J.P.J. et al "A Layered Storage Structure for Images Confronted with the Use of X-ray Images in a Hospital", in : Proc. SPIE Conf. on Appl. of Opt. Dig. Data Stor. Syst., Deese, W.M. and Carasso, M. (Eds.), June 1984, SPIE Vol. 490, pp. 49-52.
[10] De Valk, J.P.J., van Rijnsoever, R.C. et al "Simulation of a Feasible Medical Image Storage Hierarchy within the Dutch IMAGIS Project", in : Proc. Third SPIE Int. Conf. on Opt. Mass. Data Stor., Sprague, R.A., Bell, A.E. et al (Eds.), April 1985, SPIE Vol. 539, in press.
[11] Fujitani, L. "Laser Optical Disk : The Coming Revolution in On-line Storage", Comm. of the ACM, Vol. 27, 6, 1984, pp. 546-554.
[12] Reghbati, H.K. "An Overview of Data Compression Techniques", Computer, Vol. 14, 4, 1981, pp. 71-76.

APPLICATION OF PC'S IN COMBINATION WITH AN INTEGRATED HIS

W. Heijser and J.P.M. de Rie
BAZIS, Leiden University Hospital
Leiden, The Netherlands.

Abstract

In the Netherlands more than 20 hospitals use a HIS, based on the Leiden University Hospital Information System. For this HIS computer configurations with up to 400 non-intelligent terminals are being used. This paper goes (in general) into the possibilities of connecting PC's instead of common terminals to a HIS, and into the use of PC's in combination with the HIS. Consequences, pros and cons are discussed. Our plans for the future are briefly described.

The Leiden HIS-concept

The Hospital Information System (HIS), of which the development started as an experiment in the Leiden University Hospital in the Netherlands in 1972, is a grown-up HIS now. Today the concept is used by more than 20 hospitals, together about 11,500 acute beds which is almost 20 % of the total number of hospital beds in the Netherlands. The HIS has facilities for a great number of applications in a hospital, currently about 50 application packages are being used.
Further development of the system is performed in cooperation between the hospitals, which have founded BAZIS, the "central development and support group hospital information system". See for further details about the Leiden-HIS ref. [1-2] and references therein.

In the scope of this paper some details of the technical set-up of the system must be given. A computer system is being used by a large hospital, or by a group of hospitals in case of the smaller ones. The heart of the system is a duplicated central computer-configuration (at this moment are as such in use PDP 11/70, 11/44, 11/73 and VAX 11/785) with large disk storage capacity (up to 1 Gb). One configuration is available for the users in the hospital, the other system is used for back-up, software development and software quality control purposes.
The system is available 7 days a week, 24 hours per day, and has an average up-time percentage of about 99.5.
The system runs under the operating system BOS, which has been developed in-house. One of the features of BOS is the possibility to handle very large numbers of terminals, with short response times. At this moment up to 400 terminals are connected with the central computer. These terminals are either individually directly connected with the central system, or, for cost reasons, in groups via so-called (micro computer based) concentrators. The terminals are non-intelligent (and therefore cheap). All application software runs on the central computer. As a consequence, it is in principle possible to start each program on each terminal. Of course an extensive access control is performed for each use of the system.

Although also a limited number of satellite computers for special purposes are connected with the system (e.g. data-acquisition in laboratories, ECG-analysis), the concept of our HIS is a central concept. Up to now we are generally convinced that, for our purposes, this set-up is less complicated and cheaper than a network-approach, with a number of processors and/or a distributed database. Of course, the approach must not lead to capacity problems, but it does not : even for

a large university hospital the new generation of available processors has
sufficient power for many years against acceptable costs.
However, the central concept is no dogma for us. If it becomes profitable to
decentralize, we will do. With the new generation of our laboratory-subsystem which
we are writing at this moment, we anticipate on such a development : the labsystem
is designed in such a way that it can function on the central hospital computer as
well as on a dedicated laboratory computer, connected with the central system. In
the future other suited subsystems will be designed in the same way. For this
purpose the recently introduced microprocessors in the PDP 11 and VAX-line are very
interesting for us.

What is a dogma for us is the central database (as far as the patient data are
concerned). With "central" is meant at least centrally controlled.
Possibly, if such is advantageous, the database might be physically distributed,
but at this moment this has no advantages at all for us.

Which part can Personal Computers play in relation with such a Hospital Information
System ?

Personal Computers

The use of PC's is assuming enormous proportions. Everywhere in the society PC's
appear, and are used for a multitude of tasks. PC's are available now in all sorts
and sizes, varying from small, simple home/hobby computers (not more than a CPU, a
keyboard and some K memory) till powerful professional ones (with an advanced CPU,
more than 1 Mb RAM-memory, a Winchester disk, etc.).
In this paper we will merely focus on PC's of the type : 16 bits processor, some
100 K's RAM-memory, 1 or 2 floppy disk units, possibly a small Winchester, standard
operating system (MS-DOS, possibly CP/M), and, last but not least, facilities for
communication with other computers (you can take in mind a PC like the IBM-PC). For
this type of PC's an enormous amount of software is becoming available.

Of course the PC has also entered into hospitals. Rather soon this entrance brings
with it the question of PC-users to connect their PC with the HIS. With what
purpose ? Generally this question is not answered very clearly by the users. Only a
few have in mind a clear picture of the way in which they want to use their PC in
combination with the HIS. In most cases it concerns a "dedicated" application for
which only a few data must be retrieved from/stored into the HIS-database. Most of
the users however give loose answers like "we want to retrieve all kinds of data
from the HIS", and "we want to play with some HIS-data", without being able to
become more concrete.
Putting this question to suppliers of PC's, and asking them for examples of
application of PC's in comparable situations, generally does not get you any
further.
Is it possible to become more concrete at this point ? Let's try it, somewhat
systematically.

Possibilities for use of PC's

We can classify the use of PC's in a hospital which has a HIS to its disposal in
the following way.
1. Stand-alone use of PC's, without any relation with the HIS.
2. Use of the PC as a HIS-terminal. This requires that the PC can emulate a
   terminal, which means in our case the asynchronous VT52/VT100-protocol, in other
   cases e.g. behaviour of a block-mode terminal.

Because PC's are more expensive than common terminals, use of PC's only for this purpose has no advantages. But, of course, combination of 1 and 2 has. Instead of a PC plus a common terminal you only need a PC ("equipment-integration").
3. Record/file-transfer between PC and HIS.
   According to a certain protocol/mechanism the PC can send data which have been prepared by the PC to the HIS, e.g. for storage into the HIS-database or for further processing or distribution by the central system (example : data-acquisition, -reduction and -preprocessing in laboratories).
   Vice versa, and even more important, the PC can ask for HIS-data, and process and manipulate them (example : analysis and graphical presentation of data which have been archived in the HIS-database).
   Although somewhat arbitrary, the PC (-software) is not considered to be a part of the HIS.
4. The HIS is designed in such a way that typical HIS-functions are carried out by PC's. Workfiles and possibly local copies of central files are located at the PC (example : a PC on a nursing-ward, with data concerning the admitted patients present in the PC).
   In this set-up, which requires more advanced communication-facilities between HIS and PC, the PC is really an integrated part of the HIS.

The boundaries between these four classes are not always very sharp, and of course all kinds of combinations of PC-use are possible.

Discussion

Let's now discuss a number of aspects of the use of PC's in hospitals, especially in relation with a hospital information system, with in mind as the most important question : when (and why) is it possible and advantageous to apply a PC instead of using central HIS-facilities.
Flexibility for the user.
PC's offer a high degree of flexibility to the user. He can select, install, modify his software, without being dependent on a central data processing department and heavy HIS-procedures.
Experiments can easily be performed. If adjustment turns out to be necessary, it is rapidly possible.
Software development by the user himself.
You have to be very careful if you let users develop their own software within the hospital information system. To avoid disasters you have to establish very severe procedures, which are attractive nor for the users nor for the DP-department. With a PC you can let the user have his way, without being anxious that he will disturb the HIS-production. This holds as far as PC-use of classes 1-3 is concerned, and supposed that adequate HIS-access control measures have been taken. Both at this and the previous point things become different when you start using PC's for class 4-purposes. Because in this case the PC is an integrated part of the HIS, an own software development by the user brings much more risks with it, and you have to apply the same severe procedures as to the software development at the central system.
Tools for software development.
Generally the development-facilities which are available on a big system in a professional environment are much better than those with PC's. This is not very important for the person who incidentally writes a program, but it is for professional software-development.
Available software.
For the current types of PC's a lot of software is available (of which the quality is strongly varying !). The amount of commercially available software is growing rapidly. Besides, it is quite simple to copy and to implement programs which are written by friendly colleagues.
At this point a PC gives much more possibilities than big computer systems.

Integration.

Sometimes software-packages function purely "stand-alone", but very often programs require data from other software, deliver results for further processing by other packages, or contain "excursions" to other programs: a hospital itself is just an integrated system ! This type of communication between software is frequently very difficult or even impossible with commercially available or other "foreign" software, because it has no or insufficient standard facilities at this point, while the source-code is not available. This is a very complicating factor for a smooth integration of PC's within a HIS. Of course within a (central) HIS this type of communication is much easier to perform.

Let me give a very characteristic example at this point. For PC's a number of excellent word processing packages exist. Word processing is very valuable e.g. for patient correspondence. However, many of the data which are inserted in a patient letter are already present in the HIS (patient-name, -number, -address, physician, results of investigation and treatment).

If you want to use a PC (or a common word processor) coupled to the HIS for this purpose, it is generally impossible to insert the already available data automatically in your document (by using commands, function keys and such).

In practice it is also impossible to modify the word processing software yourself because the source code is not available.

This example is one of the reasons we have developed our own word processing facilities within the HIS [3-4].

Data definition.

One of the largest risks of the introduction of PC's in hospitals is that people are going to use in their programs their own definitions of all kinds of hospital quantities, and compare their results with results based on other definitions.

This may lead to an enormous confusion of tongues.

It is also for this reason that a central database is very important for us.

Software control

Round a HIS you must have good control procedures. It must be clear who controls the program-sources, with which source the (only!) current load-module corresponds, etc.

It needs no explaining that this requires much more attention in case of an extensive use of PC's with own storage facilities, than for a (central) HIS.

Data-protection.

Especially in hospitals a very important subject.

A (central) HIS can be supplied with a good access control mechanism. With the sending of data to a PC, they disappear from sight of the hospital authorities. Of course the same holds for printed information in the centralized set-up, and even in the non-automated situation (in which privacy aspects often get much less attention than in the automated one). An important difference however is the scale in which undesirable use of (patient) data (systematically) becomes possible if no adequate measures are taken.

This point needs much attention.

Calamities.

In a HIS, housed in a professional computer centre, it is possible to offer effective back-up and recover-facilities, as well as protection against fire and theft. Again it needs no explaining that comparable facilities in a distributed approach are more complicated. Besides they require much discipline of the user. But of course the size of the disaster is generally much smaller in the PC-case.

Cost aspects.

From application to application should be considered whether a central or a PC-solution is more profitable. A general rule cannot be given. Besides that, you often compare solutions which are (functionally) not equivalent.

You can say that, because the price-difference between PC's and common terminals is going down, and because PC's can also be applied as a terminal, it becomes more attractive to install PC's.

Concerning the software, again no general rules can be given. Frequently it is stated that the commercially available software is cheaper than an own development, but such statements must be looked at suspiciously. Probably it holds if the software is only used by one PC, but things may become different when you have to

pay for more than one licence.
Finally, the hidden costs as a result of software development by the user himself should not be forgotten.

Conclusions

Application of PC's instead of or in combination with central facilities has pros and cons. As pointed out it is certainly not true that the PC is the solution for all your problems, as is frequently suggested these days. On the other hand, for certain applications use of PC's may be very valuable. But be very careful, and try to avoid uncontrollable developments.
According to this advice, in our hospitals we are introducing PC's for use in combination with the HIS little by little. The PC's are used for application in the classes 1, 2 and 3 as mentioned before, for the present not yet in class 4.
It is foreseen that the number of connected PC's for a large hospital (1000 beds) will increase with about 20 per year, which means that at the end of the eighties about 100 PC's will be connected with the central computer, that is 15 % of the total number of terminals. After the goregoing it will be obvious that, with this development, we will hold to the concept of a central database.

References

[1] A.R. Bakker, The development of an integrated and co-operative hospital information system, Med. Inform. 9 (1984) 135.
[2] A.R. Bakker and J.L. Mol, Hospital Information Systems, Effective Health Care 1 (1984) 215.
[3] R.J.A. Dujarding and W. Heijser, Hospital Information Systems and Word Processing, in Proc. MEDINFO 83, J.H. van Bemmel et al., eds, p. 100 (North Holland, Amsterdam, 1983).
[4] R.J.A. Dujardin, Experiences with word processing integrated in a hospital information system, these proceedings.

AN APPROACH TO THE DEVELOPMENT OF A COMPLEX INFORMATION SYSTEM

FOR THE WROCŁAW PROVINCE HOSPITAL

I. Klimek–Grzesiak,   J.B. Lewoc,   J. Lorenz,   W. Minta

Voivodeship Wrocław, Health and Social Care Dpt., Pl. Powstańców Warszawy 1,
50–951 Wrocław;   POLAND.

Computer Systems and Computer Section, Polish Electrical Engineers Society, Wrocław Region,
ul. Świerczewskiego 74,   50–020 Wrocław;

Hospital of 40 th Anniversary of the Polish People's Republic, ul. Kamieńskiego 73a,
51–124 Wrocław,

Central Hospital CKP WAM, 00–909 WARSZAWA 60, ul. Szaserów 128

In Poland, several hospital information systems have been developed or are in progres. They are oriented towards solutions of specific fragmentary problems and developed on various home and imported hardware. This way is not preferable for a country in a down economy period and in 1984 a project was initiated for development of a reproducible complex information system which should constitute a sound basis for a global Health Service Information System in our country.

The aim of the present paper is to discuss our approach to the development of the System in order to obtain advice, criticism and/or approval of our ideas at the instant that it is still possible to make the best of them in our job.

THE APPROACH TO DEVELOPMENT OF THE SYSTEM

The basis for defining the approach to development of General hospital system topology Ghost are its objectives:
– utilitary goal: improvement of medical care results due to development of tools facilitating data acquisition and collection for health Service;
– Didactic goal: training of experts in design, development, implementation and use of computer systems and networks for Health Service;
– Research goal: development of novel medical techniques in the domain of studies on large populations and of computer system and network development.

Local bonds are another premise: we do not possess information on successful implementations of similar global systems; economical troubles of our country make it necessary to develop Ghost on home hardware and exclude high initial investment; there is an experienced staff or computer experts and doctors capable of solving big problems; there is no global public communication network, a severe lack of communication links and lack of effective experience on local raea networks.

The above premises imply a safe approach: a new hospital (Hospital) was chosen and the first lane along which a patient suffering urinary tract illness passes in a typical case (the Thread) was defined. At the points where lanes of many patients cross facilities are to be provided for all of them; thus the Computer facility initial topology is being created. The Thread is dedicated to one and only one user: a ulorogist and the only criterion of Comfit quality is if the User uses the facilities along the Thread. In our opinion, system quality must not be assessed basing on more or less arbitrary technical characteristics and/or measures or by voting (usually with discrimination) in a multiuser collection.

A team of people involved in the development of the Thread, starting from the first User via representatives of all units along the thread.

The Patient enters the Urology (department) where he may pass any of the following treatment actions: determination of illness cause (lithiasis cause, urodynamical measurements of pressure), instrumental treatment (electroresection, Zeiss loop), operational treatment (determination of chronic formotherapy), conservation cure of lithiasis and urinic acid. Typical examples of long—term treatment may be: care of Patient suffering from papillomatous tumor (cystoscopy, cytological examination of urine, feeding of cytostatics); care of the Patient suffering from tumor (examination, liver action testing, X—ray examination of bones).

For Urology two new files are foreseen: Patient (data on patients in the Department, ca. 150,000 characters) and History (history of treatment file — ca 5 mln characters per year).

From Urology the Patient may enter again the Ambulatory. Data files are then the same as those described heretofore.

MEDICAL RESEARCH WORK

Computer data acquisition and retrieval should add new quality to the User's work by enabling real research work covering: automatic locating of ward infections, analysis of complications, hazard source locating and/or analysis, etc.

HOSPITAL ADMINISTRATION

Hospital administration provides services very important to Patient's comfort and, consequently, to results of medical treatment. In spite of that administration has not been included into the Thread. This job is being done by another group involved in computerization of Health Service.

HARDWARE ENVIRONMENT

Designing hardware environments is, like freedom, a realized necessity. The two types of rather big computers manufactured in our country cannot be considered for the application because of economical and/or technical reasons. Low stability of private companies production excludes many microcomputer systems available now. Therefore, a PDP—11/40 compatible minicomputer SM—4 and Intel 8080 based microcomputers MK 4501 and/or PSPD 90 were chosen and a star topology was proposed for Comfit (Fig. 1). Doubled SM—4 configuration was chosen to ensure higher availability factor and to remove off—line jobs from the basic minicomputer.

Further development of Comfit (increasing number of terminals, change to discs of higher capacity) will be limited for several years by computing capabilities of the minicomputers and by low reliability of the star topology. We do hope that in some five years governmental computer manufacturers will be delivering hardware enabling easy development of local computer networks. Therefore, it is planned to change back to the topology worked out in hospitals for centuries but, of course, using microcomputer facilities. Thus, the Hospital network system will be developed (Fig. 2). We have chosen a ring type network (probably based on Cambridge Data Ring [1] because of simple technical solutions required) since bus type networks or Ethernet [2] like ones are inacceptable because of technical and/or operational reasons [3] according to the leading designer and project menager. Inclusion of the User to actual work from its very beginning and medical services is intended to increase gradually their xonfidence in computer experts and to enlarge chances for positive results.

Urology was chosen because of two reasons: objective reason — urology covers a wide range of medical specializations; subjective one — experience of the leading designer as a urology user (dissectio renis arcuatus). The latter is even more important because it is easy to find a common language with the User as well as because of an individual view upon activities of the Urology Department.

46

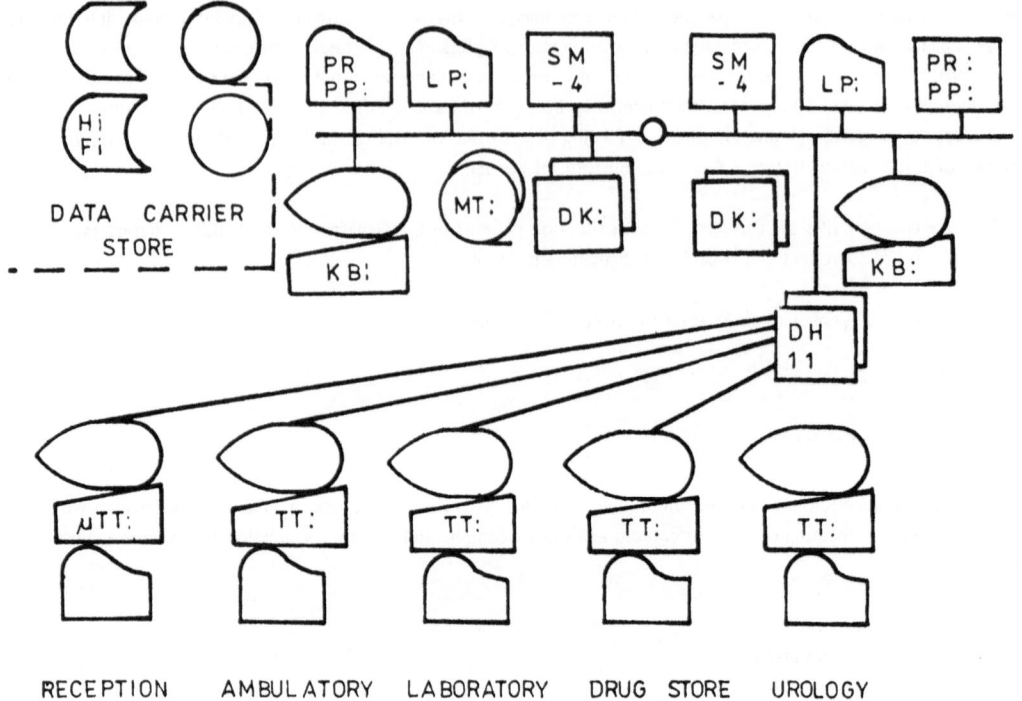

RECEPTION   AMBULATORY   LABORATORY   DRUG STORE   UROLOGY

Fig. 1. System Comfit
Legend: DK: − disks, KB: − keyboard and screen, LP: − printer, PP: − taper punch,
PR: − paper tape reader, MT: − magnetic tapes, DH11 − multiplexer, TT: − terminal, μTT: −
intelligent terminal

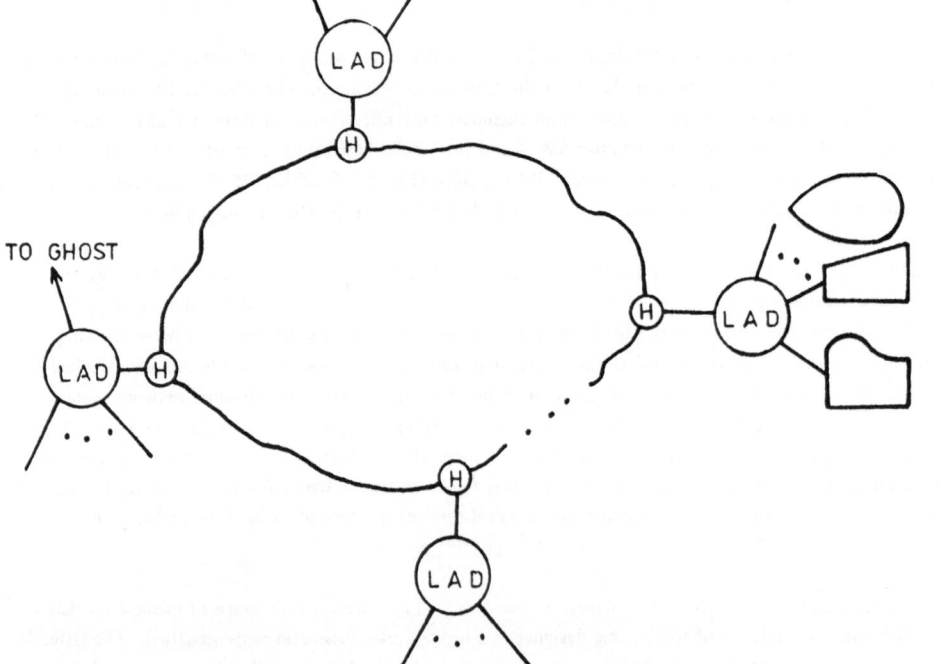

Fig. 2. Local area network Honey
Legend: H − Honey network node. Lad − Local data processing centre

REQUIREMENTS FOR COMFIT

In a typical case the Patient is under pre—hospital care of the Ambulatory of typical throughput 60—80 visits per day times ca. 300 working days per year, which gives up to 24,000 visits per year. Typical activities of the Ambulatory include: interview, medical testing, specialized testing, conservative cure (including minor operation measures).

In the Ambulatory, the Patient is to be registered and data referring to pre—hospital care (if any) retrieved for a Doctor as well as the Doctor and visit time established. Thus the following data files should be used: Precare (data on ealier care), Registration (data on registered patients) and Dates (data on visit dates and doctors). To Precare low speed (L) and medium speed (M) access is required, to Registration — H (high) or M, while to Dates — M or L.

In accordance with the upper mentioned throughput rates, and assuming 400 characters of information per visit, 1000 per the first visit and ca 25% income of data from external sources, capacities of individual files are assessed as follows: Precare ca 15 mln characters per year Registration — ca. 0.1 mln chars and Dates ca. 0.1 mln characters.

The above figures are, in no case, limit values. When defining the target version of Comfit and, in particular, Honey appropriate facilities should be provided basing on the worst case method.

Laboratory. Along the Thread, the Patient usually passes a series of Laboratory examinations. The most typical are: general—purpose laboratory — general examinations of urine, urine pH; biochemical laboratory — concentrations of various components in serum, gasometrical examinations of serum; pathohistological laboratory — cytological examination of urine, tumor, biopsy; X—ray laboratory — X—ray examination, urography, etc.

The files to be processed by the laboratories and their capacity reserved for the Patient are as follows: Findings (laboratory) — 1 mln characters, HiFi (Historical laboratory Findings) — 12 mln characters year, Larum (Laboratory records for usage monitoring) — 0,2 mln characters. The User should have H access to data in Findings.

Drug store. The Drug store is to mantain the following three basic files of data: Panacea specifying data about drugs covered by the store (capacity ca. 1 mln characters), Dingo (Drug information and general contradictions) specifying data on interactions,etc. (capacity ca. 1 mln characters) and Drift (Drug inventory friendly tome) for drug store inventory control (capacity ca. 1.5 mln characters).

Network Honey should be developed in various hospitals and other Health Service utilities all around our country and combined into a global computer network enabling full realization of the target goals (Fig. 3).

We have not decided if a public X.25 network should be used for Health Service purposes or should we develop our own global network like that used in power industry. For instance, Tv transmission links may be used. Irrespective of the final choice, considerable attention should be paid from the very beginning to identification data security. We have developed a data protection method basing on "alive" passwords agreed upon two talking persons and on random number generators.

CONCLUSIONS

The computer systems for Health Service should be developed by the bottom—up method, starting from the first thread facilitating treatment of patients by the first user (doctor). The target solution of such systems should base on local area networks combined into a global computer network.

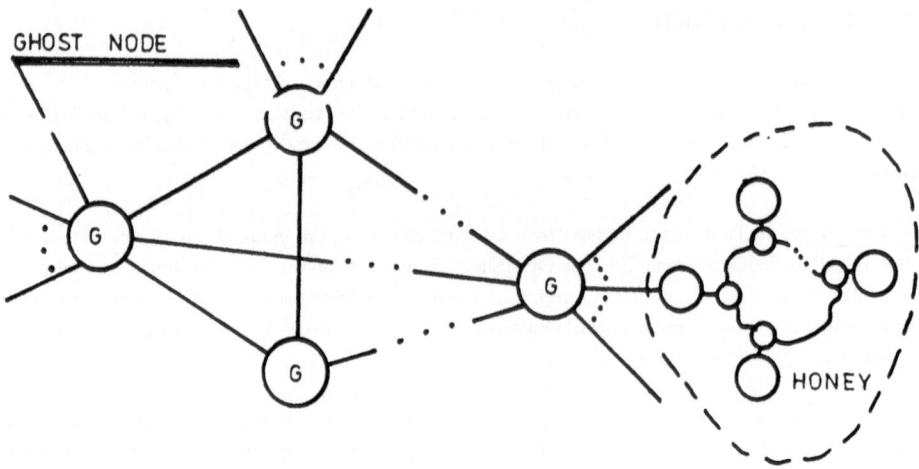

Fig. 3.   Global network Ghost

Ask for help.   The paper was written in order that our approach might be discussed when eventual criticism might be actually taken into account. Also any supporting voice and/or action will be welcome.

Acknowledgement.   The authors acknowledge unpaid share of the Hospital staff and of the Polish Electrical Engineers Society in working out the Concept of Hospital computerization which formed the base for present paper.

References

1.   University of Cambridge, Cambridge Ring 82, 1982.

2.   Digital, Intel, Xerox, Ethernet Specifications,   1982.

3.   J.B. Lewoc, R. Sibilski, Some critical remarks on studies limited to mean values, Adv. on Modelling and Simulation, vol. 4, no. 2,   1985, pp. 43–53.

DISTRIBUTED APPLICATIONS IN THE HOSPITAL INFORMATION SYSTEM

J. Burrichter, R. Göhring

Klinikum der J.W.Goethe-Universität

ZINFO/ADD

Theodor-Stern-Kai 7

6000 Frankfurt am Main 70

Federal Republic of Germany

1. Introduction

For the information system at the J.W.Goethe University Medical School
at Frankfurt it was planned from the beginning to decentralize well defined tasks into function specific subsystems /3/. This decision was
based on two main ideas:

- The load of transactions is to be handled right where it arises. It
  is disadvantageous to concentrate it at one point in a centralized
  system.
- Moreover, the end user should be able to choose his own system and
  retain the responsibility for "his" application and "his" data.

Experiences made with strictly centralized solutions later confirmed this
approach /9/. In the past, centralized systems were used because they
were considered to be economical. Mainly the validity of the Grosch'
law /7/ was cited according to which the performance of a computer increases with the square of its price; for this argumentation /1/ is
cited as an example from the field of medical information systems. Considering the technical development of the hardware, the Grosch' law is
no longer valid /10/. Moreover, for micro-computers the performance/
price relationship is by far better than even for super computers. Due
to this technological development a decentralization in function specific
subsystems makes sense not only for economical reasons. Chapter 4 will
treat the subjects availability, data protection, and privacy requirements.

2. System Layers

The hospital information system is built as a hierarchical system. **The**

relational patient data base is in the center of the system. The subsystems transmit all information of general interest concerning the patient into this data base from which they also receive all information
regarding the patient. Centrally stored are e.g. patient identification,
actual ward, key data files etc. (for details, vide /5/). Well defined
and limited tasks such as admission, medical documentation using the BAIK
system /4/, organization in the radiology etc. are carried out in the
subsystems. The relational data base system runs on a Tandem system
TNSI; the subsystems are either logical subsystems - running also on a
Tandem system -, or physical subsystems - running on their own hardware.
It is essential, however, that each subsystem, be it logical or physical,
communicates via one general interface with the data base.

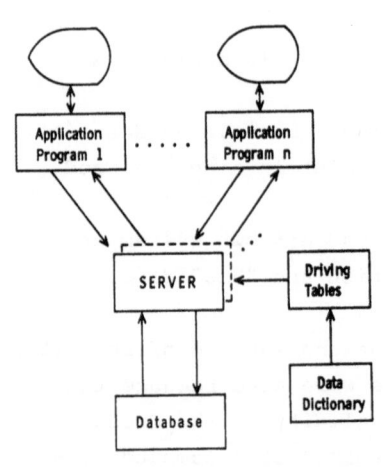

Figure 1

Figure 1 shows the different layers of
the application system and its interface -
called "server" in the figure. Server
just means a relational data manipulation
language (DML) /8/. It enables the four
general data base operations - retrieve,
insert, update, and delete - in application dependent schemata of the data model
of the relational patient data base. Due
to our specific requirements - realization
of specific tasks to be carried out by
function specific subsystems - a data interface (request and reply) was chosen
for the server (DML) rather than a language interface.

The definition and realization of this data interface is the prerequisite
for realizing concrete tasks in physical subsystems or for moving out
existing logical subsystems into a hardware of their own without major
modifications. Whatever is communicated by means of an interprocess communication between the logical subsystem and the data base in the Tandem
system is communicated identically via a communication line between the
physical subsystem on a specific computer and the data base on the Tandem.
Thus, a distinct separation between transport layer and application layer
as stipulated in the ISO reference model /11/ is possible.

The ADT subsystem is a subsystem which communicates with the relational
patient data base via the described interface. At present it is realized
as logical subsystem in the Tandem system. In order to guarantee a rea-

sonable response time for each user, according to our experience up to 12 dumb terminals can be handled per processor of the Tandem system with this application. To move this application into intelligent terminals would greatly relieve the processor. We think that 40-50 intelligent terminals could be handled by one processor.

The programming system MUMPS is available on micro-processors. It is thus possible to move the ADT system written in MUMPS to an intelligent system. In order to be able to put this solution into practice and mainly also to make it economical, these intelligent terminals must fulfil certain requirements which will be discussed in the following chapter.

3. Requirements for the subsystem

Three requirements have to be fulfilled for a successful application in the subsystem:
- user friendliness
- technical requirements regarding the hardware and software
- economical point of view.

Run time of the application is a main factor regarding user friendliness. Disengaging the central system by moving the application into intelligent terminals must not hamper the user, i.e. he should have the same good response time on his intelligent terminal that the application would have on the central system. This fact naturally influences the design of the hardware and software of the intelligent terminal. The data transfer between subsystem and central system is also important. The necessary handling for an intelligent subsystem must be about the same as it would be for a dumb terminal. Not a playground for hackers is to be installed but a device for daily routine for which also the ergonomic aspect is essential. According to German standards, a 15" CRT and a flat keyboard are required - normally not a standard equipment for micro-computers or PCs. The fact that a MUMPS interpreter is to run on an intelligent terminal makes certain requirements necessary. The operating system of the PCs must consequently be either MS/DOS or CP/M. For economical reasons it does not make sense to connect a Winchester disk to the intelligent terminal. This means, however, that the MUMPS interpreter must be able to manage a sufficiently large area of the main memory for programs and data in order to avoid program loading from floppy disks. Whether the distributed data processing as described so far will be economical depends on many factors.

According to more detailed economical analyses /6/, the leeway for the prices for an intelligent terminal is rather small. Due to the present market situation we feel certain, however, that an economical solution will be found for the distributed processing. The number of systems fulfilling the prerequisites is limited intentionally. Longterm delivery and maintenance further reduce the list of possible suppliers who are above all IBM (AT), Olivetti (M24), Siemens PCD), and Tandem (Dynamite). Among the existing MUMPS interpreters we are thinking of Micro MUMPS by the University of California at Davis or MSM by Micronetics. Each system of the different suppliers has to pass a thorough benchmark test with each of the two MUMPS interpreters. For this benchmark the dynamic frequencies of the MUMPS operations of the entire application system are analysed in detail and a corresponding benchmark program is then generated. The run time results are a decision parameter for a certain system. The results of the benchmark tests will have to be reported.

4. Availability and security of the system (and data protection)

It is not intended to discuss in detail the entire subject of "availability" and "security" for an application in distributed systems. Only certain points will be mentioned which constitute design criteria and which must, by all means, be considered.

The ADT system is realized as logical system on the Tandem NonStop system. For performance reasons, however, it is not realized as NonStop-program itself - the financial means available establish the priority for the aspect of total availability. The user in the patient admission realizes an availability of his application which is made up of the availabilities of the terminals (CRT), the line and the subsystem (ADT system) of the Tandem. If this subsystem is moved into an intelligent terminal, we want to achieve at least the same availability for the end user.

Equally important is the data consistency of the application. In order to avoid uncalculable risks, no data are stored in the intelligent terminal. All necessary data are retrieved from the data base by means of the interface, all received data are immediately transferred into the data base.

The security of the system entails special requirements; i.e. the application in the intelligent terminal must meet the same requirements for data protection as the application in the Tandem system /2/. That means e.g. that the user of the intelligent terminal must by no means be able to enter into the programming mode. As soon as the application is moved to an intelligent terminal, the interface has to be especially protected; in order to carry out the data base operation, the line-control-program receives the data and transfers them to the requested server. Thus, the usual LOGON-procedure of the operating system is bypassed. Theoretically and provided the interface is known, one could connect a micro-processor to the line and tap the data base. Appropriate means of protection must be found in order to prevent such abuse.

5. Conclusion

Due to the modern computer technology, special systems can be used for special tasks within a hospital information system. This distributed application is an economical alternative and meets the justified wish of the end user to be responsible for his own data and procedures. The market analyses carried out so far show that despite these severe requirements intelligent terminals are available which are able to carry out distributed data processing on a wider scope.

References

/1/ Bakker A.R.: Centralized versus Decentralized Hospital Information Systems
                 in: Shires, Wolf (Edrs.): MEDINFO 77, North-Holland Publ. Comp.
                 1977, pp. 895-899
/2/ Deier D., Göhring R.: Data Privacy within the Patient Database of the Frankfurt
                 University Medical School, in Bemmel, Ball, Wigertz (Edrs.):
                 MEDINFO 83, North-Holland Publ. Comp. 1983, pp. 971-972
/3/ Giere W.:   Gesamtkonzept 1976, Veröffentlichungen der ADD, Frankfurt 1976
/4/ Giere W.:   Foundations of Clinical Data Automation in Cooperative Programs
                 in: Heffernan (Edrs.): Proceed. 5th Symposium on Computer Applica-
                 tions in Med. Care, Computer Soc. Press 1981, pp. 1142-1148
/5/ Göhring R.: Die relationale Patienten-Datenbank der Universitätsklinik Frankfurt.
                 Das Umfeld bei Konzeption und Implementation.
                 in: Berger, Hoehne (Edrs.): Methoden der Statistik und Informatik
                 in Epidemiologie und Diagnostik. Medizinische Informatik und Stati-
                 stik Bd. 40, Springer-Verlag 1983, pp. 208-214
/6/ Göhring R.: Wirtschaftlichkeitsuntersuchungen für Verteilte Datenverarbeitung,
                 to be published
/7/ Grosch H.:   High Speed Arithmetic: The Digital Computer as a Research Tool
                 J. Opt. Soc. Amer. 53 (1953) 4
/8/ Hesse S.:   A Data Independent Manipulation Language for a Relational Database
                 in: Bemmel, Ball, Wigertz (Edrs.): MEDINFO 83, North-Holland Publ.
                 Comp. 1983, pp. 1102-1105
/9/ Klonk J., Reichertz P.L.: The development of the software environment and data base
                 concept in the Medical School Hannover, Med. Inform. 8 (1983) 4,
                 pp. 243-253
/10/ Meuer W., Wacker H.M.: Gilt noch das Grosch'sche Gesetz? Elektron. Rechenanl.
                 25 (1983) 5, pp. 234-240
/11/ Zimmermann H.: OSI reference model - the ISO model of architecture for open
                 systems interconnection. IEEE Trans. Commun. COM-28 (1980), pp. 428-432

USERS' ROLE IN DEVELOPMENT AND IMPLEMENTATION OF A PATIENT INFORMATION
SYSTEM WITHIN HELSINKI UNIVERSITY CENTRAL HOSPITAL

H. Kalpa, T. Pesonen, S. Ripatti
Department of Data Processing
Helsinki University Central Hospital
Helsinki, Finland

Background

Helsinki University Central Hospital (HUCH) is the largest hospital in
Finland with 2700 beds and 25 clinical departments in five areas of
Helsinki. HUCH is owned by municipalities of Uusimaa Province and the
University of Helsinki. It is a teaching and research hospital and the
population of its catchment area is 1.3 million. The largest groups of
departments are Meilahti Hospital with 800 beds and 110000 out-patient
visits a year, the Department of Gynecology and Obstetrics with 320
beds and 48000 out-patient visits and the Department of Pediatrics
with 280 beds and 32000 out-patient visits.

In the late seventies new solutions were sought to replace the old
batch-processing patient information system in HUCH. Several health
care information systems in use were studied and the Finnish health
centre system Finstar was chosen to be the basis of development for
the new information system.

In the first phase it was decided to develop an information system of
the out-patient department. The work was started in 1980 and at the
moment the system is implemented in the Departments of Gynecology,
Obstetrics and Pediatrics. All the projects were carried out using the
same methods.

In this paper the development methods and especially the significance
of the users' contribution in this work are described.

Objectives

The following objectives were set for the development of the
information system:

- to create an information system which can be transferred to other
  departments of HUCH with minimum amount of changes
- to replace some old pieces of office machinery like typewriters and
  label printers
- to alleviate paper work of the nurses and other staff
- to improve nursing services
- to avoid double book-keeping of patient data
- to create a base for laboratory, pathology and follow-up systems

In daily routines the new system should not need EDP personnel in the
department.

System description

At the moment the out-patient information system in use includes
following features:

- processing of referral letters
- room schedules
- appointment scheduling
- lists and labels
- registration
- in-patient admission and inquiries
- billing information
- encounter data
- utilities
- reports and statistics

The prototype of the laboratory system is in test use and the in-patient information system will be implemented in the beginning of 1986.

Both in the Department of Gynecology and Obstetrics and in the Department of Pediatrics the computer system consists of a PDP- 11/44 with ISM- 11 stand-alone MUMPS operating system and with approx. 30 VDU's, 4 printer terminals and several auxiliary printers. The computers are situated in the EDP centre and operated by its staff. The system is an interactive database system. For the follow-up of special patient groups the File Manager database system is used. The linkage between these two databases was made and the first system implemented was the follow-up of patients with cervix dysplasia.

Project team

The patient administration system has been developed as a joint project between research and planning division, edp-department and the clinical departments concerned. The managerial group of the clinical department in question and the data processing manager form the steering committee of the project.

A comprehensive representation of the personnel of the clinical departments was considered of great importance when choosing the members of the project team. Also plenty of attention has been paid to selecting persons who are interested in developing hospital services. Physicians, nurses and office staff of e.g. the out-patient departments, bed wards, operation theatres, delivering room, financial department, i.e., the persons whose daily routines the system concerns, have been represented in the project team. When selecting nurse members of the team we preferred to choose specialized nurses because they have a more comprehensive knowledge of the clinical speciality and they usually hold their office more permanently.

It is very important to release members of the team from daily routines to work full time in system design and training. In actual practice this has been most difficult because of lack of trained nurses. When the desired arrangements have succeeded the system has been adopted rather quickly and there are always persons who manage the system present.

Design method

When describing the system a simplified ISAC-method (Information System Work and Analysis of Changes) was used (1). Using this method the functions, information and relations between these are described, tested and rectified. This structural design method is rather troublesome and takes time but results in an unambiguous description of the system. It is also a useful tool of communication between the end-users and the edp-analysts. (Fig. 1).

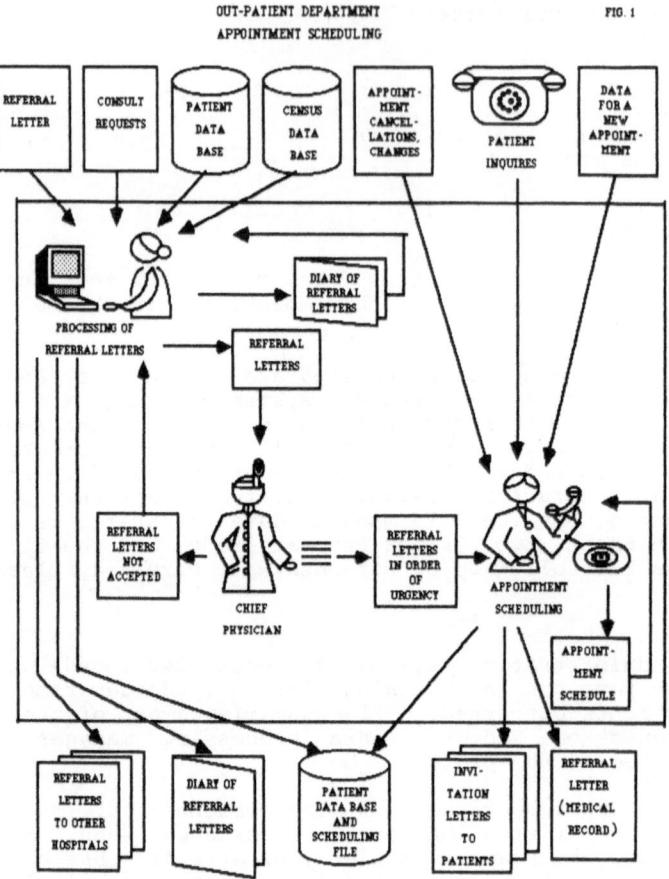

OUT-PATIENT DEPARTMENT   FIG. 1
APPOINTMENT SCHEDULING

Inventory of the existing conditions

All details and problems attached to manual data processing and data
transfer were documented. In this work the contribution of the
representatives of the users has been:

- to describe the data processing tasks of the work units of their own
  specialities
- to document the data transfer between units
- to make a list of forms in use
- to collect activity statistics for the system design
- to make a list of the existing reports
- to document the data processing problems

Also the problems not actually connected to data processing were
analyzed (e.g. problems in timing of tasks and in work environment).
The report of the existing conditions was produced jointly between
edp-analysts and users.

Design of the new system

The design of the new system has been based on the analysis of the
problems in the manual system. We have tried to solve these problems
by edp as well as by other rationalizing methods. The planning,

describing and documentation of the new system have been done in keen collaboration between users and edp-analysts.

In this phase of the system work the users were responsible of the following tasks:

- to apply the nomenclature of diseases (ICD-8) to this system
- to create other nomenclatures and codes specific to the department in question e.g. operations and non-medical treatments
- to design the report models
- to write help responses and instructions for the use of the system

Training

Every project was introduced with a training period of one week. The programme covered principles of the project work, methods of system analysis, methods of rationalizing one's work and an overview of the hospital's edp-systems and development projects.

The general principle in training the users of the patient information systems has been that one or two persons of every work unit have been trained in small groups by the data processing staff. The training period of these users was about 40 hours. After this period these users train the rest of the staff and new personnel to operate the system. They also should be able to maintain and develop the system together with the data processing staff. Most of these trained users are nurses.

The project design, implementation and training took approx. ₊17 person-months in the out-patient department of Gynecology and Obstetrics and 20 person-months in the out-patient department of Pediatrics and 70 person-months in edp-department for the three departments combined. (Fig.2)

THE DEVELOPMENT OF THE PATIENT INFORMATION SYSTEMS WITHIN HUCH

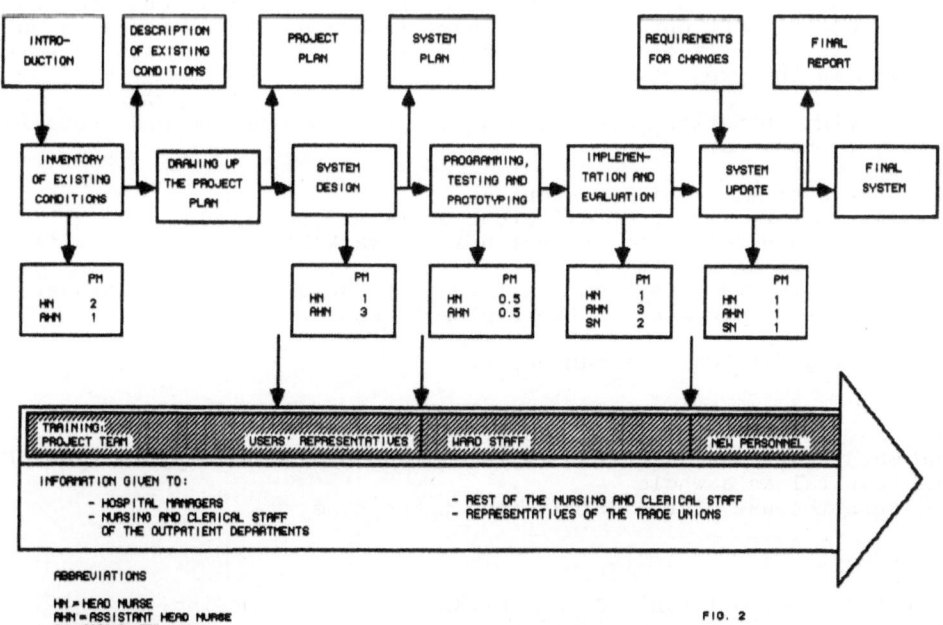

FIG. 2

Evaluation of the new system

To evaluate the effects of the information system a survey in the out-patient department of Gynecology and Obstetrics has been done both before and after the implementation of the system. The goal of the survey was to describe the quantitative and qualitative effects of the system on the data processing tasks in the out-patient departments. The study consisted of the following parts:

1. A survey of users' opinions concerning the effects of the system on the different data processing tasks, on the nursing services, on the work routines etc.

2. A work structure analysis, based on the staff's own estimate of the distribution of work time between the most essential data processing tasks during a period of one week.

3. A work time analysis, in which the time elapsed in some essential tasks was measured.

Before the implementation of the system, the share of data processing tasks in the nurses' work was about 10 per cent, measured in work time. After the implementation it was two per cent units less, which means 30 hours per week. The method of the survey was quite rough, but the result shows the same trend as the survey of the users' opinions and the work time analysis. The weakness of the analysis was, that it was not clear how the remaining work time was used. It would have been interesting to know, to what extent time was used for patient care.

Conclusions

For a successful implementation of an edp-based patient information system an extensive participation of the end-users in the system design and training is necessary. The system must be built on the conditions of the end-users. The edp-training has become a natural part of hospital routines. We are happy to find out that the administration of our hospital has realized the importance of releasing the members of the team from their daily routines to work full time in the project.

The following benefits are gained if the role of the end-users is properly emphasized:

- the new system is quickly adopted
- details characteristic of different units are observed
- working in a development project has a remarkable educational effect and influence on attitudes
- the end-users and dp-system staff learn to speak the same language
- the further development of the system is easier

The following difficulties can occur:

- the hospital staff is not necessarily interested in development and they may object to changes in daily routines
- the ward staff works quite isolated and has an incomplete view of the hospital as a whole
- to learn the use of the ISAC-method takes time

References

1. Lundberg, M., Goldkuhl, G. and Nilsson, A., Systemering.
   Studentlitteratur, Lund, Sweden, 1979.

FIVE YEARS OF TOTAL HIS COST ACCOUNTING, ANALYSIS AND PROGNOSIS

A.R. Bakker and H.G.M. van der Zanden
BAZIS, Leiden University Hospital
Leiden, the Netherlands

Abstract

In earlier MIE-papers was reported on a cost allocation model used around Leiden University Hospital Information System and results obtained. The figures are extended now to a five years period and it is found that, notwithstanding an average growth rate in HIS use of about 20% per year, total HIS costs at Leiden are not increasing and almost stable at 1.4% of the hospital budget.
This result is contradictory to what is often expected.
Especially for the US market projections on cost levels are available. A growth of HIS cost is predicted to 3-4% of the hospital budget.
In this paper the phenomenon (constant cost level, combined with considerable growth of HIS use) is studied in more detail and it is concluded that under certain assumptions on the growth of HIS use and the growth of the co-operative around Leiden University Hospital Information System, the cost level can be expected to remain constant for the next 5 years.

Introduction

Adequate information handling is an essential aspect of a modern hospital. The application of computers to support this activity may potentially be of great help, especially when set up as an integrated system. After initial failures nowadays more or less sophisticated hospital information systems are in use and they are rapidly expanding.
Around Leiden University Hospital Information System a cooperative structure has grown covering some 20 hospitals now with together over 11,500 acute beds.
Within this cooperative, the careful monitoring of the further development of the HIS was considered to be necessary. Such an analysis not only should cover functionality and benefits but also costs of the system. For that reason already in 1981 a cost allocation model was developed [1]. With this model all costs can be allocated to the various aspects of HIS usage (development, production and implementation/support) and specified for the different application packages within the system.
Results for the 4 years period 1980 - 1983 were already reported [2] and are extended now with some data about the year 1984. Earlier analysis of figures indicated that the percentage of the total hospital budget that was spent anually on HIS costs was not increasing, notwithstanding an average growth in intensity of HIS use of about 20% per year. The figures for 1984 confirm this finding.
Since this trend is different from what is indicated in literature for the US-market, in this paper cost components are analysed in a prospective sense.

The cost allocation model

The model is aiming at quantifying the costs of the aspects:
development, implementation/support production.

Costs on the user side, either for specification, implementation or routine usage are not taken into account.

Cost contributions are mainly caused by:
- costs for salaries of personnel and direct overhead,
- depreciation of equipment,
- maintenance of equipment,
- housing,
- material,
- general overhead.

Within the model it is irrelevant whether development was sponsored by an external agency. All costs are taken into account, also sponsored costs are fully attributed to HIS subsystems.

In the model certain rules are used for the allocation of costs. Basically in a first step costs are assigned to two groups:
- Costs of activities of personnel in development, support/implementation. By dividing the total costs in this group by the total number of manhours produced the average cost per manhour is determined.
- Costs of the computercentre inclusive of operational personnel costs.

From a registration of manhours spent both the development effort and the implementation and support effort per year per application package can be determined. Development efforts are depreciated in 5 years. These development costs are attributed to the various participants. Implementation/support is a typical local activity of participants and counted directly in the year manhours are spent (no depreciation).

For the HIS operational system an accounting system exists where by means of a tariff the use of the system is charged to the endusers. From this accounting system operational costs per application package are derived. The tariff is set in such a way that the total operational costs are covered.

Although some parameters are involved in the model (e.g. the tariff structure) different parameter values will have only a small effect on the distribution of the costs over the various application packages. It is emphasized once more that the total costs are not influenced by this choice.

During the 5 years to which the model was applied, only the percentage of computer centre costs that was attributed to development was changed, from 20% to 15%, the percentage attributed to operational costs was by consequence increased from 80% to 85%.

Some results

For the Leiden Universital hospital the model was applied for 5 consecutive years (1980 - 1984). The figures for 1984 are preliminary (based on available data by the end of January 1985).

In table 1 some overall results as to the cost level are combined with average intensity of HIS utilisation.

In the first row the total hospital budget is given in millions of Dutch guilders. Initially there was some increase of the budget, in the later years it is almost constant. In the second row the total HIS-budget (the sum of the 3 cost components: development, implementation/support and production) is shown, again in millions of Dutch guilders. In the third row the HIS costs are given as a percentage of the total hospital budget. It is found that this figure is not increasing and almost stable at 1.4%.

In the fourth row the intensity of HIS use is given as the average number of messages input into the HIS in the dayshift of a workingday. We see a gradual growth of HIS utilisation, the annual growth rate is given in row 5.

The figures of table 1 demonstrate clearly a not increasing costlevel (1.4% of the hospital budget) combined with an average growth rate of HIS use between 15 and 20%.

Table 1.
Some results of the cost model for Leiden University Hospital Information System.

	1980	1981	1982	1983	1984
Total hospital budget(MDFL)	225.5	238.0	251.3	255.8	259.6
Total HIS-budget (MDFL)	3.28	3.31	3.57	3.28	3.09
Total HIS costs as percentage of hospital budget	1.46	1.39	1.42	1.28	1.19
Intensity of HIS use (k messages/day)	190	225	280	315	375
Annual growth of HIS use (in %)	-.-	19	24	13	19

The results found over the past 5 years deviate from what is often assumed to be the trend. Especially in studies on the U.S. market it is found that the average percentage of the hospital budget being spent on dataprocessing is steadily increasing and already well above 2%. It is expected that this percentage will grow to 3-4 % by the end of the eighties. In the next chapter the results found will be analysed slightly further and future trends will be considered.

Expectations as to further development of HIS costs

Considerations in this chapter on further developments in HIS costs to be expected are concentrating on the situation in our Dutch cooperative structure. Although a part of the arguments presented here will be generally applicable one should be careful, conclusions are not simply transportable.

Findings from the application of the cost allocation model can be summarized as:
- the HIS scene is one of average growth of use by 20 % per year, this growth is only partly caused by more intensive use of existing application packages, a major part of the growth is due to introduction of new application packages.
- The percentage of the hospital budget spent on HIS costs is stable at about 1.4 %.
- The major cost aspects are development (35 %), implementation and support (20 %) and production (45 %). The contribution of each of these aspects is stable with a tendency of a slight increase of the production component combined with a decrease of the development component.

For the years to come a steady further increase of HIS usage is expected. In the medium term plan of the cooperative around Leiden University Hospital Information System this growth is estimated at an average of 20 % per year.
For each of the cost aspects it will be tried now to give a prediction of effects to be expected in the coming 5 years.

Development costs

As to development efforts to support certain functions in a hospital three effects play a part :
- the wish of users for an ever more complete product. Over time the functionality of an application package will increase. This often appears in the form of new generations of application packages. In the clinical laboratories for instance we are nowadays in the phase of development and implementation of third generation packages. This effect complicates application software development considerable.
- Software methods are improving gradually; better tools become available, this has a reducing effect on the effort involved in the development of a application package.
- The further development of computer technology, both hardware and software, combined with experience gained in present applications leads to a request for development of additional application packages.

The first two effects in our expectation will compensate each other. The third will lead to a further increase of total development efforts required.
At present hardly any standards exist in HIS development. There is e.g. no standard demarcation of application packages, no standard data description and no standard HIS interface. As a consequence every HIS development has to define almost all new data-elements and application packages of other manufacturers can hardly be transported. Although IMIA installed a working group with among others as task to propose standards in this field this is a long term activity and for the next 5 years no significant improvement is expected. If one intends to keep the development cost component stable an extension is necessary of the number of hospitals that use the packages to be developed. For that reason our cooperation intends to grow to 17,500 beds in 1990. If we hit this target we expect the development cost component to remain stable.

Implementation/support

Nowithstanding the rapid growth of HIS use we see over the past 5 years no increase in the effort for implementation and support. This phenomenon is probably caused by the following effects :
- the software is becoming gradually more userfriendly; less implementation effort is necessary.
- Since the application software is used in many hospitals the quality of the software is improving. Each hospital has to deal with less software problems (they share the burden).
We feel both effects will continue to have effect and will compensate the further growth in HIS use for the coming years. So the costs for implementation and support are also expected to be stable.

Operational costs

To be able to give a prediction of production costs we split these up in the following groups:
- Costs for hardware (depreciation and maintenance) (45%),
- Costs for computer centre personnel + overhead   (35%)
- Costs for system software   (5%)
- Costs for the computer centre (floor space,
  airconditioning, entrance control etc.)   (5%)
- Costs for material and energy   (10%)

In brackets the contribution of each group to total operational cost is indicated for Leiden University Hospital in 1983.

With respect to the various groups the following comments can be made:

- The contribution for system software is limited. Since system software is an own development within the cooperative, a moderate increase of total cost of development in this area can easily be compensated by the anticipated growth of the number of participating hospitals.
- As far as costs for materials and energy are concerned, a further shift of output from the central lineprinters to terminals at the workinglocation can be anticipated. This effect will compensate the growth of HIS use. Of course this costgroup is heavily influenced by current prices of materials (especially paper). Apart from such effects no significant change in cost level is expected.
- Development of hardware technology leads to a steadily growing capacity for the same price. The volume and energy consumption is reducing rather quickly. The present computer centre can be expected to offer sufficient floor space and cooling capacity for the next 5 years. As long as normal twisted pair telephonelines can be used also the growth of costs for the network will be moderate and have no significant effect on total operational costs.
- Over the past 5 years we've seen no increase in operational staff. The userfriendliness of HIS software increases, reliability of equipment (especially terminals) increases and a part of operational activities is moved to the user site. For the coming 5 years it is expected that these effects will continue to keep operational staff at the same level.

So far we found no indication for growth of operational costs, however hardware costs still have to be considered.

Is is a well-known fact that price/performance of hardware has been improving considerably over the past 10 years. Typical examples are magnetic disc memories, where the price per Megabyte storage capacity (for the largest units) drops with some 30% per year. For terminals and direct memory we've seen a price reduction of some 20% per year. For CPU 's we've also seen a considerable improvement. The capacity of the HIS configuration must be geared to the intensity of HIS use.

For most of the hardware components almost continuous growth can be realized (terminals, dc equipment, disc storage). However for CPU's the steps in capacity when introducing a larger model are significant and so is the price effect. At Leiden production will switch early 1985 from a double PDP11/70 configuration to a double VAX 11-785 configuration. At the same time high performance tape units will be introduced. This switch will have an increasing effect on hardware costs, + 35%. At first sight this price increase may be surprising, however it can almost completely be explained by the present unfavourate dollar exchangerate.

The total HIS costs are expected increase by 8-9% due to this introduction. Total HIS costs are expected to stay below 1.4% of the hospital budget. Such significant replacement effects can be expected every 4-5 years in the set up with one duplicated CPU. In case the workload could be distributed over more CPU's this effect might disappear to a large extend.

For the next 5 years no significant further increase in the price of the central configuration is expected, however, the average price per terminal may well be constant or even increase because of the introduction of personal computers as intelligent terminals. At Leiden we expect that by 1990 10 - 15% of all terminals will be a p.c.

Taking everything together as a trend a slight increase of the hardware cost component can be expected. The total HIS costs will not pass the 1.5% mark.

This prediction is given for a situation of HIS growth by 20%/year (both in number of messages processed per day and in number of terminals installed). In case the growth would be significantly bigger or in case a higher percentage of terminals will be p.c.'s, costs might pass the 1.5% mark. It should be realized that the growth perspective used implies that by 1990 over 750 terminals will be operational in Leiden University Hospital (940 beds).

[1] Bakker, A.R., Hoogendoorn, C., van der Zanden H.G.M. "Cost aspects, cost allocation and cost figures for an integrated hospital information system", In: Proc. MEDINFO '83: J.H. van Bemmel et al.,eds., Amsterdam, Augustus 1983, North Holland Publ.Comp., pp. 214-217

[2] Bakker, A.R., van der Zanden, H.G.M., "Trends in Costs of a Hospital Information System", In: Proc MIE '84, F.H. Roger et al, eds., September 1984, Springer Verlag, Berlin Heidelberg New York Tokyo pp. 61-65

PLANNING, IMPLEMENTING AND INSTALLING A MUTUAL PATIENT ADMINISTRATION
SYSTEM FOR THE MEDICAL SCHOOLS IN BAVARIA
- EXPERIENCES AS VIEWED BY THE COMPUTING CENTRE OF THE UNIVERSITY OF
  MUNICH -

L. Gierl, R.L. Greiller and H. Kristin
Computing Centre of the University of
Munich for the Medical School

Klinikum Grosshadern, Postfach 70 12 60
D-8000 Munich 70, FRG

1. Introduction

In the past the Bavarian universities' medical schools have pooled their
efforts and developed a mutual computerized patient administration system.
Two of these medical schools are located in Munich, one in Erlangen and
one in Wuerzburg. The system's main aim is to support the hospital administration for three comprehensive centralized hospitals and about 30
smaller hospitals with a total of more than 8.000 beds. The total patient
admissions amount to about 170.000 inpatients p.a. and 600.000 out-
patients p.a. A modular, four level scheme was developed and implemented with a centralized data base for each medical school [1-10]. The
concept avoids the draw-backs of total centralization as well as the
problems incurred by total distribution of data storage and processing.
The mutual effort provides for compatible hardware at all four medical
schools, a common operating system and uniform applications software as
far as possible. Most of the hardware planned is in operation by now.
The applications software is presently being installed. It is mainly
concerned with patient admission, patient data base, statistics, billing
etc. There are interfaces to the bookkeeping programs and to medical
data base systems. What experiences have we gained in the course of this
project?

2. The organizational basis for developing and implementing the system

The medical schools of the state of Bavaria are (within normal legal
restraints) free to choose their own structures in the university board
and in coordination with the ministry of culture. It was therefore a
prerequisite for mutual planning to find a common platform, able to
coordinate the diverging views and interests of the partners concerned.
This job was undertaken by a working group set up to develop a "Skeleton

Plan for the Utilization of Electronic Computers in the Medical Schools of Bavaria". At completion of this general scheme two teams were commissioned with the accomplishment.

The team for administration laid down in a rough draft the requirements to be fulfilled and outlined the resulting administrative procedures in a detailed report.
The EDP-team elaborated the plans drawn up by the other team into precise DP drafts and coordinated the programming, tests and documentation. It was responsible for the development of extensiviley uniform software using mutual guiding principles. The implementation was done by the EDP-departments of the medical schools participating in the project.

3. Experiences with the team for administration and the phase of elaborating the concepts

The main task of the team for administration was to state the administrative concept for the system on a common basis. The delegates of the four medical schools had to agree as far as possible on a single solution and in consequence on a unique concept. Of course, minor modifications and adaptions to local requirements had to be accepted.

In our opinion this situation had the following positive aspects:

- it was the first chance for the administrative personnel of the four medical schools to meet in a working group and to discuss problems of mutual interest;

- those experts for patient administration were forced to agree on a common interpretation of debatable administrative rules.

There were however also negative aspects, impeding the progress of the project:

- a trend to overemphasize minor details;

- the attempt to maximize aims, especially as regards a comprehensive user interface, quite often beyond the possibilities of efficient technical implementation;

- the extreme difficulties administrative personnel had formalizing the results of their work, so that in effect the members of the EDP-team had to write most of the administrative concepts themselves;

- the unwillingness of the administrators to accept evolutionary procedures for the realization and installation of the project.

A further very problematic aspect arose during the introduction of the system in the hospitals:

- the demands stated by the working group did not always meet the requirements of the subordinate personnel that actually had to work with the system.

4. Experiences with the EDP-team

This team's main purpose was to elaborate the DP-concept on the basis of the administrative concept and was responsible for programming, test and documentation of the system. Further it had to support the installation of the system in the hospitals. It had to make sure that common standards and rules were used during the EDP-oriented phases. Thus it was possible to standardize system structure, user interfaces and use of software tools to a large degree. The development of standardized procedures binding the different medical schools was particularly important for the exchange of programs and documentation as well as instructions for the system's installation.

The experiences with this team's work revealed that the transfer of the seperate parts of the system to the other medical schools were made easier by

- defined interfaces to cope with local modifications necessary in just one university;

- parametric adaption to accomodate for functional differences;

- common system architecture;

- detailed documentation for all processes and for all user groups entailed.

On the other hand the consideration of nearly all user demands, the independence of the software regarding organizational environment (decentralized or centralized structure of the administration) and the lengthy process of coordination had enough disadvantages:

- the program systems developed are very large and complex;

- sometimes the user demands were modified in parallel to the implementation phase, thus requiring multiple changes in programs already developed.

5. The installation of the system in the hospitals of the university of Munich

The strategy of installation started with a pilot installation of the different administrative procedures in one of the decentrailzed hospitals thus achieving a genuine environment for exhaustive final tests.

As soon as this phase was successfully completed the system was transferred to other dezentralized hospitals one at a time. Finally the system was introduced to the large centralized hospital in Grosshadern (1.500 beds), that had up to this time been supported by older software. Because of the centralized organization and the existence of a previous DP environment the exchange of software procedures hat to ensue within a margin of 12 hours.

Another characteristic feature of the strategy was the forming of small groups with two or three experts out of the administrative and the DP fields in order to accelerate the installation process. These groups introduced the administrative staff to the use of the peripheral equipment.

The administrative personnel was mainly trained in the hospital chosen for the pilot installation. At the outset the hospitals were supported by an expert of the administrative side and by a DP specialist and experience with this strategy have shown, that these partners really are essential in the phase of installation. It took many weeks to overcome the personnel's initial reserve against the new equipment and procedures. Administrative procedures had to be introduced one at a time and in adequate intervals. Generally some weeks passed studying the effects of the new system on other areas of the hospital, such as wards and medical departments.

It proved most important that the leading staff of the site chosen is willing to further and accelerate the introduction process. The operative staff should, on the other hand, be capable of standing the inevitable stress caused by the problems encountered in installing a newly implemented software system.

In Grosshadern the replacement of the current dialogue system by new software was especially difficult, because it is practically impossible to run old and new in parallel. However, the old system has to be kept in a state enabling immediate reactivation in case of the new system's failing unexpectedly. It is much easier to replace a manual system step by step by a newly developed computerized one.

6. Conclusion

The following objectives of the mutual project of the medical schools in Bavaria were achieved:

- a unique hardware and system software has been installed at favourable conditions;

- the software system for patient administration was planned, implemented and installed in a mutual effort;

- the project was optimized for all partners by involvement of the experienced staff for both administration and data processing in all the medical schools, thus reducing the total number of people required for the project;

- the administrative personnel's work has been substantially reduced by the new dialogue oriented software system;

- the process of patient administration has been accelerated;

- a common software maintenance group has been installed, so that the costs can be kept to a minimum.

References

1. HORBACH, L.; ÜBERLA, K.:
   Rahmenplanung zum Einsatz der elektronischen Datenverarbeitung für die medizinischen Fachbereiche der Bayerischen Universitäten,
   München, 1977

2. GREILLER, R.:
   Das EDV-System für die Medizinischen Fachbereiche der Universitäten in Bayern
   DSWR 8 (1979) 7, 165-168

3. MEYER-BENDER, B.A.; GREILLER, R.; HORBACH, L.; LANGE, H.J.; SEIDEL,H.;
   ÜBERLA, K.:
   Interfaces in a Computer Network for the Medical Schools in Bavaria.
   Proceedings of Medical Informatics Berlin, 1979,
   Springer-Verlag Berlin, 1979

4. GREILLER, R.:
   Verteilte Datenverarbeitung in den Medizinischen Fachbereichen der Universitäten in Bayern: Aufgaben, Planung, Vorteile und Nachteile.
   Das Rechenzentrum 3 (1980) 1, 4-12

5. GREILLER, R.; ÜBERLA, K.:
   Data Security and Data Safety in Distributed Systems exemplified by the Medical Data Processing System Munich.
   Proc. MEDINFO '80 TOKYO, North-Holland
   Publ. Co. Amsterdam 1980, 292-298

6. GREILLER, R.:
   Zusammenarbeit zwischen Medizin, Verwaltung und Rechenzentrum in der Medizinischen Fakultät der Ludwig-Maximilians-Universität München - Erfahrungen aus der Sicht eines Rechenzentrumsleiters
   In: 9. Jahrbuch der EDV (1980), HEIDI HEILMANN (Hrsg.)
   Forkel-Verlag Stuttgart 1980, 125-143

A MICROCOMPUTER SYSTEM FOR
EMERGENCY UNITS

L-H BARTHELEMY*, P. LE BEUX*, J-M FONTANELLA**
*C.I.T.I.2, **S.M.U.R. DE MONTLUCON

The information processed by emergency units (S.A.M.U., S.M.U.R. in France) are extremely various and useful if they are timely processed.

The emergency unit professionals were keen to have computer processed data in order to improve the quality of their intervention as well as accurate and aggregative data regarding their activities.

The National Association of emergency units (S.N.A.M.U.) has defined a set of requirements for computer processed data for the field. The software has been developed by a group of engineers and physicians cooperating during several months.

1) THE HARDWARE AND SOFTWARE SUPPORT

The hardware had to be choosen in order to be able to execute several simultaneous tasks on several terminals sharing some files. Thus we needed a multiuser system.

For these reasons, we choose a MICROMEGA 32 (FORTUNE) microcomputer running under the UNIX operating system (1).

The configuration is : 1 Mbyte of central memory with hard discs going from 20 Mbytes to 40 Mbytes.

The system can support from two to six terminals.

In order to be able to share the data in the files in a multiuser environment we looked for a data base management system and we choose the INFORMIX DBMS (2).

It is a relational type of data base (3) which is quite comprehensive and it is useable for insuring data security with a minimum of redundancy.

2) THE SOFTWARE TOOLS

The SGBD system enables the user to define several views of the data base and the data entry is done via a sequence of screen frames.

These frames can be activated to store, modify or read the data contained in the data base.

During the data entry, systematic control and coherence checking of the data base can be made.

The data consultation can be required for any field of the screen frames.

The user can enter the values or the keys that he wants to select in the data base.

Automatic print outs can be build by using the form generator given with the Informix system. Some other print outs have been implemented direct- ly in the C language (4).

3) THE APPLICATION

The application software can be divided into three main software packages :
- a regulation module,
- a medical module,
- a ressource module.

These three modules can be run in real time and each of them can access the data base and generate print outs.

3) - 1 THE REGULATION MODULE

This module keeps the record of the calls to the emergency units and the decision of the regulation physician.

It uses the data proposed and contained in the national regulation form defined by the Ministry of Health and the S.N.A.M.U.

The real time management is insured by two views :
- a call form which enables the storage or the consultation of the call : identity and coordinates of the caller, the place of the call (accident, ...) the typology of the call, the medical query, etc...,
- a decision form which enables the storage or consultation of information concerning the decision which has been taken (intervention of regional emergency unit, general practitioneer, private ambulance, ...) and the summary of the intervention.

The operator can record several decisions for one call if necessary.

Several print outs can be generated from the data stored in the data base.

3) - 2 THE MEDICAL MODULE

This module keeps the records of the medical activity of a regional emergency unit (S.M.U.R.).

The principal views which enable the real time management are :
- Intervention Frame which contain the following characteristics of each move of a mobile unit : (call reference, vehicle used, medical staff, hours, place of intervention, ...),
- Identity Frame : this frame is used to keep track of the identity of the patients treated by the S.M.U.R.,
- Summary Frame : it gives a summary of the medical problems relating to the case : clinical data, therapeutic given, results and other necessary data.
A link is made by a summary record between the intervention and identity records.

This structure enables to take into account all the interventions of the S.M.U.R. especially :
- several interventions on the same patient,
- several patients on a given intervention,
- several print outs can be given by this module :
- print outs for statistics on S.M.U.R. activity,
-print outs for each physician : patients treated, pathology, time spent for each patient, ...
- pathology typology.

3) - 3 THE RESSOURCES MODULES

This module helps the regulation physician to consult all the data concerning the health ressources of a given department.

The following information can be consulted :
- Profession file : it enables the finding of a health professional
(physician, nurse, dentist, pharmacist, ...) in a given place (commune
or city). It gives also the professionals which are "on call". Some
other administrative data are available : police, city hall, landing
zone for helicopters, ...
- Intervention means : it gives all the ressources in a given locality
in the department : S.M.U.R., emergency unit, ambulance, the responsible
persons, the telephone and radio frequency to call these responsible
units and a complete catalog of the available vehicles and their charac
teristics,
- Hospitals and avalaibility of beds : it gives the address and places
of each hospital, their speciality equipment and number of beds,
- Remarquable place : it is a catalog of the factories or places which
present an identified risk factor and the access to these places.

This module enables the output of several print outs. They insure the
continuity of the follow up in case of momentary break down of the system.

These catalog are sorted according to different criteria.

4) EXPERIMENTATION AND EVOLUTION OF THE SYSTEM

A three months experimentation has been set up in two regions : the province of Auvergne (Center of France) and Picardie (North of France).

The system is now completely operational and a national diffusion is
planned after january 1985.

News extensions are planned :
- decision aid to help inexperienced physician,
- a collecting and aggregating of data for epidemiological purposes,
- an integration in the hospital information system where this system
is installed.

5) CONCLUSION

The elaboration of such a software is the result of close cooperation between physicians, users and computer engineers with the help of the administration.

The system gives an improvement and better accuracy of the data processed by the emergency unit which in return helps the professionals to give better advice and better care to the patients.

The flexibility and evolutivity of the software is also a quality of the system which enables the progressive installation and diffusion of such systems on a national level.

REFERENCES

(1) R. THOMAS, Jean YATES
A USER GUIDE TO THE UNIX SYSTEM.

(2) RELATIONAL DATABASE SYSTEMS, INC.
INFORMIX V 3.2
REFERENCES MANUAL

(3) E.F. CODD
RELATIONAL MODEL OF DATA FOR LARGE SHARED DATA BANKS.
Comm. ACM, vol. 13, n° 6, June 70, pp 377-387.

(4) B. W. KERNIGHAN - D. M. RITCHIE
THE C PROGRAMMING LANGUAGE.
PRENTICE HALL.

EXPERIENCES WITH WORD PROCESSING INTEGRATED IN A HOSPITAL INFORMATION SYSTEM

R.J.A. Dujardin
BAZIS, Leiden University Hospital
Leiden, the Netherlands

From 1983 on word processing has been available as an integrated function within the Leiden HIS. At present a considerable amount of experience is available. The functional advantages of integration of dataprocessing and wordprocessing (use of data from the database, one terminal at the working location, use of the HIS network) are presented as well as figures on cost and system load.

1. Introduction

In a hospital there are many activities that might be supported by wordprocessing facilities. One can think of the recording of radiodiagnostic results, reports by laboratories to wards for in- and out-patients, but also information to the general practitioner about treatment in clinic or outpatients ward. Beside these patient related applications there are also many non patient related applications, e.g. research and financial reports, notes, memos etc.
To meet this demand for word processing facilities several approaches are possible. We have considered three models : stand-alone word processors, word processors connected to a Hospital Information System (HIS) and software fully integrated in a HIS. We decided to realize the third model for those applications where there is a relation between dataprocessing and wordprocessing. For applications where such a relation does not exist stand alone word processors may suffice, the choice will be heavily influenced by cost considerations [1].
Arguments for this choice are :
- integration of word processing and data processing will result in a much greater efficiency and a consistent and consequently more correct handling of data.
- in work situations in which documents are processed without any relation to the HIS stand alone word processing may suffice very well. However, for terminals that are used by the same persons and/or in the same room integrated software will be the solution to be preferred.
- a HIS with a large central database can easily answer the need for fast search and retrieval facilities. In addition, data stored a such a database are available on every terminal.
- a HIS offers advantages in the area of data protection, e.g. security arrangements and privacy protection, protection against calamities (fire and water damage) and recovery facilities.
- a HIS is equipped with a terminal driver that is capable of handling all different types of terminals that are known to the system. Because of the absence of standardization in this field, use of different types of commercially available word processors would cause substantial problems in the area of special characters and putting emphasis on texts by underlining or bold printing.
In this paper a report will be given on our experiences with this framework, where the integrational aspects will be worked out in detail for a number of subsystems of a HIS.

2. Hospital Information System

By a HIS we mean a total, integrated, information system by means of which most of

the data processing in the hospital can be handled, i.e. a system [2] as is now in use in the Leiden University Hospital. Our HIS is built around one large central database, and equipped with one terminal network that provides for communication in every ward of the hospital (in Leiden over 350 terminals).
This HIS includes a broad range of subsystems, e.g. for patient administration (in- and out- patients), examination- and treatment- departments (e.g. laboratories, radiology), medical, financial and personnel administration, nursing, auxiliary services (e.g. stock control, kitchen), etc.

3. Word processing. Advantages and facilities

For the concept of word processing a number of definitions is used. A narrow definition is
- working with a word processor.
A wider definition is
- the entire proces from conceiving an idea up to the finished product of a typed document (via the different stages of making a draft, collecting the necessary data and finally using a word processor).
The most comprehensive definition is
- all the activities concerning texts and documents, which also include, in addition to the activities already mentioned, the duplication, storage and even the distribution of documents.

In this paper the last, most comprehensive, definition of word processing will be used.
The main advantages of the use of word processors may briefly be summarized as follows :
- increase in productivity and efficiency (the extent of which strongly depends on the type of application);
- improved quality (invisible correction, lay-out facilities etc.);
- improved service (e.g. storage and retrieval facilities, the use of wordprocessors by the authors themselves, a more flexible secretariat).
Facilities which we incorporated in our software are :
- basic functions such as creating, correcting and printing of documents as well as their retrieval
- manipulating (parts of) documents
- use of standard paragraphs (easily generated text segments)
- use of standard forms (any kind of standard document that can be assembled from prerecorded text and may require variable information to be inserted before it is printed).
These functions are not only implemented as a stand alone subsystem for reason of integration of hardware, but also as modules that can be embedded in other subsystems of our HIS.

4. Some examples of applications within a Hospital Information System and their relation with word processing

4.1 GUIDE Information System

General description of this subsystem
With this system a source of information for users of the HIS is created. It concerns a facility for consulting the system on non patient related information through a video terminal in a way that is somewhat comparable to the teletext systems well known from television.
The information stored originates from handbooks, hospital regulations, bulletins,

etc. Examples are data relevant to requests for laboratory research, descriptions of medicine, nursing protocols and publications of the information service.
The authors themselves take care of structuring, editing and updating their data. Free text is handled by word processing functions.
The retrieval of data is realised by using a table of contents or with the use of keywords. Again a word processing facility of the system is activated for either showing (parts of) the documents on screen or for making a hard copy of documents.

Word processing features of this subsystem
In view of the general arguments mentioned above for developing word processing software, for this subsystem a number of specific arguments were valid. All documents are available on-line not only for information retrieval from any terminal connected to the HIS, but also for modification or updating by authorised users. Because authors process text only incidentally and in most cases already use the HIS (for instance the laboratory system or pharmacy system) the possibility to use the HIS-hardware for word processing purposes turned out to be very economical. This system has been in production in approx. 8 hospitals since 1983.
Some figures about the Leiden University Hospital:
Number of documents produced : 850 (jan. 85)
Users authorized to create documents : 30
In Leiden 2500 users are authorized to retrieve data from the system using over 250 video screens.
The average document length is 1500 characters.
The costs of creating one information item (one document) amounts to approx. Dfl 0.50 (US $ 0.15)
The costs of retrieval of one information item (one document) amounts to Dfl 0.10 (US $ 0.03).

4.2 Histo-pathology

General description of this subsystem
This subsystem supports the administration on the histo pathology laboratory by means of processing of requests, production of reports and storage of diagnoses and reports.
To create and to update reports the HIS word processing functions are used.
The archive function of this subsystem is of great importance: the archived examination data are available on-line via patient data, histo-pathology number or diagnosis.

Word processing features of this subsystem
Here we are confronted with a need for the integration of dataprocessing and wordprocessing in every stage of the examination. Data and free text have to be mixed during the recording of the request for examination, the results of different examinations and drawing a final conclusion. When reports are retrieved several subreports have to be distinguished. It concerns a large number (65,000 a year) of relatively small documents that are fully integrated in the histo pathology report. A complete report of a histo pathology examination consists of subreports like macroscopy, microscopy and conclusion. The different documents like macroscopy, microscopy and conclusion are created in different stages of the examination of a sample. It is desirable that these documents can be retrieved separately.
Reports are sent to the printers on the various wards. The report stays available on-line to all authorized personnel in the entire hospital. In this case an alternative might be stand-alone word processors exclusively used for editing the free text, coupled with the HIS for storage in the database. Arguments against this solution are the frequent switch of off-line editing to on-line transporting, the load on the transportlines, and the availability of a lot of rarely used functions that nevertheless have to be paid for.
An example of a histo-pathology report (the bold printed characters are created with the help of word processing functions) shows what is meant by integration of data and text.

HISTO PATHOLOGY REPORT

```
DOCTOR'S NAME : DAM V        PATIENT NUMBER: 123456    HP NUMBER: A84-80
WARD CODE     : BETK         NAME : SMITH
DATE ANALYSIS : 07-01-1985   DATE OF BIRTH : 01-03-1936
DATE ARRIVAL  : 05-01-1985   SEX : FEMALE
TYPE MATERIAL : conisation portio
DIAGNOSIS     : serious dysplasia in the glands
MACROSCOPY    : conus biopt slide, surface granular, slightly red-coloured  on  the
                edges.
MICROSCOPY    : No signs for malignity found. No microscopic confirmation of a
                clinically malignant tumor.
CONCLUSION    : Skinbiopt without any sign for malignity
```

06-01-1985   DR. JANSEN, PATHOLOGIST

This system has been in production in approx. 4 hospitals since 1984.
Some figures about the Leiden University Hospital:
Number of documents produced : 65,000 (Jan. 85).
Number of users authorised to create documents : 20.
In Leiden 100 users are authorized to retrieve this type of data from the database
using over 250 video screens.
The average document length is 2000 characters.
The costs of creating one report (including several documents) amounts to approx.
Dfl 3.00 (US $ 0.90).
The costs of reading one report (including several documents) amounts to Dfl 1.00
(US $ 0.30).

4.3 PATIENT LETTERS subsystem

General description of this subsytem
Hospital doctors and specialists report to colleages about treatments when a
patient is discharged from the hospital or has been treated in an outpatients
clinics.
Frequently a standard framework is used. The letter contains a number of fixed
components, together giving a sketch of the treatment.
This subsystem offers support to these activities by using data on the patients
treatment, his personal data such as name, address, date of birth, and name and
address of his general practioner stored in the HIS and by using word processing
facilities. Moreover the process of creating, updating and sending the letter is
managed, by automatically initiating a letter when a patient is discharged and
giving information about the status of letters per doctor, ward etc.

Word processing features of this subsystem
Here we are confronted with probably the most important subsystem for
wordprocessing in a hospital. In university hospitals we estimate that about 50% of
the total word processing concerns this type of correspondence.
In general hospitals this percentage is probably higher. As these letters contain
data that are stored in the HIS database, it is obvious that an integrated approach
best suits the demands of this subsystem. When we consider that a letter of
discharge itself should be stored in the central database to make it possible to
retrieve the letter at a later stage, it is even more clear that this subsystem
should make use of the advantages of integrated word processing software.
In the Leiden University Hospital approximately 300,000 letters a year are typed
and posted. For 1985 we expect to handle one third of these letters with the use
this subsystem.
For this system special standard paragraph functions have been built:

type A   standard paragraphs that pass information from the subsystem through to the
         word processing system. They contain texts such as the patient's correct
         name, date of birth, mailing list, date or period of visit to the hospital
         etc. These texts can be moved into the letter which is under construction
         by simply activing function keys.

type B   standard paragraphs that retrieve information from the database about the
         patients treatment (e.g. laboratory results, medical diagnosis, radiology
         conclusions, ECG, etc).

This system has been in production in approx. 6 hospitals since 1984.
Some figures about the Leiden University Hospital:
Number of letters produced : 1400 (Jan. 85).
Users authorised to create documents : 15
In Leiden 100 users are authorized to retrieve this type of data from the database
using over 250 video screens.
The average document length is 2000 characters.
The costs of creating one letter amounts approx. Dfl 0.50 (US $ 0.15).
The costs of retreaving one letter amounts Dfl 0.20 (US $ 0.06).

4.4. Other sybsystems

With our word processing software we also constructed a stand alone subsystem to
manipulate text. About 25 secretariats, including 100 users use this facility. In
1984 4500 documents were created. Other subsystems that make use of word processing
functions are radiology, ECG, operation history, and in the near future medication
and the chemical lab system.

5. Conclusion

In 1982 we decided to develop word processing software. Now we have realized
functions for word processing within subsystems of the HIS and stand alone using
the HIS hardware.
Experiences with implemented subsystems justify our choice in view of the
advantages of integrated processing and the advantages of integration of hardware.
In the context of our experiences with an integrated system it may be of interest
to note that calculations show that the load of the average word
processing-terminal is equal to the load of an average HIS terminal. However,
because of the large number of candidates within a hospital one may expect a
substantial growth of the system load and database. In view of the positive
experiences with integrated wordprocessing sufficient hardware capacity will be
reserved.

References:

1. Dujardin, R.J.A.; Heijser, W.
   Hospital Information Systems and Word Processing
   in : van Bemmel/Ball/Wigertz (eds),
   Medinfo 83 (North-Holland, 1983)

2. Bakker, A.R.,
   Scope and limitations of a mini-based centralized Hospital Information System
   in : Lindberg, D.A.B., and Kaihara, S. (eds.),
   Medinfo 80 (North-Holland, 1980)

ORGANIZATION AND INFORMATION TOOLS OF A MENTAL HEALTH DEPARTMENT INFORMATION SYSTEM

M. Rafanelli

Institute for Systems Analysis and Computer Science

I.A.S.I. - C.N.R.

Viale Manzoni 30 - 00185 Roma, Italy.

1.INTRODUCTION

The approval of national laws on Health Reform and on Psychiatric Assistance (L.180/78) has caused a profound change in health and (in particular) in psychiatric assistance. The law L.180/78, among other things, "abolished madhauses, intended as places of segregation rather than social rehabilitation". Before such law psychiatric services were organized in such a way as to strongly favor "hospitalization structures" rather than clinical or consultant services. In particular, in the period 1974-1977 (look at these last ten years) the psychiatric hospital represents the principal assistance service and users are notably without differentiation; patients are composed primarely by "long term in-patient care" and "obligatory treatment". Treatment is focused on bio-medical therapy and rehabilitation is scarcely considered.

In the period 1978-1980 law L.180/78 was approved. The urgent cases are treated predominantly by psycho-pharmaceutical therapy (with a brief hospitalization) and are received new hospital treatment centers./1/6/

In the period from 1980 to until the present the Mental Health Services (intended as the set of services) and the Health Service Centers (HSC) that carry out preventive, curative and rehabilitative functions are organized on departmental base by the institution of "Mental Health Department".

2.THE MENTAL HEALTH DEPARTMENT

In such Information System the Mental Health Department (MHD) is considered as "a complex system, ordered temporally with respect to the population, through the development of its structure, with regard to inter-

nal and external requests". The system is focused on the "care"and
the goal of this research is to allow for a system with a better capacity to elaborate information on the state of its use, and to furnish
aggregate information on the state of the population's health. These
indicators will be refered to both users and the resident population
(incidence and prevalence).

The MHD performs the following functions: a) prevention activity, to
prevent psychological disability; b) diagnosis and treatment activity;
c) rehabilitation activity and social reintegration./2/

The most important MHD parts are (Fig.1):

1) Territorial Multi-Surgery Center (or Mental Health Center (MHC));
it provides both medical-pharmaceutical interventions and psycho-ther-
apeutic and social assistance interventions.

2) Hospital service; it includes the "Diagnosis and Treatment Service"
(DTS), that is addressed particularly to "acute patients".

3) Rapid Intervention Service for Psychiatric Emergencies (RISPE); this
responds to the requirement for an emergency intervention, trying to
avoid hospitalization.

4) Intermediate Services; these can be subdivided as a)Crisis Center;
b)Family-hauses; c)therapeutic Communities; d)Day Hospital.

We are using, at present, two types of "data file cards"/3/4/.

The first card is located at each Departmental Center and is called
"Request for Services Module" (RSM). It defines a "personal contact"

In it different parts are present: anagraphic data, type and modality of both the request and the response; the second part of RSM is the
"Medical Recors" of the patient and is completed only if the user is
processed.

The second card is called "Individual Departmental Form" (IDF). It
is only one for each user, is filed in the Departmental Central Archive
(DCA) and it is without name of the patient (it is used an opportune
"code").

3.OPERATION MODALITY AND INFORMATION FLOW OF THE DEPARTMENTAL I.S.

The detailed operation modality of the Departmental Information System (DIS) is described in /5/. Briefly, the MHD operator, who receives

a request by user (for which there is not already a treatment in progress) compiles the RSM (in three copies), if both a treatment continuation is necessary, and it is not necessary that. The first copy is sent
to the DCA at the beginning of the care; the second copy, filled also
in the Medical Record part, is sent to the DCA at the end of the care.

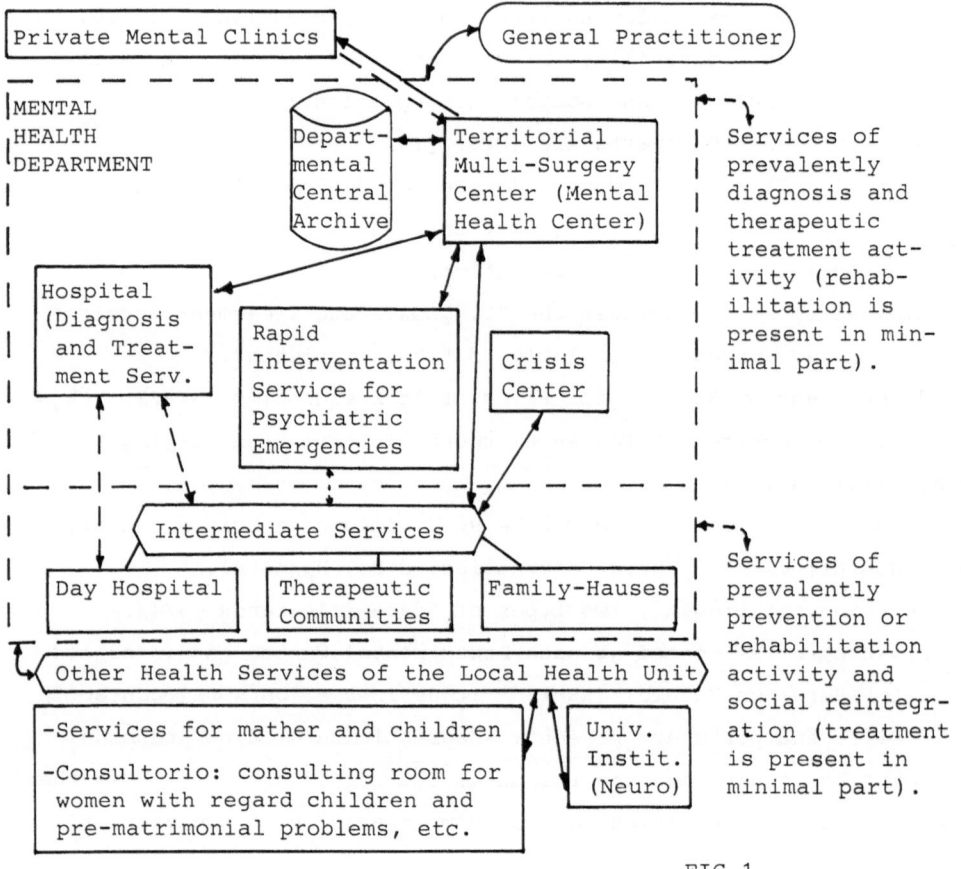

FIG.1

If the user is not resident in the area under juristiction of such
MHD, hardcopy of RSM will be sent to the relative Local Health Unit (LHU)
of residence.Finally, the third copy will form (with others) the Center
Users File at every Center of the MHD.

4.INDICATORS OF THE STATE OF THE POPULATION'S HEALTH

From the departmental level an information flow will go toward the
government organs of the LHU and of the Region. It is a matter of ag-

gregate information, able to form indicators of the state of the resident population's psychical health, resident in such Department's territory and indicators of the efficiency of Centers and Services in the Department.   The population indices, _incidence_ and _prevalence_, are defined and determined as:

a) _incidence_: number of new requests in a year to the psychiatric services (it corresponds approximately to the incidence of disease in the population).   In this D.I.S. it is: $I = Nr/P \times 10{,}000$ where Nr is the number of new requests of resident users and activated in a year, and P is the average resident population in the LHU during the same year.

b) _prevalence_: number of patients in treatment at the MHD services at a given point in time. In this D.I.S. it is: $P = Nt/P \times 10{,}000$ where Nt is the number of individual files of residents that have a treatment in course and P is the same of point a).

5. INDICATORS REGARDING THE UTILIZATION OF THE SERVICES

Certain indicators of the efficiency of the services and certain rates relative to the modality of the service'suse have been identified.

They are:

a) Correlations. These are indices that have as numerator characteristics of user and as denominator data on availability of the Department.   In such a way it is possible to define:

a1) Distribution of the users by Center, sex and age: $Du = Skt/W \times 1{,}000$

where Skt is the number of individual files of resident and non-resident users with effected or in course treatment during a year, and W is the average number of hours of service per week provided by the Department operators in the same period.

a2) Distribution of requests by Center, sex and age: $Dr = Mrp/W \times 1{,}000$

where Mrp is the number of requests per services in a year and W is defined as above.

a3) Distribution of the type of response by Center, sex and age: $Dtr = N_{1-2}/W \times 1{,}000$ where N_{1-2} is the number of responses for each type of response and W is defined as above.

b)<u>Ratios</u>. These are the percentages which (together with the preceding correlations, clarify the way in which the services are used.   Then it will be possible to know "rates" : b1) of the requests of resident users, which treatment is continued, as to the total number of requests; b2) of requests by resident and non-resident users, as to the total number of requests for every center; b3) of the treatments that are obligatory, as to the total number of treatments.

The used indicators are (with regard to a certain year):

1) number of in-patients per year (total and per hospital bed);

2) number of in-patient days per year (total and per hospital bed);

3) Average duration of hospitalization (in total and per 100 hospital bed);

4) Number of in-patient days per in-patient.

At the end of every year, by extracting a sample, the distribution of the diagnoses of all the patients will be evaluated.

BIBLIOGRAPHY

/1/ M.RAFANELLI, F.L.RICCI:"A Socio-sanitary DBMS for epidemiological researches on psychiatric hospitalization" III World Conference on Medical Informatics, MEDINFO 80, 29-9/4-10-1980, Tokyo.

/2/ D.DE SALVIA, P.CREPET:"Psichiatria senza manicomio" Ed. Feltrinelli, Milano, 1982.

/3/ E.VISANI, V.MIRIZIO et al.:"La prima consultazione in un servizio psichiatrico: studio e proposta di un modello di rilevazione" Riv. di Freniatria, vol.106, 307. 1982.

/4/ P.MANACORDA:"Strumenti informativi per la medicina di base" Ed. La Nuova Italia Scientifica, Roma, 1983.

/5/ M.RAFANELLI et al.:"Organizzazione e strumenti informativi di servizio di un sistema informativo di un dipartimento di salute mentale" Tech.Rep. IASI RI.28, Aprile 1984.

/6/ M.RAFANELLI et al.:"A DBMS for an epidemiological research about mental diseases and relative hospitalization" III Intern. Congress of the European Federation for Medical Informatics, MIE 81, 9-13, 3,1981, Toulouse, France.

AN APPROACH TO THE MICROCOMPUTER-NETWORK SYSTEM IN THE HUNGARIAN NATIONAL INSTITUTE OF CARDIOLOGY

P. Kerékfy, M. Ruda   M. Csukás
Computer and Automation Institute   National Institute of
Hungarian Academy of Sciences   Cardiology
Budapest, P.O. Box 63. H-1502   Budapest, P.O.Box 88. H-1450

1. Introduction

On the last MIE meeting (Brussels, 1984), the authors presented some microcomputer-based systems [6-8] . Based on those and similar results [2-5, 11] we have initiated the development of a hospital microcomputer network [1,9]. A network of 8-bit microcomputers is installed in the Hungarian National Cardiological Institute. This network (presently, as a first phase of development) covers two inpatient departments and the admission as well as the personnel department and a fifth workstation dedicated to the developments.
In the next phases, the laboratories, the operating theatres and the intensive care units will be connected to the network.
This hospital system is composed of a set of microcomputers connected to cluster controllers. The cluster controller provides the necessary networking functions. This local network system has the following characteristics [1]:
- the topology of the system can be modified easily,
- the system is transparent, i.e. the user need not know anything about the topology and functions of the network,
- it allows interprocess - task-to-task- communications,
- each remotely connected device (printer, disk, etc.) can be accessed as if it were locally connected,
- it includes a gateway function which allows accessing public data networks or IBM compatible host computers from all stations within the network system,
- high speed (1Mbit/sec) data transportation,
- CP/M compatible operating system,
- the cluster controller belongs to the "MS" network controller family,
- microcomputers are based on Z80 microprocessor, operative storage capacity is 64-128 kByte RAM,

- floppy disk storage: 2 ✱ 1 MByte at each workstation.

In our hospital system the main software tool is the micro-SHIVA form editor and data management system [5,8]. The form editor is an extended full-screen editor with the aim of meeting data input and query requirements. Its usage is intended to be easy for people without previous experiences in work with computers. The system micro-SHIVA is a visual tool: the results of a command are visualized immediately and the user can judge them easily. The form editor serves as a communication interface to the data management subsystem. The database is accessed through forms used in everyday practice. The forms are filled in on the screen and are used for data input, modification and query. Forms are managed (defined and filled in) through the micro-SHIVA form editor.

2. Nursing systems

The Institute of Cardiology not having utilized computers before, will be equipped with our local computer network system. Consequently, this system should be easy-to-use, effective and fast. It must not consume more time and labour than the traditional methods or disturb the normal way of life in the hospital, and must be introduced gradually.

For this reason, first a relatively small department (the children department) and the most important one (the surgery) will be partially supported by computers.

The user-friendliness of the system is based on the visual tools of micro-SHIVA and the transparency of the microcomputer network. Homogenity of the network is a source of the easy usage. The system should be homogeneous in the sense that the workstations are on equal rank i.e. any workstation can be a controlled element as well as a controlling element. Transactions initiated at any of the workstation should bring about changes at other nodes, too. E.g., discharge of a patient from the hospital results in a final report at the department, while in the central register and in the statistical database it should produce a hew record, and it has an effect on food and medicine supplies, too.

Another important matter in healt-care systems results from the private character of medical data. On personal computers professional secrecy can be assured by simple means. Micro-SHIVA assures both comfortable data processing and data security through utilization of forms. Any user can perform operations only on data that appear on

forms that he has access to. While defining new forms he can use
names of data that are known to him. Since names of data fields are
never displayed for general users, this method assures data security.
Only the system manager disposes of subsystems for database definition
and modification.

3. Inpatient admission

The inpatient admission handles administrative data of patients. It
schedules patients waiting for operation, maintaines hospital bed
registry and produces statistical data.
This system releases the department from a significant percent of
administrative duties since data collected by the admission can be
transmitted to any department. For the same reason, data of out-patients can be managed easily in the nursing systems.
Beside treatment of the patients, it is necessary to supply the local,
regional and national managing bodies with statistical data. These
data are useful in scientific research, too (mobidity statistics,
study of effectivity of treatments). Statistical data are needed for
planning food, medicine and chemicals supplies, too.
A nation-wide complex data system is useful and fit for life only if
the data to be processed are recorded and checked at their very source,
i.e. in the hospitals (e.g. at the inpatient admission). Otherwise,
a rather worthless mass of data is obtained only. And we know that
management based on inadequate data is useless, even destructive.

4. Outpatient registers

Registry of out-patients is motivated in various respects. One of its
tasks is the support of the out-patients' department. In this respect,
we will solve the following problems (as a first step):
- storage of the most important particulars and diagnoses of some
  thousand out-patients,
- the event and concise results of laboratory tests and examinations
  (e.g. X-ray, haemodynamics, echocardiography, etc.) are stored,
- through the network, data of admitted patients can be transmitted
  to the admitting office.
Another important task is scheduling of patients waiting for hospital
treatment, examinations or operations. Such systems have been reported

in 8 . (Infarction register, patients waiting for cardiac operation, IHD register.)

The out-patient systems are overlapping with the nursing systems since some out-patients are occasionally in the hospital (for medical care or operation). Therefore, data of out-patients must be stored in the same computer network as data of the admitting office, the laboratory and the other departments.

5. Personel department

As a model, we have developed a personnel data system. It is to illustrate microcomputer usage in fields different from the nursing systems. In this case, instead of micro-SHIVA, we have made use of the system pDMS [10]. It has already been utilized when developing a drug register [1]. The system pDMS is able to store and query the data and it is very flexible since the data storage structure is ISAM and auxiliary files are used. The I/O layer for pDMS is provided by the form management procedures of micro-SHIVA.

References

1. Bakonyi P., Békéssy A., Demetrovics J., Kerékfy P., Ruda M. A Microcomputer-Network Based Decision Support System for Health--Care Organizations, Preprints, IFAC 9th World Congress, Budapest, Vol. XI., eds. J. Gertler, L. Keviczky, pp. 85-92, 1984.

2. Kerékfy P., Ruda M., Microcomputer-Based Medical Information Systems, Proceedings, MEDINFO 83, Part 2., eds. M. van Bemmel et al., North-Holland, Amsterdam, p. 733, 1983.

3. Kerékfy P., Ratkó I., Ruda M., Patient Registers on Microcomputers, Cybernetics and Systems Research 2., ed. R. Trappl, Nort-Holland, pp. 519-522, 1984.

4. Kerékfy P., Ruda M., A System Model for Microcomputers in Health--Care Applications, System Science in Health Care, ed. W. van Eimeren et al., Springer-Verlag, Berlin, Heidelberg, New York, Tokyo, pp. 1419-1422, 1984.

5. Kerékfy P., Ruda M., Micro-SHIVA Editor, System Science in Health Care, ed. W. van Eimeren et al., Springer-Verlag, Berlin, Heidelberg, New York, Tokyo, p. 1439, 1984.

6. Kerékfy P., Ruda M., Data Management Tools on Microcomputers in Medical Information Systems, Medical Informatics Europe 84, eds. F.H. Roger et al., Springer-Verlag, Berlin, Heidelberg, New York, Tokyo, p. 241, 1984.

7. Kerékfy P., Ratkó I., Ruda M., Csukás M., Microcomputer Based Cardiological Patient Registers, Medical Informatics Europe 84, eds. F.H. Roger et al., Springer-Verlag, Berlin, Heidelberg,

New York, Tokyo, p. 240, 1984.

8. Kerékfy P., Ruda M., Micro-SHiva, User Friendly Information System
   Development in Medical Applications, Medical Informatics Europe 84,
   eds. F.H. Roger et al., Springer-Verlag, Berlin, Heidelberg, New
   York, Tokyo, pp. 235-239, 1984.

9. Kerékfy P., Ruda M., Distributed Systems on Simple Microcomputer
   Architecture, Proceedings, IFIP'84 Symposium, Sofia, pp. 444-447,
   1984.

10. Kovács K., pDMS, a Data Management System in Health Care Application
    (manuscript for MIE 85), 1985.

11. Ratkó I., Ruda M., Csukás M., Computer Systems in Cardiology,
    Proceedings, MEDINFO 83, Part 2., North-Holland Amsterdam, p. 1286,
    1983.

COMPARISON OF DATA

GATHERED WITH HELP OF AN AUTOMATED QUESTIONNAIRE

AND MEDICAL HISTORY DATA OUT OF THE MEDICAL RECORD

M.J.Quaak
Free University, Department of Medical Informatics
Van der Boechorststraat 7, 1081 BT Amsterdam
The Netherlands

INTRODUCTION

In an outpatient clinic of internal medicine patients themselves answered an automated questionnaire. Thereafter an extensive medical history was taken by a medical student. Similarities and differences of the data are presented and discussed.

Earlier comparisons between paper questionnaire and nurse interview[1], between a paper questionnaire and an extensive medical history[2], or between a patient interviewed by a nurse using a terminal questionnaire and the traditional medical history[3], showed that questionnaire data is more complete and accurate in comparison with the medical record data.

PROCEDURES

Using the system described in [4], patients answered an automated questionnaire on a computer terminal. By presenting them a broad scala of answeroptions they were able to express their complaints as freely as possible. After answering the questionnaire, the answers were printed on paper. The patients got their own copy of the printed answers and they were asked to check the given answers and add comment to it if needed.

Thereafter the patients were questioned by a medical student. In the fifth year of their education the medical students are in training for the internal medicine field: such as medical history taking and examining patients physically. At the end of their three months practise in internal medicine they work in the outpatient clinic. Patients coming for the first time to the clinic are contacted first by these students who take an extended history and do a general physical examination. These patients were asked to answer the automated questionnaire before they met the students. In this way two registrations of the complaints of 99 patients were gathered. NB. The students were not able to see the answers given to the automated questionnaire before or during their history taking. The recordings of the student are checked by physicians who are in training for internist (registrars).

In order to compare the two registrations, the automated questionnaire was answered by the researcher using the medical history data in the medical record. In this way for each patient two answer series were present in the computer. With help of a computer program the answers were counted and compared.

COMPARISONS

The questionnaire contains 179 items which are questioned with 402 questions. The questionnaire asks more questions when a question is answered positively in a certain degree. See for the description of the different type of questions and the reactions to the answers <4>. The items in the questionnaire are general items belonging to the internal medicine field.

Here the items are presented that are used to question the circulation tract:

- Pain and/or shortbreathed during:
  - Staircase ascending
  - Walking
  - Sitting
  - Emotions
- Palpitations
- Pain in calves
- Varicosis
- Thick ankles
- Nightly urinating
- Nightly awakening

These items are initially questioned concerning the frequency of their occurrence. They might be answered with one of the next answer options:

Never, Once, Seldom, Sometimes, Regularly, Often, Always

Also 'escape' options are available, "No answer", "Don't know" or "Don't understand". Dependent of the given answer, relating questions are asked to gather more specific information concerning the questioned item. In the comparison here described only the comparison is given for the first frequency question. For each item and for each patient the answer of the patient on the questionnaire by the patient themself and the answer based on the medical record were compared.
The number of similarities and differences were counted per item and per patient.

Because the frequency answers have some overlap in their subjective meaning, some of them are combined with each other.
In figure 1 the codes are given that are used for the combinations used in the comparison tables of figure 2.

```
           |Never|Once|Seld|Some|Regu|Ofte|Alwa|Dnun|Dnkn|Noan|

             NS | - DL - Denied - DM - - DS -
Never       Neg | .Light     |  Moderate|  .Strong     .     .     .

Once       PNR | . LPS. |PLD | . PBD. Big.        .           .
           Not |  Light |    |          Dif              PNE
Seldom      .  |.Positive . |PLD |      . fer       .     .     .
           Re  |        |    |             en               Not
Sometimes   .  |RLD  . | . MPS. |PLD |.ce          .           .
           cog |        |  Moderate|              Expressed
Regularly   .  |Big  RLD|Positive |    . |PLD       .     .     .
           ni  |Dif     |         |
Often       .  |.fer . |RLD |  .  | . SPS.         .     .     .
           zed |  en   |         Strong
Always      .  |  . ce. RBD.|RLD |Positive        .     .     .

Don't know  - - - - - NI No Information - - -          US
           Neg| Light  | Moderate|  Strong         .           .
           NN |  NL    |   NM    |   NS               Unknown
```

Figure 1: Ordering of combinations of compared answers
Horizontal rows: Answers of the patient
Vertical columns: Answers based on medical record data

The itemgroup Circulation is formed by the item groups "Pain and/or shortbreathed" (94 patients), part of item group "Limbs" (92 patients) and the item group "Nightly complaints" answered by 89 patients. In figure 2 the result of the comparisons is presented.

CIRCULATION

Pain and/or shortbreathed during:	Numbers	Similar						Different			
	Tot	NS	LPS	MPS	SPS	US		PLD	PBD	RLD	RBD
:Staircase ass	63	41	3	18	1	–	–	1	2	1	1
:Walking -----	65	54	1	9	1	–	–	–	2	–	–
:Sitting -----	54	50	–	4	–	–	–	–	–	1	–
:Emotions ----	21	10	1	8	–	2	–	1	1	2	–
Palpitations -	62	40	2	18	2	–	–	1	–	1	–
Pain in calves	36	24	1	9	1	1	–	1	1	–	–
Varicosis ----	15	3	1	2	1	8	–	–	–	–	–
Thick ankles -	67	49	2	12	4	–	–	3	–	3	–
Nightly urinat	44	21	1	19	3	–	–	3	–	1	1
Nightly awake	28	3	4	15	5	1	–	8	–	1	1
SUM ----------	455	295	16	114	18	12	–	18	6	10	3
Mean percent -	49	32	1.7	12	1.9	1.3	–	1.9	0.6	1.1	0.3

Numbers Circulation --	Denied				No Information Record						Patient	
	DL	DM	DS		NI	NN	NL	NM	NS		PNR	PNE
:Staircase asc	7	10	3	–	2	–	–	1	1	–	4	–
:Walking -----	3	10	2	–	8	6	2	–	–	–	3	1
:Sitting -----	5	9	1	–	16	11	1	4	–	–	7	1
:Emotions ----	1	3	–	–	63	39	2	22	–	–	2	–
Palpitations -	8	3	–	–	11	3	2	5	1	–	6	2
Pain in calves	1	4	2	–	46	28	6	12	–	–	1	–
Varicosis ----	–	–	–	–	77	61	5	5	6	–	–	–
Thick ankles -	3	5	–	–	8	5	1	2	–	–	1	2
Nightly urinat	12	10	1	–	17	2	3	11	1	–	–	–
Nightly awake	5	6	1	–	38	4	10	21	3	–	1	–
SUM ----------	45	60	10	–	286	159	32	83	12	–	25	6
Mean percent -	4.9	6.5	1.1	–	31	17	3.5	9.0	1.3	–	2.7	0.6

Figure 2: Number of similarities and differences of compared data, see for the meaning of the codes figure 1.

The itemgroup Circulation is answered on an average of 49% with similar answers, especially the items: 'Thick ankles'-67, 'Pain and/or shortbreathed during Staircase ascending'-63 and 'during Walking'-65, and 'Palpitations'-62 cases. In these cases the majority of the similarities are negative statements.
A total average of 12.5% of the comparisons were positive statements (once-always) of the patient that was denied on basis of negative

information in the medical record (DL+DM+DS).
An average of 31% of the comparisons were items that could not be
answered on basis of the information in the medical record (NI). 10.3%
were positive answers (sometimes-always,NM+NS) of the patients such as
for the items: 'Pain and/or shortbreathed during Emotions'-22, 'Nightly
awakening'-24 and 'Pain in calves'-12 cases. So information about these
items is lacking for a great deal in the medical record.

The result of the comparisons between all the patient answers and
the whole medical history registration is about the same or somewhat
worse for the whole record as presented here for the itemgroup
circulation. Characteristic items are frequently questioned by the
student and give great similarity with the patient answers. Other less
questioned items differ a lot in some cases. Overall in 43% of the
questioned items no information was present in the medical record.
Although the majority was answered negatively (never-23%), patients
also answered 'sometimes' or 'regularly' in 11% and 'often' or 'always'
in 2.3%. In 37% of the compared items the information in the record
indicated that no complaints were present concerning a certain item
while the patient indicated that in 9.4% the complaint was present
'sometimes' or 'regularly' and in 1% 'often' or 'always'.

Overall one might say the patients direct answers to the automated
questionnaire differ in some cases for a great deal with the
information in the medical record. To get reliable and extensive
information about the medical history it seems to be relevant to ask
the patient several times and in different ways about their complaints.

References:

<1> Aspinall M.J. Development of a patient-completed admission
questionnaire and its comparison with the nursing interview, Nurs Res
1975;24:377-81.
<2> Pecoraro R.E. and others, Validity and reliability of a
self-administered health history questionnaire, Pub Health Rep
1979;94:231-8.
<3> Lilford R.J. and others, The development of on-line history-taking
systems in antenatal care, Meth Inform Med 1983;22:189-97.
<4> Quaak M.J. and other, Design of and experience with an automated
questionnaire for medical history taking, Proc. MIE-84, F.H.Roger and
other eds. Springer-Verlag Berlin, 1984:140-5.

A MINICOMPUTER BASED CLINICAL PHYSIOLOGICAL LABORATORY SYSTEM FOR THE OFF-LINE COMPUTATION AND DOCUMENTATION OF THE STUDIES

S. Hyödynmaa, E. Länsimies and M. Eloranta
Department of Clinical Physiology
University Central Hospital
SF-70210 Kuopio, FINLAND

Modern trend to use a special purpose, dedicated microcomputer for each measurement in clinical physiology is expensive for a medium-size or small hospital. In addition, the documentation of each analysis-program and reference values is insufficient in most cases. Various recorders and processors have different types of reports producing difficulties in organization of hospital journals.

In this work we report our minicomputer and graphic digitizer based system for computing and reporting the results of most common clinical physiological function studies. The system is mostly nurse-oriented and output form is organized similarly for all studies allowing easy handling, photocopying, microfilming and archiving in primary care and hospitals.

MEASUREMENTS AND COMPUTATIONS

The system is presently used for computing the results of the following studies:

- cardiac systolic time intervals
- ultrasound echocardiograms
- heart rate beat-to-beat variation
- autonomic nervous control of circulation
- invasive cardiology
- peripheral circulation
- spirometry (including flow-volume loops)
- urodynamic studies

The measurements produce recorder outputs from strip chart recordings to full-size XY-recorder plots with varying individual calibrations. Many instruments also produce results that have to be written down from displays (e.g. blood pressure). The recorded signals are most commonly ECG, respiratory flow or volume, physiological pressures, doppler blood flow, plethysmographic volume signals etc. The computation system consists of a minicomputer (Eclipse S/130) with two 5 Mb disks and two-user operating system together with a 25x25 cm graphic digitizer pad and a printer.

The computation program has the modules sketched in Figure 1.

ANAIN
input of administrative
and anamnestic information

STI	ECHO	AUTO	BEAT	CATH	SPIR	UROD	PERI
syst.	echo-	auton.	beat-	invas.	spiro-	urody-	peri-
time	cardio-	control	to-beat	cardio-	metry	namic	pheral
intv.	graphy	of circ.	variat.	logy		meas.	circ.

ANAOUT
output of administrative
and anamnestic information

RESOUT
output of results and
reference values

INTPRE
output of interpretation
(if available)

Fig. 1. The modules of the computation program.

For ANAIN the administrative information of the patient (name, ID#, height, weight etc.) are fed in. It computes the body surface area and body mass index, which together with sex, age, height and weight are used for calculating the reference values. In addition, information about occupation, smoking habits and medication are given. The given data may also include diagnosis, reason for study, referring department and physician and investigator.

For various computation modules different recordings are fed in. The individual amplitude and time calibrations are given preceeding the either pointwise or continuous curve input of the signals: heart R-to-R-intervals, spirometric volume curves, echocardiographic diameters, times, or slopes, urodynamic pressure curves etc.

Module ANAOUT prints the topmost part of the output form having all the relevant administrative information in fixed order. RESOUT prints the measured and computed values from each examination comparing them to reference values. INTPRE prints the interpretation, if the analysis has been done by a physician, or an interpretation form for checking by the physician, if the analysis has been done by a nurse. Number of reports to be printed is freely selectable (filing in the laboratory, in-patient departments, research files etc.).

DISCUSSION

This type of system has been proven flexible and may be transferred to hospitals and primary care units with limited resources and various needs for clinical physiological measurements. The experience of almost five years has shown that nurses were easily motivated and the threshold from conventional calculations to this computerized off-line system was low. The system easily allows the use of own or national reference values, if such values are available.

The computation system has also been used for producing files of the number and type of examinations performed in the laboratory for minthly and yearly reports. In the future some independent microcomputers (such as the ergospirometric measurement system and ambulatory ECG analysis) are to be connected to the minicomputer for uniform reporting. Presently no results of the patients are stored by the system. In the future this might be necessary for comparison of successive tests.

The contents and form of the reports produced by the system complies also with the reports printed by the automatic ECG-analysis system that runs on a larger computer in the near-by university computing centre (Jokinen 1977).

REFERENCES

Jokinen Y: Computer assisted ECG analysis system as part of regional cardiovascular information system. Computers in Cardiology, IEEE, 1977.

X-RAY DATA PROCESSING AS A PART OF A PATIENT INFORMATION SYSTEM.
A radiologist's point of view

P. Virkkunen
Finnish Student Health Service
Töölönkatu 37 A, Helsinki, Finland

1. The patient information system

At the beginning of 1980, a minicomputer-based, real-time patient
information system was implemented in Finnish Student Health Service
(FSHS). During the first phase in 1978-79 the system was developed
and built mainly for administrative purposes. During the second
phase in 1980-84 the system has been developed also to handle the
medical information of the patients. The system contains time
scheduling and patient information activities.

Patient information includes all the personal medical history and
visit data of the patients, such as health examinations, medical
consultations, dental services and mental health services. X-ray
data processing is a part of the whole system. This presentation
describes the data processing of X-ray treatments from a
radiologist's point of view.

2. The objectives of X-ray data processing

When the development of X-ray data processing started at the end of
1983, the main objectives were:
- -X-ray treatment requests and results to be made by terminals
  (without paper documents)
- -Real-time access to the results
- -Statistics on diagnosis and number of treatments to be produced
  automatically from the treatment information

3. Daily utilization of the X-ray system

X-ray data processing as a part of the patient information system
was implemented in Helsinki health centre in September 1984. All the
X-ray activities of FSHS in the Helsinki area are concentrated in
the same department headed by one radiologist. The annual number of
treatments is about 14.000 and represents a normal range of primary
health care treatments.

When there are terminals in all the consultation rooms the

physicians will key in the X-ray requests on the terminals when recording the other patient information of the consultation.

The radiologist can see the requests on his own display and retrieve the other patient information (symptoms, allergy, clinical results, etc) he needs for the X-ray statement. When making statement he keys in the patient's social security number (which is used as the patient's identification). He gets on the display the X-ray information layout, where he keys in the data, the treatment and the diagnosis. The diagnostic codes of the American College of Radiology (ACR: Index for Roentgen Diagnosis. 3rd edition, 1975. Illinois, USA) are used. The first two numbers of the code indicate the organ (lung, wrist, etc) and the following two numbers the sickness (pneumonia, fracture, etc). If no affection is found in the organ, the next two numbers are .00. If the sickness is so exceptional that it has not yet been included in the diagnosis database (about 130 diagnoses), it can either be included or the numbers .90 (other) can be used. Every treatment has a diagnostic code. When the diagnosis numbers are recorded at the terminal, the name of the diagnosis is diasplayed. For the commonest X-ray diagnoses the database has ready made statements (about 25). When statements with free texts of different lengths are recorded the wordprocessor is used as an integral part of the X-ray system. The statements are stored in the same database as the other patient information.

There are three different ways of recording the X-ray statement:
1. The diagnosis is keyed in with a ready made statement from the database and accepted without change. The ready made statement is displayed at the terminal.
2. The diagnosis is keyed in with a ready made statement and the necessary changes are made in the text with help of the wordprocessor.
3. The diagnosis and the statement are made in the normal way in free text without the help of the prepared text. Again, the statement is written with the wordprocessor.

The acceptance of the text is always made by giving the signature. After acceptance, the X-ray treatment and result can be displayed on the physician's terminal. Statistical facts on the diagnosis and numbers of treatments are produced at the same time.

The radiologist himself can key in the statements for about 75% of the treatments: In the cases in which no sickness is detected in the radiographs or for which there are ready made statements in the database. In other cases he can dictate the statement and the nurse or typist can key it in later. Recording the statement does not take much longer than dictating it for the radiologist himself.

4. The advantages of the system

When the system is in full use its advantages are:

1. The physician does not write a separate request and the radiologist can obtain from the display all the information he needs about the patient.
2. The time spent on writing the statement is saved and the statement is available immediately on the physician's terminal, which improves the service for acute cases.
3. The work load of the X-ray department is reduced by eliminating the typing and preparing of statistics.
4. Interesting radiographs are easily found for scientific work (Nuutinen P, Kataja M, Soila P: Computer analysis of accuracy of roentgen diagnosis based on a large verified material. Proc. of the third conference on computer applications in radiology. Univ. of Missouri-Columbia, 1972) or presentations at meetings.

CLINICAL INFORMATION SYSTEM FOR URGENT SURGERY AND TRAUMATOLOGY

J. Münz, M. Dvořák, O. Gotfrýd and M. Peštál
Dept. of Medical Informatic
Research Institute of Traumatology
Ponávka 6, 662 50 Brno
Czechoslovakia

Introduction

There is no doubt, that the application of an automated information system in any institution and particulary in a hospital could be successful only, when the hospital is extremly well organised. This situation allows, most of functions and interactions between departments to be planned and controlled.

Due to the fact, that in traumatology and acute medicine in general is no chance to forecast the numbres of critically ill patients or their condition. It is therefore even more difficult to build an automated information system, than in general hospital. Nevertheless after five years experience with an Automated monitoring and information system development and practical application on ITU we decided to develop a clinical information system (CIS) as a patient oriented multiuser database information system suitable mainly for urgent surgery clinic or traumatology department. The first version supported by a traumatological knowledge base CIS-1.T is now in routine use in our institute. The concept of CIS-1.T is based on collection, processing and retrieval of all relevant data, which may be used for:

  a) diagnostic decision procedures
  b) therapy control and optimalization
  c) optimal ward control
  d) research

All necessary data are stored in a patient oriented data base. The
basic applied principle of data collection and retrieval is an active
dialogue of medical and paramedical staff with the information stored
in data base. The basic means of dialogue is an alphanumeric display
with a clasical keyboard. Up to 16 terminals are installed not only
on clinical wards, but also in operating theatre area, emergency
dept., central biochemistry and haematology laboratory etc. ITU forms
a special subsystem of the CIS-1.T. Beside dialogue data collection
a microcomputer monitored signal preprocessing was developed and
connected to the central computer PDP 11/34.

Program development conception and data base structure
──

The complete software of CIS written in MUMPS language could be devided to the following program groups:

        a) system programs supporting DSM 11 operating system
        b) system programs supporting data base CIS functions
        c) universal communication program library
        d) user's communication and print programs
        e) real time programs for signal processing

The most important atribute of the developed software is maximal
unification of input-output communication, storage and use of common
data structures. The patient oriented data base consists of information records. Type and structure of information records is described
in separated structures called "descriptors". Information records
form patient oriented data base ^CZ and their structure is described
in the descriptor tree ^DES. Beside these two main dynamically
changing structures some fixed supporting structures exist as well.
Fixed structure ^FIS contains information about clinics, wards, rooms,
patient-doctor interactions and technical configuration of computer
system as well. Another structure called ^PRG is in fact a patient
register. It is a part of ^CZ data base information contents, which
is disc resident and remains on the disc permanently.

Another structure ^PRC contains all necessary information about
authorized persons to communicate with the system CIS. Hierarchy of
user's programs and their mnemonic four alphanumeric character names
are described in global ^SNP.

The medical knowledge base is a set of ^Pn structures, which contains all necessary information about drugs, laboratory methods and extending tree structure of terms allowed to construct and automatically coded diagnostic, patient history and other necessary sentences for patient's state description.

As we already mentioned the CIS-1.T is a dialogue oriented interaction system. For non technical users (medical staff) it is necessary to construct a dialogue as follows:

- fast (especially in data collection mode)
- understandable for non trained persons
- as standard as possible

Medical care in todays state of art level is extremely complicated process. To support all necessary processes of acute surgery diagnostics as well as treatment and management of the clinic more than 500 programs had to be developed. To make communication in such an extended system more friendly and fast enough, any of the user programs may be activated directly by a four character program name. So more than 250 mnemocodes exist. However a doctor during his daily diagnostic and treatment procedures requires less than 20 different programs, which may easily be memorized. It is possible to find a program by searching in the program menu as well.

Another very useful tool, which made a dialogue more friendly and flexible was an application of softkeys. Up to ten standard communication control function can be selected by numeric keys 1,2,...,0 corresponding to ten displayed strings on the last screen line of alphanumeric terminal. The soft keys allow to change the program, to proceede the same program for another patient data or initialise hard copy of data etc.

Structure of the system and information flow

Clinical information system CIS-1.T was implemented in the specialized traumatology centre in following configuration. Two terminals and line printer are located on each clinical ward, another two terminals with a special hard copy device are located on emergency and casualty, one in operating theatre area and one in central laboratory. Ten terminals is the maximum which could be effectively connected to the computer

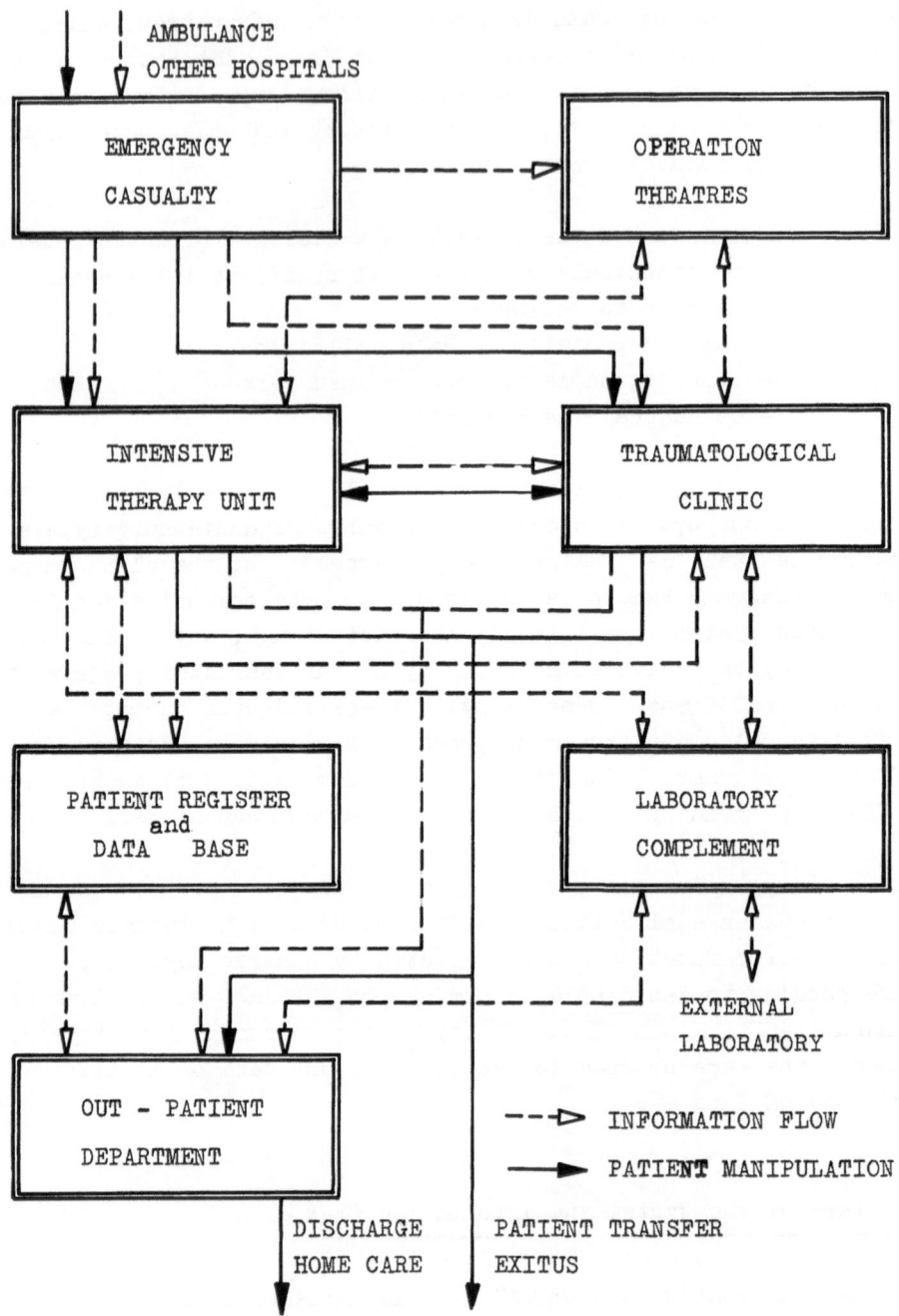

Fig.1 The configuration of CIS-1.T implementation

of this type running under DSM 11 operating system. System
configuration, data and information handling and transfer, patient
manipulation and department interactions can be seen in the figure 1,

Discussion and practical experience

An active dialogue between medical staff and data base is the only
prospective way for a clinical departmental system development.
However some serious contradictions exist as well, particularly in
acute medicine where in a period of treatment of a patient in critical
state, there is no time to insert necessary data to the computer and
thus no computer support can be used. The number of terminals is
limited as well. Medical staff have to record the information of
patient state and current treatment continously and at this time the
terminal is occupied. Also the doctor needs the information at the
time of patient examination. The terminal is not usualy situated
in patient's room.

Our experience shows, that it is extremly useful to combine active
dialogue with periodicaly or on-demand printed information. Partially
filled up forms serve for manual data collection over a time period.
Collected data may be input later on.

The periodically printed documents in CIS which have been found moust
useful are daily printed patient reports, time schedule of drug and
infusion therapy and other comments for nurses. Automatically printed
final (discharging) reports, which save a lot of very expensive
doctor's time are also very well received.

The combination of dialogue input and manually printed filled up
forms seems to be the only practical way of implementation of clinical
information system until new man-machine intercommunication are
available.

References

1. Bakker, A. R. Costers, L. Mol, J.L.: Concluding report on
   the Nobin-Zis-Project Leiden 1978

2. Peterson, H. E.: Hospital and health system., In: Van Bemel, J. H.,
   Ball, M. J. Wigertz, O. (Eds) Medinfo 83, North Holland
   Amsterdam 1983, 2 - 5

3. Greenberg, A. G.: Computer in emergency system, surgery and
   intensive care units: An overview., In: Linberg, P. A. B.,
   Kaihara. S. (Eds) Medinfo 80, North Holland Amsterdam 1980
   1184 - 1189

4. Tannebaum, A. S.: Computer networks, Prentice-Hall New Jersey 1981

A PHARMACY MANAGEMENT SYSTEM BY AN ONLINE COMPUTER SUSTEM DESIGNED TO FACILITATE
DISPENSING FUNCTIONS, CLINICAL AND PHARMACY MANAGEMENT.

Christiane Arriudarre   Dr. BERNARD GARRIGUES
Hopital Pharmacist   MEDICAL DOCTOR
General Hopital   GENERAL HOSPITAL
Avenue des Tamaris   AVENUE DES TAMARIS
13616 AIX EN PROVENCE CEDEX   13616 AIX EN PROVENCE CEDEX
France

This communication is about a computer system " Pharmacy Management System " cou-
rently use in U.S hostital Pharmacy and its adaptation in European Hospitals.
This system is a comprehensive hospital pharmacy system designed to enhance pharmaceutical services by facilitating all dispersing functions, management functions
and clinical functions.
Pharmacist's objectives are drugs' efficiency and security for patients. This informatic system can actuelly help Pharmacists in their functions if its capacities in calculating, memorizing and communications are used

I) The prescription

The physician's prescription is the first step in the entire cycle of drug dispensing. To assure an upmost security the order entry programs have different
characteristies.

1) The order enttry is done in the care unit. All partners, physicians, pharmacists, nurses having access to the informations. The use only one document is
very important. There is a decrease in the time required to fill and check mé-
dication carts and errors are minimized. Pharmacists can immediately see on the
sceen physicians orders.

2) Security codes are assigned to each user to prevent unauthorized entry.
Security codes are confidential.

3) The entry of prescriptions is easy and user oriented. For example the operator
type the drug generic name or the drug trade name as he wants

4) Physician's orders are complete

It is possible to find: the date
                              the physician's name
                              the patient profile
                              drug characteristics
(name, form, dose, route, first dose date en time, duration, rate, contraindications

5) The entry of the physician order is swift.

a) Patient profile is entered only one time and after automatically appears onthe screens and papers.

b) When entering physician's orders the pharmacist simply enters a mnemonic code for the drug and a second code for the dosing interval. Immediately all other information relating to the order automatically appears in the order entry from displayed on a CRT. This same procedure is used for intermittent or continuous IV.orders as well.

c) In using the first dose date and time the frequency and the treatment duration the system automatically calculates and writes all times of administration.

d) It is possible to suspend, discontinue,or modify a prescription lign in entering a significant letter to the left of the lign in question.

e) Clinical data as protocols, side effects entered in memory automatically appear.

II) System help in a care unit

1) The physician can see on the screen the available list of drug and their cost.

2) One of the major features of the Pharmacy management system is a comprehensive clinical screening that occurs when the order is entered.
These quality control checks include screening for appropriate dosing for the patient, potential drug interactions, duplication of therapeutic intent, incompatibilities and potential allergic reactions.
For IV orders the system screens for potential drug concentration problems.
A unique feature of the Pharmacy Management System is the ability to have to a drug monograph during the entry process to review information describing the clinical use of the drug (indications, doses, contraindications, side effets, treatment supervision)

3) The systel allows to retrieve easily anterior prescriptions. It is interesting to establish statistics for our patients.

4) Print reports.

The system provides:

– Doctor's standing order list

- Medication fill list
- Medication catch up list
- Medication administration record list

freeing nursing personnel from the time consuming tasks of manually maintaining the Medication administration record.

Piggybags administration schedule (24 H clock graph with times of administration high lighted), a stop order report may be automatically generated to list all patients and medications for which orders will expire unless physicians reorder them.

III) Helps of the system in a Pharmacy

Pharmacists play an important part in hospitals by providing accurate, clinically relevant drug information and efficient drug distribution for the care of hospitalized patients.

To facilitate this work and to entrance the accuracy of the pharmacists activities, computers are taking over many laborious and time consuming tasks

The results are not only an improvement in the efficiency and productivity of the hospital pharmacy, but perhaps still offer a major improvement in the quality of patient care

1) The most important point concerns the swift, surely precise transmission about physicians' orders.

2) The system provides to the pharmacist all necessary informations. He can provide unit dose drug distribution and IV admixture services (he can daily prepare IV admixture in a sterile room)

3) Print reports

a) As the patient's medication profile is updated the system automatically prints a Medication Delevery Envelope with the patient's demographics and the pertinent drug information. At tht timt of dispensing the medication is sealed in the envelope and delivered to the care unit. The envelope can contain an update label to be place on the nurse's medication administration record which facilitates nursing administrative work.

b) When extempoaneous preparation or intravenous orders are entered the system automatically generates labels entered releasing pharmacy personnel from time consuming label preparation and increasing patient safety in providing labels with accurate and complete patient, drug and dosage information

c) The system provides preparation list

The user can check drugs in preparation time, storage place, care unit...as he wants.

" Total medications " lists the total number of bags, generic drug name and the total amount of the drug needed within the dose period.

Total solutions lists the solution names and total volume needed per dose period

4) Management functions

The system facilitates the management of pharmacy in terms of productivite and utilization.

a) Whenever Medication Delivery Envelopes, Medication Fill List and IV labels are printed, appropriate charges are automatically generated.

Medications which have not been used by the patient can be credited by posting on the Post Credits/Charge program.

b) Order entries generate automatic patient charging based on the codes used in the Master file and the prices entered into the Charge Description Master File.

c) Twelve months or five years utilization information for selected drug is displayed numerically and graphically.

Today the computer offers the promise of liberatory doctors, pharmacists, nurses from clerical tasks as well as automatory their critical links of communication with each other.

The result is an enhancement of their therapeutic efficiency and a new level of quality patient care.

- AMERICAN SOCIETY OF HOSPITAE PHARMACISTS :
  UNIT DOSE DRUG DISTRIBUTION SYSTEM
  1972 WASHINGTON

- A. G. HOLEN :
  EDT IN THE PHARMACY AT RADBOUD
  HOSPITAL NIGMEGER
  PROCEEDINGS OF THE SECOND A PIS CONFERENCE 1977, p 8
  FK SCHATTAVER VERLAG STUTTGART

- K. ROSENKRANZ , K. KRAGELOH :
  SYSTEM FOR DRUG INFORMATION
  MEDCOMT 77 PROCEEDINGS BERLIN
  EDITION AMK BERLIN

- A. VAN SORGE, N. MULLER. M. MASS :
  COMPUTER ASSISTED DRUG DISPENSING IN HOSPITAL PHARMACIES
  MEDIN JO 83 PROCEEDINGS ISIP IMIA
  NORTH HOLLAND

- D. SWANSON. R. BROECKEMEIER, M. ANDERSON :
  HOSPITAL PHARMACY COMPTER SYSTEM
  DEC. 1982 VOL 39 AMERICAN JOURNAL OF HOSPITAL PHARMACY

- CARLIER, DESCOUTURES, GERARD, MALICKI :
  PRATIQUES DE BONNE DISPENSATION DES MEDICAMENTS EN MILIEU HOSPITALIER
  MAI 84

- COORDONATEUR CHAST PARIS :
  PROPOSITIONS RELATIVES A LA DELIVRANCE DES MEDICAMENTS DANS LES ETABLISSEMENTS
  DE SOINS
  JUIN 1984

- ROBERT ZALESKI
  DIRECTOR OF PHARMACY OF WORCESTER :
  AN AUTOMATED PHARMACY MANAGEMENT SYSTEM MAKES A DIFFERENCE

- P. JEFFREY AND J. GALLINA :
  PHARMACY SERVICE UNITS
  THE EVOLUTION OF A CONCEPT
  AMERICAN JOURNAL OF HOSPITAL PHARMACISTS
  VOL 37 JAN. 80

- P LACHEZ . PASQUET
  L'INFORMATISATION DES HOPITAUX
  TECHNIQUES HOSPITALIERES FEV. 84 N° 461

- FEDERATION HOSPITALIERESDE FRANCE
  VERS UNE FUSION DES INTERACTIONS MEDICO-ADMINISTRATIVES
  A PARAITRE EN 1985

A MICROCOMPUTER SIMULATED INTERACTIVE CLINICAL PROBLEM

W. A. Corbett & M. J. Taylor*
Departments of Surgery and Computer Science*
University of Liverpool
Liverpool. L69 3BX UK.

Introduction   Conventional clinical teaching uses real-life problems, often at
the bedside itself, to demonstrate correct diagnosis and patient management. Clearly
bedside management requires an appropriate patient at a time when clinical teacher
and student are together so that teaching can occur.   There is always responsibility
to the patient for correct diagnosis and management.   Therefore, teaching is
necessarily channelled towards the correct solution. In principle students cannot
be allowed to find the correct diagnosis by making and understanding their own
mistakes yet a learning environment which would simulate clinical problems and
allow the student to test his own ideas would provide a valuable tool in medical
education.

In essence there is a need for a simulated interactive clinical problem that
progresses in time, whether or not decisions are made, incurs penalties for
incorrect decisions yet shows benefit from correct choices (with appropriate
changes in the patient's condition). Essential information regarding the
patient's clinical condition must be available on demand as must details of
special investigations such as X-Rays and blood tests. Specific clinical
rules need to be followed and other clinicians may be introduced into the overall
equation each bringing their specific requirements that the student must fulfil
in order to gain benefit.

The criteria for successful management and diagnosis must be clear and allowance
made for the possibility of error and complete failure with the option to try
again or view a 'correct' solution.

To cope with these demands we have used the dialogue programming language Microtext
(Bevan & Watson, 1983) implemented on a BBC model B microcomputer (Coll, 1982).
Microtext (Barker, 1984) Lends itself to structured, frame-based, information that
allows branching between frames in response to user input of numbers or free text.
Full use can also be made of colours, sound and teletext graphics to improve the
presentation for the user.

The Problem   The clinical problem selected for simulation by Microtext was based
on an actual event encountered by one of the authors. A young man out for the night
on the town had been involved in a knife fight and sustained little external evidence
of injury, a small wound in his right side. The subsequent clinical events provided
a good example of the need for prompt and essential evaluation of the situation with
speedy resuscitation with intravenous fluids and blood.   Surgery was necessary to

repair major damage to main blood vessels and associated injuries to liver, kidney and bowel. The clinical progress of this patient was predictable in the light of these internal injuries which were not immediately apparent on his arrival in the casualty department. Appropriate action was taken in this particular case but in real life little room for error is allowed as incorrect decisions will lead to an immediate deterioration in the patient's condition. Thus he represents a difficult clinical problem to assess that requires special attention to reach the correct diagnosis and appropriate action to retrieve the situation and successfully treat the patient.

Clinical Simulation   The system designed starts with an introductory module to explain the purpose and mode of operation of the simulation programme. This is followed by the central controlling module. Three time bases are used within the simulation. Microcomputer system time allows the programme to run for a maximum of twenty minutes. Hospital time is computed from the system time and makes allowances for delays over investigations or operations so that apparent hospital time may progress three hours during the twenty minutes of the programme. In addition there is the physiological time of the patient which determines and enables selection of appropriate values in accordance with hospital time elapsed but with allowance for positive, supportive, measures that improve the patient's condition and change the physiological status. Thus hospital time is inexorably progressive, physiological time tends to progress but can be reversed by appropriate action. The physiological parameters are recorded in relation to hospital time so that graphical representations of blood pressure and pulse may be displayed. In principle the student determines the pathway which is moved against the clock which alters the parameters of concern.

The central module is used to select either by a free text entry format or by single-key entry numeric menus to opt for investigations that will elucidate the patient's problem or for actions that will help improve the patient's condition. There are seven sub-modules for investigative action:

     1. History and examination   Relates the story as is known at the time plus the pertinent clinical findings on examination of the patient. A choice can be made between a brief synopsis and full details and appropriate hospital time penalties incurred of 10 minutes and 30 minutes respectively.

     2. X-rays   A choice is allowed for high quality X-rays in the main department or for emergency quality films in the casualty department. More information is gained from the high quality films but a heavy hospital time penalty is incurred (45 minutes).

     3. Blood pressure chart   The progress of the patient in response to clinical care can be mapped in physiological terms by recording the patient

parameters of pulse and blood pressure as the simulation progresses, which can then be displayed graphically on the microcomputer screen.

4. Fluid balance chart can be inspected at any time for a time related summary of urine output and fluids given in ½ hourly periods with accumulative totals. (No hospital time penalty incurred).

5. Blood tests Emergency blood tests that are routinely available out of hours are allowed as is the cross-match of blood for transfusion. After selection there is a period of waiting before either results are available or cross-matched blood can be transfused which amounts to 20 minutes of hospital time.

6. Peritoneal lavage is a diagnostic test which necessitates the insertion of a catheter through the abdominal wall into the peritoneal cavity for the instillation and withdrawal of one litre of 0.9% saline solution. This is a critical test which is sensitive to intra-abdominal damage with bleeding and gives important information for diagnosis and treatment. The small hospital time penalty incurred (10 minutes) is more than offset by the diagnostic benefit.

7. Observation In cases of difficulty it is reasonable to observe clinical progress over a period of time (30 minutes). A changing clinical picture can be of great help when the single observation is equivocal. However, in this case the rate of deterioration of the patient's condition because of continued bleeding does not allow such luxury and risks a fatal outcome for the patient.

There are six sub-modules providing direct action on the patient:

1. Insertion of an intravenous line. A critical step to take as no blood can be transfused without it. If the seriousness of the injuries is appreciated or suspected this will be an early option to take up. Failure to do so until a later stage may adversely affect the outcome as a hospital time penalty is necessarily involved (10 minutes).

2. Insertion of a urinary catheter. Another standard procedure in accordance with the gravity of the patient's injuries. Again failure to implement this at any early stage will have consequences as no urine output can be displayed in the fluid balance chart without a urinary catheter.

3. Insertion of an intercostal drain. From the site of the injury it is possible that the knife may have entered the chest causing damage to the lung with entry of air and internal haemorrhage. The appropriate line of action in this case is the insertion of an intercostal drain but this is quite unnecessary if a chest X-ray has been performed and so hospital time penalties are incurred by this action (20 minutes).

4. Blood transfusion. And the transfusion of other fluids such as

0.9% saline or 5% dextrose in water are the positive short term measures that will improve the patient's condition by restoring pulse, blood pressure and urine output to normal values. This module can be used repeatedly to improve the patient's status.

  5. <u>Exploration of the wound under local anesthesia</u>. This is a very time consuming and limited action. Nothing can be done about the internal injuries from this approach and the patient is left worse off because of the hospital time penalties incurred without benefit (30 minutes).

  6. <u>Operation under general anaesthesia</u>. Without doubt the patient will require surgical intervention to stop the bleeding and repair the damage. In order to reach this stage an anaesthetist must be recruited who will put the patient to sleep. However, the anaesthetist is most critical of management and requires you to produce a patient who has been resuscitated with intravenous fluids to relatively acceptable levels of pulse and blood pressure, has cross-matched blood available for transfusion and in whom you have some idea of the extent of the injuries within the body cavities. Satisfying all these criteria will lead to the revelation of the horrendous intra-abdominal injuries that are responsible for the patient's changing condition.

Successful patient mangement, the end of three hours' hospital time or the death of the patient completes the simulation. At this stage a higher level of the problem may be entered (currently under development) or the student may be given the opportunity to try again.

<u>Experience</u> Initial trials were performed within the University Department of Surgery for final system trials prior to release of system for general use.

Experience with the system by undergraduate medical students and surgeons in training has shown it to give a realistic and absorbing simulation of the clinical problem. Of particular note is the marked preference for users inexpert with keyboards to prefer simple numeric input rather than the more elegant and potentially more powerful free text allowed by Microtext. Currently further developments to provide a higher level of the clinical problem and improve the graphic displays are underway and it is hoped that it will be possible to merge Microtext programs and VCR display information that will extend the usefullness of the system.

<u>References</u>

BARKER, P.G. 1984. Microtext - A New Dialogue Programming Language for Microcomputers. Journal of Microcomputer Applications, <u>7</u> (2), 167-188.

BEVAN, N, and Watson, R., (eds) 1983. Microtext for the BBC Microcomputer Cambridge: Acornsoft Ltd.

References (Continued)

COLL, J., 1982. The BBC Microcomputer User Guide. London : British Broadcasting
Corporation.

PROBABILISTIC PROGNOSTIC DECISION MAKING : A CLINICAL EXAMPLE

Jos L. Willems, J. Pardaens, E. Lesaffre, L. Dekeyser and H. De Geest*
Div. Medical Informatics and Cardiology*, Univ. of Leuven
49, Herestraat, 3000 Leuven, Belgium

1. INTRODUCTION

The major tasks of medical consultation can be summarized as follows :
- sequential collection of findings and testing of their consistency
- interpretation of these findings in terms of a diagnostic model
- extrapolation of the natural course that is likely to follow (prognosis)
- formulation of therapeutic management plans and selection of initial therapy
- explanation and justification of the above
- reassessment and possible modification of diagnosis, prognosis and therapy.
The applications of formal methods of decision making have until now mostly been
concentrated on problems of diagnostic reasoning (1-4). Only few investigators have
applied decision analysis and other techniques to treatment selection problems and
even fewer have focused on the prognostic phase of the medical consultation process.

We have established a data base and coronary-care information system to estimate
survival of early and late deaths after acute myocardial infarction using clinical
findings gathered routinely in most CCUs (5-9). The purpose of the present paper is
to illustrate the use of statistical techniques for prognostic decision making.

2. METHODS

2.1. Data Collection

As reported previously (5-9) special forms were used to collect over 250 different
historical, biochemical, ECG and X-ray data, as well as data related to complications and therapy in the CCU for each patient admitted to the Univ. Hospital of
Leuven with the diagnosis of suspected myocardial infarction. According to WHO
criteria 2312 proved to have a definite (85 %) or possible (15 %) acute myocardial
infarction in the period between October 1, 1973 and April 30, 1979. The alive status of the patients was gathered from official community registers at two-year intervals. At the latest survey, in the summer of 1984, only two patients were lost
to follow-up. For the prediction of death within 1 year after discharge, patients
admitted before December 31, 1977 were used as learning sample (N=1724), those admitted later as test group (N=588) (7). For long term prognosis odd and even admissions were used for learning and testing respectively (8-9).

2.2. Variable selection and transformation

Through a plausibility program, checks were made for inconsistencies and missing
information. The data were stored in an IMAGE data base on an HP1000 minicomputer
and were transferred to an IBM 370/158 computer for further statistical analysis.
Descriptive, uni- and bivariate analysis techniques were firstly used to examine and
if necessary, transform the variables (7,8). Clinical judgment and the results of
the bivariate analysis served as a basis for the preselection of a total of 35 variables, including so-called compound items. For example the compound item intraventricular conduction defects includes all patients with either complete left,
right or other intraventricular conduction defects with QRS duration > 120 msec.

2.3. Data Analysis

In order to predict CCU, 28-day and 1-year mortality, stepwise linear discriminant
analysis was applied using the SPSS statistical package. The SAS- and BMDP-packages
were used for long-term survival analysis. Each individual patient entered into the
study at the moment of admission to the CCU, i.e. the starting event. Death from
any cause was used as terminal event. When this end point was not reached, the date
of last check-up was taken as censoring date. The statistical analysis techniques
were first applied to the learning population. The prediction formula and goodness
of fit of the hazard model were next examined in the test group in order to check
the reliability of the results. Allocation of patients to different risk categories
was further examined according to deciles and quintiles of obtained risk scores.

3. RESULTS

3.1. Prediction of short term mortality

Twelve variables proved to have a significant ($P < 0.05$), independent contribution
to 28-day mortality, which was 21 % for the total population (N=2312). A maximal
classification of 89.3 % could be obtained with a cutt-off discriminant score of
1.27 in the training sample. The predictive values for survival and early death
prediction were respectively 91.8 % and 77.9 %. By lowering the threshold more early deaths could be predicted, but specificity decreased similarly. When the formula
were applied to the test set, the overall accuracy figures dropped only slightly by
1 to 2 %. Eighty per cent of the early deaths (286 out of 359) in the first population occurred in the 3 upper deciles of the risk score distribution. The 28-day
mortality in the 3 lowest risk deciles equalled 2.7 % in the training set (14 out of
522). The 50 % lowest risk patients in the test set (N=588), had a mortality of
only 3.0 %, against 39.4 % for the remainder.

3.2. Prediction of one-year mortality

Factors related to the extent of the infarction, the severity of left ventricular dysfunction as well as to pre-existing vascular disease showed a significant relationship to one-year mortality in the patients who survived 28 days (N=1829). Patients with a second infarction, signs of heart failure or unusual dyspnoe in the past, those with cerebral or peripheral vascular disease and diabetes, high peak enzyme levels, arrhythmias, conduction disturbances, all had significantly higher one year mortality rates. Discriminant analysis formula derived from the learning set, predicted correctly one-year mortality with a total accuracy rate of 73.3 % in the learning sample, against 75.6 % in the validation or test set. Consistent sensitivity (68 versus 65 %) and specificity (74 versus 77 %) figures were obtained in the learning and test sample respectively.

Table 1 demonstrates that patients in the lowest 3 risk deciles, based on discriminant function scores derived from the learing set, presented only a one-year mortality of 2 %, against 40 to 54 % in the highest risk decile.

3.3. Long-term prediction based on survival analysis results

Fitting of the Cox-Breslow model yielded 11 significant (P < 0.01) covariates for long-term survival : age, peripheral vascular disease, X-ray signs of cardiomegaly or lung congestion, Killip class III or IV, previous infarction, digitalis or diuretics therapy during CCU stay, under- or overweight, low systolic blood pressure at admission, ventricular arrhythmias, diabetes and abnormal precordial pulsations.

Table 1 : One year mortality after acute MI   Fig. 1 : Survival of Risk Quintiles

Risk Decile	Learning Set		Test Set	
	Number	Mort %	Number	Mort %
1 - 3	410	2.4	147	2.0
4 - 5	274	6.6	99	7.1
6 - 7	271	12.9	95	12.6
8	138	21.0	28	21.4
9	136	26.5	58	25.9
10	136	40.4	37	54.1
Total	1365	13.4	464	13.6

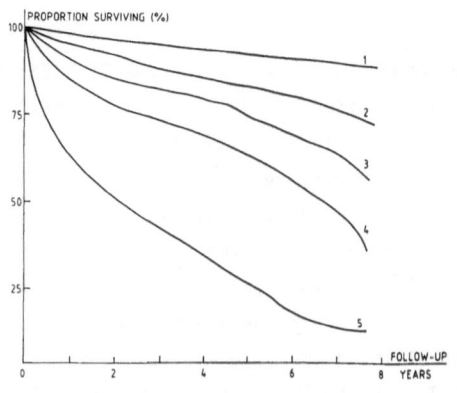

Extensive validation of the goodness of fit and model predictions was carried out in the learning and test set. Survival curves stratified by risk quintiles are shown in Fig. 1 for the total group. The log-rank test comparing these curves was highly significant. When risk ratio's were calculated for 5-year survival (N=1014 patients in total, 672 censored and 342 uncensored) similar mortality rates were obtained in both sets.

4. DISCUSSION

Various statistical, logical and pattern-recognition techniques have been introduced for medical decision making in the early sixties (1-4). However, only few investigators have applied these techniques for prognostic purposes. The main reason may be due to the fact that the probabilistic approach requires a large data base to obtain reliable prediction formula. Aid in prognostic decision making for patients with acute myocardial infarction is of considerable interest to clinicians. Indeed objective methods which enable to identify high risk patients for prolonged intensive care and low risk patients for early discharge, may have great socio-economic and financial benefits due to the high incidence and treatment costs of this disease. Not only early risk stratification, but also prediction of middle and long-term survival remains a major aim in view its potential impact on long-term treatment with beta-blockers and other medications. In order to be of widespread clinical interest the prediction model should be applicable to the patient population at large. For this reason we have focused our attention on non-invasive, clinical findings which are gathered routinely in most CCUs. We have demonstrated that a fairly good estimation of prognosis can be made by means of discriminant function analysis of such clinical data.

Prediction of 28-day, and also of CCU mortality, could be made with almost 90 % accuracy using 7 to 12 routine clinical variables. In the lower half of the risk distribution only 34 out of 1156 patients (2.9 %) died within on average 72 hours after admission. Similarly, patients who survived 28-days and which were classified in the lowest 3 risk deciles presented only a one-year mortality of 2.0 %. From a statistical point of view one would need a very large population to demonstrate a significant improvement by any therapy in a group with a starting mortality of only 2 or 3 %. Those in the upper 3 risk deciles, on the contrary, showed mortality rates which were 10 to 20 times higher. They form an ideal set to test new therapies. Results obtained in the learning set have been extensively validated in the test set which is another important point of our investigations (5-9). This was possible due to the very large number of patients examined.

Other investigators have recently used hemodynamic monitoring, radionuclide studies, echocardiography, ECG stress tests and ambulatory monitoring, as well as cardiac catheterisation for prognostic stratification. These techniques provide more direct information of left ventricular dysfunction, the extent of coronary artery disease, residual myocardial ischemia or ventricular arrhythmias which are the most important determinants of survival. However, these methods are either expensive, invasive or can for logistic reasons or contra-indications not be applied to the patient population at large. The costs and benefits of these techniques should in our opinion be evaluated against non-invasive clinical risk scores, such as those derived from our investigations. The sample size in most investigations of the prognostic value of hemodynamic, scintigraphic or exercise stress testing, has been rather small. Although comparison between different studies should be made with caution, data that we obtained for 28-day, one-year and long-term prediction using clinical data collected during the CCU stay without further tests and additional costs compare favorably to results of these studies.

We may therefore conclude that multivariate, probabilistic techniques using routine clinical data gathered during the CCU stay may be very helpful for risk stratification and individual patient management after myocardial infarction.

5. REFERENCES

1. Lusted L.B. Introduction to Medical Decision Making. Charles C. Thomas, Sprinfield Ill., 1968
2. de Dombal F.T. and Gremy F. (Eds.). Decision Making and Medical Care : Can Information Science Help ? North-Holland Publ., Amsterdam, 1976, pp. 1-603
3. Clancey W.J. and Shortliffe E.H. Readings in Medical Artificial Intelligence. The First Decade. Addison-Wesley Publ. Comp., 1984, p. 1-512
4. Feinstein A.R., Rubinstein J.F. and Ramshaw W.A. Estimating prognosis with the aid of a conversational mode computer program. Ann. Int. Med. 76 : 911-921, 1972
5. Willems J.L., Ector H., Pardaens J., Van Poecke G. and De Geest H. Use of the computer in determining prognostic determinants in acute myocardial infarction. Transactions Eur. Soc. Cardiol. 1 : 63, 1978
6. Willems J.L., Dekeyser L., Pardaens J. and De Geest H. A data base for the assessment and prognosis in acute myocardial infarction. MEDINFO 80 (Lindberg D.A. and Kaihara S., Eds.), North Holland Publ. Co., 1980, p. 1024-9
7. Willems J.L., Pardaens J. and De Geest H. Early risk stratification using clinical findings in patients with acute myocardial infarction. Eur. Heart J. 5 : 130-9, 1984
8. Pardaens J., Lesaffre E., Willems J.L. and De Geest H. Multivariate survival analysis for the assessment of prognostic factors and risk categories after recovery from acute myocardial infarction. Amer. J. Epidemiology, (In press).
9. Pardaens J., Dekeyser L., Lesaffre E., Willems J.L. and De Geest H. Robustness of prediction and influence of sample size, age and sex on prognostic factors for long-term survival after myocardial infarction. In Computers in Cardiology 1984 (Ed. Ripley K.L.) IEEE Computer Society, Long Beach (In press)

A FLEXIBLE RULE BASED SYSTEM FOR THE INTERPRETATION OF THYROID FUNCTION TESTS

P. Brosnan+, G. Boran*, Jane Grimson+,
A. Cranny*, J. McSweeney* and R.R. O'Moore*.

*Department of Clinical Biochemistry, St. James's Hospital.
+Department of Computer Science, Trinity College Dublin.

1.   INTRODUCTION

There has recently been a growth in the development of expert systems for the assessment of thyroid function (1,2,3,4). The reasons for this include the wish to:- a) increase diagnostic accuracy by improved test strategies; b) provide an internal laboratory tool to reduce the numbers of tests carried out; c) to provide interpretative reports for the majority of users of the laboratory who are non specialist physicians.

In parallel with this development the number of potential thyroid function tests available has rapidly increased over the past five years. Furthermore considerable controversy exists concerning the usefulness of the individual tests and which of the various batteries of tests are the most effective (5). Thus there is no universally accepted diagnostic strategy for the investigation of thyroid function. The result of this is that most of the present computer aided decision support systems for thyroid function are not easily transportable and have a tendency to be local curiosities.

In an attempt to overcome this problem we have developed a rule based system which incorporates all of the most commonly used thyroid function tests into its logic. The facility for each user to stipulate the decision and reference ranges for the tests used in the local laboratory is also provided.

2.   PROGRAM OPERATION

The program is intended to be an 'expert system' for interpretation of thyroid function test results. It requires a first line test of thyroid function to be always available and the tests chosen are

the total thyroxine (TT4) level or the immunoradiometric assay of
thyrotropin (TSH-IRMA), which has recently emerged as a possible
first line test (6,7).   The program accepts any combination of the
following supplementary tests:-

    1.   Total triiodothyronine
    2.   Free thyroxine (or Free thyroxine index)
    3.   Free triiodothyronine
    4.   Thyroxine binding globulin (and T4:TBG ratio)
    5.   Thyrotropin radioimmunoassay (TSH-RIA)

The decision ranges for these variables are stipulated by the local
user.   One of the following clinical information codes is required:-

    1.   Suspected hyperthyroidism
    2.   Suspected hypothyroidism
    3.   On maintenance T3/T4 therapy
    4.   Treated thyrotoxicosis
    5.   Not specified or other indication for thyroid
        function tests.
    6.   Drug therapy.

This information, as well as the age and sex of the patient, is
taken into account in the interpretation.

3.   PROGRAM DESIGN

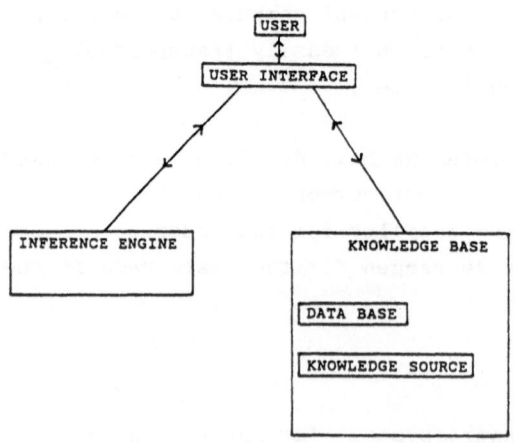

Figure. 1   Program Design.

An overview of the program
is illustrated in Figure 1.
The program contains an
inference engine which
interacts with a knowledge
base.   The knowledge base
consists of a knowledge
source and a database.   The
knowledge source is
expressed as a tree
structure containing over
1,300 decision points/rules.
The database comprises over
300 comments.

Based on the results of either of the two first line tests there are
fourteen main branches. As one progresses down one of these branches
successive branching decisions taken are based on the results of
subsequent tests. At appropriate points in the branch a suitable
comment module is referenced. The combination of all the comment
modules constitutes the final interpretation module which is reported.
the comments which are age and sex related may support or refute a
clinical suspicsion and suggest further appropriate tests if necessary.

4.   IMPLEMENTATION

The software is coded in FRANZ-LISP and is currently running in an
interactive mode on the University VAX mainframe computer. It is
presently being translated into a subset of Common LISP for
implementation on a DEC 100 microcomputer which is interfaced with the
main laboratory PDP 11/44 MUMPS system (8). It is intended that
batches of test results with be downloaded from the PDP and the
interpretative comments generated and printed together with the
test results on the microcomputer. The system has been extensively
tested and modified using patient data from the endocrine laboratory.
A specimen report is illustrated in Figure 2 and the corresponding
logic in Figure 3. We are about to embark on a more extensive
clinical evaluation prior to implementing the system in the routine
service.

SURNAME SMITH	**FORENAME** JOHN	**ST.JAMES'S HOSPITAL**
LOCATION BIOCHEMISTRY	**SEX** M **D.O.B.** 12/03/45	CENTRAL PATHOLOGY
CONSULTANT O'MOORE		LABORATORY
RECORD NO. 50/125000		
LAB NO. C0125718	**REQUESTED** 21/03/85	**BIOCHEMISTRY**
ADDRESS		
CLINICAL DETAILS SUSPECTED HYPOTHYROIDISM		

```
          TOTAL T4      227    nM/1   (50 - 157)
          FREE T4       44     pM/1   (10 - 32)
          TSH-IRMA      0.05   mU/1   (0.08 - 7.5)
```

INTERPRETATION

Suppression of TSH-IRMA indicates that your patient is
hyperthyroid. (COMMENT 1)
The markedly elevated TOTAL T4 strongly suggests
hyperthyroidism (COMMENT 2)
The elevated FREE T4 suggests clinical hyperthyroidism
(COMMENT 3)

In summary although you suspected hypothyroidism the
markedly elevated TT4 with raised free hormone and
suppressed TSH confirm hyperthyroidism. Your patient
may be a case of apathetic thyrotoxicosis (COMMENT 4)

```
Received                              Reported
21/03/85  12:00                       24/03/85 12:00
```

FIGURE 2 Specimen report with comment number inserted
         (vide infra)

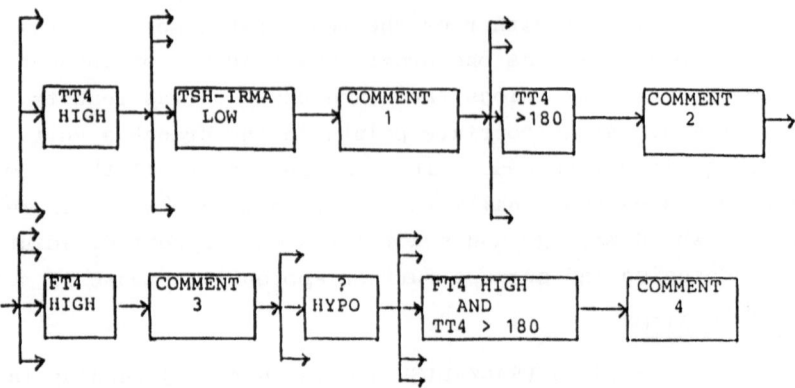

Figure 3   Algorithm corresponding to the report in Figure 2.

5.   REFERENCES

1. Hyde, T.A.   The interpretation of In Vitro tests of Thyroid
   Function with a Minicomputer. Am. J. Clin. Path (1981) 75,
   70 - 74.
2. McConnell, T.H. et al.   Algorithm derived computer generated
   interpretative comments in the reporting of laboratory tests.
   Am. J. Clin. Path. (1980) 72, 32 - 41.
3. Kulikowski,C.A.   Expert systems for Thyroid Function Testing.
   Diagnostic Medicine (1981) 99 - 102.
4. Sator, H. et al.   On the development of a computer assisted
   diagnostic strategy.   Lecture Notes in Medical Informatics
   Vol. 16 1982 470 - 476. Springer Verlag.   Ed. R.R. O'Moore,
   B. Barber, P. Reichertz and F. Roger.
5. Ray, R.A. et al. Controveries in Thyroid Function Testing.
   Clinics in Laboratory Medicine (1984) 4, 671 - 682.
6. Alexander, W.D. et al.   First line tests of Thyroid Function.
   (Lancet (ii) (1984) 647.
7. Seth, J. et al, A sensitive immunoradiometric assay for serum
   thyroid stimulating hormone: a replacement for the thyrotrophin
   releasing hormone test?
8. O'Moore, R.R. et al. Experience with a MUMPS Based System for
   Clinical Chemistry.   Lecture Notes in Medical Informatics
   Vol. 16.   Proceedings 'MIE 82', Dublin (1982) 82 - 88.
   Springer Verlag.

HELP: A Medical Information System With Decision Making Capability

Paul D. Clayton, T. Allan Pryor, Reed M. Gardner, Peter J. Haug,
and Homer R. Warner. Dept. of Medical Biophysics and Computing,
LDS Hospital/University of Utah, Salt Lake City, Utah 84143 USA

HELP is a medical information system which is routinely used to collect and review patient data, to provide financial, administrative and management information and to produce computer generated medical decisions. Although the HELP system was developed at the LDS Hospital and University of Utah in Salt Lake City, it has now been successfully transported to other institutions. The system (see figure) consists of three main components: 1. A comprehensive clinical database for all patients in the hospital. 2. A separate, modular medical knowledge base which contains criteria necessary to make specific medical decisions (alerts, interpretations, diagnoses, or therapeutic suggestions). 3. The HELP interpreter. This module provides the control function to decide which logic modules should get evaluated and then evaluates the appropriate medical logic. In the following sections, each of these components will be described in greater detail.

HELP DECISION SUPPORT SYSTEM

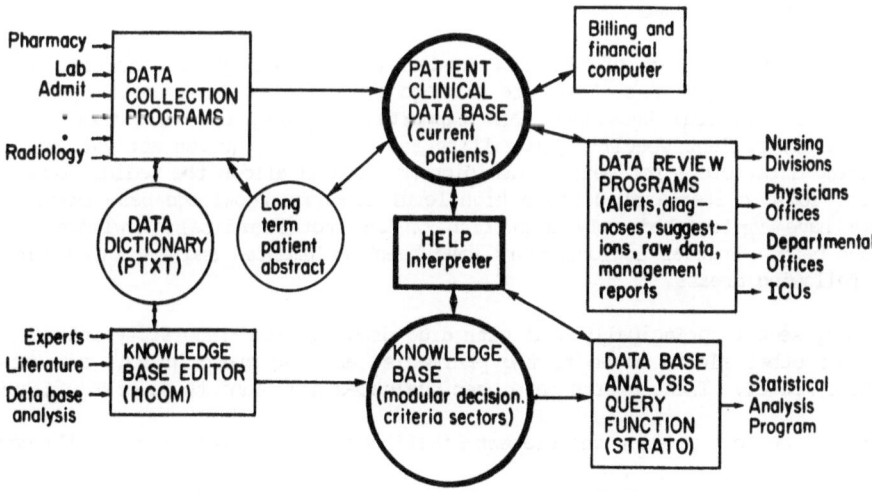

The On-line Clinical Database

The clinical data base consists of two elements: long term abstract of demographic and clinical information likely to be useful if the patient is readmitted to the hospital and a short term comprehensive collection of all data gathered during the current hospital admission. All data are stored in coded form (as opposed to free text) so that data can be retrieved and analyzed for use in research and decision logic. Hierarchal codes are defined using a system called PTXT which is basically a computer based dictionary. Using this program, a user defines the codes for a data item, as well as the associated text to be used for reports and terminal display, and key words which are appropriate for the data item. Key words enable users who are constructing data retrieval items for decision logic sectors to easily specify the codes which should be sought.

The data are entered automatically in many instances through digital or analog interfaces (ECG, catheterization laboratory, pulmonary function laboratory, clinical laboratory, etc.) or by interaction with a terminal (pharmacy, radiology, nurses notes, etc.).

A general question asking program (GQAP) makes it possible for technical personnel without programming skills to construct data entry questionnaires. To develop a questionnaire, it is necessary to type a free text question, specify the type of answer expected, and define codes which should be associated with the answer. Follow-up questions which depend on previous answers and error-detecting logic are system capabilities which are routinely used to construct branching type questionnaires for data entry.

The database generated while the patient is in the hospital is generally complete except for physician derived data such as a complete history and physical examination. We are currently attempting to develop ways in which the physician can conveniently enter these missing data. Because the database is presently hospital oriented, information from the private physician's office and post-discharge outcome measures are generally not available except in specific research areas.

The Medical Knowledge Base

The most unique aspect of the HELP system is the ability to construct modular decision sectors. These sectors are analogous to frames in symbolic processing systems. This medical knowledge base supports a variety of logic models (If... Then... rules, patient specific probability revision, data driven activation, query for missing data, etc.) for medical decision making and allows the medical expert to enter the logic criteria by using a high level language knowledge base editor. To date we have implemented only a portion of the total medical knowledge in our knowledge base. However logic sectors have been implemented and are in current use in the following areas:

Pharmacy sectors principally deal with drug-drug and drug-laboratory interactions as well as other alerts given to the pharmacist as drug prescriptions are entered into the computer. These alerts have been evaluated and found to be cost effective.

Radiology sectors predict the pretest likelihood that a given finding will occur.

Blood gas sectors interpret the measurements and indicate whether there is hypoxemia, hyper-or-hypoventilation, or respiratory or metabolic acidosis or alkalosis and the direction of any change in the patient's status.

The ECG sectors interpret parameters derived from the waveform to assess morphologic abnormalities, arrhythmias, and serial changes.

Clinical laboratory sectors generate alerts and interpretations based upon electrolytes, blood chemistries, hematology, and drug levels.

Decision analysis is used to assess decisions regarding treatment of patients-with suspected coronary artery disease.

Diagnostic sectors have been written for specific areas of internal medicine, the most detailed emphasis to this point has been upon pulmonary disease.

Pulmonary function tests in pre-admission screening and the pulmonary laboratory are analyzed and interpreted using HELP logic.

Hemodynamic and cardiac function measurements in the intensive care units are also interpreted using HELP logic.

HELP logic is used to determine which specific history questions to ask an individual patient.

HELP logic is used to ascertain when a candidate satisfies explicit criteria for admission to a research protocols.

To objectively assess the status of patients in the critical care unit, criteria have been defined to create a multi-organ failure index.

Dietary and diabetic alerts based upon a brief history, pharmacy and clinical-laboratory information are run daily.

HELP logic has been developed to recognize patients with high risk pregnancies and prescribe management protocols for these patients.

Pathologic findings obtained by electron microscopy are classified according to explicit criteria defined in HELP sector logic.

When arrhythmias occur in patients in the cardiac intensive care unit, the extent to which the arrhythmia is judged to be life threatening and suggestions for appropriate conversion are presented.

Triage sectors based upon recently published protocols for deciding when an emergency room patient should be admitted to the cardiac intensive care unit have been developed.

Infectious disease/antibiotic monitoring sectors have been developed. The computer reminds physicians when there is a cheaper or more appropriate antibiotic.

Therapeutic suggestions and requests for diagnostic tests are made in a broad range of the applications which have been described. Requests for bronchodilators during a pulmonary function test, or a serum creatine measurement for patients receiving the drug gentamicin, and the suggestion that a specific drug be discontinued are examples of this feature. Most of the applicatations that have been discussed are used routinely in day-to-day clinical service. A few of the areas are being used only by one or two physicians to test feasibility of widespread application and to develop more extensive and sophisticated logic.

The HELP Interpreter

A HELP interpreter (the third major component of the system) acts as the interface between the knowledge base and the clinical database. It evokes the appropriate subsets of the knowledge base and interprets the logic found in each individual logic module. The sectors themselves contain the logic which determines how they are evaluated, e.g. if....then..... rules or statistical probability calculations. An arithmetic item can be used to perform tasks ranging from Boolean logic to calculation of a value for a discriminant function. Chronologic statements can be used to retrieve the time of certain specified events so that these times can be used for search limitations or action flags. Existence items use the presence or absence of a piece of data rather than the value of the data as the basis for logical or arithmetic calculations. Search items are used to retrieve specific data within prescribed time limits from the clinical data base. Modifiers such as frequency, minimum, maximum, mean etc. may be appended to the search item as appropriate. Search items may also request the evaluation of additional HELP sectors by asking for the results of that sector. Because of the frequent use of Bayes' formula in some types of HELP decisions, this function has been explicitly defined; the logic for other types of statistical decision models is performed using arithmetic items.

Radiologist Assistance

As an example of the capabilities which the system provides, we shall describe a recent project in which the computer assists radiologists as they read chest roentgenograms. We developed medical logic which is used to present the radiologist with a synopsis of clinical information about the patient in the form of a differential list of likely diagnoses. After entry of the radiological findings, this list is re-evaluated to show the impact of the information obtained from the current examination.

We used a probabilistic model (sequential applications of Bayes' Theorem) to develop medical logic for diagnosing 29 different pulmonary diseases. The logic modules (HELP sectors) for each of the diseases consist of 4 parts: 1) the a priori probability of the disease, 2) a group of search items which direct the computer to ascertain the presence or absence of data items specific to the disease under consideration (history, physical exam, chest radiograph findings, and laboratory data), 3) a set of conditional probabilities for those data items referenced in the search items, and 4) a series of Bayesian constructs which generate posterior probabilities sequentially using the results of one data item as the prior probability of the next calculation.

Forty-one pulmonary diseases were identified in the discharge summaries of 82 control patients. Fifty-one of these patients fell into the category of "No Pulmonary Disease". An initial analysis of the disease modules was done prior to the addition of the x-ray findings to the patient records. Based on historical and clinical data which were available before the initial chest x-ray, seventy-eight percent of the diseases found in this group of patients appeared on the diagnostic lists generated by the computer. Sixty-three of 82 (77%) diagnostic lists were completely accurate i.e. contained all pulmonary diagnoses recorded for that patient. After the findings from the initial chest x-rays were added to each patient record the diagnostic modules were run again. 80% percent of the disease states were correctly included in the differential diagnostic lists. Sixty-seven of 82 lists (82%) contained all recorded diseases.

Summary

In summary, Help is a routinely used system for automated medical decision-making. A specific study of the alerts for contraindicated drugs showed that the system is cost-effective and that physicians normally agree with the computer generated decisions. Another study of electrolyte abnormalities showed that patient care was improved when the computer alerted nurses and physicians to abnormal values. General purpose tools exist for entering clinical information and expert medical logic into the respective databases. Increased availability of the system will hopefully result in the development of additional amounts of appropriately formatted medical logic as well as improved patient care.

References:

1. Pryor TA, Gardner RM, Clayton PD, Warner HR. The HELP System. J of Medical Systems 7:87-102, 1983.

2. Gerard MJ, Haug PJ, Morrison WJ, Tocino I, Frederick PR, Crapo RO, Harada SK, Clayton PD. A computer system for diagnosing pulmonary disease. Proc. Am. Assoc. Med. Inform., San Francisco, p. 119-123, May, 1984.

MEDICAL DECISION MAKING VIA SIMULTANEOUS CONFIDENCE
INTERVALS BASED ON SELECTION PROCEDURES

G. Giani

Department of Medical Statistics and Documentation
Technical University Aachen
F.R. Germany

1. Introduction

Just in medical decision making a major problem is to compare several treatments with regard to their efficiency. One intends to separate *good* from *bad* treatments. But since in real situations the mechanism of the influence of a treatment is full of complexities every final decision is made under uncertainty. We have to accept the fact that decisions may be wrong. To control the error being made if a wrong statement is given one has to design a clinical trial according to statistical requirements. In the preceding situation the classical approach to decision making suggests to make inference for all pairwise comparisons of treatments via simultaneous confidence intervals or tests. This method however is at best indirect since the comparisons between only good or only bad treatments are included in the resulting statements. So they do not contribute to the solution of the task stated above. Rather it would be better to turn one's attention to simultaneous inference between all treatments and the unknown best. In this paper we intend to give an introduction to statistical methods for latter inference taking into account newest developments in this area. Finally medical applications are presented.

2. Notations and assumptions

Suppose there are $k \geq 2$ competing treatments numbered from 1 to k. Further, assume we can get relevant information about their effects from only one clinical parameter. Otherwise, if more than one parameter has to be taken into account, it should be possible to combine this multi-dimensional information to one real-valued variable in a suitable way. Now, to get statistical inference we have to make measurements which we imagine to be generated by a normal distribution model. n independent observations $X_{i1}, \ldots, X_{in}$ - each normally distributed with mean ϑ_i and equal variance σ^2 - are assumed to be available for every treatment i . If larger means reflect greater quality, that treatment, say (k), which corresponds to $\vartheta_{[k]} = \max_i \vartheta_i$ has to be regarded as being best. In our framework all others are assessed in terms of their distances

$$\delta_i = \vartheta_{[k]} - \vartheta_i$$

from the best.

3. The indifference zone formulation of Bechhofer

In this approach the purpose is to identify the best treatment with high certainty. Generally this cannot be done for all possible configurations of true means and moreover such a wishful thinking would not even be meaningful. For if the true (but unknown) mean vector $\vartheta = (\vartheta_1, \ldots, \vartheta_k)$ has some components ϑ_i, $i \neq (k)$ which are very close next to the best, then in real situations it is meaningless and clinically irrelevant to distinguish among the corresponding treatments. There is some indifference in the decision which of these treatments should be named the best. They all have to be considered as equally good. More precisely, for given ϑ the definition of the set G_ϑ of *good* treatments is commonly based on a critical value $\delta_1^* > 0$ specified by the clinician for practical reasons. This threshold value reflects the maximum amount in which the means of any two treatments are allowed to differ to be regarded as being undistinguishable. We write $G_\vartheta = \{i: \delta_i < \delta_1^*\}$. Note that this set always contains the best treatment and that only if its cardinality $|G_\vartheta|$ is greater than one the corresponding mean vector ϑ gives rise to the mentioned indifference in decision making. Therefore the subset

$$\Omega_I = \{\vartheta \in \mathbb{R}^k : |G_\vartheta| > 1\}$$

of the entire parameter space $\mathbb{R}^k$ is called the *indifference zone* by Bechhofer (1954). Over Ω_I there is no strong preference to select an unique best treatment.

If the mean vector ϑ lies in the complementary *preference zone* $\Omega_P = \mathbb{R}^k \backslash \Omega_I$ then there is substantial interest to select the best treatment with high probability, say with at least probability P^* ($P^* > 1/k$) . For this purpose in the normal case Bechhofer proposed the "natural" procedure

> B : select the treatment that yields the
>
> largest mean $\bar{x}_i = n^{-1} \sum\limits_{j=1}^{n} x_{ij}$.

The probability requirement regarding a correct selection (CS) now states as follows:

(1)   Pr (CS using procedure B) $\geqslant P^*$ whenever $\vartheta \in \Omega_P$.

Given P^* and δ_1^* this is a condition for the sample sizes n . Easyly it can be seen that for the validity of (1) we have to choose $n \geqslant (d\sigma/\delta_1^*)^2$, where d is given by

(2) $\int\limits_{-\infty}^{+\infty} \phi^{k-1}(x+d) \, d\phi(x) = P^*$

and ϕ denotes the standard normal distribution function.

Even though B is designed to quarantee a CS over the preference zone nevertheless it is of interest how the procedure behaves when ϑ lies in the indifference zone. It is not astonishing that in this case the selected treatment, say S , can be shown to be good (i.e. $S \in G_\vartheta$) with at least probability P^*. Thus, we obtain at level P^* for all $\vartheta \in \mathbb{R}^k$

$$\delta_S \leqslant \delta_1^* .$$

Fabian (1962) has even proved that without decreasing P^* it holds

(3) $\qquad \delta_S \leqslant D_S \overset{!}{\leqslant} \delta_1 \quad$ where $\quad D_i = \max(\max_{j \neq i} \bar{X}_j - \bar{X}_i + \frac{d\sigma}{\sqrt{n}} , 0) .$

Hsu (1981) strenghened this result and showed that (1) is equivalent to the set

(4) $\qquad 0 \leqslant \delta_i \leqslant D_i \qquad i = 1, \ldots, k$

of simultaneous confidence intervals for all δ_i .

4. The subset selection formulation of Gupta

Here the goal is to select a subset of treatments which contains the best. The procedure G proposed by Gupta (1956) is

(5) $\qquad G:$ select subset $M = \{i: \bar{X}_i \geqslant \max_{j \neq i} \bar{X}_j - d \frac{\sigma}{\sqrt{n}}\} .$

Given d by (2) we get

(6) $\qquad Pr$ (CS using procedure G) $\geqslant P^*$ whenever $\vartheta \in \mathbb{R}^k$.

Note that the probability of CS is controlled over the entire mean vector space $\mathbb{R}^k$. Again Hsu (1981) showed that (6) is equivalent to (4) . The statements also remain true in the more interesting case of unknown variance. Only σ has to be replaced by the estimate $\hat{\sigma} = \left[k(n-1)\right]^{-1/2}\left[\sum\sum_{ij}(X_{ij}-\bar{X}_i)^2\right]^{1/2}$ and d has to be choosen according to

(7) $\qquad \int_0^\infty \int_\infty^\infty \phi^{k-1}(x+dy) \, d\phi(x) dX_{k(n-1)} (y) = P^*$

where X_ν is the distribution function of $X_\nu/\sqrt{\nu}$.

5. Two-sided simultaneous intervals for δ_i

We consider the case of unknown σ only. Thus, in the previous terms one has to replace σ by $\hat{\sigma}$. Recently Edwards and Hsu (1983) have obtained the following result. If d fulfills

(8)
$$\int_{0}^{\infty}\int_{-\infty}^{+\infty} \left[\Phi(x+dy) - \Phi(x-dy)\right]^{k-1} d\Phi(x)\,dx_{k}\binom{y}{(n-1)} = P^{*} \; ,$$

a set of two-sided simultaneous inverals for all δ_{i} at level P^{*} is given by

(9)
$$d_{i} \equiv \max(\min_{j\in M} \bar{X}_{j} - \bar{X}_{i} - d\,\frac{\hat{\sigma}}{\sqrt{n}} , 0) \leqslant \delta_{i} \leqslant D_{i} \qquad i=1,\ldots,k$$

Moreover, it is also guaranteed that $(k) \in M$.

6. Decision making

For a posteriori decision making we can use the confidence intervals (4) or (9) in the following way.

Suppose first we are interested in selecting good treatments only or, using above notation, in selecting treatments contained in G_{ϑ}. Then, given d according to (2) or (7) depending on whether σ is known or unknown it follows from (4) that $M_{1} = \{i: D_{i} \leqslant \delta_{1}^{*}\}$ is a subset of all good treatments. The set M_{1} is consistent in the sense that at least for $n \to \infty$ M_{1} equals G_{ϑ} . If the true mean vector ϑ lies in the preference zone and M_{1} contains only one treatment, this treatment is the best at level P^{*} . But also it may happen that M_{1} is empty. This case reflects the situation where there is no evidence in the data for identifying good treatments. Further investigation with larger sample sizes has to be done. However, in any case we can establish that the best treatment is controlled to be in M at level P^{*} .

Suppose secondly we want to seperate good from bad treatments where *bad* ones are those which are too far apart from the best or, more specifically, those treatments i for which $\delta_{i} \geqslant \delta_{2}^{*}$ for some specified $\delta_{2}^{*} > \delta_{1}^{*}$. Note that not for all configurations of means there exist bad treatments. Using (9) , with confidence P^{*} the sets M_{1} and $M_{2} = \{i: d_{i} \geqslant \delta_{2}^{*}\}$ contain only good and only bad treatments, respectively. Again M_{1} and M_{2} are consistent and with confidence P^{*} the set M contains the best treatment. The case of empty set M_{2} has to be interpreted as mentioned above.

7. Medical applications

In this section two medical applications are presented. All simultaneous one- and two-sided confidence intervals have been computed at level $P^{*} = 95\%$, where the tables of Dunnett (1955) and Hahn and Hendrickson (1971) were used to determine d in (7) and (8).

a) After aorto-coronary by-pass operations 36 patients were treated in a prospective randomized study with 3 types of hypocaloric parenteral nutrition consisting of the same content of amino acids (70g/day) but different amounts of carbohydrates : 120 g dextrose (treatment 2), 120 g dextrose/fructose/xylitol (1:2:1) (treatment 3)

and 200 g dextrose/fructose/xylitol (1:2:1) (treatment 4). The control group
(treatment 1) consisted of 12 patients having received only 75g/day of dextrose. The
main variable of interest was the nutrition balance $[gN]$ cumulated over 4 days,
where the best treatment should show largest values on average. Note, the cumulative
nutrition balance always has to be negative after such serious operations. The data
including confidence intervals are summarized in Table 1.

Table 1: Cumulative nutrition bilance data $[gN]$ (n=12)

treatment	mean	standard deviation	Simultaneous confidence intervals	
			one-sided	two-sided
1	-48.19	13.87	$[0,39.78]$	$[12.54, 41.41]$
2	-19.76	10.49	$[0, 9.01]$	$[0 , 10.64]$
3	-22.10	13.44	$[0,13.78]$	$[0 , 15.41]$
4	-22.76	14.22	$[0,14.26]$	$[0 , 15.89]$
			$M = \{2,3,4\}$	$M = \{2,3,4\}$

Since $1 \notin M$, we see that with confidence 95% treatment 1 can be excluded to be
the best. This statement is also supported by the non-zero lower bound of the cor⁻
responding two-sided confidence interval. If we accept $\delta_1^* = 10$ as a threshold value
for defining good treatments we can conclude from the one-sided intervals that
$M_1 = \{2\}$,i.e.only treatment 2 can be identified to be a good treatment.For $\delta_1^* = 15$
M_1 equals M what means that in this case all treatments elected by Gupta's subset
selection procedure have to be regarded as being good.

b)   Still today the malignant hyperthermia is a dread complication of an anesthesia.
Clinical symptoms among others are increased creatinphosphokinase (CPK) values. There-
for the choice of the adequate anesthesia should also be governed with the object of
keeping the CPK-gradient low. Six anesthesic methods frequently used in the children
surgery for diseases in the area of nose, ear and throat were randomized to 48 otherwise healthy children in equal proportions. The main variable of interest was the
CPK-difference: CPK-value before intubation minus CPK-value measured 30 min after
intubation.That method with the largest expected CPK-difference was defined to be the
best. The data are given in Table 2.

The set M of treatments eligible to be best is different depending on whether
it is based on one- or two-sided intervals. Note that even though method 4 is not
included in M the lower bound of the corresponding two-sided interval is zero. So
it is not possible to detect method 4 as being bad whatever the choise of δ_2^* may
be (i.e. $M_2 = \emptyset$). Statements concerning good anesthesic methods can be made in the
same manner as in the first example.

In a critical way of looking at the presented evaluation one has to admit that

Table 2: CPK-differences (n=8)

anesthesic method	mean	standard deviation	Simultaneous confidence intervals	
			one-sided	two-sided
1	- 1.13	12.88	[0, 69.70]	[0, 78.16]
2	-22.50	30.25	[0, 91.07]	[0, 99.54]
3	14.25	10.14	[0, 38.95]	[0, 47.41]
4	-77.75	84.68	[0,146.32]	[0, 154.79]
5	-13.13	21.90	[0, 81.70]	[0, 90.16]
6	-44.75	66.62	[0,113.32]	[0, 121.787]
			$M = \{1,2,3,5\}$	$M = \{1,2,3,5,6\}$

instead of having based the confidence intervals on empirical means it would have been better to use robust intervals taking into account the possiblity of outliers. Just the extreme differences in the standard deviations support these arguments.

8. Concluding remarks

Clearly to give confidence intervals for δ_i the restriction neither to a balanced one-way layout nor to the normal distribution model is necessary. For instance, for a block design exact nonparametric intervals have been given by the author and will be published elsewhere.

References

BECHHOFER, R.E. (1954). A single-sample multiple decision procedure for ranking means of normal populations with known variances. The Annals of Mathematical Statistics 25, 16-39.

DUNNETT, C.W. (1955). A multiple comparison procedure for comparing several treatments with a control. Journal of American Statistical Association 50, 1096-1121.

EDWARDS, D.G. and HSU, J.C. (1983). Multiple comparisons with the best. Journal of the American Statistical Association 78, 965-971.

FABIAN, V. (1962). On multiple decision methods for ranking population means. The Annals of Mathematical Statistics 33, 248-254.

GUPTA, S.S. (1956). On a decision rule for a problem in ranking means. Ph. D. Thesis (Mimeograph Series 150). Institute of Statistics. University of North Carolina, Chapel Hill.

HAHN, G.J. and HENDRICKSON, R.W. (1971). A table of the largest absolute value of k Student t variates and its applications. Biometrika 58, 323-332.

HSU, J.C. (1981). Simultaneous confidence intervals for all distances from the *best*. The Annals of Statistics 5, 1026-1034.

AN EXPERT CONSULTATION SYSTEM TO AID CLINICAL DIAGNOSES

Vladimir Srdanović[*] and Branko Limić[**]

University of Belgrade

* Center for Multidisciplinary Studies

** Institute of Rheumatology

ABSTRACT An expert consultation system to support clinical decision making has been developed. Medical expert knowledge and data from clinical practice are combined to comprise the knowledge base of the system.

The system has originally been designed to deal with problems in rheumatology, and it has been tested successfully.

1. INTRODUCTION

The system presented has been under development for five years as a joint effort of the two institutions of the University of Belgrade: Center for Multidisciplinary Studies and the Institute of Rheumatology. The original task was to design a decision supporting system which will help physicians diagnose diseases from a group of so called seronegative arthropathies.

The artificial intelligence approach was taken in developing strategies to combine data from clinical practice and the expert knowledge.

Excellent reviews of the applications of the artificial intelligence in medicine as well as discussion of the main problems of the field are given by Pople /1/, Shortliffe /2/ and Barr and Feigenbaum /3/.

Our research has given satisfactory results /4,5/, but has also led to a design of an domain-independent expert consultation system.

2.TRANSFER OF EXPERTISE

To facilitate communication, a natural language interface was developed, letting the clinician define his data himself.

Also, the consultation system allows the expert clinician enter his knowledge about associations between entities in the knowledge-base in a form of production rules (see Example 1).

IF Morning pain is not alleviated &

   Swelling is present &

   Skin redness is present   (Example 1)

THAN Character of pain is inflamatory

3. REPRESENTATION OF KNOWLEDGE

Knowledge of the specific medical domain is represented in such a way that manifestations are linked with each of the disease categories (and among themselves) by associations of various strenghts. This is expressed by an integer between 0 and 10 (0 meaning that manifestation does not occur with the particular disease and 10 that it is pathognomonic for the disease). Statement presented in Example 2 thus expresses the possibility of ankylosing spondylitis (AS) being present with diagnostic strenght (DS) equal 7, given that character of pain (CP) is inflamatory (I).

$$DS\ (AS,\ CP = 1) = 7 \qquad\qquad (Example\ 2)$$

Some of this knowledge is provided to the system by the expert, reflecting the theoretical criteria and practice unanimously accepted by rheumatologists, and some of his own experience and/or believes. Typically, it is given in the form of IF-THAN rules (see Example 1).

On the other hand, analyses performed on a clinical data base, to which the consultation system is linked, provide the knowledge about associations between entities in the knowledge-base and the estimates of their strenght in cases where no explicit medical knowledge is existing and/or recorded /6/. (See Example 3.)

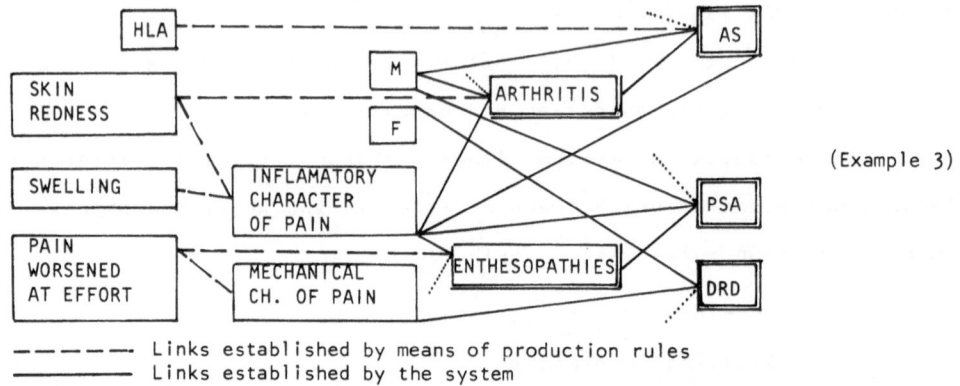

(Example 3)

– – – – – – Links established by means of production rules
——————— Links established by the system

After the knowledge-base is so formed the system employs a heuristic procedure to extract the key features (manifestations) for particular
diseases, i.e. differential diagnoses. The procedure has proven to be
efficient in practice and much less computationally complex than the
corresponding methods of multivariate statistics.

The notion of "cost" is also introduced in the knowledge-base, manifestations ranging from those requiring invasive and/or expensive and
lenghtly procedures in order to be established ("most costly"), to those
readily observable ("least costly").

4. CONSULTATION PROCESS

After initial data are entered about the patient for whom consulting
help is needed, the system establishes the working hypothesis of the possible disease(s) encountered. It takes on by directing the further information-gathering procedure.The system proceeds by first asking questions
about the patient that would discriminate the most among the alternative
diagnoses. Also, the "less costly" questions are asked first.

The data are then evaluated and scores are formed for each disease
category considered. The system terminates consultation by suggesting the
most likely diagnosis when data provide sufficient evidence for it (score
above predetermined treshold). Otherwise, or in cases when no single diagnosis can be reached by a predetermined margin, the system would suggest

performance of the additional, "more costly" tests.

Also, the system is capable of "explaining" its decisions by displaying portions of its knowledge base that were used in the consultation process.

5. EVALUATION

The physician in charge is frequently faced with the problem of differential diagnosis between the rheumatic and pararheumatic process. Therefore, the consultation system is used as a vehicle to test the possibility of patients screening based upon the existing symptoms, signs and available findings.

Presently, clinical data base adjoint to the consultation system contains data on over 600 patients hospitally treated at the Institute of Rheumatology in the period from 1965 till 1980, whose cases were thoroughly reviewed and diagnoses confirmed. Also, included in the base are data on about 100 out-patients suffering from various degenerative rheumatic disorders mainly affecting spine.

The system was then tested on a group of 242 patients treated at the Insitute of Rheumatology in Belgrade. The system´s performance, based upon clinical data on cases presented, was the following.

Out of 100 patients confirmed by human experts to have ankylosing spondylitis, the system has diagnosed correctly 99 of them (99% accuracy). Out of 98 patients suffering from degenerative rheumatic disorders, the system has correctly diagnosed 93 (95%). Out of 24 patients suffering from Reiter´s disease, the system was correct at 22 (92%). Finally, out of 20 patients suffering from psoriatic arthritis, the system was correct at 18 (90% accuracy).

6. CONCLUSION

Consultation system supporting clinical decision making was presented. It has been realized in MUMPS-11 language on a PDP 11/70 computer.

The system allows medical expert to enter his knowledge of the domain directly and combines this knowledge with data from clinical practice to form its knowledge-base.

The consultation system has been tested on a group of 242 patients and has shown satisfactory results. It has to be noted that no expensive and/or pathognomonic tests (like HLA B-27, for instance) have been used by the system in the consultation proces, thus providing evidence for its possible future use in educational environments or by general practitio ners in medically underserved areas, where no specialist consultation, or more complex, pathognomonic tests are available.

Authors share the opinion that the application should be expanded to include other rheumatic diseases and the system should be tested aga- inst the average population of rheumatic patients.

Applications of the consultation system to some other medical domains are also considered.

REFERENCES

1. Pople, H.E., Heuristic methods for imposing structure on ill-structu-red problems: the structuring of medical diagnostics. In Artificial Intelligence in Medicine (P. Szolovits, ed.), Westview Press, Inc.1982.

2. Shortliffe, E.H., Hypothesis Generation in Medical Consultation Sys-tems: Artificial Intelligence Approach, MEDINFO-83, van Bemmel/Ball/Wigertz, eds, North-Holland, 1983.

3. Barr, A. and Feigenbaum, E.A., The Handbook of Artificial Intelligence, Vols. 1 & 2, Heuristech Press, 1981 (V.1) & 1982 (V.2).

4. Srdanović, V. and Limić, B., Decision Supporting System for Screening Patients for Certain Rheumatic Disorders, Lecture Notes in Medical Informatics, MIE-82 Proceedings, Springer-Verlag, 1982.

5. Limić, B. and Srdanović, V., Consultative Computer System as an Aid in Medical Decision Making, MEDINFO-83, van Bemmel/Ball/Wigertz, eds, North-Holland, 1983.

6. Srdanović, V., Integrating Knowledge and Data Bases in a Medical Expert System, presented at CAS International Seminar on Artificial Intelli-gence, Dubrovnik, 1984.

THE USE OF CENSORS AND REASONING BY ANALOGY TO AID
IN THE DIAGNOSIS OF THYROID DISEASES

M
Hormoz Mansour   USA

Massachusetts Institute
of Technology

Harvard Medical School

Address for reply:

Artificial Intelligence
Laboratory
545 Technology Square
Cambridge, Massachusetts 02139
Telephone: (617) 253-5871
Arpanet: HORMOZ at MIT-OZ

Topic: Expert System, Clinical
Decision Making.

Keywords: Censor, Thyroid
Analogy, Causal Reasoning,
Learning.

Abstract

A patient rarely has a single, isolated disease.
The situation is usually much more complex since
the different parts of the human organism and
metabolism interact with each other on multiple
levels and follow several feedback patterns.
These interactions and feedback patterns become
more important with the addition of the external
environment. When several diseases are present,
the first steps of a medical diagnosis should
be to research and determine whether one of the
diseases interacts with ("Censors") or changes
the significant symptoms, syndromes, or the
results of the laboratory tests of the other
disease. We will try, within this paper, to go
beyond the scope of the first generation of
Artificial Intelligence systems in medicine to
see the effect of two diseases on each other.
One important part of the effect of two diseases
on each other is the entrancing effect of what
we call "Censors." In addition, causal reasoning,
reasoning by analogy, and learning from precedents
are important and necessary for a human-like
expert in medicine. Their application to thyroid
diseases, with an implemented system, are considered in this paper.

1. INTRODUCTION

Over the last ten years, we have seen the birth of applications of Artificial
Intelligence in medicine; among these were Casnet/Glaucoma (1974), Mycin (1976),
Digitalis Therapy Advisor (1976), Pip (1976) and Internist-1 (1977); [8].

Until now, most of the methods of diagnostic aid which were used in medicine
seem to have been based on a purely phenomenological approach. With the help of a
formal method, one tries to draw conclusions of known diagnoses from the data observed about the patient. Such is the case, for example, with "bayesien" statistical methods, which utilize conditional probability matrices based on the biomedical data and the diseases. To go beyond these systems, although there have been
some attempts (Caduceus [8] and Abel [7]), we should consider a specific medical
situation where several diseases are present. These diseases could have an inhibiting
or an amplifying effect on each other, such as when the second disease has a blocking
effect on the symptoms of the first disease. This blocking effect, which we call a
"Censor," will be analyzed and developed in this paper. In addition, we will talk
about the cause/effect concept and a type of learning and reasoning ability by analogy
in medicine.

2. CAUSAL ANALOGY

Diagnosis is a problem-solving process based on the information supplied to the
machine; here it is in the form of medical descriptions. This sort of medical diagnosis is based on a description already acquired as a precedent by the system and in
the case of a new patient. If there is a correlation (matching) between (1) the
findings and the causal relation of one description, and (2) the findings and the
causal relation of the case of a new patient, there is a solution to the problem,
a diagnosis for the disease, and a principle for the system to learn. The descriptions, as well as the patient cases to be diagnosed, are described in an English-
like input.

The sample below shows the chain of causality between the thyroid secretion T3 and hyperthyroidism.

DESCRIPTION-1. There is a patient who has hyperthyroidism. The patient has hyperthyroidism because the patient's T3 is increased. The patient's T3 is increased because the patient's thyroid has high-thyroid-hormone-secretion.

Each diagnosis is deduced in the form of an if/then/else rule, with the symptoms as the "if" part. The successive generation of these rules creates the knowledge base of the system. The following description and related exercise from the system show a proper analogical situation between a precedent description and the case of a patient. This situation leads to a diagnosis and generates a rule:

DESCRIPTION-2. There is an alcoholic patient.* The patient has hyperthyroidism. The patient has hyperthyroidism because the patient's T3 is increased. The patient's T3 is increased because the patient's thyroid has high-thyroid-hormone-secretion and causes the patient to have sleep-disturbances, diplopia, hyperpigmentation, hyperphagia, profound-delirium, erythema and palpitations.

Now we have the case of a patient with a number of symptoms characteristic of hyperthyroidism:

EXERCISE-1: Jacques who is a patient has sleep-disturbances, diplopia, hyperpigmentation, hyperphagia, profound-delirium, erythema and palpitations. Jacques has high-thyroid-hormone-secretion.

The case of this patient corresponds to the factual precedent already expressed above. Therefore, this case properly matches the precedent causal network and the findings, and the system is able to make the diagnosis that Jacques actually has hyperthyroidism.

```
IF        [THYROID HAS HIGH-THYROID-HORMONE-SECRETION] is TRUE
          [THYROID CAUSES [PATIENT HAS SLEEP-DISTURBANCES]] is TRUE
          [THYROID CAUSES [PATIENT HAS DIPLOPIA]] is TRUE
          [THYROID CAUSES [PATIENT HAS HYPERPIGMENTATION]] is TRUE
          [THYROID CAUSES [PATIENT HAS HYPERPHAGIA]] is TRUE
          [THYROID CAUSES [PATIENT HAS PROFOUND-DELIRIUM]] is TRUE
          [THYROID CAUSES [PATIENT HAS ERYTHEMA]] is TRUE
          [THYROID CAUSES [PATIENT HAS PALPITATIONS]] is TRUE

THEN      [PATIENT HAS HYPERTHYROIDISM] is TRUE

UNLESS    [T3 INCREASES] is FALSE

BASED ON THE EXERCISE:  EXERCISE-1

AND THE PRECEDENT:  DESCRIPTION-2
```

At this stage, creation of the rule, nothing indicates what inhibits T3 from increasing. This will be the role of Censors; they indicate the appearance of particular constraints on the typical causal chain. From a theoretical point of view, the introduction of the operator "unless" is related to Censors and relies on nonmonotonic logic [10] which will be explained further in the next section.

3. CONCEPT OF "CENSOR"

One of the most important stages of diagnosis is to pinpoint the eventual existence of an inhibiting mechanism (internal, external or psychological), which is capable of entirely modifying the typical interpretation of the observed findings, symptoms, syndromes, or results of laboratory tests. Specifically, a Censor often

---

*The fact of "alcoholism" does not intervene in the process of reasoning by analogy. The relevant facts are the findings which do interfere with the chain of causality and consequently with the analogy. The findings are sleep-disturbances, diplopia, etc.

expresses the interaction between two diseases or between one disease and a specific context. The absence of Censors may lead to the neglect of certain inhibiting causes of the hormone secretion and to the inability to interpret certain apparently paradoxical clinical situations.

If we try to analyze the natural medical reasoning (at least its logical part), it seems that the doctor explores his medical knowledge to determine the causes of the symptoms that he observes about the patient. With this approach, he must also research the causes that would block the functioning of the habitual causes.

The cases of hyper- and hyperthyroidism are the most characteristic of the neuro-endocrinological diseases. We have classified into two categories the whole range of factors and diseases that have the effect of blocking or censoring hyper- or hypothyroidism.

The two categories are:

1-Conditions which cause a decrease in T3 and T4 levels of blood:

SURGERY
STRESS
EMOTIONAL STRESS
HIGH BLOOD PRESSURE
INTERACTION WITH GLUCOCORTICOIDS
RENAL DISEASES
HEPATIC DISEASES
ANDROGEN USE
INFECTIONS
MALNUTRITION

2-Conditions which cause an increase in T3 and T4 levels in blood:

PREGNANCY
ORAL CONTRACEPTIVE
OVEREATING

3.1 SYSTEM WITH CENSORS

The rules for a diagnosis that the system creates are supplied with an "unless" condition that is a type of augmenting diagnosis. For example:

IF   THRYOID SECRETION IS HIGH

THEN   PATIENT HAS HYPERTHYROIDISM

UNLESS   T3 IS NOT INCREASED

The previous rule is blocked by one of the Censors that has a rule-like form as follows:

IF   PATIENT HAS HYPERTHYROIDISM
            PATIENT HAS AN INFECTION

THEN   T3 IS NOT INCREASED

This previous rule becomes a Censor with a blocking possibility over the first rule and there is not way to conclude hyperthyroidism. This type of augmented diagnosis with an "unless" condition is not an ordinary rule of inference and is based on nonmonotonic reasoning. The blocking factor itself could be blocked and the diagnosis again follows the appropriate pattern. The following rule or Censor blocks the first one:

IF   PATIENT TAKES ANTI-BIOTICS

THEN   PATIENT WILL NOT HAVE AN INFECTION

When infection (the first Censor) is present, the principal clue to the diagnosis of hyperthyroidism, T3 blood level increased, is no longer true. When the patient takes antibiotics, the infection disappears and T3, again increasing, allows us again to diagnose for hyperthyroidism. To better understand this approach and the way that the Censors interact with each other, we will examine the following case from the system. In this case stress is the first Censor and end-of-stress is the second. The first Censor that concerns stress, has the following description:

CENSOR-1. C1 is a Censor about a patient. The patient has hyperthyroidism. The patient's T3 is not increased because the patient is depressed. The patient is depressed because the patient is stressed. Make C1 a Censor using the patient's T3 is not increased. The Censor in its rule-like form is:

```
IF        [PATIENT HAS HYPERTHYROIDISM] is TRUE
          [PATIENT IS STRESSED] is TRUE

THEN      [T3 INCREASED] is FALSE

UNLESS    [PATIENT IS DEPRESSED] is FALSE
```

Now we have the case of a patient who is stressed.

EXERCISE-2. Jacques who is a patient has sleep-disturbances, diplopia, hyperpigmentation, hyperphagia, profound-delirium, erythema and palpitations. Jacques has high-thyroid-hormone-secretion and he is stressed.

With the Censor present, we are not able to proceed to any diagnosis. As we saw previously, the system observes many symptoms which are due to hyperthyroidism. In addition, the system is aware that if hyperthyroidism is the correct disease diagnosis, the patient's T3 level should be increased. However, the principal cause is blocked and we are not able to find T3 increasing. The final messeage consists of the determinant message that T3 is not increased and a diagnosis is not available. If we now have a second Censor with the following description:

CENSOR-2. C2 is a Censor about a patient. The patient has hyperthyroidism. The patient is not depressed because the patient is at the end-of-stress. Make C2 a Censor using the patient is not depressed.

This second Censor also has a rule-like form:

```
IF        [PATIENT IS AT THE END-OF-STRESS] is TRUE

THEN      [PATIENT IS DEPRESSED] is FALSE
```

We consider again the case of the previous patient but this time at the end-of-stress.

EXERCISE-3. Jacques who is a patient has sleep-disturbances, diplopia, hyperpigmentation, hyperphagia, profound-delirium, erythema and palpitations. Jacques who was stressed, has high-thyroid-hormone-secretion and is now at the end-of-stress.

With the second Censor present the reasoning is the following: first of all, because of the second Censor and secondly, because the patient is at the end-of-stress, the patient is not depressed any more. Because of the first Censor, not being depressed any more allows T3 to increase again. Now we are again presented with all of the symptoms mentioned previously. Also, the increasing levels of the thyroid secretions finally make the system diagnose for hyperthyroidism again and the following rule is created, which looks like the first one, except that it is based on Description-2, and Exercise-3, and Censor-1, and Censor-2 as follows:

```
IF        [THRYOID HAS HIGH-THRYOID-HORMONE-SECRETION] is TRUE
          [THYROID CAUSES [PATIENT HAS SLEEP-DISTURBANCES]] is TRUE
          [THYROID CAUSES [PATIENT HAS DIPLOPIA]] is TRUE
          [THYROID CAUSES [PATIENT HAS HYPERPIGMENTATION]] is TURE
          [THYROID CAUSES [PATIENT HAS HYPERPHAGIA]] is TRUE
          [THYROID CAUSES [PATIENT HAS PROFOUND-DELIRIUM] is TRUE
          [THYROID CAUSES [PATIENT HAS ERYTHEMA]] is TRUE
          [THYROID CAUSES [PATIENT HAS PALPITATIONS]] is TRUE

THEN      [PATIENT HAS HYPERTHYROIDISM] is TRUE

UNLESS    [T3 INCREASED] is FALSE

BASED ON THE EXERCISE: EXERCISE-3

AND THE PRECENDENTS:   DESCRIPTION-2, CENSOR-1, AND CENSOR-2
```

The use of Censors, as shown above, could give a new perspective to clinical observations and clinical decision-making: a systematic study of the problem or secondary disease (related to the first disease), which has an important effect on the causality and leads to a false diagnosis.

4. CONCLUSION

Within this work, concepts such as blocking points or Censors, as well as the cause/effect relations and reasoning by analogy within an implemented system, were considered for diagnosis of thyroid diseases. Our primary idea was based on a clinical observation of the way that a certain number of diagnoses related to these diseases in a medical environment. Therefore, we considered this work to be based on our observation of medical practice. Later on, we systemized a set of the so-called Censors for all thyroid diseases. The next step would be to generalize this crucial part of the medical diagnosis, the mechanism of Censors or blocking points, to other medical domains and to establish a systematic numer of Censors for each diagnosis. Another step and extension of the actual work would be the study of the system with two basic aspects of reasoning by analogy: causal reasoning and contextual reasoning [3]. The combined effect of these two types of reasoning with the Censors and the blocking points is a powerful one. Our observations within the medical environment related to the diagnosis of thyroid diseases confirms these ideas.

5. REFERENCES

[1] DeGroot, L.J., Stanbury, J.B. The Thyroid and Its Diseases, Fourth Edition, J. Wiley and Sons, 1975.

[2] Ingbar, S.H. and Braverman, L.E. Active Form of the Thyroid Hormone, Annual Review of Medicine, 1975, Vol. 26, pp. 443-449.

[3] Mansour, H. A Structural Approach to Analogy, MIT AI Memo No. 747, November, 1983.

[4] Martin, J.B., Reichlin, S. and Brown, G.M. Clinical Neurendocrinology, Contemporary Neurology Series, 1977.

[5] Minsky, M. Jokes and the Logic of the Cognitive Unconscious, MIT AI Memo November, 1980.

[6] Newell, A. and Simon, H. A Human Problem Solving, Prentice-Hall, Inc., Englewood Cliffs, New Jersey, 1972.

[7] Patil, Ramesh, Causal Representation of Patient Illness for Electrolyte and Acid-Based Diagnosis, PhD Thesis, MIT, Cambridge, MA, 1981.

[8] Szolovits, Peter (editor), Artificial Intelligence in Medicine, Westview Press, Boulder, CO, 1982.

[9] Werner, S. and Ingbar, S.H. The Thyroid: A Fundamental and Clinical Test, Fourth Edition, Harper and Row, 1978.

[10] Winston, P.H. Artificial Intelligence, Second Edition Addison-Welsey, 1984.

The physician's needs versus the system features in the design of an effective Knowledge Based System

F.L. Ricci[1], A. Rossi - Mori[2]

[1] Istituto Studi Ricerca e Documentazione Scientifica CNR, via C. De Lollis 12, 00185 Roma (Italy)

[2] Istituto Tecnologie Biomediche CNR, via Morgagni 30/E, 00161 Roma (Italy)

1. Introduction

Computer applications are more and more spreading in the doctor's environment, but remain limited to minor tasks in his professional activities, such as accounting, agenda management or data processing in complex instruments. In other fields, as in the industrial environment for example, Information Systems (IS) aim at a full support of the information flows within the structure; methodologies for the analysis and the design of such ISs were developed, to model at the same time both informational and organizational features of the structure.

The main obstacle in the use of computers in medicine is the inability to capture the main aspects of the physician's work, - those related to his process of decision making.

The first generation of Knowledge Based Systems (KBS) fostered strong expectations about the possibility to fill in this gap, but they have not lived up to the expectations they had generated, and the same will probably happen with the present generation of experimental KBSs.

Nevertheless, these systems (even those abandoned, such as MYCIN) show features which are not usually found in the 'traditional' techniques for decision aid: 1. experts can express their deep and invaluable subjective knowledge in a (relatively) easy way during the system design; 2. modifications and upgrades are inherently modular; 3. the end - user interacts easily and friendly with the system; 4. the system can explain its 'behaviour' in nearly natural language, using concepts familiar to the user.

At first the KBSs will result efficient in the most specialized fields of medicine. As a paradox, these involve more complex and advanced knowledge. But they require less 'common sense' (the human feature that is difficult to model into present KBSs), because the problems are less ill-structured.

Future applications cover 'intelligent' instruments, teaching drills, and interfaces towards complex hardware or software in research environments.

Many methodologies (developed in various settings) are currently available, for the analysis of procedures and for IS design. Description languages were built as a support to specify the behaviour of a process. The actual design of an IS requires the combinatrion of different methodologies, each for a specific aspect of the whole system. Such methodologies were mainly conceived for applications in the private sector, related to the production of goods; they must be therefore deeply adapted and upgraded to catch also the decision making aspects in the (public) medical field.

Here we examine the problem of a gradual inclusion of more 'intelligent' components into the IS that should support the current work of a doctor, and in particular we outline an analysis of KBS features in view of extending the present design methodologies to consider such decision aids.

2. The KBSs as components of an Information System

Until now, KBSs were built for research purpose; so they isolate (often artificially) a single decision topic, with little regard for the environment in which they will operate, or to the multiplicity of decision aspects that a physician meets in his daily work. As a matter of fact, a large number of problems contribute to the definition of the real activity of the doctor (interacting among themselves and with decisions made by other decision makers), but often they result of relatively limited complexity.

The construction of a KBS by the current tools may be looked at from a number of points of view. As far as design methodologies are concerned, we may focus on two topics: the rationale supporting the building of a KBS, and the complexity of the decision problem.

Within the IS, a KBS (as the other components do) must support **the physician's daily activities** and provide a decision tool at the bedside, helping to identify components of complex problems (possible choices, causal relations, different scenarios, ...); from the point of view of the KBS architecture, emphasis is on the short term memory and in its management (facts related to the single patient and his environment).

The rationale of the present experimental KBSs are different:
- **research on medicine**: the study of the decision process in itself; with respect to a KBS, the interest is in the inference engine and in the global architecture, to assess the validity of a theory. The aim is to identify the features of the intellectual process that experts use in the clinical judgement, observing and simulating the ability of reasoning in medical terms and the 'art' of using attainable information to get a diagnosis and suggest the suitable therapy.
- **research in medicine**: the analysis and formalization of medical knowledge on limited topics; the KBS stresses the long term memory, and the assessment is based on some form of agreement from medical community on new formalization (or on by-products as standardization hints). The aim is to help the medical scientists to analyse their own knowledge on specific fields.

3. The appropriate level of complexity

According to the amount of knowledge present in the system (the complexity of the overall architecture is normally coherent with that quantity), three rough levels can be distinguished : simple (100 - 500 'elements of knowledge', such as concepts and parts of rules), medium (from 1000 to 5000 'elements'), complex (more than 10000 'elements').

KBSs in the first class may be used as drills or toy systems. Similarly to 'traditional' decision aids (that are however more powerful and less expensive in dealing with this kind of problems), they can also be applied as examples or for highly structured problems.

On the other hand, ISs are exacting by themselves and Lisp Machines have been too recently put on the market, for considering a 'common' diffusion of complex KBSs within the scope of present IS technology.

As a result, the class of effective use nowadays seems the intermediate one. They constitute a progress compared to more traditional ISs, even if strong limits were noticed about their utility and possibilities of application.

At least for the next few years, only modest tasks can be entrusted to single knowledge based subsystems, with flat architecture and low use of metaknowledge. This intermediate class of KBSs deals with partially structured problems, thus needs an irreplaceable physician's intervention to form a man - machine system. The features of both components are brought out: human capabilities, as common sense and experience, are combined to the memory and the systematic behaviour of the machine.

4. Physician and computer as a combined decision 'system'

Let us consider the physician together with a 'partner' that can help him (person or object, from a consultant to a book) as a combined decision 'system' (in a broad sense).

We can observe different patterns of cooperation:

1- the physician is **a higly qualified user.** He receives non-processed knowledge (handbooks, flow charts, non-'intelligent' instruments), and his experience is directly compatible with that knowledge, for an adequate use. The 'inference engine' of the system is nearly all in the physician;

2- the physician is **a partially experienced user.** He may directly reach a partially organized knowledge (as numerical systems for modeling and decision analysis). This pattern is common mainly in the medical research. Reasoning is performed partly by the user, and partly by the decision aid;

3- the physician is **not necessarily an expert.** He needs an interface toward decision aids of tipe 1, to deal with ill-structured problems (it is the field of medium - complex KBSs or human consultants). Most reasoning is entrusted to the 'partner'.

5. Changing established roles in the doctor's environment

KBSs will cause a gradual shift of the IS towards the latter form, influencing competences and responsibilities in an existent structure. The actual nature of this influence is difficult to predict. Let us take the example of a doctor who esitates whether he should treat a patient he feels difficult, or entrust other colleagues. The KBS advice may produce two contrasting outputs: the doctor may feel enough confident to treat the patient himself, or he may acquire more competence in re-routing the patient to a collegue.

As every technological innovation does, KBSs will affect the work organization in different ways:

- replacing higher level functions (of physicians, skilled technicians), widening the possibilities of intervention for less qualified personnel;
- replacing (routine) functions of lower level, hence allowing experienced personnel to by-pass the help from other people on previously delegated tasks;
- creating new functions, when the introduction of the subsystem in the structure give rise to completely new tasks.

The project of a KBS must therefore be inserted in the context of the whole IS, considering also the organizational aspect.

6. The design methodologies from a Management IS to the IS 'for the physician'

Present design methodologies already offer advanced features: allow modular analyses of subsystems while preserving an overall view of the system; assure flexibility of use and updating; find out authorities and responsibilities during the project development and the following operation; involve users from the beginning of the project; finally, they cover the complete life cycle of the system. The most important shortcoming concerns precisely the definition of decision problems, seen as an ordinary function, like data management.

The methodologies need to be extended, so that the most relevant decision nodes (where a computer based decision aid can be useful) are identified, before the 'internal' definition of each single decision procedure in itself. Then possible flows of information and control (i.e. the interaction among nodes) are to be modeled. As a result, the requirements about the global architecture should have been specified, and the design details and the interface of each subsystem should have been outlined.

Possible implementations of decision aids through different classes (for complexity, portability and cost) must be considered: in the near future hybrid systems are predictable, which will include, under the doctor's supervision: i) the ability in problem structuring of expert systems, ii) the capability of dealing with uncertainty of decision analysis, iii) the formal simplicity of numerical modeling, iv) the familiarity (and low cost ?) of paper support, for flow charts and handbooks.

7. Conclusions

In the future, Knowledge Based Systems will be of common use. The daily activities of the physician will be affected, as their introduction will modify not only a single decision - making process, but also the whole organization of the physician's work.

They represent powerful interfaces between clinical problems and the physicians' mental structures and knowledge; they help their decision making through hints of new hypoteses and checks for completeness of the observed ones.

It is therefore reasonable to foresee that in the future it will be routinely possible to' design powerful and efficent KBSs from previously defined requirements, as a function of physicians' needs, and to integrate them into advanced medical ISs.

The design of such ISs in actual medical settings will require a powerful methodology to work out the organization (task changes, time allocation, alteration of the patient - physician relations) and the information flows of an integrated man - machine decision process and to specify the interdependent roles of the Knowledge Based Systems, the other decision aids and the physician himself.

References

D.Ballow, S.W.Kim: **A Systems Life Cycle for Office Automation Projects.** Information and Management 7, 1984, 111-119

W.J.Clancey, E.H.Shortliffe: **Readings in Medical Artificial Intelligence: The First Decade.** Addison - Wesley, Reading, Mass. 1984

A.S.Elstein, L.S.Shulman, S.A.Sprafka: **Medical Problem Solving: An Analysis of Clinical Reasoning.** Harward University Press, Cambridge 1978

F.Hayes-Roth, D.A.Waterman, D.B.Lenat (ed.): **Building Expert Systems.** Addison - Wesley, Reading, Mass. 1983

E.A.Patrick: **Decision Analysis in Medicine: Methods and Applications.** CRC Press, Boca Raton 1979

W. Reitman (ed.): **Artificial Intelligence Applications for Business.** Ablex Publ.Corp. Norwood 1984

A.Rossi-Mori, F.L.Ricci, O.Stock: **I sistemi esperti come possibili strumenti per l'aiuto alla decisione in medicina.** Medicina e Informatica, 1, 2, 1984, 87-102

P.Szolovits (ed.): **Artificial Intelligence in Medicine.** AAAS Selected Symposium 51. Westview Press, Boulder, Colorado 1982

B.T.Williams (ed.): **Computer Aids to Clinical Decisions, vol.1 & 2.** CRC Press, Boca Raton 1982

___ , **Structured Analysis and Design,** State of the Art Report, Infotech, 1978

This work was partially supported by the Working Group on KBS Applications in Medicine, through a grant of the Technological Committee of the National Research Council.

AN EXPERT SYSTEM FOR STATISTICAL APPLICATIONS IN MEDICAL RESEARCH

Wittkowski, Knut M.

Eberhard-Karls-Universität, Institut für Medizinische Biometrie
Westbahnhofstr. 55, D-7400 Tübingen, Bundesrepublik Deutschland

Statistical analysis in medical (clinical and laboratory) research is predetermined by the experimental design. Corresponding information, however, is neglected by common data base management systems. It is shown, how an expert system (implemented on a laboratory-site PC within a network) can help physicians to use statistical analysis systems and to avoid erroneous application of statistical (graphical or analytical) methods to medical data.

Key words: artificial intelligence, software packages, experimental design, data base management systems, method base management systems

INTRODUCTION

Common statistical analysis packages (BMDP, GLIM, SAS, SPSS) are designed to be used exclusively by experts in applied statistics (LUCE 1980). They provide little advise to the medical user what type of (implicit) problems the statistical methods have been developed for, i.e. how a "significant" result has to be interpreted, provided the assumptions implicit to the method are not met; recommendations in the documentation and applied literature are often misleading or even wrong: E.g. the aproach of CONOVER and IMAN (1981) who suggested that analysis of variance methods should be generally applied to "rank transformed" data even in factorial designs.

On the other hand, clinical and laboratory research aims at combinations of treatment effects. Differences between those effects typically require sensitive measuring techniques that are sensitive also to uncontrollable sources of variation. The wealth of methods currently available in modern statistical analysis systems, where the appropriate methods have to be selected from, consequently, often leads to erroneous applications of statistical methods in clinical and laboratory research (ALTMANN 1982): Either the user chooses a method whose interpretation of treatment effects is not identical to the medical interpretation or the data are not arranged in a suitable way.

EXPERT SYSTEMS FOR MEDICAL DIAGNOSIS

Since LEDLEY and LUSTED (1959) discussed the reasoning process of clinicians and proposed the use of computers to aid clinical decisions various approaches to the application of artificial intelligence to medical problem solving processes have been proposed. In the Seventies the first programs for solving problems that require expert knowledge (expert systems, ES; BUCHANAN 1982) were developed for applications in medical diagnosis: i.e. MYCIN, CASNET, PUFF, and INTERNIST (c.f. SPIEGEL-HALTER, KNILL-JONES 1984). Their knowledge bases consist mainly of heuristic rules of the form "IF (condition) THEN (conclusion) WITH (degree of certainty)" and "probable" conclusions are drawn by means of inexact reasoning. Only few routine applications of these programs, however, have been documentated, mainly because the lack of meta-knowledge about medical knowledge results in a difficult and time-consuming process of knowledge acquisition (DUDA, SHORTLIFF 1983).

EXPERT SYSTEMS FOR MEDICAL RESEARCH

Application of artificial intelligence to statistics was introduced by HAJEK and IVANEK (1982) for applications in the field of exploratory data analysis, where inexact reasoning is similarly adequate as in medical diagnosis. Knowledge of analytical statistical methods and knowledge of experimental designs in clinical and laboratory research, in contrast to knowledge of medical diagnosis and EDA, can be sufficently structured as described in WITTKOWSKI (1984):

- Variables can be divided into factors (treatment, dose), nuisance variables (sex, patient, replication), and observations with respect to problems and into dependent and independent variables with respect to methods.

- Observational units are defined by the hierarchy of variables, i.e. whether the meaning of a value depends on the meaning of the values of another variable.

- Theoretical relations between these observational units can be described by e.g. sampling strategy (fixed or random) and scale types (discrete or continuous; nominal, ordinal, interval, or absolute).

- Hypothetical relations between observational units can for a wide range of methods (l.c.) be described by influence types (expectation, linear regression, tendency, monotone regression, distribution).

As a consequence, choosing a statistical method for the analysis of a clinical and laboratory experiment reduces to a special pattern recognition process which consists of

(1) representing problems by their experimental design, a formalized question (theoretical and hypothetical relations) and the data,

(2) representing methods by their implicit problems,

(3) choosing a subdesign by means of projecting and restricting the (conceptual) data structure,

(4) normalizing the resulting (external) data structure, and

(5) selecting a method with a corresponding implicit problem type.

When a number of variables and corresponding influence types is selected i.e. when a subproblem is defined (typically by a physician) its design and theoretical relations can be derived (by the expert system) from the conceptual question (defined typically by a biometrician before the experiment is started).

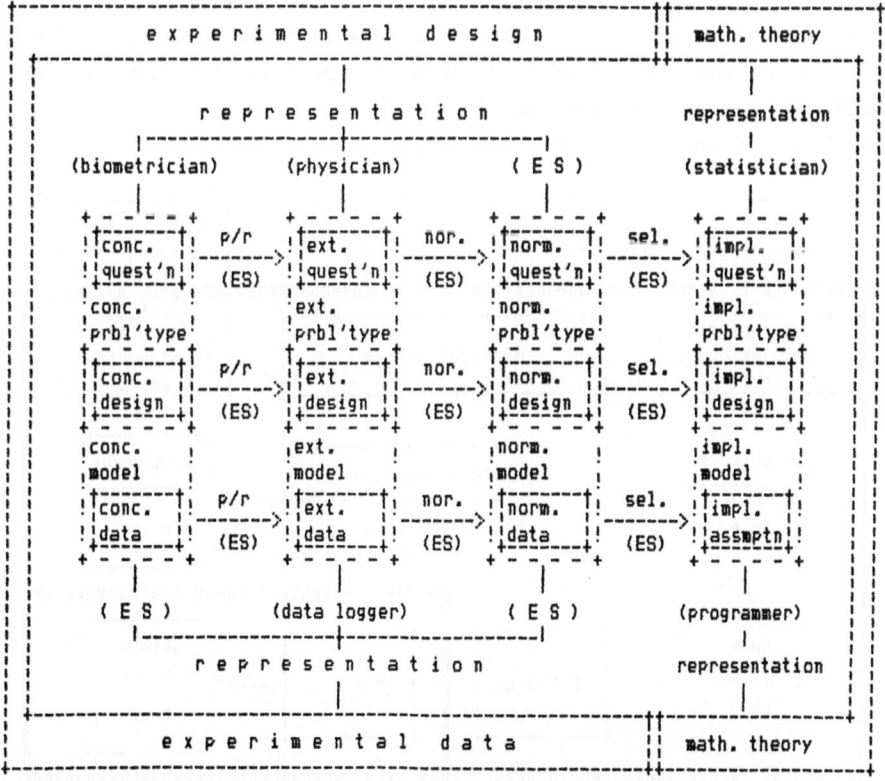

Fig. 1: Choosing statistical methods as a pattern recognition process
(p/r = projection/restriction, nor. = normalization, sel. = selection)

DISTRIBUTED INTELLIGENCE IN MEDICAL RESEARCH

The expert system, including the problem and methods knowledge bases, may be logically separated from the analysis systems. This logical separation allows for implementing the expert system on a laboratory-site PC and letting the expert system call methods from statistical analysis system(s) implemented on a host. The purpose of this physical separation is two-fold:

(1) The laboratory staff does not need to update statistical method bases and

(2) the hosts CPU and memory capacity can be utilized without increasing its I/O activities (WITTKOWSKI, KLAR 1982).

Although the data (separated from the knowledge) could similarily be handled by a host-site data base management system, this is not recommended for medical data: Sensitive data is best protected if access is physically inhibited. Since data in clinical and laboratory research is often needed only at certain times by a small group of physicians, this protection can be effectively guaranteed by storing media i.e. in a laboratory lock-box. This protection is effective even during analysis at the host, because typically only a small part of the data and few knowledge about this data are utilized by a single method. Note that linkage of values of different variables requires the knowledge independently stored within the problem knowledge base.

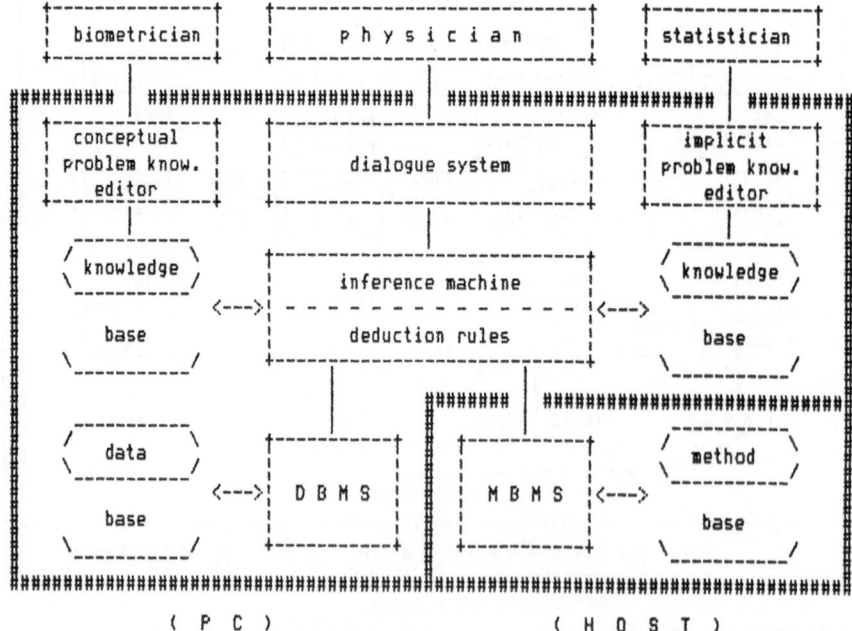

Fig. 2: Distributed processing in clinical and laboratory research

CONCLUSIONS

The major advantages of the proposed expert system approach to statistical analysis in clinical and laboratory research can be summarized as follows:

(1) Utilizing knowledge of the conceptual problem type, defined typically by a bio-metrican, the amount of necessary information to be entered by a physician during statistical analysis of subproblems is significantly reduced. This reduction allows for short menu-driven dialogue procedures and results in fewer erroneous applications of statistical methods.

(2) Instead of choosing certain test procedures and defining a complete subset of relevant information for each sub-problem, the physician can concentrate on the formulation of questions (selection of variables and definition of corresponding influence types). This shift in paradigm facilitates interpretation of statistical answers in terms of medical questions.

(3) The separation of data, knowledge of the data, and methods allows for more protection against unauthorized access to medical data.

REFERENCES

ALTMANN DG (1982) Statistics in medical journals. Statistics in Medicine 1:59-71

BUCHANAN BG (1982) New research on expert systems. Machine Intelligence 10:269-299

CONOVER WJ, IMAN RL (1981) Rank transformation as a bridge between parametric and nonparametric statistics. The American Statistician 35:124-133

DUDA RO, SHORTLIFF EH (1983) Expert systems research. Science 220:261-268

LEDLEY RS, LUSTED LB (1959) Reasoning foundations of medical diagnosis. Science 130:9-21

LUCE SR (1980) A conceptual analysis of SPSS and BMDP. In: Barritt MM et al. (Hrsg.) Compstat 1980. Physica, Wien

SPIEGELHALTER DJ, KNILL-JONES (1984) Statistical and knowledge-based approaches to clinical decison-support systems, with application in gastroenterology. J R Statist Soc A 147:35-77

WITTKOWSKI KM (1983) On the use of structural information for a statistical expert system in medical reasearch. In: VAN EIMEREN W, ENGELBRECHT R, FLAGLE CD (Hrsg.) Springer, Berlin:1140-1143

WITTKOWSKI KM, KLAR R (1982) The use of a computer network for simulation and application of nonparametric statistical methods. In: CAUSSINUS H et al. (Hrsg.) Compstat 1982. Physica, Wien:275-276

IDEA - INTEGRATING EXPERT SYSTEMS WITH APPLICATIONS.

J. van der Lei, H.Y. Kwa, A. Hasman, M. Waage
Dept. of Medical Informatics
Free University
van der Boechorststraat 7
1081 BT Amsterdam.

1. Introduction.

The Department of Medical Informatics has been involved in the construction of a variety of departmental information systems. In order to facilitate the development and to provide an uniform structure for such systems a software toolkit has been constructed: AIDA (Applied Interactive Design of Applications (1,2)). AIDA gives the (end-)user the opportunity to develop (medical) database systems virtually without any programming effort and it offers the possibility to maintain and adapt the system in a dynamic environment.
Amongst the users of these systems there is a rapidly growing interest in the use of expert systems, not as independent systems but as a logical extension of their already existing information system. AIDA, however, does not provide facilities for constructing and maintaining expert systems. For this reason a research project was initiated with the aim to develop a set of utilities for the construction of an expert system within the context of an AIDA application. To emphasize this we named the project IDEA: Integrated Design of Expert systems within an Application.

In this paper the interaction between an expert system and already operational AIDA applications is discussed. The validity of our approach will be demonstrated by a prototype system which has been built. This system does not excel in sophisticated knowledge representations nor in search strategies (the development of which was not our primary concern) but is able to demonstrate that the facilities provided by AIDA together with the IDEA facilities result in an expert system which is characterized by a high degree of integration with the already operational information system.
Since AIDA is written in MUMPS and most AIDA applications are operational in environments which do not allow the use of another programming language concurrent with MUMPS the choice was made to develop IDEA also in MUMPS and not for example in LISP or PROLOG.

2. Knowledge representation.

A fact is an attribute and associated value (e.g. age over 20 yrs, medication is propranolol, etc.). A hypothesis is a concept that can be inferred using facts and/or other hypotheses, its value ranges from -1 (absolutely false) to +1 (absolutely true). A short (often cryptic) name is stored, along with a longer (in general more meaningful) name. The short name is used during the definition of rules, the longer one in explanation facilities. Textblocks describing the hypothesis more in detail and an identification of the expert who has defined the hypothesis are also stored.
Three basic operations are allowed on a hypothesis: consider the hypothesis (which can be seen as an initial focussing process), reject the hypothesis and

accept the hypothesis. These operations involve the evaluation of production rules. Consider rules define the circumstances under which the hypothesis is a valid goal to be pursued (if all consider rules fail then the hypothesis is not further persued). Accept rules provide support for the hypothesis, reject rules deny the hypothesis. Along with each hypothesis a list of pointers is stored to the rules which mention that hypothesis in their THEN-clause. For combining the results of accept and reject rules the model for certainty factors as suggested by Shortliffe is used (3). Consider rules do not effect the certainty factor of the hypothesis. With each rule an import value is associated. The order in which rules will be evaluated is determined by their import value: the higher value has priority over a lower. It is also possible to associate a question to a hypothesis which may be asked either if the evaluation of the rules does not yield sufficient information (which is defined as a threshold the certainty factor fails to reach) or to query the user directly concerning a given hypothesis, followed by evaluation of the rules only if the the user is not able to provide an answer.

A hypothesis also contains a "command" segment. This section enables the user to issue commands such as 'run an external routine' or 'place new goals on the agenda' (see section 3.); each command is to be preceeded by a threshold the hypothesis has to reach before the command is to be executed.

The premise of the rules consists of references to attributes and/or hypotheses, any combination of AND and OR clauses is allowed. The THEN-clause is separated in two sections: the first section draws conclusions concerning a hypothesis, the second section enables the user to issue commands (see section 4). The commands are executed if the premise of that rule is true.

In order to facilitate the definition of rules a keyword parser is available. This parser has access to the data dictionary of the expert system and performs some syntactical checks (e.g. the detection of references to not existing attributes or hypotheses, impossible attribute values, etc.). This input is translated into a postfix notation. The postfix is stored along with additional information such as the author of the rule, references to the literature, import value and certainty factor.

Attributes are defined in the data dictionary of the expert system. The attribute name is stored together with: a text to be displayed when the attribute is requested from the user; helptext (to be displayed when the user enters a "?"); type of attribute (listvalue, numeric, date, etc.); possible answers (the listvalues, possible and plausible ranges of numeric values, etc.); and block membership (if one attribute of a block of attributes is requested all attributes in that block will be asked from the user).

When the value of an attribute can be obtained by querying the database of the AIDA application additional information is stored: references to one or more elements in the data dictionary of the AIDA application and, since AIDA supports a relational database, relationname(s) and key(s). This information enables the controller to perform a query on the database of the AIDA application. It is also possible to store a segment of MUMPS-code that describes how the result of the query has to be translated into the attribute values used in the expert system.

3. Control structure.

A control language was defined to guide the inference process and to handle the interaction between IDEA and the AIDA application (see fig. 1). It consists of elementary commands which are executed and global commands which are first expanded into elementary commands and then executed as a sequence of elementary commands. All commands to be executed are placed on the AGENDA. The AGENDA is processed by the controller according to the last in first out principle. If the execution of a command produces new commands these are added to the AGENDA. Each finished command is removed from the AGENDA.

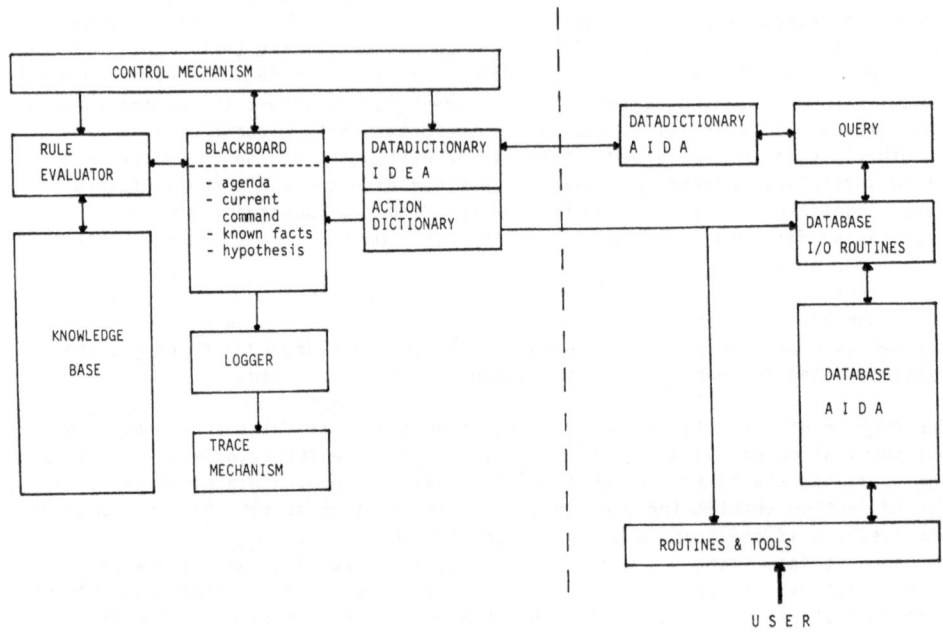

Figure 1: The interaction between IDEA and AIDA.

A summary of the commands is given below.

Elementary commands:
    <CONSIDER><HYP> : evaluate the consider rules of that hypothesis
    <REJECT><HYP> : evaluate reject rules, if necessary query user
    <ACCEPT><HYP> : evaluate accept rules, if necessary query user
    <ASK><ATRR> : ask user the value of an attribute
    <ACCESS><ATRR> : retrieve attribute from database
    <PERFORM><ACTION> : execute the string ACTION as MUMPS-code
Some global commands:
    <EVAL><HYP> = <REJECT><HYP><ACCEPT><HYP>
    <ALL><HYP> = <EVAL><HYP><CONSIDER><HYP>
    <REQUEST><ATTR> = <ASK><ATTR><ACCESS><ATTR>
    <REQUEST><HYP> = <ALL><HYP>
    <REFINE><HYP> = <ALL><HYP>

Additional commands may be defined in terms of already existing commands. A logger stores a record of the tasks performed; this record is used by the trace mechanism. The controller is responsible for invoking the different routines of either the expert system or the AIDA application. A consultation is initiated by placing one or more commands on the AGENDA and handing the control over to the controller. A session is terminated by an empty AGENDA.

Suppose the controller encounters <ALL><HYP> as the most recently introduced command on the AGENDA. It will be parsed to <EVAL><HYP><CONSIDER><HYP> which will be parsed to <REJECT><HYP><ACCEPT><HYP><CONSIDER><HYP>. The consider rules are evaluated and an attribute value is requested by the rule evaluator: <REQUEST><ATTR>. This command is added to the AGENDA and is parsed to <ASK><ATTR><ACCES><ATTR>. The AGENDA then contains <REJECT><HYP><ACCEPT><HYP><CONSIDER><HYP><ASK><ATTR><ACCES><ATTR>. The last command, <ACCES><ATTR>, is executed resulting in a query on the AIDA database. If this is not successful the command <ASK><ATTR> will cause the attribute value to be requested from the user.

Different global commands may be parsed into the same sequence of elementary commands. This is for example the case for <REQUEST><HYP> and <REFINE><HYP>. This is caused by the fact that although for the controller they may represent the same sequence of basic operations they may be radically different from the experts viewpoint and therefore require different explanations.

The rule evaluator is invoked when the controller encounters <CONSIDER><HYP>, <REJECT><HYP> or <ACCEPT><HYP>. The rule evaluator retrieves the rules in question. First a scan is made to see if any of the rules has a premise which is already satisfied. These rules are executed first. If after execution of these rules the hypothesis is not yet absolutely true or false the rule with the highest import value is evaluated. A preview mechanism determines whether or not the premise still can be satisfied and determines the "shortest way" (the smallest number of variables) that allows the premise to become true. The response of the rule evaluator will be either <REQUEST><HYP> or <REQUEST><ATTR>, and control is handed back to the controller. The controller adds the command(s) to the AGENDA, looks for the most recently introduced command and executes that command.

On the blackboard the AGENDA is stored, together with the command which is presently executed, the status of the already evaluated hypotheses and the known facts. The logger keeps a record of the modifications on this blackboard.

The command <PERFORM><ACTION> may be used to initiate routines within the AIDA application. The actions are defined in the action dictionary which contains segments of MUMPS-code provided by the knowledge engineer.
Through the action dictionary database I/O routines can be initiated for storing the results of a session.

Only limited explanation facilities are available: with the aid of a trace mechanism we can show the present rule or a trace of rules and commands executed prior to the evaluation of the present rule.

4. Discussion.

The idea behind IDEA: integration with existing information systems might be a conditio sine qua non for the successful implementation of expert systems. The AIDA/IDEA package is therefore aimed at those environments which are characterized by the need to develop and maintain a large (medical) database and to provide expert systems facilities using that same database.

The first version of IDEA is used within our department. For several AIDA
applications expert systems are under development (primary care, hospital
pharmacy). Experience so far indicates that the integration of IDEA with AIDA is
successful: IDEA uses the relational database provided by AIDA both for
retrieving data and storing the results of a session; IDEA does not have an
independent user interface but again uses the AIDA facilities; as a matter of
fact, any routine within AIDA can be initiated by IDEA. This integration was
achieved by defining a control language which contains commands for both AIDA and
IDEA and by constructing a controller which can be seen as an interpreter for
this control language.
Also problems have been encountered. Virtually any routine is able to add any
command to the AGENDA. This encourages an unstructured approach involving
procedural knowledge which is not made explicit.
Other problems center around the oversimplified knowledge representation scheme
we adapted for our first version. The most urgent problem in this respect is that
facts and/or hypotheses cannot be assigned to a context.
Our present developing efforts are therefore aimed at a further development of
the control language together with a definition of what commands may be added to
the AGENDA by the different modules and the introduction of contexts.
MUMPS deserves a special comment. Though, in contrast to LISP or PROLOG, it was
not specially designed for the construction of systems like IDEA, it provided a
convenient programming environment. MUMPS is an interpreter thus allowing rapid
testing and modification of programs and, more important, allows us to use data
structures as if they were executable code. Also the database facilities provided
by MUMPS coupled with good string handling facilities proved valuable. For a
comparison of MUMPS with LISP see (4).

5. References.

(1) J.H. van Bemmel, J.S. Duisterhout, B. Franken. Fourth generation software for
    Medical Information Systems (AIDA). 8th Annual SCAMC, 1984.
(2) B. Franken, J.S. Duisterhout. Clinical support with AIDA. in: J.H. van
    Bemmel, M.J. Ball and O. Wigertz, eds. MEDINFO 83. Amsterdam: North Holland
    Publ. Comp., 1983:818-21.
(3) E.H. Shortliffe. Computer-based medical consultations: MYCIN. New York:
    Elsevier, 1976.
(4) F.M. Brown. A comparison and synthesis of MUMPS and LISP facilities. MUG
    Quaterly 1983:52-57.

TWO FLOWS OF APPROXIMATIVENESS IN DIAGNOSTIC EXPERT SYSTEMS

M. Popper and F. Gyárfáš
Research Institute of Medical Bionics
Jedľová St. No. 6
833 08 Bratislava, Czechoslovakia

Introduction

Several methods for approximative diagnostic problem solving under uncertainty have been adopted for expert systems (ES). Usually, however, no difference is made in application of those methods in controlling a c t i v a t i o n of diagnostic concepts for evaluation and in concept e v a l u a t i o n itself. Two different and independent control flows of approximative inference have been incorporated in our diagnostic expert system CODEX [1,3]. Their principles are introduced briefly in our contribution.

The notion of a diagnostic ES knowledge base (KB) may correspond with a net of diagnostic concepts. The concepts, in terms of data structures, can be seen as frames. The notion of inference (the reasoning) performed by the ES can be then seen as a p r o p a g a t i o n of concept a c t i v a t i o n s for evaluation and as a p r o p a - g a t i o n of t r u t h - v a l u e a s s i g n m e n t s to e- valuated concepts in the net. Each propagation is based on a separate generate-and-test principle in which different and separate approximative evaluations occur:

(a) in activation - due to modally weighted associations among diagnostic concepts reflecting variable degree of their correspondence (e.g. specificity, sensitivity, etc.)

(b) in evaluation - due to modality of matching concepts against the facts available about patient status.

The computational processes related to approximative inference in ESs, as they are published, are based on pragmatical approaches as theoretically sound and complete underlying principles do not exist [2,5]. In our contribution we do not intend to deal with corresponding theories neither, we rather tend to present also a pragmatical but in a way refined approach to approximative inference.

A s s o c i a t i o n

The concepts which are to be evaluated in the course of inference are
activated for different reasons: on users´ demand, as a consequence
of backward or forward chaining, and by association. It is on the latter that we shall focus our attention in this section.

Under the term ´association´ we mean a case in which evaluation of a
concept and its truth-value assignment may cause activation of other
concepts for evaluation due to some sort of correspondence among them.
It should be stressed that association, in contrast to other kinds of
activations, is an extension of the inference process as it is usually understood. The association activity in ESs serves to imitate such
human mental acts in the course of reasoning in which a concept or
concepts occur that may appear to deserve consideration. The association strength of these concepts may depend on the concept giving
rise to the association, as well as on the whole context in which association takes place.

The association connections between concepts are modal in their nature. Both positive and negative associations should be considered.
They can be well represented by proper weighting values related to
activated concepts. The numerical weighting values from the closed interval $\langle -1,1 \rangle$ may be admitted to represent the association modality.
The weight -1 stands for elimination of the concept evaluation and 1
for categorical requirement to evaluate it. If a concept is several
times associated (possibly with various weights) in different steps
of inference (in evaluating different concepts) all the involved
weighting values are accounted for and combined. For the combination
of those values the MYCIN-like combination function [6] can be well
employed (considering the ´aggressivity´ of 1 over -1). Note however that unlike MYCIN only the association modality is based on
those weighting values, not the inferred truth-values of concepts.
The resulting weighting values are of significance for setting up
priorities in evaluating assocociated concepts.

Both, specificity and efficiency of problem solving on expert level
may be influenced by proper filtering the associated concepts for
actual evaluation. This can be achieved by an adequately selected
threshold for association weighting values in a given context: only
those concepts whose resulting association weighting value   exceeds

the threshold would actually be evaluated.

The described association approach is not so sensitive for establishing weighting values as it is in case of certainty factors specification used for modal concept evaluations. This is due to the fact that
those values serve for ordering the associated concepts only. Even
when inadequacies occur in those values, no fatal inconsistency results as only the subsequent concept evaluation is responsible for
truth-value assignment.

Evaluation

A physician has no need in his real decisions for any continuos certainty factor interval. He has only a finite, discrete, and rather
small repertoire of real clinical actions available. Therefore he
needs only to qualify the truth-value assigned to the evaluated concept by some discrete modality (certainty factor). Mostly this qualification is sufficient for positively evaluated concepts (i.e. to
which the TRUE value had been assigned) yielding only one possible
clinical action. For example, if a diagnosis can not be definitely
confirmed or excluded, then it is practically sufficient to qualify
the TRUE valued diagnostic concept so as it is related to some class
of available and legally defendable medical action. In real clinical
situations physicians use various criteria for this classification. The same criteria can be used also by the ES.

Different criteria for diagnosis classification, enabling for example
to quality the diagnosis as e.g. DEFINITELY-TRUE, LIKELY-TRUE,
POSSIBLY-TRUE, with corresponding and mutually different actions,
can be categorically specified to qualify the resulting evaluation
unambigously as falling into one and only one of the classes. Every
criterion can by expressed as a set of alternatives. This then enables to formulate a whole range of conditions for every diagnosis
qualification: the alternatives, representing different conditions,
can be ordered monotonically in a criterion from the strongest (most
rigorous) to the weakest but still sufficient for the given class.
For each class a range of conditions can be designed in this manner.

Each concept representation in the KB may contain individually as many criteria as needed for sufficiently detailed (fine grained) qualification of its truth-value within the range from DEFINITELY-TRUE to
DEFINITELY-FALSE. It has, however, no sense to construct more detail-

ed evaluation criteria than appropriate for a feasible scale of clinical actions. The scaling in different concepts need not be uniform in the whole KB. If necessary a stronger criterion can embody or refer to a weaker one. Sequential ordering of criteria and their evaluation from the weakest to the strongest, or in the opposite direction, corresponds to inference approximativity. The result of concept evaluation is always given by the strongest (most rigorous) TRUE valued criterion. A combination of truth-value modalities should be rendered possible by proper criteria design. The criteria design enables stepwise referencing to other modally qualified truth-values of concepts.

The described approach enables the ES to avoid the use of numerically expressed certainty factors for approximative inference and for qualifying the attained results modally.

The expert system C O D E X

CODEX [1,3] is an empty expert system designed primarily for medical diagnostics. However its capabilities are more general. The CODEX knowledge representation is based on frame-like data structures. Each frame is a concept representation in the sense of a conceptual scheme [7]. The whole KB is to be considered as a conceptual network over which the concept activations and truth-value assignments are autonomously propagated in order to obtain a semantically relevant subnet corresponding to a causal-associative closure [4]. To this purpose the frame representation of concepts consists (among others) of two distinct parts for concept evaluation and for concept association.

The evaluation part may consist of an ordered set of criteria corresponding to a scale of modalities (classes) by which the assigned TRUE value is qualified. The association part may consist of a set of concepts connected individually or in groupings with criteria and corresponding weighting values. In evaluating this part each positively evaluated criterion yields activation of the corresponding concept or concepts with the prespecified weighting value.

The control mechanism of the CODEX inference engine uses a controlling agenda which consists of data reflecting the course of solving a given problem and its current state. The agenda involves three dynamic data structures serving the different concept activations: initial plan, deductive stack, and association priority queue. The concepts activated under user demand, in the inference chain, and by association are placed into the initial plan, deductive stack, and the priority queue, respectively. A concept association always evokes a procedure for priority queue organization.

The CODEX architecture is in concordance with those ones mostly used in ES design. It comprises modules for interactive communication, inference and its control, explanation, and result integration. The data the system works with are organized in the KB, database (acquired and inferred facts), and the agenda. In addition the KB design modules are provided. CODEX has been written in the MUMPS language. It requires about 50 Kb of disc storage and only 8 Kb memory partition to run. The size of KBs, limited only by disc capacity, does not influence significantly the systems response time.

Conclusion

We have indicated the possibility to carry out two flows of approximativeness in diagnostic ESs in general and some of the related CODEX implementation principles. Although no sufficient theoretical basis has been employed in our contribution, our empirical results had demonstrated that the choosen approach makes the KB design more feasible and that the CODEX performance yields convincing results.

References

1 GYÁRFÁŠ, F., POPPER, M.: CODEX: Prototype driven backward and forward chaining computerized diagnostic expert system. In Trappl, R. (ed.): Cybernetics and system research, North-Holland, Amsterdam, 1984, (821-824).

2 HÁJEK, P.: Combining functions in consulting systems and dependence of premisses. In Plander, I. (ed.): Artificial intelligence and information-control systems of robots, North-Holland, Amsterdam, 1984, (163-166).

3 POPPER, M., GYÁRFÁŠ, F.: CODEX: A computer-based diagnostic expert system. In Plander, I. (ed.): Artificial intelligence and information-control systems of robots, North-Holland, 1984, (297-300).

4 POPPER, M., KELEMEN, J.: An attempt to formalize the medical diagnostic problem solving. Computers and Artificial Intelligence, 5, 1984, (423-435).

5 SHORTLIFFE, E.H., BUCHANAN, B.G.: A model of inexact reasoning in medicine. Mathematical Biosciences, 23, 1975, (351-379).

6 SHORTLIFFE, E.H.: Computer-based medical consultations: MYCIN. Elsevier/North-Holland, New York, 1976.

7 SOWA, J.F.: Conceptual·structures: Information processing in mind and machine. Addison-Wesley, Reading, 1984.

A TRADITIONAL CHINESE MEDICAL EXPERT SYSTEM
BASED ON COMPUTER — GUDES

Yuke Wang, Dehying Bian and Qinglin Gao
Institute for Artificial Intelligence
in Beijing Institute of Technology,
Beijing, China.

ABSTRACT

GUDES is a Traditional Chinese Medical (TCM) expert system.

There are two basic features of TCM diagnosis, one is the organic conception of the human body, viewing its various parts as forming an organic whole; the other is that diagnosis and treatment are based on an overall analysis of the patient's condition and illness. Developing a famous TCM doctor's diagnosis system about many kinds of diseases can integrally simulate the procedure of doctor's diagnosis.

This system is designed to understand and employ expert knowledge flexibly.

In the system, inferential net is used for representing expert knowledge, a blackboard for data buffer of program communication, heuristic search for simulating thought procedure of expert. GUDES is equiped with an explanation subsystem which explains its own behaviour whenever the system pauses to wait for user's response.

So far GUDES can make diagnoses of respiratory tract, hepatitis, alimentary canal, coronary heart disease and gynecological diseases. it will contain all the clinical experience of Prof. Guan Yupo in the near future.

The whole program is written is both PASCAL language and PROLOG language, and has been run at PRIME 550 and IBM PC-XT.

Since sept. in 1983 the system has been operated about 1600 person-time in hospital of B.I.T. . the effective rate reached 97%, the cure rate is up to 35.4%.

A TRADITIONAL CHINESE MEDICAL EXPERT SYSTEM
BASED ON COMPUTER - GUDES

Yuke Wang, Dehying Bian and Qinglin Gao
Institute for Artificial Intelligence
in Beijing Institute of Technology,
Beijing, China.

1. INTRODUCTION

Expert systems are one of the major achievements in the application
of Artificial Intelligence (AI) since 70'. Encouraging progress has
been made in the field of medicine, physics, chemistry and geology,
etc. from the begining of 80', research on expert system has a tendency
towards big system and working on advanced programming environment,
such as PROLOG, FP, etc.

A traditional Chinese Medical (TCM) expert system has been developed
in The Institute for AI in B.I.T. It is named Guan Youpo Diagnosis
Expert System (GUDES), following the name of the famous TCM doctor.

2. AQUISITION OF EXPERT KNOWLEDGE

The TCM is such a field where decision making is mainly based on a
doctor's rich clinical experience and subjective judgement upon patient's symptoms.

A doctor collects the information concerned with patient, by using
four methods of diagnosis (observations, auscultation and smelling, interrogation, pulse-feeling and palpation). Nowadays, test, check and
photofluorography are sometimes used as the supplimentary methods. There
are two basic features of TCM diagnosis, one is the organic conception
of the human body, viewing its various parts as forming organic whole;
the other is that diagnosis and treatment are based on an overall analysis of the patient's condition and illness. Developing a famous TCM
doctors diagnosis system with many kinds of diseases can integrally simulate the procedure of doctor's diagnosis.

Prof. Guan Youpo is a famous old TCM doctor who is very experience
and has abundant original ideas about human diseases. His method of
choosing drugs also possesses a distinctive style. In the development
of GUDES, his valuable ideas and experiences (the knowledge) are sys-

tematized in order to be feed into computer and used in certain from by the system.

3. REPRESENTATION OF EXPERT KNOWLEDGE

Knowledge representation is the combination of data structures and related interpreting procedures. It is considered as key issue in building expert system.

The knowledge of TCM doctors focuses on the diagnosis and treatment. Referential net and blackboard are used to represent knowledge in GUDES.

a. General description about inferential model.

An inferential model is defined as six-tuple

$$M=(L,so,Q,T,f,g)$$

where

    L: set of the characters.

    Q: set of states.

    so: Initial state. so is belong to Q.

    T: set of terminal states.

        T is contained in Q. $T \cap \{so\} = \phi$

    f: function of state transformation.

        f: $L \times Q \to Q$

    g: mapping.

This mapping is held for reducing symptoms which are redundant.

b. Data structure

The prime foundations which are used for diagnosis diseases by TCM doctors are set of symptoms. These symptoms are interrelated in three ways, causality, compatibility and exclusion. These relations can be represented by a network. In GUDES the network is changed into a binary tree for convenience of implement.

The levels of nodes in the tree are arranged based on the TCM principle that to seek temporary relief for treating acute disease, to give drugs mainly according to the pathogeny for treating chronic disease. Each node is composed of following information,

SORT KEY	KEY	DATA	ATTRIBUTE	MARK	POINTERS

c. Blackboard.

The blackboard in GUDES is dynamic database established in execution for system to store the user's data, record the reasoning line, communicate with knowledge base, etc.

4. CONTROL STRATEGY

GUDES employed heuristic search method of state space including binary tree cut-off. Rules about cut-off are very simple.

a, Satisfy rule (general rule)

For a node which satisfies the condition the right subtree is cut off
and the left subtree is followed in the further reasoning.

b, Backtrack rule (special rule)

For a node which does not satisfy the condition the left subtree is
cut off and the right subtree is followed in the further reasoning.

If the system backtracks twice and can not terminate, it will ask the
user to supply new information. If the user fails to offer, the system
will try to produce a probing prescription. For each searching a subtree is always produced.

5. EXPLANATION SUBSYSTEM

To make the system acceptable for doctors, GUDES is equiped with a
explanation system. A record-list, RL, is used to take down every step
in the system's line of reasoning. During the operation, whenever the
system pauses to wait the user's response, the user could ask the system questions about its behaviour, such as "Why do you ask me such question?" or "How do you come to this conclusion?", etc. In this way,
GUDES can also be used as a assistant teaching system for training no-
vices at TCM.

The following is the diagram of the system.

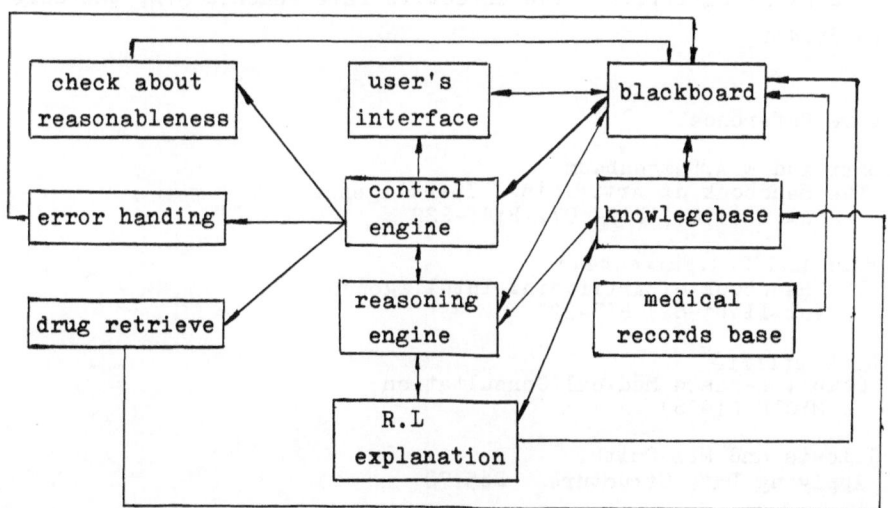

fig. The relation of parts in the system

6. THE ESSENTIAL FUNCTIONS AND FEATURES OF GUDES

GUDES possesses the following functions and features:

a. Many kinds of diseases can be diagnosed with this system. So far the system accomplished can deal with respiratory track, hepatitis, alimentary canal, coronary heart disease and gynecological diseases. It will contain all the clinical experience of Prof. Guan Yupo.

b. GUDES can produces a reasonable prescription according to diagnosis. In a prescription there is diagnosis based on an overall analysis of the illness, type, method of treatment, a group of medical herbs and doctor's advice.

c. GUDES can give 7 alternative groups of medical herbs for the same symptom, which makes prescription various and flexible.

d. GUDES is capable of checking and handling error to ensure that data into system is correct.

e. The system can explain its own behavious on a certain working step.

f. The control strategy of GUDES is simple and flexible.

g. GUDES is can interactive system which responds the user's requirements very quickly.

h. In GUDES the program and the data are seperated from each other, which makes it easy for the system to be created, modified and expanded.

The whole program is written in both PASCAL language and PROLOG language, and has been run at PRIME 550 and IBM PC-XT.

Since sept. in 1983 the system has been operated about 1600 person-time in hospital of B.I.T. The effective rate reached 97%, the cure is up to 35.4%.

Literature Reference

1. A.Barr and E.A.Feigenbaum
        The Handbook of Artificial Intelligence
            vol.I (1981) P19-107, P141-222

2. A.Barr and E.A.Feigenbaum
        The Handbook of Artificial Intelligence
            vol.II (1982) P77-222

3. E.H.Shortliffe
        Computer-Based Medical Consultation
            MYCIN (1976)

4. T.G.Lewis and M.Z.Smith
        Applying Data Structure   P65-70

5. C.A.Kulikowski

Methods and Systems for Medical Consultation IEEE Transactions
on Pattern Analysis and Machine Intelligence
PAMI-2 NO.5 Sept. 1980 P465-476

6. N.J.Nilsson Principle of Artificial Intelligence (1980)

7. C.A.Kulikowski
      Progress in Expert AI Medical Consultation System
      (1980)
      MEDINFO-83 IFIP IMIA North-Holland
      (1983) P499-502

8. H.R.Warner and P.Haug
      Medical Data Acquisition Using an Intelligence Machine
      MEDINFO-83 IFIP IMIA North-Holland
      (1983) P582-584

9. P.Szolovitz and S.G.Paunker
      Categorical and Probabilistic Reasoning in Medical Diagnosis
          Artificial Intelligence vol.1,2 P115-144 (1978)

Appendix

About Treatment Situation and Clinical Example

1. The General Situation of Treatment

a) About Patients:

Most of patients are teachers or staffs in the university. The age
range of patients is basically 45 to 55, and a few of patients is over
60. There is no significant difference between male and female.

b) About Histories:

Most of patients have chronic disease histories. The courses of disease varies from a few years to a few ten years.

c) About feature of the diseases:

Most of these patients has been cured by chinese and western medicine
in various hospitals. Some of them were in-patient department of hospital for several times, but the states of their illness sometimes took
a favourable turn, sometimes got worse. Whenever spring or autum was
coming, the weather alternately changed, their cases got worse. Among
these cases, cough and bronchial asthma, loose stools and diarrhea were
often encountered.

2. Curetive Effect

a) The Statistics of curetive effect: See attached Table.
b) Typical Case of Illness:

. Miss. Wu, Age: 58, Occupation:staff, NO.: 1533

She has suffered from cough and asthma for a few ten years. In spring or autum seasons, her ill states got worse. While illness was sho-

wing its effect she couldn't lie down whole night, and couldn't walk daytime. Although she was cured by in-and out-patient departments of hospitals, the states sometimes got better, sometimes worse. She has been treated by computer doctor since October, 1983. After she had taken 45 dose of medical herbs, her symptoms basically venished, and she was able to sleep soundly at night and able to do work daytime. During The Spring Festival of 1984, she went home to visit her family in the Northeast. Though she had cold during a trip, she had only a little cough. Since then bronchial asthma hasn't shown effect no longer.

. Mr. Chen, Age: 53, Occupation: worker, NO.: 3803

He had diarrhea before dawn for twenty years. Every early morning, he was urgent desire for immediate lowel movements, and couldn't control himself at that time, there was yellow mucoid and fetid in his stools. He was very thin and weak in physique. In addition someting else went wrong with him, such as nadai, tireness, fear cold, gastralgia, abdominal pain, etc. He was only able to work a half-day. After he had been treated by computer doctor for three months, the symptoms above gradually venished. There was no mucous in his stools. He has recovered in physique. Since he stopped taking drug ten months ago, The curetive effect has been steady. Nowdays he's already able to work a whole day.

Statistical Table of Curetive Effect about Partial

Diseases in Outpatient Department

Diagnose		The number of samples	Person-time on outpatient service	Curetive Effect			
TCM	Medicine			Recovery	Obvious effect	Effect	Inefficiency
Ache of gastral cavity	Gastric ulcer	6	27	1	3	1	1
	Gastritis	42	447	19	14	8	1
	Enteritis	31	333	14	14	3	
	Cholecystitis	2	11	1	1		
Cough and Asthma	Tracheitis	22	251	10	5	7	
	bronchial Asthma	8	136	2	5	1	
	Pulmonary emphysema	2	42			1	1
	Pneumonia	1	3	1			
	Others	16	339	7	3	6	
Total		130	1589	55	46	26	3

Attached table

MAN-MACHINE COMMUNICATION IN NATURAL LANGUAGE
FOR AN EXPERT SYSTEM IN MEDICAL CONSULTATION

P. Trigano, P. Le Beux, D. Fontaine

Compiègne University (U.T.C.)

Génie Informatique B.P.233   UA 817

60206 Compiègne Cedex FRANCE

I INTRODUCTION.

Nowadays, a lot of computer programs are used, for medical applications, by clinicians, students, or health professionals. However, it is usely difficult to interact with the machine, and, generally, people need to answer the computer program by using artificial languages to be understood. Such a solution becomes irritating for the user, who is not always a computer litterate.

Improvement of man-machine communication is one of the aims of artificial intelligence (1). In this paper, we are especially concerned with expert systems, and natural language study, using automatic deduction and knowledge representation technics. Today, several applications of expert systems have been chosen in the medical field (4,9). These kinds of programs behave like a human expert in a given domain, for clinical consultations or teaching applications. They can deduce facts, find conclusions, explain their way of thinking, and act more intelligently than in classical computer programs. But to be widely used by any kind of people, these programs need to be interactive, and able to communicate in a way very close to the natural language.

Natural language study can be found in fields such as psychological human behavior (14), data bases interrogation (13,15), or expert systems (3,8). We present a natural language system, implemented on a medical expert system (SUPER) (7), developped for clinical consultations or teaching applications. It is written in PASCAL language, and runs easily on any micro computer system.

II THE PROGRAM.

Our system is based on three separated parts :

- the lexico-semantic base (network associated to the knowledge base)
- the interpretor (independent on the application - expert system, data base, or even any program using keywords)
- the executor (wich executes specific tasks, depending on the main program - here the expert system SUPER).

2.1. The network.

2.1.1. Structure.

The base is composed of two kinds of elements : terms (nodes of the graph) and relations (semantic relationship between these terms). There are three kinds of terms : words, expressions, and concepts.

Words can have a semantic meaning or not, for a given application (for example, we will say that articles have no semantic meaning). So, there is a difference between a word taken as a lexical term, and the meaning of that word. On an other part, a set of words (expression) can have a meaning different from a word taken separately (for

ple, *hair dresser* and *hair*). It is also possible to have different words to repre-
. a same idea (or concept), for example in the case of synonyms. Thus, each word,
xpression, if it has any semantic meaning, will be associated to a concept, by a
ationship of synonymism. If different words or expression have the same meaning,
y will be linked to a same concept . Then we will say that words and expressions
resent the external language (human natural language), and concepts represent the
ernal language (semantic ideas), useful for the system. Words, expressions and con-
ts are structured in a tree, ordered like in a dictionnary, to improve the speed
search.

Our system uses a semantic network (5,10) to associate a meaning to the words, and
prove the dialogue by using synonyms. Such a representation is organized as an
riented graph, where the nodes are words, and the arcs are relations between these
rds. By running over the network, it is possible to find the semantic link between
wo words,like in an ensemblist data base (2). The shortest path between two nodes in
he graph gives the semantic proximity between the two words (6).
Two kinds of relations are present in the network : lexical relations (towards
words, expressions, concepts), and semantic relations (such as *"is a kind of*, "con-
tains", "is the contrary of",...). Each relation has a number to describe its category. It is possible to associate to a term a property of separator, like *if... then*
(to cut the sentence in different parts), of negation, like *not, lack of, no*,...(to
give a positive or negative meaning), or to use the term as a variable, and assign
values to it, like *pression = 7.5*

2.1.2. Automatic deduction.

It is possible to deduce relations from the given data of the network owing to a
certain transitivity between some relations. For example, if SOCRATE is a kind of MAN,
and MAN is a kind of HUMAN BEING, it is then possible to say that SOCRATE is a kind
of HUMAN BEING. Similarly if A MAN has LEGS, and if A LEG is a kind of MEMBER, it is
also possible to deduce that A MAN has MEMBERS. But it is not possible to apply these
deductions to all the relations. For example if UP is the contary of DOWN, and DOWN
is the contrary of UP, we may not conclude that "UP is the contrary of UP" !

The deductions are made by a finite state automata associated to the semantic properties. So, for a given concept, it is possible to know all the semantic relations
directly associated or deduced at any level.

At the creation of the network, an optimization of the graph is done, using all
the different possible deductions. For example, if we have A BOY is a kind of HUMAN
BEING, and HUMAN BEING is a kind of LIVING CREATURE, and we want to introduce A BOY
is a kind of LIVING CREATURE, this relation will not be taken, because the system
knows that it will be possible to deduce it from the network. On an other hand, if we
have A BOY is a kind of HUMAN BEING, and A BOY is a kind of LIVING CREATURE, and we
give the new relationship HUMAN BEING is a kind of LIVING CREATURE, then the third
relationship will be taken, and the second one removed automatically, to simplify
the network.

2.2. The interpretor.

The module translates the external language (words and expressions) to an internal
configuration (concepts). It represents the lexical part of the analysis (scanning),
as in a compiler. This analysis is done in real time.

2.2.1. Search of words.

First, a normalization is done, to convert each letter in capital character, and to search for a word in the tree. If it is not found, then the interpretor checks if it is possible to find a word included or containing a part of that word. This method enables the system to find directly any word at the plural mode, or any conjugated verb, only from its initial form written in the dictionnary (11).

If the word is still not found, then the program uses a pattern recognition algorithm with dynamic comparaison of words, in order to check if any character was missed, added, or inverted (12). Each word of the dictionnary is compared to the unknown word, and a cost is associated to the word. If the cost exceeds a given threshold, the word is rejected, otherwise, the word is put into a stack, where the nearest word will be the one on the top.

If the word has not been found even after these tests, the system asks different questions to the user (to define this new word), and the word is inserted into the network.

2.2.2. Translation.

Once all the words got (found or inserted), the program acts in four parallel steps to normalize semantically a sentence. First, all the words without any semantic meaning (like articles, etc....) are discarded. Then the system checks if a word is contained in an expression (left to right analysis) by looking for a relation "*is contained in the expression...*" issued from that word. The expression will be pointed by that relation, and will have relations "*contains the word...*"pointing to the different words contained in it. A technics close to the <u>A.T.N. (Augmented Transition Network</u>) (16) enables the interpretor to rebuild the expression, if possible.

If an expression is recognized, it is converted to its concept. Otherwise, all the different words pointing to that expression are translated into their concepts. Such an operation is possible owing to the relation "*means...*" pointing from a word or an expression to a concept. If any word or expression has a relation "*is a separator*", it cuts the sentence in two parts. If a word or an expression has a relation "*is a negation*", then the part including that term is put to a negative meaning.

For example, let us assume that the user writes the following sentence : *if the oxygen pressure does not go over 45 then there is a risk*. The interpretor will translate it into two parts :

Part 1 : non (PO2$>$ 45)   Condition

Part 2 : DANGER   Action

Here, *if* and *then* are separators, so the sentence is cut into two parts, one from *if*, and the other one from *then*. The expressions "*oxygen pressure*", "*does not*", "*go over*", and "*there is*" have been recognized. "*does not*" gives a negative meaning to part 1, and "*there is*" has been discarded because it has no semantic meaning (in this context).   "*oxygen pressure*" and "*go over*" have been translated into their concepts, "PO2" and "$>$", and the word "*risk*" to its concept "danger".

2.3. <u>The executor.</u>

2.3.1. Summary of medical description.

The first application of the executor is the introduction of facts into the data base. A little description is given by a user to the system, in an application of clinical consultation. The interpretor simplifies and normalizes the sentences (as seen above).   The executor has to find the different rules concerned by this description of facts. Each rule is a set of propositions (several premisses and one action), composed of keywords. The system will find a proposition owing to these keywords.

When an unknown word is found, the system tries to find the semantic link between the good answer and the user's answer. To realize such a thing, the program finds the shortest path between the two concepts (the good one and the other one) in the network, taking into account the different possible deductions for a given concept (as explained in chapter 2.1.2.). The length of the path and the kind of relationship found defines the quality of the recognition. When no rule is found, questions are asked to the user, who can always give new facts.

2.3.2. Inserting a new rule.

The second application is the introduction of a production rule into the knowledge base. The interpretor localizes the different premisses and the action of a rule owing to the relation "*is a separator*". If they do not exist yet, the executor creates them. Then, they are linked to the concerned concepts. A sentence written in the external language (human natural language), is associated to the proposition, for a better dialogue with the user. The insertion of a production rule can be done either in a special mode of knowledge building, or during an interrogation in the consultation mode.

2.4. Example of dialogue.

We present here an example of dialogue between the user (U) and the program (S), for a mediacal application (a "rubella advisor") (7).

The user can give facts to the system, or answers to the different questions asked by the system.

U : This is a consultation for a diagnosis in rubella infection. The patient is consulting for a contagious risk. There is no observable skin eruption.

S : HAS THE PATIENT HAD A CONTACT WITH A SUSPECTED PERSON DURING A PERIOD SPANNING FROM 8 DAYS BEFORE AND 16 DAYS AFTER AN OBSERVABLE ERUPTION ?

U : Why ?

S : I AM TRYING TO SEE IF THE FOLLOWING RULE IS APPLICABLE. IF CONTACT WITH CONTAGIOUS PERSONS THEN POSSIBLE CONTAMINATION.
SAME QUESTION AS ABOVE.

U : Yes.

S : THEN THERE IS A POSSIBLE CONTAMINATION. YOU MUST IMMEDIATELY TAKE A BLOOD SAMPLE FOR SERUM ANALYSIS (S1). WAS THE S1 TAKEN IMMEDIATELY AFTER THE SUSPECTED CONTAMINATION ?

U : No, but a first serum sample has been taken before the 16th day after the presumed contamination. A second serum sample has been taken 15 days after.

S : THE WORD "PRESUMED" IS UNKNOWN. PLEASE GIVE A SYNONYM.

U : Suspected.

S : OK. WERE THE SERUM SAMPLE S1 AND S2 EXAMINATED SIMULTANEOUSLY BY THE LABORATORY ?

U : No, but we still have taken a sample 4 weeks after the presumed contamminattion. The result of the analysis goes over 20.

S : THE WORD "CONTAMMINATTION" IS UNKNOWN. IS IT POSSIBLE TO WRITE IT AS "CONTAMINA-TION" ?

U : Yes.

S : OK. THE PATIENT HAS BEEN IMMUNIZED EITHER BY AN ANCIENT RUBELLA OR A RECENT ONE. WAS THE SERUM SAMPLE TAKEN LESS THEN 6 WEEKS AGO ?

U : Yes, a fractionning has been made, and there was no antibodies in the IGM fraction.

S : DO YOU MEAN THAT A FRACTIONNING OF IMMUNOGLOBULIN HAS BEEN MADE ?

U : Yes.

S : OK, THEN IT IS NOT A PRIMOINFECTION. ARE THERE ANTIBODIES IN THE FRACTION IGG.

U : Yes.

S : IT IS A REINFECTION. IN PRINCIPLE, THERE IS NO RISK.

III CONCLUSION.

III <u>CONCLUSION.</u>

The purpose of our system described above was primarly to improve the interface between a user and the expert system SUPER.

It is possible to communicate with the program in natural language. During the consulting mode, people can describe the facts, check at any time the knowledge base, and eventually modify it, by introducing new production rules. So, the system learns at any time, and can increase its dictionnary and its knowledge base. The semantic network is mostly used for answer analysis, but it is also very useful for the expert program itself, to represent knowledge. It is possible to use variables, by associating a numerical or an alphanumerical value to a concept.

The system has been implemented in PASCAL language, and therefore can be transported immediately on any micro computer. A new version running on MACINTOSH and LISA micro computers is being developped now.

<u>REFERENCES :</u>

(1) A BARR, E FEIGENBAUM : The handbook of Artificial Intelligence 1983.
(2) JP BARTHES, M VAYSSADE, MZ MIACZYNSKA : Property driven data bases, Tokyo 6th IJCAI
(3) A BONNET : Baobab, a parser for a rule-based system using a semantic grammar, Stanford Computer Science Dept, Report STAN-CS-78-668, sept 1978.
(4) R DAVIS, B BUCHANAN, E SHORTLIFFE : Production rules as a representation for a knowledge based consultation system. Artificial Intelligence. 8:15-45. Spring 1977.
(5) N FINDLER :Associative networks.Representation and use of knowledge by computers. Academic press, 1979.
(6) F FODDA : Sur le problème d'accès dans les bases de données de type ensembliste, Thèse de docteur ingénieur, UTC France 1982.
(7) D FONTAINE, P LE BEUX : An expert system for rubella consultation, Medinfo 1983 P 529-532.
(8) M JOUBERT, M FIESHI, M ROUX : Framed knowledge for medical man machine communication with computer programs, Medinfo 1983.
(9) E SHORTLIFFE : Computer based consultation in clinical therapeutics explanation and rule acquisition capabilities of the MYCIN system. Computers and biomedical research. Aug. 1975.

(10) R SIMMONS : Semantic networks : their computation and use for understanding english sentences . "Computer models of thought and language". R SCHANK & KM COLBY (Eds) San Francisco : Freeman.

(11) P TRIGANO : Reconnaissance de mots clés conjugués et mots voisins pour une application système expert, Rapport interne UTC, France 1983.

(12) R WAGNER, M FISHER : The string-to-string correction problem, ACM vol 21, n°1, jan 1984.

(13) D WALTZ : Natural language to a large data base. Computers and people 25, april 1976, 19-26.

(14) WEIZENBAUM : "ELISA", a computer program for the study of natural language communication between man and machine. Communication ACM, vol 9, n°1, 36-45.

(15) M WOODYARD, V HAMEL : A natural language interface to a clinical data base management system. Computers and biomedical research 14, 41-62, 1981.

(16) WOODS : Transition network grammars for natural language analysis, ACM vol 13, N°10, 1970 591-606.

AN EXPERT SYSTEM IN NEUROPSYCHIATRY

A. GIRON, M. EINIS, P. LE BEUX, L-H BARTHELEMY, G. LANTERI-LAURA
CITI 2, 45 rue des saints-pères 75270 PARIS CEDEX 06

Since 1962 there have been numerous applications of computer techniques in the field of psychiatry (1-2-3). These have concerned the psychometric as well as diagnostic aspects, and have even included endeavours in therapy. Although the clinical problems remain the same, the approach we suggest is appreciably different, both as regards to the methods we use and our definition of the field to be tackled.

OBJECTIVES AND ENVIRONMENT

The project's practical goal is to put a diagnostic technique at the disposition of residents on duty in emergency services, which will help them with patients who have serious consciousness troubles. Cases of troubled consciousness are very frequent in emergency medecine, and the etiological diagnoses are scattered over a very broad nosological field. Also when the diagnostic is essentially psychiatric, it usually leaves the resident on duty, helpless. This system permits to make use of the knowledge of specialists experts, and thus makes for a quick diagnostic approach, so that the patient can be directed to the specialist service best suited to his case.

The interdisciplinary team which has developed this system consists of seven members. It includes two computer experts, two psychiatric doctors, two neurologists and one general practitioner. The knowledge base was devised on the expert system "SUPER" (University of Technology of Compiegne)(4). It is a system built around an inference engine, whose rules are organised into a network, which has the distinctive feature of updating and completely optimising the network every time a new rule is inserted. Written in PASCAL

language, it is available on large computer (DEC 10) and also, in a smaller
version, on micro-computer (IBM-PC - LISA MAC INTOSH). The knowledge base
now contains nearly 300 rules.

First, we define the syndrome of mental confusion by producing a
differential diagnosis of a whole series of psychiatric pathologies revealing a
deeply troubled consciousness. If the diagnosis of the syndrome of mental
confusion is confirmed, the system then proceeds to an etiological research, and
can distinguish, not only the mental confusion itself (psychiatric syndrome) but
also the syndromes of confusion whose origin may be TOXIC NEUROLOGICAL,
INFECTIOUS, METABOLICAL, ALCOHOLIC. If the diagnosis of the syndrome of
confusion is not retained, the system then explores the other pathological fields
including consciousness troubles (DEMENTIA, CATATONIC SCHIZOPHRENIC
SYNDROME, STUPOROUS MELANCOLY, HYSTERICAL STATES), until it obtains a
likely diagnosis.

The development of a knowledge base in a domain like psychiatry imposes
additional constraints besides the usual criteria of homogeneity of knowledge
and classification of reasoning :

- the patient's confusion means that any information obtained during the
interview cannot be considered out of context : the form of the answer is as
important as its content.

- the patient's total or partial mutism, sometimes makes any attempt at
differential diagnosis, very difficult.

- the relative ambiguity of the signs and the very great complexity of the
psychiatric terms have obliged us to elaborate several stages in the
interpretation of the data : from a simple description, given in everyday
language and not interpreted, to the definition of syndromes and illnesses.

METHODOLOGY

The above mentionned constraints have led us to the strict definition of a
six-stage methodology, in order to build up a network of rules :

1 : DELIMITATION OF THE FIELD OF RESEARCH

2 : <u>THE SEMANTIC TREE</u>   Every physician, member of the team, must
therefore draw up a semantic tree, showing the different symptoms, as well as
the etiological forms, of a diagnosis. The root of the tree consists of the
diagnosis, the leaves represent the symptoms and regrouping of symptoms,
which lead to that diagnosis. The tree must, moreover, be built in such a way
that the semantic links, which compose it, may be made operational by a
preliminary systematisation. It will serve as a frame for the future rules.

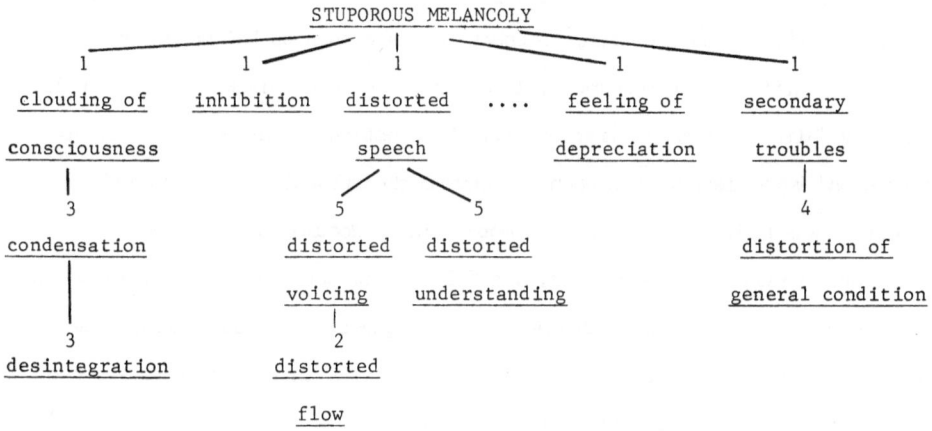

EXAMPLE OF A SEMANTIC TREE

3 : <u>DETECTION OF THE CONTRADICTIONS AND REDUNDANCIES AMONG THE</u>
<u>SEMANTIC TREES.</u> The duty composed trees are introduced into a relational data
base, with a view to testing the model's coherence and eliminating any possible
contradictions. The semantic nature of the links which join the elements is
naturally not taken into account.

4 : <u>CONSTRUCTION OF THE LANGUAGE - IN DIRECT CONTACT WITH THE</u>
<u>USER</u>. Due to the complexity of the nosography and the ambiguity often inherent
in certain psychiatric terms, general practioners may often interpret these in a
number of ways. The unequivocal nature, necessary for the apprehension of the
phenomenon obliged us to translate all the psychiatric terms into everyday
language. For example instead of "Does your patient reveal anxious perplexity",
a sign which, in itself, may pass unnoticed or be interpreted by the general
practioner in several ways, we would ask : "Does your patient seem unable to

understand what is happening to him and make any effort to overcome his condition ?". Thus the sign becomes significant and is integrated into the "syndromic sphere". So we can distinguish three levels :

- the "observable phenomenon", questionned in everyday language

- the psychiatric interpretation of the "observable phenomenon", which may vary according to the syndromic sphere considered

- the symptoms or regrouping of symptoms

5 : <u>VALIDATION OF THE LANGUAGE</u>. Once the questions had been expressed by each expert, it was necessary to check that a consensus had been established between the different team members. In order to achieve this we settled on the following "blind system" : first of all, the questions relating to "observable phenomenon" were listed, then each one became the subject of a form on which no mention was made of the related symptom. These documents were then distributed to each of the doctors, who filled them out individually, and wrote on the symptom and various syndromes which the question called to mind. The pooling of the results then showed up any ambiguities in the interpretation of certain signs, and this is turned to discussion.

6 : <u>CONSTRUCTION OF THE RULES</u>. The network is then constructed by translating the semantic links of the differents trees, itemized beforehard, into the form of rules of production. This translation gives rise to new kinds of rules, able to call on sets or sequential processes.

7 : <u>EXPERIMENT ON REAL CASES</u>. The final part of the project which will validate the first knowledge base, is to run the expert system on real documented cases. If the validation of this step is positive, then we will proceed to use it in a real clinical environment.

<u>CONCLUSION</u> :

The development of a system which facilitates decision making, in the field of neuro-psychiatry, imposes a certain number of specific constraints which oblige us to make innovations of particular interest to the development of knowledge bases. Indeed the experience and heuristics of the practitioner come into play here, even before the construction of the rules : both when the field is structured by the semantic trees, and when the "user's language" is established.

EXAMPLE : (in fact there are 25 questions in all)

Does your patient seem to be "in the clouds" ?	NO
Would you say that your patient seems "hypnotised" ?	YES
Is he making any effort to overcome his condition ?	YES
....	.....
Do the objects around your patient seem strange to him ?	NO
Does he has trouble recognising his parents or those who are looking after him ?	YES
Does your patient sometimes speak incoherently ?	NO
....	.....
Does he remember if he has been visited that every morning ?	NO
Does he has trouble remembering things about his own past ?	YES
Does he has trouble concentrating on a particular object ?	YES
Does he seem incapable of reading or carrying out simple operations ?	YES

AS A RESULT OF SUCH A DIALOG THE SYSTEM WOULD CONCLUDE THAT THE PATIENT HAS PROBABLY : A SYNDROME OF MENTAL CONFUSION.

REFERENCES :

(1) GREIST J.H, KLEIN M, ERDMAN H, JEFFERSON J.
    "Clinical computer applications in mental health"
    Computer in psychiatry, psychology, NH, 1983 - vol 2.

(2) SCHMID W., BRONISH T., VON ZERSSEN D.
    "A comparative study of PSE/CATEGO and Diasika : two computer diagnostic system"
    Br. J. psychiatry 1982, sep. ; 141 : 292 - 5

(3) COLBY K.
    "Computer simulation and artificial intelligence in psychiatry"
    Method of behavioural research - 1979

(4) FONTAINE D., LE BEUX P.
    "An expert system for rubella consultation"
    Medinfo 1983 proceedings, vol 1, p 529-532

(5) HENRI EY, BERNARD P., BRISSET C.
    "Manuel de psychiatrie"
    PARIS - MASSON 1969

(6) American psychiatric association
    DSM 3
    PARIS - MASSON 1983

EARLY DIAGNOSIS PROGRAM OF BREAST CANCER

L. Fernández, M.L. Buch, M. Caraballoso, A. Martín, M. Pardo and
M.V. Carreras

National Oncologic Institute, Havana, Cuba

In this paper we show the organizative, scientific and computer bases
for the beginning of the Early Diagnosis Program of Breast Cancer in
an Urban Health area of Havana City. This program was planned together
with Swedish collaboration also to serve in comparative studies in both
countries.

INTRODUCTION

In Cuba, in the period from 1979 to 1981 the Breast Cancer occupied
the first place among the malognant neoplastic diseases of female patients both in incidence (18,7 of the total) and in mortality (15,5
of the total) (1). The rate of incidence increased to 23,5 per 100000
women in the period 1979-1981. The rate of mortality increased from
11,9 to 13,5 per 100 000 in the same years in the whole country.

The Havana City province presented the highest figures with an incidence rate of 51 per 100 000 women in 1982 according to the Cuban National Cancer Registry. These figures show that urgent actions have
to be started in order to improve the situation of Breast Cancer.

In this context, epidemiological and statistic studies using computers
have been carried out (2). The computer system for the National Cancer
Registry (3) and risk factor studies by multivariate analysis (4) have
been used for this purpose. To decrease mortality, to increase survival rates and to improve quality of women life are the objectives of
the National Control Program of Breast Cancer. The program has two main
activities; Diagnosis and Treatment.

An important experience in massive use of mammography in Early Diagnosis of Breast Cancer is gained in Sweden since 1969 (5,6). In Cuba we
will start a similar study with Swedish collaboration as an experimental task of diagnosis activities in the program.

A computer system using a Cuban minicomputer CID 300-10 was designed
in order to guarantee reliability and smooth process. The system was
written in Pascal programming language.

PROCEDURES

The figure 1 shows the main procedures of the system. The first computer process is to select women from a file where names, addresses and
ages of all women between 40 and 70 years are stored. Appointment
scheduled for the diagnosis Centre are produced. The Centre uses these

Computer Centre   **Diagnosis Centre**   **Women**

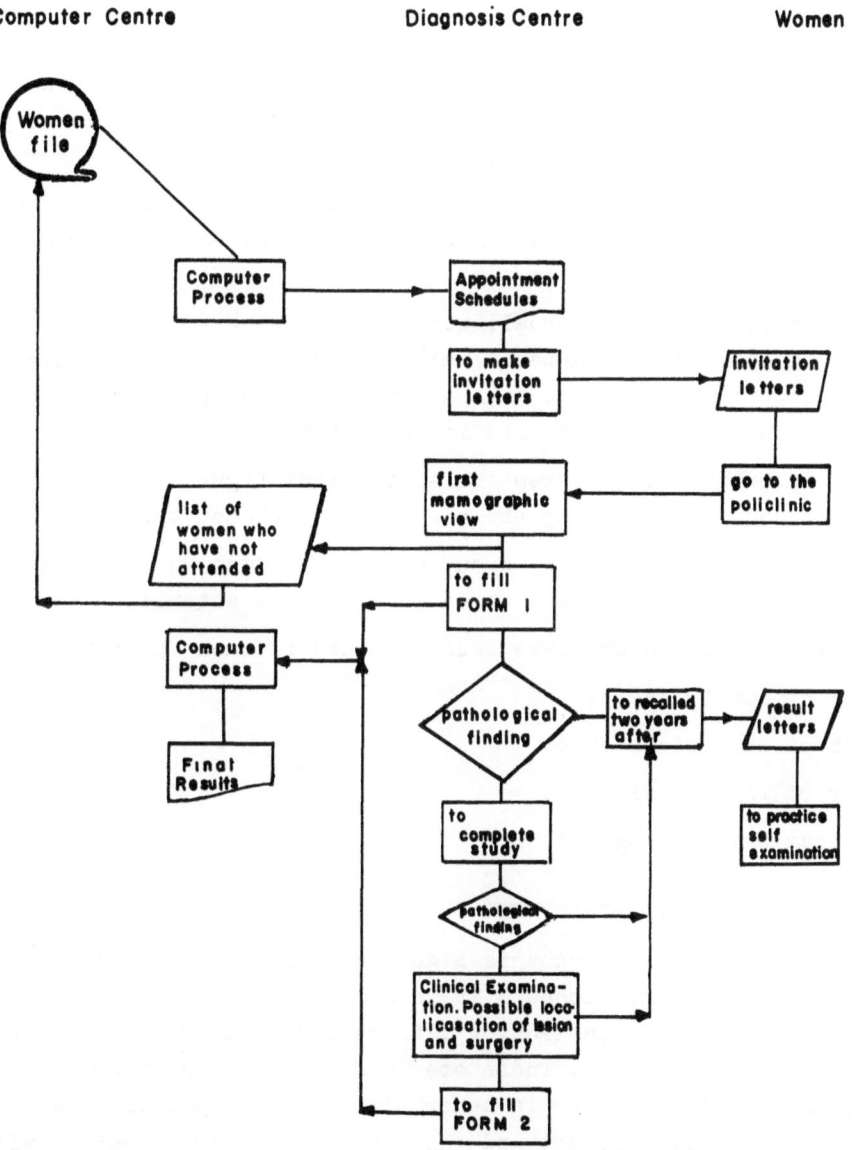

FIG 1. Main procedures of the system. Inputs, outputs, process in
Computer Centre and in Diagnosis Centre.

schedules to send an invitation letter to each woman. Each day seventy women are checked with a first mammographic view and the primary forms are filled. This form contains general identification, anamnesis and mammography results.

Result letters are send to the women if there were no pathological findings ("NOT"). They will be recalled after two years. The women are recalled to make them a complete study if the mammographic results were positive. These studies may be negative in which case result letters are send to the women and they will be recalled two years after. Clinical examination, localization of lesions or surgery would be possible when the results are suspicious, bening or cancer.

Each day a list of women that have not attended the appointment is send to the computer centre. The women who have not attended are recalled two times.

The second form is filled for all women who require surgery. It contains clinical and pathological data, final mammography results, clinical stage and treatment. All the data are stored in order to make statistical and epidemiological studies in the future.

The final outputs of the system are statistical figures for evaluating the program and for comparing the results in both countries:

- numbers and percentages, by group of age of women who have been invited, women examined and women who have not attended.

- percentage of women who have been attended in each appointment.

- number of cancer cases.

- number of suspicious cases.

- number of false positives.

- mean examinations per day.

DISCUSSION AND FUTURE DEVELOPMENT

The massive use of mammography is a good auxiliary in the Early Diagnosis of Breast Cancer. Although it is an expensive study for a developing country. The comparison of different methods used in Early Diagnosis is recommendable. Therefore Self examination Program and Clinical examination Program in other similar municipalities have been planned. Cost, social impact and the clinical stage of lesions will be analyzed, too.

REFERENCES

1. Caraballoso M., Fernández L. Cáncer en Cuba, trienio 1979-81.
   En prensa.

2. Caraballoso M., Fernández L. Las primeras localizaciones en Cáncer
   en Cuba. En prensa.

3. Fernández L., Caraballoso M. et al. Project for a New System of the
   Cuban National Cancer Registry. Medinfo 83, Van Bemmel, Bal, Wigertz
   (eds). IFIP-IMIA. North Holland Publ. Co. 1983.

4. Fernández L., Martín A., Buch M.L. Diagnóstico Precoz de Cáncer
   Mamario II. Selección de Variables relacionadas con el Riesgo de
   Cáncer Mamario. Rev., Cub., Oncol., En prensa.

5. Lundgren B., Jakobsson S. Repeat Screening by single oblique view
   mammography. Breast Cancer Research and Treatment 1, (1981) 273-280.

6. Lundgren B. Breast Cancer Screening. Expected and Observed Incidence
   and Stage of Female Breast Cancer in Gavleborg Country, Sweden, and
   Implications of Mortality. Recent Results in Cancer Research. Vol.
   90 (1984).

A GENERAL ARCHIVE MANAGEMENT AND LENDING SYSTEM IN A HOSPITAL INFORMATION SYSTEM
ENVIRONMENT.

W.A. op het Veld and M.L. Koens
BAZIS, Leiden University Hospital
Leiden, The Netherlands

Abstract

The described system provides the different departments of a hospital organization
with facilities for archive management and lending administrations. It can be used
for different kinds of collections of objects e.g. X-ray folders, medical records
and non-patient related objects as books etc. By interfacing to other subsystems of
the HIS, the flow of the objects within the organization can be monitored and
controlled.

1. Introduction

The registration of information and the fast accessibility of this information is a
main condition for the adequate functioning of a hospital.
Therefore in every hospital a lot of different collections of information can be
found, e.g. medical records, X-ray folders, pathological specimens, books, employee
files.
For the storage of this information various media are used, e.g. paper, film
(alphanumerical as well as images), computer files. The last category has
undeniable advantages, such as accessibility, the possibilities for processing and,
of course, the cost. Evidence for this is the increasing tendency to register
information in computer files. With alphanumerical data considerable results have
been attained. Due to fast progress in the development of automation one can expect
that image registration will be viable within the coming decade, technically as
well as economically [1].

However at present, hospital organizations will for a great extent depend on
conventional media. This means huge archives. The management of these archives is
no small task. Often there is little insight into the contents of such archives and
access is in general reduced to the sequence in which the objects have been stored.
The distribution of objects in different (physical) archives increases the
difficulty of retrieval. To increase the control over these problems a
comprehensive administration is a necessity. Due to the enormous effort required,
this is often neglected.

An additional problem is introduced if objects from an archive are made available
to other groups of users.
Partly due to the fact that a user is not fully informed as to which objects are
available, requests by users are often not sufficiently defined. Besides this
requests are unstructured (i.e. not in file sequence). Effective handling
necessitates the preprocessing of the requests; this can for instance mean a
division into sub-archive level and sorting into archive sequence. This process
also includes the tracing of requested objects which have already been borrowed
and, of course, possibly the reclaiming of these objects. To be able to locate
these objects a lending administration is required.
The lending administration must also provide the possiblity of producing reminders
for users for which the borrowing period of objects is overdue. Nevertheless,
experience shows that these administrative tasks are only partly executed or
completely ignored. Where an administration is maintained, this is not always found

to be correct; objects can be wrongly booked.

Experience proves that the size of these problems progressively increases with the volume of the collections of objects.
The above mentioned problems can be illustrated with an example. The Leiden University Hospital is an averaged sized university hospital, with 25,000 admissions and 350,000 outpatients visits each year. The total number of medical records in the various archives is about 4 million. An estimated number of 500,000 are borrowed each year, resulting in one million transfers. The X-ray archives of the radiology departments contain about 2 million X-ray folders. Here the number of folders borrowed is slightly smaller (+ 350,000 per year). In these archives a more or less reduced administration is maintained. Although no measurements have been made, it is estimated that a great deal of time is wasted in tracing lost objects. One could assume that the quality of the patient care suffers due to this problem.

Considering the extensive problems with which the archive management, as well as the users, were confronted, it was decided in the beginning of 1983 to develop an automated system. The aims of this system were formulated as (1) the supporting of the tasks of the archive management and (2) the coordination of the movements of objects among the archives and users.
The decision also implied the integration with the already existing Hospital Information System (HIS). Actually a HIS has been under development since 1972 and is currently being used in a cooperation of 20 separate hospital organizations. It currently administrates approximately 11,500 hospital beds.
On the one hand the most important advantage of this approach is that the system can use the subsystems of the HIS and their collected data, moreover the costs of development could be shared by all participants in the HIS cooperative. On the other hand the system had to be extended to support all kinds of archiving methods as used by the various participants.

Section 2 reviews the activities supported by the system and the way in which it will be realized. Section 3 describes the available facilities in a HIS environment. In section 4 the aspects of introduction of the system in a hospital environment will be discussed. Finally in section 5 some concluding remarks.

2. Description of the activities to be supported by the system.

To reach the objectives described in the introduction, the following activities have to be supported by the system :

2.1 Cataloguing the collections of objects.

In order to give the management, as well as the users, insight into the available objects, a catalogue has to be created of all existing objects. This catalogue includes the patient-related objects, e.g. medical records, X-ray folders, pathological specimens, ecg's, eeg's, etc., as well as non-patient related objects such as employee files, books etc.
By means of an adjustable user authorisation a window can be created making only the relevant part of the catalogue accessible to the user.
Identification of objects in this catalogue will be possible by using different keywords. Optionally this can be done by using data which has been registered by other subsystems.
For example : the patient registration system allows patients to be identified using several different keys i.e. surname, birthdate, sex and/or patient identification number. After the identification all the patient-related objects are retrieved. A detailed selection can then also be carried out on this collection (for example, only medical records). Another example : in the subsystems for radiology support is registered which X-rays are stored in each X-ray folder. Identification of these X-ray folders can be done by using this subsystem (see figure). One final example : the library subsystem allows books to be easily

identified by means of author and/or title.

```
┌─────────────────────────────────────────────────────────────────────┐
│  ███████████        ████████     --              W        X.Y.Z.     │
│  GEB: 08-06-49      LEIDEN         ███████████        M       PAG. 1  │
│  ─────────────────────────────────────────────────────────────────   │
│  18-01-85  - RADIODIAGNOSTIEKVERRICHTINGEN - TOTAALOVERZICHT          │
│  ─────────────────────────────────────────────────────────────────   │
│  1    31-03-78    X1    5002    THORAX        RONP    LONP            │
│  2    08-06-79    X2    7002    B.O.Z.        RONP    LONP            │
│                         5002    THORAX                                │
│  3    05-12-80    X3    2002    AANGEZICHT    RONC    CHIB            │
│  4    16-11-84    X4    7211    MAAG          RONC    CHIP            │
│                         7711    GALBLAAS                              │
│                                                                       │
│  WELKE FOTOMAPPEN WILT U AANVRAGEN? : 1 4                             │
└─────────────────────────────────────────────────────────────────────┘
```

Figure: Identifying X-rays folders using the radiology information subsystem

Some collections of objects are related to each other by means of a hierarchical structure (e.g. masterfolder and subfolder). These methods of archiving are also supported. The number of levels is unlimited.

2.2 The registration of the actual location of the objects.

It is obvious that each object always has a particular location, either at a user or an archive location. To retrieve each object these locations must be known by the system; only then can the system give a true representation of the actual situation. This is a requisite to guarantee a quick delivery of the requested objects.
In order to keep the registration of transfers as easy as possible various facilities are available; e.g. each object is labelled with a barcode. Furthermore, all terminal locations throughout the hospital equiped with a barcode reader are provided with a list containing all potential users with their relevant barcodes. A simple movement with the barcode reader on both the object barcode and the user barcode is sufficient to register the new location.

Each organization has to consider how detailled the network of users and/or locations should be. It seems clear that the more detailled the network is, the more exact the actual location of each object can be determined . On the other hand more effort is required in keeping track of the actual location of all the objects. Depending on its needs, each hospital has to determine the initial degree of location detail necessary. After the system has been used in practice for some time the necessary degree of location detail can be refined (e.g. the number of locations within a single department).
In connection with this it is also necessary to determine whether objects will only be lent to seperate users or only to physical locations within the organization. Combinations of the two will also be possible.

2.3 Allocation of objects to the locations where they belong.

In the previous section it was stated that each object has a specific location at any particular moment. As soon as a request is presented it can be said that a desired situation comes into force. From this point of view a request means that an object should be at a certain place at a certain moment. Often such a request also implies that the object has to be there for a certain period; i.e. a reservation. The requests c.q. reservations for all objects together represents, as it were, a desired future situation.
To realize this desired situation, which is of course continuously changing, is one of tasks of the system.

Requests for objects can be presented as follows :

- Conversationally.
  Requests for objects can be input via any terminal connected to the system. As described in section 2.1. the data collected by other subsystems of the HIS can be used for identifying objects. Besides the identification code of the object and the user also the reservation period and the reason for borrowing can be registered.
  For each request it is checked if the borrower is authorized for the specified object. For patient-related objects one of the checks is the medical relationship between the borrower and the patient.
  It is also verified whether the requested reservation period conflicts with any other outstanding request for the object.

- Automatically by other subsystems.
  In carrying out certain activities within an hospital a number of objects are always required. For example : during an outpatient appointment at least the medical record is required; during a clinical admission a number of documents (e.g. medical record, X-rays) are required; during the review of an X-ray, earlier X-rays are required. Some of these activities are already registered within the HIS (patient scheduling, admittance). As far as possible the system tries, with the aid of these subsystems, to generate requests for the desired objects without intervention by the users.

- Automatically by the lending system.
  One of the tasks of the archive management is to support the timely return of borrowed objects. The lending system automatically produces requests to return objects.
  The moment for reclaiming the objects depends on a number of adjustable criteria; e.g. reclaiming takes place after the expiration of the period of reservation, taking into account an adjustable margin, or reclaiming takes place after the completion of an activity e.g. discharge of a patient. As long as there is only one archive for a collection of objects it is obvious that the objects have to return to this location. In the case of more than one archive the system has to determine which archive is preferant. For each object it can be registered whether this archive is dependant on the object to be reclaimed (e.g. return to the archive where the object originats) or on the borrower (e.g. return to the nearest archive). Due to the lack of space some archives have to be thinned out periodically. Objects are then transferred to a non-active archive. This activity is also to be supported by the system. Periodically the system generates requests to achieve these transfers. By staggering the desired transfer dates the thinning out process can be integrated into the daily activities of the archive staff.

Requests generated for an object in any of the above mentioned ways must, of course, be respected.
Periodically (e.g. twice a day) the system selects all requests which have to be honoured within a certain, adjustable period. To each borrower or archive, in possession of one or more of these objects, a so-called mailing list is dispatched. Each mailing list instructs the receiver to send the relevant objects to the stated new borrowers or archives. Each mailing list is printed on a receiver adjustable printer. The requests can be sorted in any way the recipient of the list wishes (e.g. in filing sequence).

With the help of the above mentioned functions it is quite clear that the activities of the archive staff in particular are lightened. To summarise :
- The users generate directly the requests for objects without intervention of the archive staff. The number of telephone calls are therefore considerably reduced.
- The requests are more structured, e.g. in filing sequence.
  The requests for already borrowed objects can, if desired be routed directly to the relevant borrowers.
- Registration of transfers is simplified by barcode wands.
  Transfers, mentioned on a mailing list, can be confirmed in a single action.

- Reclaiming of objects is automatically controlled by the system.
- Thinning out the archives is also automatically controlled by the system. This activity has been integrated in the daily work.

2.4 Management information

As stated before one of the main tasks of the archive staff is to place the material managed by them, at the disposal of the necessary persons or departments. In supplying these needs several means are available e.g. manpower, file space, administrative tools. To make the most efficient use of these assets there should be sufficient insight into how, and in which quantity, the objects are used.
The number of objects, the number of objects lent, the volume of the borrowing population and the urgency with which the objects have to be available are determinate magnitudes. To provide more insight into these magnitudes reviews can be produced such as :
- diagram of transfers.
  These diagrams provide the number of movements of objects between each borrower and each archive within a certain period.
- review of discrepancies between planned and real transfer time. This review can be seperated into different reviews per borrower or per archive.

3. Integration in a HIS.

The general archive management and lending system is developed as a part of a still expanding Hospital Information System (HIS in development since 1972) [2].

Integration of this system in a HIS has many advantages, such as :

- Accessibility
  The hardware configuration includes an extensive network of terminals (up to 350) connected to a central database by means of a central processor.
  All the lending data in this database is retrievable and processable from any terminal (vdu or printer).
  A dedicated and adjustable authorisation procedure will, of course, ensure that only authorised users have access to these files. Due to the size of the terminal network the lending facilities can be used from practically any work location within the hospital.

- Integration
  From the description of the system in chapter 2 can be seen that other subsystems of the HIS make extensive use of the lending system and visa versa.
  These subsystems can be categorized as follows :
  . Subsystems supporting the identification of the objects. In determining further information regarding the contents of the object the following subsystems are used.
    E.g. - patient registration system
         - radiology information system
         - library system
  . Subsystems describing patient activities.
    From these subsystems information can be determined as to when and where activities take place whereby objects are needed.
    E.G. - appointment scheduling system for outpatient departments and supporting services such as radiology.
         - admission scheduling system
         - admission and discharge system

- Reliability and availability
  The reliability of the HIS is high. The HIS is operational 24 hours a day, 7 days a week with an average availability of over 99.5 %. This is due to the fact that

the essential hardware is duplicated and the switching from one computer to the other is a simple matter.
The HIS runs an in-house developed operating system, tailor-made for a hospital environment and incorporating recovery facilities. Every evening a copy is made of the complete HIS database.

A long period of system failure would cause a chaotic lending administration, which is difficult to recover. This makes a high degree of reliability indispensable.

4. Introduction aspects

Apart from the normal introduction aspects, such as user training and installation of terminals the following aspects are of interest:

- The building-up of the object catalogue.
  With the introduction of the system already existing objects have to be catalogued. A conversion requires a huge amount of manpower, which is financially difficult to realize, therefore, a gradual conversion is preferred.
  Only active objects will be catalogued in the system. However, requests for not catalogued objects must also be possible. To prevent garbling of the catalogue a authorisation procedure is essential.
  Instead of a seperate function this authorisation is implied in the transfer function of the system, this to prevent the increase of activities of the archive staff. (A transfer is a physical action which implies the existence of the object).

- Building the borrower and archive file.
  Each organisation has to determine a more or less detailed list of borrowers and archives as stated in section 2.2.

- In a situation before the introduction of this sytem where only a part of the tranfers are registered, it has to take into account that registration of all the transfers will increase the workload of the archive staff.

5. Concluding remarks

At the present time (january 1985) the development of the described system is in full swing. The first step by step introduction of this sytem in some of the cooperating hospitals in the BAZIS foundation will take place soon.
It is, therefore not yet possible to present any experiences concerning the introduction of the system, and neither is it yet possible to predict if the objectives will be reached.
The fact that the described system is embedded in a integrated hospital information system makes it, in our opninion, a powerful tool in solving archiving problems.

References

[1] De Valk, J.P.J., Bijl, K. et al "Imagis : relation between PACS and HIS" in : proc. MIE 1985, Springer, in press.
[2] Bakker, A.R., Scope and limitations of a mini-based centralized Hospital Information System" in : Proc. MEDINFO 1980, Lindberg/Kaihara, eds. (1980) p. 505.

THE AGK-THESAURUS - FICTION OR REALITY ?

Volker Loy, Michael Möhr
Institut für Pathologie, Klinikum Steglitz, Freie Universität Berlin
Hindenburgdamm 30, D 1000 Berlin 45, Germany

Peter Röttger
Institut für Pathologie, Krankenanstalten Düren

1. SUMMARY:

The AGK-Thesaurus is one of the most important tools for free text analysis of pathology reports in German-speaking countries. Several update
systems had previously been used on large computers, which, however were
not at all portable and could only be employed sporadically. Moreover,
the update systems operating hitherto did not always check the complex
relations of the thesaurus adequately, which led to many self-perpetua-
ting incosistencies. Further difficulties arose from the original concept to keep all inflexional forms of each word as a separate entry in
the thesaurus, which grew to a size incompatible with most smaller computers. In the Department of Pathology at Klinikum Steglitz in Berlin,
a new update system has been developed which avoids all the former disadvantages and can be used interactively or by batch processing. Communication with the user is handled via the former standardized and easy-
to-use interface format. The files are checked thoroughly to eliminate
inconsistencies as far as possible. The removal of inflexional forms has
reduced the size of the thesaurus considerably. The update programs
(ANSI-COBOL) can be used anywhere. It is to be hoped that this new
possibility will revitalize the seemingly fading interest in free text
analysis of pathology reports.

2. INTRODUCTION:

The AGK-thesaurus is the most comprehensive and most widely used thesaurus for free text analysis in pathology in both the F.R.G. and Austria.
It has been supported by Swiss pathologists as well. The principles
of the thesaurus, the first edition and the first 'field-trial' had been
prepared by (1) in 1969. Afterwards many pathologists and members of departments of medical informatics joined the working-group on free text
analysis ('Arbeitsgemeinschaft Klartextanalyse'). Some parts of the thesaurus were adopted by (2) in 1973 in Graz, who combined them with
the SNOP. The first edition of the thesaurus had been compiled in Darmstadt using FORTRAN programs and was replaced by fast growing successors
prepared in Hannover using an interactive update system elaborated by
Wingert in PL1. It had to be supplemented by a batch mode version (3)
which had been implemented by (4) in Vienna using former propositions

of Wingert. The new programs were also written in PL1 and required large
computers. Its most important feature was a small collection of simple
statements and an easy-to-use record based on punch cards. Though far in
advance of its predecessors, it could not circumvent their major disadvantages: the need for a large computer which, even if available, was
completely occupied by the PL1 programs. The update of the thesaurus
thus became a nearly insurmountable burden, which greatly hampered
free text analysis by the pathologists. Nevertheless the thesaurus has
been used by different pathologists many times. Certainly, in the past
years, interest seemed to bee fading, partly because of the lack of
central computer facilities, partly because of the everlasting difficulties involved in free text analysis of pathology reports. In English-
speaking countries, these problems are often obscured by the similarity
between the natural language of the pathologists and the recommended
nomenclature like the SNOP. Remarkably, the most famous systems for
documentation of pathology reports in the USA, those of Lamson and Dimsdale (5) and Gaynon and Wong (6), use thesauruses similar to that of the
AGK.

3. PURPOSE:

a) To provide a portable, modular and self-explanatory thesaurus
   which can be used and updated anywhere and at any time in order to
   strengthen again the interest in free text analysis of pathology
   reports in German-speaking countries.
b) To elaborate the old statements proposed by Wingert for the batch
   mode update as a general interface for interactive and batch processing on decentralized smaller systems, like (7), for example.

4. CURRENT STRUCTURE OF THE AGK-THESAURUS:

The AGK-thesaurus consists of two files. The entry file ('E-FILE') and
the standard file ('S-FILE'). The E-FILE is a list of all words hitherto
encountered in pathology reports. Each entry refers to a number which
denominates a unique semantic concept, corresponding to a class of synonyms. In the past, most of the synonyms were derived from inflexional
forms. These have been now removed. Words to be examined are first
tested to determine, whether they could possibly represent the inflexion
of a more simple syntactic form. By this method alone, the overwhelming

size of the E-FILE has been reduced by half.

Record of the E-FILE: Entry (40 B, character); Number of the preferred term (4 B, numeric, packed).

The standard file ('S-FILE') is a sequential list of the referenced numbers of the E-FILE, but the whole record contains additional pieces of information. Any preferred term is attached to one of 6 categories: 1 localizer, upper term; 2 finding, narrower term; 3 localizer, narrower term; 4 modifier; 5 varia; 6 finding, upper term. Complex semantic concepts are broken up into facets, each of which is another preferred term and represents the implied finding (postcoordination).

Record of the S-FILE: Number of the preferred term (4 B, numeric, packed); Preferred term (40 B, character); Category (1 B, numeric); Counter of the following facets (2 B, binary); Up to 20 facets, together with their categories (4 B, numeric, packed / 1 B, numeric).

The original thesaurus is built up by these two files. In order to facilitate updating, an inverted list of the S-FILE's facets points to the records of the S-FILE in which a certain preferred term is referred to as a facet (V-FILE).

5. UPDATE-SYSTEM:

The programs have been written in ANSI-COBOL using nothing but standard features. There are 6 parts: an interactive module, the interface, the statement modules, elementary modules, an interactive module connected to the elementary modules for diagnostic purposes, and a module which checks the whole thesaurus and any step of the update. The interactive module produces statements according to the interface format. Each step is checked regularly; defaults and missing information are provided automatically. Any error encountered leads to an update proposition of the system, which is written in an errror file according to the interface format. This file can be used as input for the subsequent update.

Each statement corresponds to a module of its own, which uses elementary modules operating on a single record of the different files. Any elementary operation is checked and counterchecked. Any elementary modification of the S-FILE is followed by an immediate update of the V-FILE, its

original record beeing temporarily saved in addition to assure the completeness of the relations for the next operation! This has also been
neglected in former update systems leading to several inconsistencies.
The automatic addition of subreferences in the S-FILE is limited to
20 facets. If they exceed this number some facets have to be sacri-
ficed in the following order of their corresponding categories: 3 (localizer, narrower term, e.g. MUCOSA), 4 (modifier, e.g. LARGE), 5 (varia)
2 (finding, narrower term, e.g. CHOLECYSTITIS). It is the goal of this
rule to save the most important information of the category 1 (localizer, upper term, e.g. GALL BLADDER) and 6 (finding upper term, e.g.
INFLAMMATION).
Applications of the thesaurus have revealed that pathologists in fact
use only small but nevertheless different fractions of it. The thesaurus now can be regarded as a set of several updates and instead of distributing the whole thesaurus to different users it should be possible
to broadcast only update files, parts of which could be used selectively
according to the special needs of different pathologists.

Formal 'cleaning' of the thesaurus:
We started with 59 955 entries in the E-FILE. Using simple algorithms,
we removed the inflexional suffixes 'e', 'em', 'en', 'er', 'es', 's',
etc. and tried to find another entry identical to the remaining root
and (!) referring to the same preferred term. By this method, the E-FILE
could be reduced to 26 541 entries. In several subsequent steps, we
tried to reduce entries which referred to different preferred terms and
encountered a lot of multiple recordings of preferred terms in the S-
FILE. They have been removed. Some other entries referring to different
preferred terms have been kept, although they could have been reduced
and unified formally. 'ALLEM' (all) can be reduced to 'ALL' by removing
the suffix "em", e.g., but this would produce a synonym to 'ALL', the
abbreviation to 'Acute Lymphoblastic Leucemia'. This example shows that
the algorithm which automatically creates a term by removing suffixes
may fail in some cases! The cleaning operations have now left the
E-FILE with 26 034 entries and the S-FILE with 15 688 preferred terms.

Interface format (according to the propositions of Wingert):
(only a few examples of the most important operations can be given!)
'I' (insert a word or preferred term): 'I BOECK 2 SARCOIDOSE;' insert
the new entry BOECK into the E-FILE referring to the number of the preferred term SARCOIDOSE in the S-FILE. 2 is the number of the category
of SARCOIDOSE (finding, narrower term). ';' is the terminator.

'I SARCOIDOSE 2*' insert the preferred term SARCOIDOSE into the S-FILE, supplying it with the category 2 (finding, narrower term).

'X': supplement an existing preferred term with additional facets.

'X SARCOIDOSE 2 GRANULOMA 2;'

The insert and supplement statements are comparatively easy. More diffi-cult are the delete statements and those which change preferred terms into one another or into entries and vice versa.

'F SARCOIDOSE;' Delete the entry SARCOIDOSE.

'F SARCOIDOSE 2*' Delete the preferred term SARCOIDOSE. This means re-move all entries of this class of synonyms, delete the record in the S-FILE and delete it in each record of the S-FILE where it has been re-ferred to as a facet. This last operation cannot be restricted to SARCOIDOSE. Together with SARCOIDOSE all subreferences which have been introduced into the corresponding record of the S-FILE have to be re-moved too. But as the thesaurus has a polyhierarchic structure, some of the subreferences might also have been introduced into the record by another facet. Therefore, after deleting the subreferences of one facet, the whole record has to be reinserted into the S-FILE to assure the completeness of all subreferences of the remaining facets. These rather complex relationships were partially neglected in former update systems and lead to many inconsistencies.

'F SARCOIDOSE 2 BOECK;' In the original propositions, this statement meant: delete the preferred term SARCOIDOSE and replace it with the pre-ferred term BOECK. Unfortunately, it could be understood in several other ways and so we had to introduce further statements to avoid ambiguities. Most of them lead to even more complex update operations than the simple deletion of a preferred term.

6. REFERENCES:

(1) Röttger, P., Reul, H., Klein, I., Sunkel, H.: The automatic handling and statistical evaluation of pathologic-anatomical findings. Meth.Inf.Med.8: 19 (1969).

(2) Gell, G., Becker, H.: Free text analysis of biopsy findings by means of video-display. Meth.Inf.Med. 12: 10 (1973).

(3) Ries, P., Loy, V., Küsel, W., Fabricius, W.: Konzeption einer off-line Version der Ergänzung des AGK-Thesaurus. Medizinische Informatik und Statistik 1: 99 (1976). (Springer, 1976).

(4) Köberl, D., Dorda, W., Feigl, W., Kogler, W.: Konzeption und Reali-sation der Biopsiedatenverarbeitung im Rahmen eines allgemeinen medizinischen Informationssystems. Medizinische Informatik und Statistik 16: 565 (1979). (Springer, 1979).

(5) Lamson, B.G., Dimsdale, B.: A natural language information retrie-val system. Proceedings IEEE 54: 1636 (1966).

(6) Gaynon, P., Wong, R.L.: A retrieval system for a library of patho-logy reports, slides and Kodachromes. Meth.Inf.Med.11: 152 (1972).

(7) Loy, V.: Integrated decentralized flexible dataprocessing in pathology. Med. Inform. 7: 307 (1982).

Construction of a (semi-)automated
SNOMED - ICD code linkage

Rudolf P. BAUMANN
Institut neuchâtelois d'anatomie pathologique
Les Cadolles, CH-2000 Neuchâtel (Suisse)

Summary: The informatic system implemented on DEC VAX 11/730, programmed in MUMPS is active as efficient assistance for coding pathological diagnoses in SNOMED. Modifications were necessary to realize autonomous progression in the hierarchical capture tree for each SNOMED field. For malignant neoplasms, a fully automated transcription from pathology diagnosis (M-8...3 ; T- converted to ICD-O 140-199) is working without problems. For infectious and transmissible diseases, ICD code is found be a pointer in the D- (disease) field, generated automatically by the E- (etiology) definition. The ICD list is now systematically introduced in the system with necessary adjonctions to create an entry into the SNOMED codes.

The Pathology Institute of Neuchâtel serves a region of 160 000 inhabitants and procures autopsy, biopsy and cytology services for hospitals and ambulatory medicine. All clinical and surgical specialities are represented without the cardiac and neurosurgery specimens. The Pathology Institute works also as the principal source of data for the epidemiological Cancer Registry covering the population at risk in the same geographical area (10). An integrated informatic system was introduced in autumn 1982 (SIPAR: Système informatique pathologie et registre des tumeurs) (4)), implemented on a DEC VAX 11/730 system. Up till now, about 300 programs have been developed using the MUMPS data base (2), in the DSM-11 (Digital Standard Mumps) version 2, upgrading to version 3 is imminent. A large number of administrative clerical tasks run now in permanence, especially financial and report printing routines (automatic cytology reporting) (1).

1. Encoding the pathological diagnosis

Special attention and interest has been directed to a very efficient data acquisition for the diagnostic statement, encompassing disease entitities, morphological alterations, complete topographical definition, etiological agents, procedures and a security code for each diagnosis. This classification-orientated approach - with an 'a priori' retrieval objective - was followed, quite naturally, by the adoption of the most complete and detailed nomen-clature - SNOMED (5). As our experience with encoding biopsy diagnoses using the SNOP system (7) was fairly large (an ancient documentation routine was running from 1971 to 1976), the decision fell on a complete and exhaustive utilization of the SNOMED possibilities. Computer assistance had to fasten and to secure the encoding procedure. This goal was reached almost completely (3) with three search strategies (a: direct encoding of the correct number for the most frequent diagnoses; b: selection from a window in the main hierarchical list; c: choice of alphabetical presentation of all relevant terms). In fact, a simple term (like "appendicitis" or "thyroid hyperplasia") is encoded without delay (10 sec). A more complicated diagnosis (all malignant neoplasms with grading descriptors or "compatible" lesions like "tuberculoid granuloma") needs some waiting time for the apparition of the selection lists and the decision of the coding specialist.

Modifications of SNOMED: In order to accelerate the hierarchical search with the objective to realize a fully automated procedure, it was necessary to modify the subdivision of the chapters, headings and subheadings in each field of SNOMED (see on this subject: (11)). A special problem is the breach of the strict hierarchical concept in the many areas where an alphabetical order had taken place in the numerical list (e.g. bacteria and rickettsia, sections 1&2 in the etiology field). It was necessary to include supplementary convenient codes to realize a capture tree without gaps in the first three digits (1.... / 10... / 100..).

Our modifications are identified by special signs combined with the code, we can at any time restore the original SNOMED version. Until now, we have added some 500 codes in the T-, 100 in the M-, and 300 in the E- field (the F- and D- fields are not yet entirely introduced into the system). We expect a great advantage from this adaptation for the automated progression within the capture trees.

2. Transfer from SNOMED to ICD codes

From SNOMED T- to ICD-O (12) for malignant neoplasms: As our system was de- signed from the beginning to support the data acquisition for a cancer registry too, an automated transfer for malignant neoplasms from the Pathology Institute to the Registry has been developed. We proceed with a special "R" code, ap- pended to the M- 8...3/9 SNOMED morphology field (and ICD-O) code. This indic- ation releases supplementary coordinating routine: the T- (topography) SNOMED definition is automatically linked with the ICD-O localization list (corres- ponding to 140-199 in the 9th revision of ICD), according to an in-built conver- sion table, following the indications in the coding manual (6). As the system works at present, the transfer is fully automatic from SNOMED to ICD-O, for the inverted translation, some special features must intervene.

From SNOMED E- to ICD for infectious diseases: As our system permits an indif- ferent access to the multiaxial SNOMED codes from each field or from a pre- coordinated (home made) 4-digit code, the correct identification of diseases caused by a known microorganism is rather easy. So the encoding of "acute miliary tuberculosis" (T-00020 ; M-4470 ; E-2001) creates, with a pointer in the E- field, "D-01884" (disease: acute miliary tuberculosis). This code is linked, like the T- field in the neoplasms series, with the "018.0" ICD entity. In the case that the fourth digit cannot be automatically found, further inter- rogation in the T- field for localisation can be effectuated (see figure 1). The first chapter of ICD (001-139) can be addressed from a SNOMED E- and D- coded diagnosis without difficulty.

SNOMED - ICD - SNOMED transfer (example)

```
Ø39.      Actinomycotic infections >E-1Ø7.
Ø39.Ø     Cutaneous actinomycotic infection &T-Ø1.
Ø39.1     Pulmonary actinomycotic infection &T-2.
  .
Ø39.9     Actinomycotic infection of unspecified site
```

Figure 1: Extract from a computer-outprint of the ICD.9.CM (.) for "actinomycosis". The lists have a complete hierarchical structure. The "." triggers an automatical search (ICD, SNOMED E- and T-). The ">E" indicates a predefined entry to the E- field. The "&" is used as pointer for the T- field from ICD and as intermediary test in the case of a SNOMED - ICD transcription.

From SNOMED to ICD in general: Its quite clear we have chosen the two most convenient disease groups for demonstration, malignant neoplasms being charact- erized by the 8...3/9 M-code and topography, infectious diseases by 1...-4... E-code and topography (T-) or disease (D-) definition. The more precisely the codes have been defined, the more more accurate the transfer is made. We are now working on metabolic diseases (ICD 240-279) and have found that tran- scription can be done in almost each case by the D- (disease) definition.

3. Transfer from ICD to SNOMED codes

The interest for this pathway should not be questioned, in our opinion the SNOMED users have to take into account that ICD is the most popular classific- ation and reporting system for mass statistics, and, rather paradoxically, also for small and specialized disease related documentation. If SNOMED users communicate with ICD users (in our field of activity we are the only SNOMED based institution, some clinical departments are introducing ICD coding), it will be necessary to be able to convert one expression to another. "Compatib- ility" is, in our opinion, a goal we have to work for without abandoning some important principles of own (proper) responsability and efficiency. Our invest- igations, still in the state of conceptual framework, indicate clearly that exchanges of medical information should be possible even in the artificial and rather restricted area of diagnosis encoding.

Bibliography

(1) BALMER M.-C., BAUMANN R.P.: Documentation du diagnostic et établissement automatique du rapport en cytopathologie. Schweiz Med Wochenschr 115, (1985); to be published

(2) BARNETT O.G.: Massachusetts General Hospital computer system (Boston). In: Collen M.F. (ed.): Hospital computer systems. New York : Wiley, 1975. p. 517-545

(3) BAUMANN R.P.: Utilization of SNOMED for routine encoding of pathology and cytology diagnoses. Lect notes med inform 24, 154-159 (1984)

(4) BAUMANN R.P., BRANDON G.: SNOMED in four languages: English, French, German, and MUMPS. In: MEDINFO-83, van Bemmel, Bell, Wigertz, Editors. Amsterdam : North-Holland, 1983. p. 112-115

(5) COLLEGE OF AMERICAN PATHOLOGISTS: SNOMED: Systematized nomenclature of medicine. 2nd edition (with 1982 update). Skokie (Ill.) : College of american pathologists, 1979

(6) COLLEGE OF AMERICAN PATHOLOGISTS: SNOMED: Systematized nomenclature of medicine: coding manual. Skokie (Ill.) : Collge of american pathologists, 1979

(7) COLLEGE OF AMERICAN PATHOLOGISTS: Systematized nomenclature of pathology (SNOP). 2nd edition. Chicago (Ill.) : College of american pathologists, 1965

(8) ICD.9.CM. International classification of diseases. 9th revision. Clinical modification. 2nd edition. 3 vol. Washington, D.C. : U.S. Department of Health and Human Services, 1980

(9) MAJOR P., KOSTREWSKI B.J., ANDERSON J.: Analysis of the semantic structures of medical languages: part 2. Analysis of the semantic power of MeSH, ICD and SNOMED. Med Inform 3, 269-281 (1978)

(10) WATERHOUSE J. et al. (eds.): Cancer incidence in five continents: vol. IV. Lyon : International Agency for Research on Cancer, 1982. p. 542-545

(11) WINGERT F.: Automatic indexing based on SNOMED. Meth Inform Med 24, 27-34 (1985)

(12) WORLD HEALTH ORGANIZATION: ICD-O. International classification of diseases for oncology. 1st edition. Geneva : WHO, 1976.

CORAL: AN A.I. APPROACH OF "PROBLEM ORIENTED MEDICAL RECORD".

A.D'Angelo, F.Noventa*, A.M.Volpe**.
   Department of Computer Science - University of Udine - ITALY
* Department of Clinical Medicine- University of Padova- ITALY
**A.S.S.I.T. s.n.c. - Padova - ITALY

ABSTRACT - CORAL is a relational D.B. containing relevant clinical data, acquired following the medical
way of thinking compared with the patient's problem.
The structure of the system is based upon a theorem
prover, similar in some aspects with the well known
logic based language: PROLOG; namely, it is guided
by inference rules. Some of these can define the mo
del of the system and are transparent for the user,
who interacts with it in pseudo-natural language.

1. INTRODUCTION

There are several examples of D.B. for medical applications but they
are usually either statistical-epidemiological or administrative orien
ted. Some of these attempt to give to the physician, either specialist
or general practitioner, a tool that helps him to organize the single
patient's relative data flow. Some D.B. only handle standard screen display and in some cases they are quality and/or quantity inflexible.
   The CORAL project has been originated by the convinction that a
physician user will find out an effective advantage from a computer if
it is able to follow his way of thinking, namely, if it looks like a
focalizer of the current problem in the global context, recording every little variation of the subjective, objective, biochemical and morphological status and, summarizing them.

2. POMR

A clinical data recording method satisfying these criteria already
exists and it is universally known as the Weed's "Problem Oriented Medical Record" (for more details see 1,2,3,4).
   Many computational model has been proposed in the time by computer
scientists in the applicative field of "Clinical Medicine" but nothing
of them provides physicians with suitable implementations.

3. LOGICAL STRUCTURE OF THE SYSTEM

Any effort to implement the POMR fully flexibility paradigm yelds to
redesign the software architecture of a traditional D.B. from the point
of view of an "Artificial Intelligence Environment". In such a way the
system should be able to follow the logic flow of information by compar
ing and, possibly, modifying its behaviour continously.
   So, when the user interacts with the CORAL system, causes it to behave like an "expert assistant" who replies his information:action requests that he formulates in a pseudo-natural language processed by the
CORAL INTERFACE.
   Any request is activated either "in primis" or from other modula by

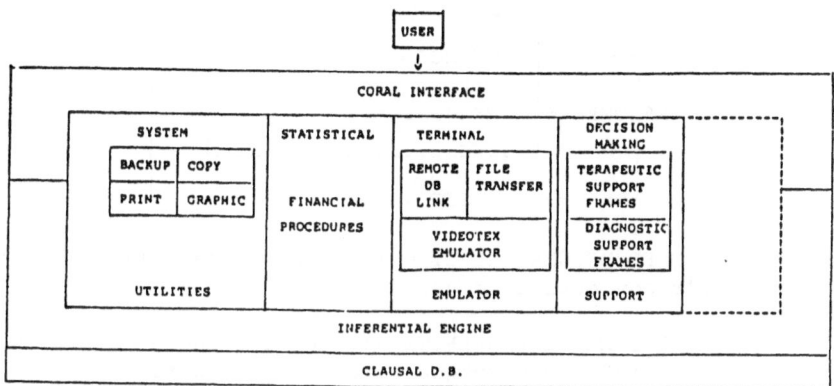

windowing.

These modula improve medical/professional productivity as such:
- linking with large bibliography Data Base - linking with legislative/
administrative D.B. - decision making support (therapeutic, diagnostic,
ecc.) - statistical analysis procedures - finantial procedures.

4. THE CORAL SYSTEM ARCHITECTURE

The architecture of a CORAL system is based upon an esperimental implementation on a sequential machine for a "Multi-Agent Planner" reason
ing on incomplete and distribuited "knowledge environment".

The kernel of the system has been originally designed for general
purpose applications in typical "Artificial Intelligence Domains", such
as Robotics, Automated Programming, Problem Solving, ecc.

In order to exploit all the features of the novel architecture a pro
totype for VAX computers is under development with the extended PASCAL
for VMS Operative System, but keeping in mind the specific application
for POMR in medical field.

Three levels of implementations are recognizable in the overall architecture of the system; namely,

      (i)   the "Inferential Engine",
      (ii)   the "Knowledge Base Organisation",
      (iii) the "Run Time Environment",

were the aim is to provide the medical user with a "programming environ
ment" friendly to use and easy to understand but powerful and efficient
enough comparably with the set of integrated tools generally provided
with standard software for D.B. applications.

The final version of CORAL will be designed by the means of a suitable "Augmented First Order Language' (QDL, see below), which can be pro
cessed using a portable C dialect.

4.1 The Inferential Engine. - Because all the activities of CORAL are
treated as queries, a general purpose "Query Definition Language" (QDL)
has been defined to schedule them. The "in-core" compiler for QDL causes
the system to produce an intermediate code to be processed by the module HORN ('Higher Order Resolution Network') which is an inferential en
gine based upon a suitable extension of standard PROLOG interpreters.

As you can see in the following figure, there are three main cycles
the inferential engine can operate with;

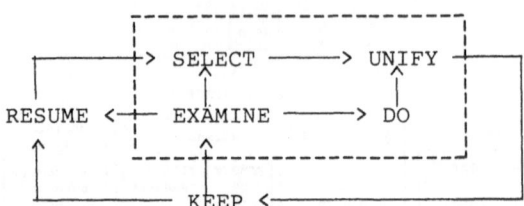

that is: 1. a KEEP/RESUME/SELECT/UNIFY cycle, where it "resumes" an
            already activated ancestor goal;

     2. a KEEP/EXAMINE/SELECT/UNIFY cycle, where it "tries to
            satisfy" a new subgoal against the current activated goal;

     3. a KEEP/EXAMINE/DO/UNIFY cycle where it "recognizes" that
            the current subgoal is more properly an action to be per-
            formed.

    Notice that here "goal" is a synonymous for query, while SELECT,
RESUME and DO are three specialised modules which perform, respectively:

     1. SELECT, a preprocessing for a "conflict resolutor" (using
            a standard terminology in the field of current expert sys
            tem terminology);

     2. RESUME, an actor invocation when "local backtracking" can
            not be executed;

     3. DO, a compiled proof evaluator if some "evaluable predica-
            te", which corresponds to some action, needs to be evalua-
            ted.

4.2 The Knowledge Base Organisation. - Since the "focusing property"
should be incorporated in every intelligent data collection, the organisation of the "Knowledge Base" in the CORAL system is "not uniform",
on the contrary, it has been grouped into "partitions" or "fragments",
each of which encloses a "Data Domain" of some specificable "topic".
    In such a way, every partition is a "knowledge base itself", which
can communicate with any other by means of the "modal operators" BELIEF
and KNOW (for more details see 5). Thus the Kripke's semantics breaks a
large and uncontrollable clause collection (notice that a "Clause" is
the way logic encodes either a "fact" or a "rule" in some given domain)
in a "partially ordered modular knowledge base" where the usual "Accessibility Relation" determines the formal way of representing the mecha
nism of "message passing" advocated by Hewitt.
    From a point of view of "Storing/Retrieving" of information, the
"knowledge base" has been partitioned into four main sections; that is:

     a) the SKELETON-TABLE, where the system finds out all the
            relevant information about atomic fact used in the K.B.;

     b) the ATOM-TABLE, used by the system as dictionary;

c)   the SEMANTIC-GRAPH, for a suitable partitioning of the
     K.B. and used by "Select/Unify" to perform efficient
     unification;

d)   the CLAUSE-BASE, where the system actually can store/
     retrieve either facts or rules about some specific domain.

4.3 The Run Time Environment. - The higher level implementation of the
CORAL system is a very sophisticated run time environment which schedu
les all the "activities" of the inferential engine by sharing them with
different "Knowledge Base" domains. To achieve such a goal the system
uses a collection of informations stored in the so called "Fragment Activation Record" (FAR) which causes the run time environment for a stan
dard PROLOG interpreter to be partitioned in order to realize an ACTOR-
like machine architecture.
   The global implementation of a CORAL system is represented in the fi
gure:

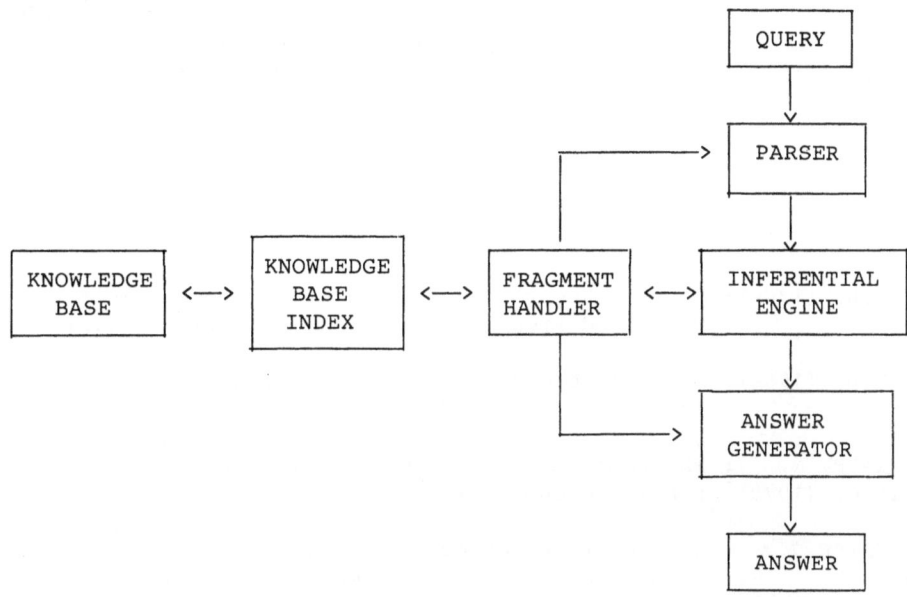

where the PARSER module performs a syntactic analysis of a "query" writ
ten in QDL and produces an intermediate codified "request" to be processed by the inferential engine; in the same way, the ANSWER GENERATOR
module returns the "answer" in a nice way.

5. USER INTERACTION - K.B.

   The higher level of the system is characterized by "Ask" and "Tell"
states, which allow the user to interrogate the system about any stored
information in conversational way.
   The "Tell" state is divided into:

1.   QUERY/INFORM, to compile POMR interactively;

2. LEARN/MAKE, to learn descriptive knowledge or actions;

3. DO, to execute predefined actions.

Some examples of knowledge base rules are the follow ones:

```
                              syntom_gen(tireness).
    One-Place predicates      syntom_gi(nausea).
      (Semantic Graph)        syntom_neu(dizziness).
                              mass_sign(hernia)

                              side_of(X,abdomen).
                              side_of(X,epigastrium).
                              volume_of(X,little).
                              subjectivity_of(X,U)  :- patient(X)
         Horn Clauses                               (syntom_gen(U);
         (clause base)                               syntom_gi(U);
                                                     syntom_neu(U)).
                        syntom(X)  :- side_of(X,Y),
                                      degree_of(X,T),
                                      type_of(X,K).
                        mass_sign(X)  :- side_of(X,Y),
                                         volume_of(X,T),
                                         ache_of(X,K).
```

REFERENCES

1) WEED L.L. (1969): Medical Record, medical education and patient care.
                 Cleveland Press of Case Western Reserve University.

2) WEED L.L. (1964): Medical record, patient care and medical education.
                 Irish J.Med.Sci. 6, 271.

3) Mc INTAYRE N.   : The Problem Oriented Medical Record.
   PETRIE C. (1979)   Longman Group Limited, London.

4) Mc INTAYRE N.   : Can we write better notes? An introduction to POMR
   (1972)   (The Weed approach).B.J.Hospital Medicine 5, 603.

5) KONOLIGE (1979) : A first order formalization of knowledge and know-
                 ledge acquisition for a multi-agent planning sys-
                 tem. Machine Intelligence n.10

6) REITER (1980)   : Reasoning by default. Artificial Intelligence n.13

7) MOORE (1979)   : Reasoning about knowledge and action. IJCAI-5.

8) NEWELL (1982)   : The knowledge level. Artificial Intelligence n.18

9) LEVESQUE (1984) : Foundations of a functional approach to knowledge
                 representation. Artificial Intelligence n.23

CONTRIBUTIONS TO AUTOMATED INDEXING BASED ON SNOMED

Friedrich Wingert
Institut für Medizinische Informatik und Biomathematik
Universität Münster, FRG

INTRODUCTION

This paper is concerned with problems and algorithms of indexing medical language data against a medical nomenclature. The algorithms are mostly independent of the special nomenclature used. As a concrete target language, SNOMED [1] has been selected because it is the most comprehensive medical nomenclature available.

In a recently published paper [2], a formal description of SNOMED has been given which will briefly be repeated in order to introduce the important notions. A **SNOMED entry** is a construct

$$c \quad t \quad [r]$$

consisting of a **SNOMED code** c, a language string (**lexeme**) t and, optionally, a **cross reference** r. The latter one is a set of SNOMED codes relating to the lexeme t information which is not contained in the SNOMED code c. E.g., a SNOMED entry is

    M40000 Nephritis (T71)

indicating that 'Nephritis' is an 'inflammation' (M40000) of the 'kidney' (T71). Because both SNOMED code and cross reference are coordinates in a 6-dimensional discrete space (except dimension "Occupations"), there is no formal reason why c and r should be distinguished. Therefore, a SNOMED entry is seen as a relation (t,p) which relates to the lexeme t the position p in the SNOMED space. p is the union of c and r. A semantic interpretation of p, i.e., the "meaning" of t, is derived from the semantic model underlying SNOMED and its partition into orthogonal dimensions.

The relations (t,p) are not definite. Two lexemes, t_1 and t_2 are **synonyms**, when there are the relations (t_1,p), (t_2,p). A lexeme t is a **homograph** when there are the relations (t,p_1), (t,p_2) and $p_1 \neq p_2$.

REDUNDANCY

The relation (t,p) can be interpreted as "t can be replaced by p". Because of the identity (p,p), **redundancy** is defined as follows:

If S is the set of relations in SNOMED then the relation $(t_i,p) \in S$ is redundant, if there is a set of transformations on (t_i,p) resulting in the relation $(t_j,p) \in S$ or in the relation (p,p).

It must be noted that this concept of redundancy depends on the content of S as well as on the available set of transformations [2] and it is inseparable from the **indexing procedure.** Thus, (Inflammation of the kidney,T71 M40000) has not been put into SNOMED because it is assumed that an indexing procedure (or a human indexer) will recognize that (M40000 of the T71,T71 M40000) is redundant because 'of the' marks the semantic relation between M and T and can, therefore, be omitted.

Let be I(u,S) an indexing procedure, transforming an utterance u into a set of SNOMED codes. This procedure should be content preserving. It is trivial that for such an indexing procedure there is the identity $I(t_i,S)=p$ for each relation $(t_i,p) \varepsilon S$. Therefore, a relation is **redundant** if

$$I(t_i,S) = I(t_i,S-(t_i,p)),$$

i.e., if the result of indexing the utterance $u=t_i$ does not depend on whether (t_i,p) is contained in S or not.

Syntactic level	Synonyms	Redundancy generating in
Sentence	Infra Sub $\rangle$ clavicular region	Skin of ...
Phrase	efferenter Ast R. efferens	efferenter Ast R. efferens $\rangle$ des ...
Word	Imbecillitas Oligophrenia	Imbecillitas Oligophrenia $\rangle$ phenylpyruvica
Word part	Nephro Nieren	Nephro Nieren $\rangle$ kalzinose
Segment	-icus -(e)alis	Rr. oesophag $\langle$ ici eales

Table 1: Syntactic levels and examples of redundancy [2]

Table 1 lists the syntactic levels of SNOMED entries together with examples of synonyms and constructions where these synonyms generate redundant entries. It also demonstrates the main strategy in redundancy recognition:

Redundant lexemes are recognized if the syntactic structures on lower levels are recognized as synonyms (or as identical).

This strategy is divided into two major steps:

(1) Morphologic analysis of lexemes below the word level and rewriting the lexemes by transformation to a new alphabet [2].

(2) Rewriting of lexemes by a recursive indexing procedure against SNOMED itself.

In contrast to step (1), step (2) excessively utilizes information from SNOMED. Each lexeme t_i is checked whether it contains parts with an independent meaning, i.e., whether it is constructed from SNOMED entries ("matches") or not. The main principles generating such constructions are:

- Refinement, i.e., establishment of the hierarchic relation, which is often reflected in the language ('Skin of head and neck').
- Established but unused orthogonality between:
  - SNOMED dimensions ('Nephrectomy'),
  - SNOMED subsections and related modifiers ('Acute inflammation').

Furthermore, there are close relations between the concepts of completeness and redundancy on the one hand and the indexing procedure on the other hand. This shall be demonstrated by the entry (Skin of head and neck,T02390).

For an approximately complete nomenclature all synonyms are missing which can be generated by replacing 'Skin' by 'Cutis', 'Head' by 'Caput', and 'Neck' by 'Collum' or 'Cervix'. Further synonyms are compound words (e.g., 'Kopfhaut' or 'Halshaut') or adjectives ('Cervical skin'). Apparently, this gives a class of more than 12 synonyms from which only one member has been listed in SNOMED.

LOADING OF SNOMED

In order to meet the above mentioned requirements, namely, to load the nomenclature free of redundancy and, more important, to make sure that the nomenclature is complete, a recursive procedure is used, loading the relations (t,p) as follows:

(1) Morphologic analysis of t and rewrite by replacing each basic morpheme by an identifier for the whole class of predefined synonymous basic morphemes, and each derivational suffix by the number of the respective suffix family. Connectors, terminal suffixes, and particles are omitted. Thus, each word part, except particles, is replaced by a symbol made up from the numbers of the basic morpheme and of the derivational suffix. Then, the symbols are sorted resulting in the relation $(t^{(1)},p)$.

(2) The relations $(t^{(1)},p)$ are sorted and redundant relations, i.e., relations which have been generated more than once, are omitted. The remainder is level I of the set S.

(3) Each relation $(t^{(1)},p) \in S$ is indexed against $S-(t^{(1)},p)$. If an index is found, then $t^{(1)}$ is rewritten by replacing the matched symbols by the corresponding index resulting in the new relation $(t^{(2)},p)$:

$$t^{(1)} = t_a t_1^{(1)} t_b \longrightarrow t_a p_1 t_b = t^{(2)}.$$

This step reveals three special types of resulting relations:

- $t^{(2)} = p$.

These are relations which are redundant due to unused orthogonality:

(Nephrectomy,T71 P11000) → (T71 P11000,T71 P11000).

- $t^{(2)} \supset p$.

These are relations which have "shorter" synonyms, i.e., which contain insignificant word parts:

(Facies med. cruris,TY9402) → (TY02 TY9402,TY9402).

- $t^{(2)} \subset p$.

These are idioms, i.e., lexemes the information of which is more specific than the "sum" of the information of its word parts, such as (Rektumblase,T68 T74 M18900). Another subclass consists of entries in the dimension "Diseases" which are supplied by cross references according to the philosophy underlying this dimension:

(Gonokokkodermie,T02 E2165 D0131) → (T02 E2165,T02 E2165 D0131).

The procedure is then repeated from step (2), using $(t^{(2)},p)$ instead of $(t^{(1)},p)$ giving the next level of S. The loop ends when no more indexes are found.

HANDLING OF MODIFIERS

Due to SNOMED, a modifier m is a language string which modifies each lexeme t if the corresponding position p is contained in the modifier range:

(t,p) corresponds to (mt,p_m).

E.g., ´acute´ modifies lexemes concerning inflammations (range M4) and changes the second digit of the SNOMED code to 1. Therefore,

(t,M40...) corresponds to (´acute´ t,M41...).

These modifiers could be handled after applying an indexing procedure. But, because SNOMED is loaded recursively, another approach has been taken:

If we have the relation (mt,p_m) in SNOMED, then step (3) results in the relation (mp,p_m). Therefore, these relations are generated from the beginning, i.e., SNOMED is supplied by all relations (mp,p_m) which can be generated for each modifier m.

INDEXING PROCEDURE

Basically, the same indexing procedure is used for loading SNOMED as well as for indexing an arbitrary utterance u. It is obvious that this procedure is the critical part of the whole strategy.

If T is the set of transformations defined on the set of utterances (e.g., adjective → noun) then an index Ind is a subset of lexemes from SNOMED ("matches"), Ind=$\{t_1,t_2,...\}$, with

$t_i \subseteq T(u)$ (i=1,2,...),

$t_i \nsubseteq t_j$,   for i≠j.

That means, each symbol of a lexeme $t_i \subseteq$ Ind must be an element of T(u) and a lexeme must not be a subset of a longer lexeme (principle of longest match). More restrictive is the exclusion of overlapping:

$t_i \cap t_j = \emptyset$ for i≠j.

A **similarity function** f is defined on all utterances u and on all subsets Ind such that

$$f(u, Ind) \begin{cases} = 0, & \text{if Ind is not an index of } u \\ > 0, & \text{otherwise} \end{cases} .$$

An index Ind* is a **best index** for an utterance u if

$$f(u, Ind*) \geq f(u, Ind)$$

for all subsets Ind.

The function f is constructed according to the following principles. **Similarity** of an index Ind with an utterance u increases, as

- the number s of morphemes of Ind increases,
- the number m of lexemes of Ind decreases.

Furthermore, similarity is assumed to be additive, i.e., if Ind_1 and Ind_2 are disjoint indexes of u, then

$$f(u, Ind_1 \cup Ind_2) = f(u, Ind_1) + f(u, Ind_2) \quad \text{for} \quad Ind_1 \cap Ind_2 = \emptyset.$$

From these principles, f is seen to be a linear function

$$f(u, Ind) = a \cdot s - m, \quad a > 0.$$

PROBLEMS

Some numbers shall illustrate the amount of data which has to be handled by using SNOMED. Level I of SNOMED contains about 86,000 relations. 62,000 relations are additionally generated from the modifiers. These 148,000 relations contain about 4% redundant relations both on level I and II. About 70% can be indexed against SNOMED itself. Because there is an average of about 2 synonyms for each relation, this number gives some insight into the degree of lexical incompleteness if indexing is done on a single level.

The most important problems under the aspect of frequency of occurrence are based on the fact that no syntactic analysis is done. These are ambiguities, generated by neglecting:

(1) the order of word parts, e.g., Caput musculi/Musculus capitis,
(2) particles, e.g., Uterus and Cervix/Cervix uteri.

Together, these two sources of error generate less than 100 ambiguous relations.

LITERATURE

1 WINGERT F (edt.): SNOMED. Systematisierte Nomenklatur der Medizin Berlin, Heidelberg, New York, Tokyo: Springer 1984

2 WINGERT F: Reduction of Redundancy in a Categorized Nomenclature In: Proc. Intern. Working Conference, WG6, Ottawa, September 26./28., 1984

AN APPROACH TO THE FREE TEXT SYNTACTIC ANALYSIS

O.Gotfrýd and M.Dvořák
Research Institute of Traumatology
Ponávka 6, 66250 BRNO, Czechoslovakia

Medical information of text type has magnificant importance and therefore its processing is necessary for statistic and research purposes.
Classical methods are time consumping and not very much suitable for
mini- and microcomputers. The paper describes a simple method of formalization and coding of free text.

One of the ways of medical text formalization is a generation of individual sentences by a formal grammar $G = \{ V_N, V_T, P, S \}$. If the used
grammar is regular, it can be represented by an oriented graph. Individual branches of this graph are marked by numbers and represent nonterminal words of set V_N and terminal words of set V_T of grammar G.
A code of sentence which is generated by grammar G is given by sequence
of numbers. These numbers correspond to the terminal words which the
sentence consist of and those nonterminal words used for derivation of
this sentence.

Figure 1 shows a part of oriented graph of grammar G_{dg} for diagnoses
coding. The diagnosis sentence FRACTURA APERTA SPIRALIS TIBIAE SIN.
has a code:

FRACTURA APERTA	– diagnostic code	1, 1, 2
SPIRALIS	– diagnostic code	1, 1, 3
TIBIAE	– local code	3, 7, 7
SIN.	– local code	20, 3

Even such a simplified example of diagnosis code shows the possibility
of searching not only the terms contained in the terminal words but
also hierarchic terms which are created of nonterminal words. There is
for example INJURIES of LEG (diagnostic code 1 and local code 3, 7) in
our example.

The practical possibilities of text coding are given by extent of V_N
and V_T sets and the structure of sentence is determined by used grammar rules P.

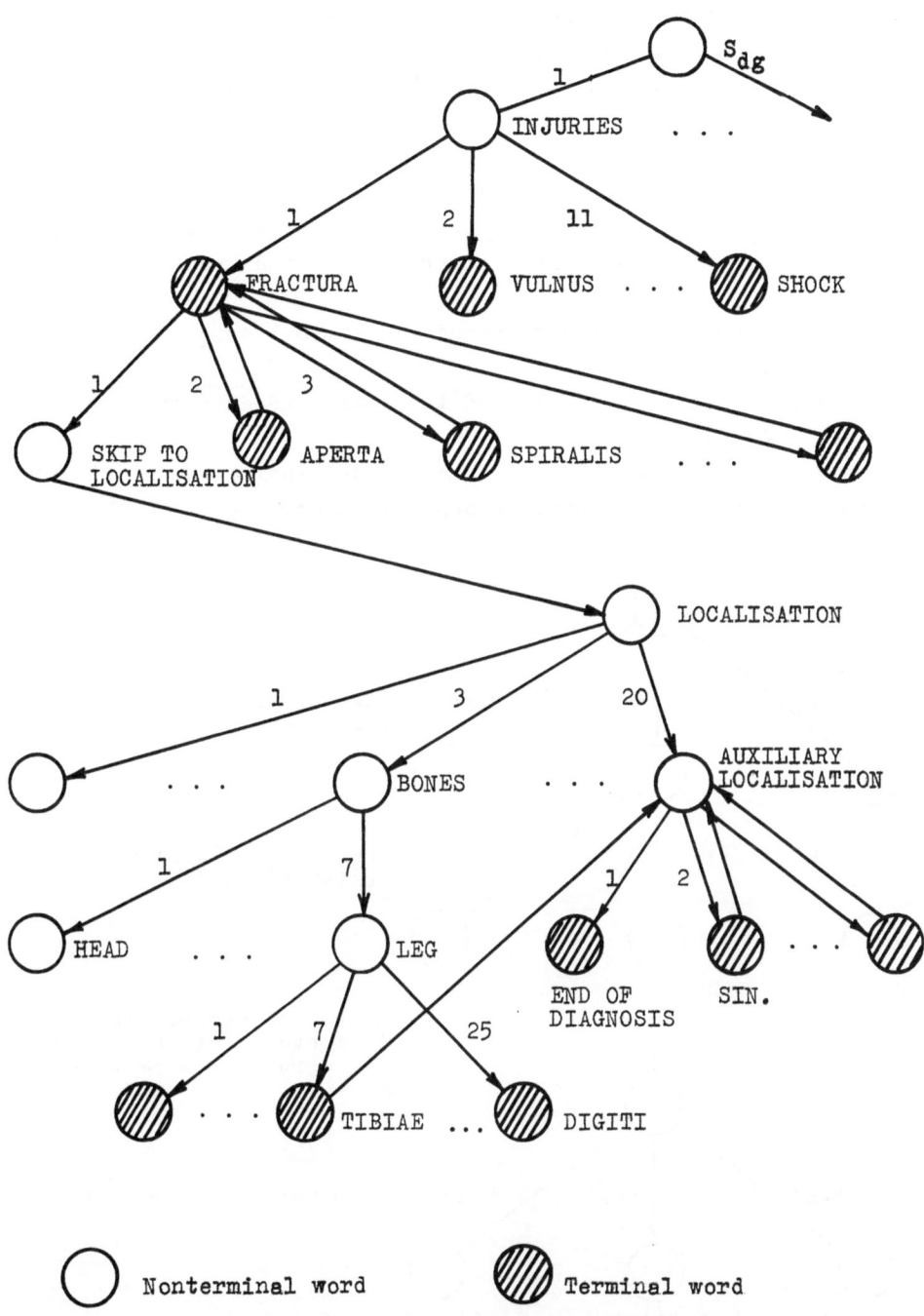

Fig.1 Oriented graph of grammar G_{dg} for generation and coding of formalized diagnosis

The realized algorithm of formalized text analysis uses a grammar in the oriented graph form (see Fig.1). Syntactic analysis used in a practice must perform extraction of terminal words from deformed or incomplete text.

For the extraction of terminal words (TW) was therefore established auxiliary structure of unambiguous abbreviations (TW - codes) of all terminal words of corresponding grammar G. TW - code has following properties:

- unambiguously substitutes corresponding terminal word in the syntactic analysis,
- quite eliminates effect of allowed terminal word deformations on the syntactic analysis,
- enables reduction of a number of checked terminal words which are processed in the given syntactic analysis step.

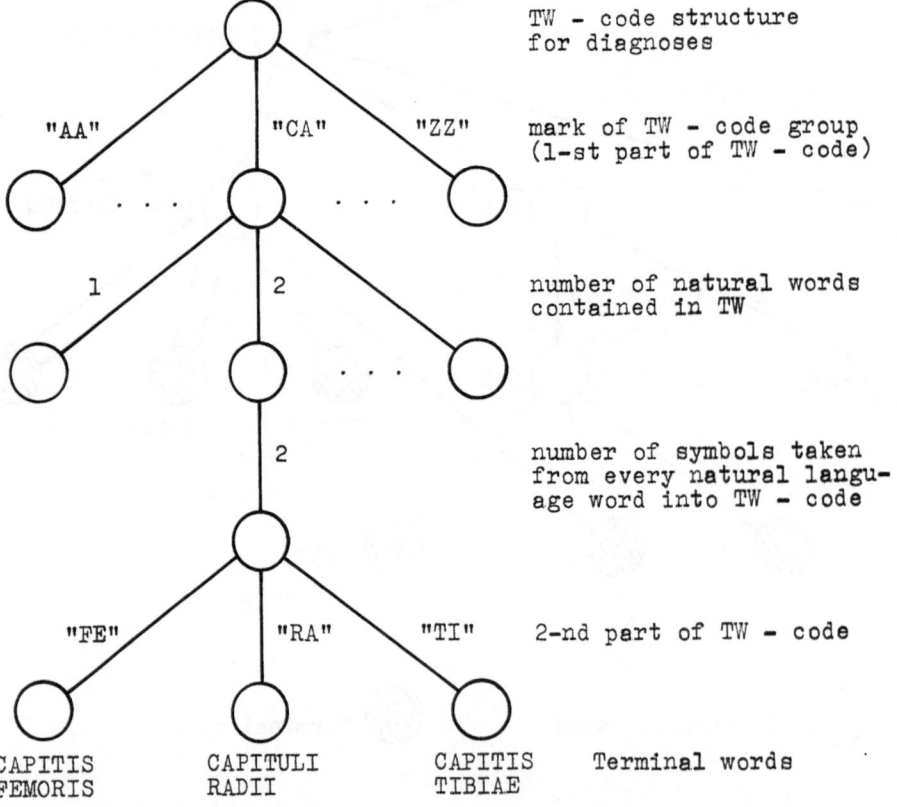

TW - code structure
for diagnoses

"AA"   "CA"   "ZZ"   mark of TW - code group
                        (1-st part of TW - code)

1   2   number of natural words
                        contained in TW

        2   number of symbols taken
                        from every natural langu-
                        age word into TW - code

"FE"   "RA"   "TI"   2-nd part of TW - code

CAPITIS   CAPITULI   CAPITIS   Terminal words
FEMORIS   RADII   TIBIAE

Fig.2   The part of possible code structure for analysis of diagnostic text (code of terminal word is in figure replaced by its text)

The TW - code structure is generated for given grammar G only once. In case of terminal word extraction TW - codes are created from the analysed text and after that it is found out if the same TW - code exists in the corresponding TW - code structure being derived from the given grammar G. If a correspondence of both TW - codes occurs, the correct terminal word is found. In the other case the checking of another TW - code construction is necessary.

There is an example of possible TW - code structure for syntactic analysis of diagnostic text in the Fig.2. There are shown three terminal words beginning with two symbols "CA" and they consist of two words of natural language: CAPITIS FEMORIS is substituted by TW - code "CA FE", CAPITULI RADII is substituted by TW - code "CA RA" and CAPITIS TIBIAE is substituted by TW - code "CA TI".

The diagnosis coding is a typical example of text processing. Fig. 1 shows a part of oriented graph of grammar G_{dg}. This grammar generates admissible formalized sentences of diagnostic text. Let us analyse for example text FRAKT. APERTA SPIRAL. TIBIE SIN. In spite of the fact that the text is written inexactly and incompletely, the analysis and coding is correct: FRACTURA APERTA SPIRALIS TIBIAE SIN.

The using of TW - codes for the analysis and coding of formalized texts accelerates the analysis considerably by reduction of permissible terminal words. The TW - code properties enable corrections of text deformations of anylysed sentence of certain degree. The formalized sentence code also contains nonterminal word codes being usually in the hierarchic structure superior to the group of terminal word codes. This can be used with advantage in statistic and research processing of information.

REFERENCES

1. Hopcroft,J.E., Ullman,J.D.: Formal Languages and their Relation to Automata. Reading (Mass), Addison-Wesley Publ. Comp., Inc., 1969
2. Manna,Z.: Mathematical Theory of Computation. McGraw - Hill, Inc., 1974

INVESTIGATIONS CONCERNING THE USE OF DIAGNOSE CODING SYSTEMS IN LARGE HOSPITALS IN THE F.R.G.

Hoffmann, W.D., Raufmann, W. and Reichertz, P.L.
Institute for Medical Informatics
(Director: Prof. Dr. P.L. Reichertz)
Medical School Hannover
D-3000 Hannover, Fed. Rep. Germany

0. Abstract

An evaluation about the use of different diagnose coding systems in the Medical School Hannover and in other large hospitals in the Federal Republic of Germany is presented. SNOMED and ICD-10 are discussed as alternatives for better comparability in terms of scientific research and health care planning.

1. Investigations on Diagnose Code Systems in German Hospitals

1973 in a publication of Gerdel (1), results from 510 German hospitals (349 with coding of diagnoses, 161 without) were analysed, the results showed that at that time ICD-8 was the most used diagnose code in German hospitals which was found in 106 cases (30 %) followed by KDS (2) in 87 cases (25 %), the remaining 156 cases (45 %) were spread over not commonly used coding systems.

In 1984 the author group evaluated responses on a questionaire which was sent out to 128 large German hospitals,(selected by number of beds ≥ 600). The return ratio was 37.5 % (48 questionaires, see Table 1).

	FREQUENCY	PERCENT	VALID PERCENT	CUM PERCENT
Acute General	20	41.7	41.7	41.7
Acute Special	7	14.6	14.6	56.3
Special Discipline	10	20.8	20.8	77.1
University	10	20.8	20.8	97.9
Other	1	2.1	2.1	100.0
TOTAL	48	100.0	100.0	

Table 1: Results from a questionaire investigation 1984
         Distribution of Type of Hospitals

The situation had changed within the passed eleven years, from 48
hospitals 35 are documenting their diagnoses, ICD is used in 26
hospitals (74.4 %), KDS in 2 hospitals (5.7 %), SNOMED in 1 Universi-
ty-Hospital (2.9 %), and other systems in 6 hospitals (17.1 %) see
Table 2).

	FREQUENCY	PERCENT	VALID PERCENT	CUM PERCENT
ICD Release ?	3	6.3	8.6	8.6
ICD Release 9	22	45.8	62.9	71.4
KDS Modified	2	4.2	5.7	77.1
SNOMED Manually	1	2.1	2.9	80.0
Others	6	12.5	17.1	97.1
ICD-8 Modified	1	2.1	2.9	100.0
Missing	13	27.1	MISSING	
TOTAL	48	100.0	100.0	

Table 2: Distribution of Diagnose Codes used in 48 large German
          Hospitals

2. Comparison of the Results

The results of the two analyses may to not be compared directly because they represent different hospitals. But at least one can observe
the trend which has developed in the periode from 1973 to 1984: less
KDS-users - more ICD-users. The reason for this can easily be found:
ICD-8 was published in 1963 and KDS in 1966, 1973, when the first
analysis was made these two code systems were the most used systems in
the FRG. Meanwhile, ICD-9 has been published, but there was no update
version for KDS. If the users wanted to keep this diagnose coding system it had to be updated by the users themselves or it would become
obsolete. These circumstances lead to the situation that nowadays many
differing - not compatible - versions of the former original KDS have
developed. So it will not surprise that newcomers in the field of
medical documentation in German hospitals chose ICD, which is revised
every 10 years by the WHO instead of KDS which must be regarded as
obsolete and can no longer be recommended. A WHO Expert Committee is
preparing ICD-10 as described by Coté (2) and the biaxial approach in

this 10th revision may probably bring solutions for many of the problems that arose in the last years.

From the results of the 1984 evaluation the aspect of therapy documentation should be regarded as a sign that in this partial field is a
need for an additional therapy classification. 22.9 % of all participating hospitals have a therapy documentation, but they all use different coding systems, most of them defined themselves (62.9 %, see
Table 3).

	FREQUENCY	PERCENT	VALID PERCENT	CUM PERCENT
ADT-Code	1	2.1	8.3	8.3
CODE self developed	7	14.6	58.3	66.7
VESKA	1	2.1	8.3	75.0
SCHEIBE	1	2.1	8.3	83.3
DONOHUE + self developed	1	2.1	8.3	91.7
SNOMED	1	2.1	8.3	100.0
MISSING	36	75.0	MISSING	
TOTAL	48	100.0	100.0	

Table 3:   Distribution of Therapy Codes used in 48 large
           Germany Hospitals

It is planned to combine ICD-10 with a 'family of classifications'
(analogue to the multi-axial Medical Nomenclature SNOMED), for example
ICPM (Procedures in Medicine), ICIDH (Impairments, Disabilities and
Handicaps) and RFE-C (Classification of Reasons for Encounter in Primary Health Care). These new additional parts of a medical coding system could satisfy the needs of the ever increasing number and variety
of professional groups in the health field, and meet the demands of
uniform assessment of health problems for decision making in prevention, in planning of health care in research on particular problems.

3. Strategie of Conversion

From the above outlined criteria one has to decide which of several
alternatives should be taken into account.

	action taken	workload	advantage/disadvantage	
a	keep the old system	none	obsolete coding no extra workload	(-) (+)
b1	introduce SNOMED manual coding	conversion of old data from KDS to SNOMED	modern coding more complicated extra workload	(+) (-) (-)
b2	automatic coding	implementation of an automatic coding system	faster input work homogeneous coding tedius input work extra workload	(+) (+) (-) (-)
c1	wait until 1990	none	obsolete coding no extra workload	(-) (+)
c2	introduce ICD-10	conversion from KDS to ICD-10	modern coding extra workload	(+) (-)
d1	introduce ICD-9 now	conversion of old data from KDS to ICD-9	modern coding extra workload	(+) (-)
d2	ICD-10 in 1990	conversion from ICD-9 to ICD-10	modern coding extra workload	(+) (-)

4. Discussion

Most of the large hospitals in the FRG use the ICD-9 for their coding
system for diagnoses, they should not alter their code until ICD-10 is
published. Only very few users of KDS or older ICD-Releases have to
consider the alternatives to turn over to ICD-9 or SNOMED or to wait
until ICD-10. Of course the final solution will depend on the different software-, hardware-, and manpower-possibilities and the background conditions in each institution. As an example Thurmayr and his
group (5) is working on a conversion matrix for an automatic translation of ICD/E codes into SNOMED codes. Just now Wingert has published a German version of SNOMED and is preparing an automatic indexing system (6). Although the medical and scientific demands for actual
and well-defined data are becoming more and more urgent the main part
of EDP-resources with over 60 % is and will in the future be consumed
by administrative programmes and functions and is utilized in less
than 5 % for medical documentation purposes (4). It is a great challenge for the medical informaticians to find an appropriate solution
for the future.

4. References

(1) GERDEL, W.: Die Diagnosestatistik in den Krankenhäusern der Bundesrepublik Deutschland, IDIS Bielefeld, Dokumentation der periodischen medizinischen Statistiken in der Bundesrepublik Deutschland (1973).

(2) COTE, R.: International Classifications for Health and Disease: the expandable common core concept. Med. Inform. (1983), 8,1, 1-4.

(3) IMMICH, H.: Klinischer Diagnosenschlüssel, Schattauer Verlag Stuttgart, (1966).

(4) LORDIECK, W., REICHERTZ, P.L.: Die EDV in den Krankenhäusern der Bundesrepublik Deutschland. Reihe: Medizinische Informatik und Statistik, Bd. 45, Springer-Verlag, Berlin, Heidelberg, New York, Tokyo, (1983).

(5) THURMAYR, R.: personal communication, (1984).

(6) WINGERT, F.: SNOMED Manual, Springer-Verlag, Berlin, Heidelberg, New York, Tokyo, (1984).

BASIC DATA SET AND LOCAL CLASSIFICATIONS

V. Lovrek[1], M. Madjarić[1] and Gj. Deželić[2]
[1] Clinical Hospital Centre, CZI, Šalata 2
[2] School of Public Health "A. Štampar", Medical Faculty of Zagreb
41000 Zagreb, Yugoslavia

SUMMARY

The paper is concerned with the use of a basic data set at the level of an integrated hospital information system covering several hospitals. The minimum basic data set of a single hospital is described in detail. The entities and attributes of a hospital information system as well as disease and drug classification systems are presented.

1. INTRODUCTION

In spite of greatly increased funds and markedly improved medical technology, modern medicine still has serious problems to face. Some authors refer to this situation as to a crisis through which medicine is currently passing /1/, thinking primarily of the inflation of information in therapeutic procedures and related activities. Abundance of information has always been the hallmark of medical science but never has there been such a mass of therapeutic and diagnostic procedures in medicine and public health care, nor have these procedures, owing to the lack of available technology, ever generated such a wealth of information as nowadays.

A good example illustrating this hyperproduction of information is the utilization of nonselective multichannel automatic analyzers where it is easier to perform a whole battery of analyses rather than select only those that apply to the case in question. In comparision to other "practical" professions (which unlike law or business science produce other effects besides information), medical procedures generate a higher proportion of useful information owing to the very nature of medical activities /2/.

It is obvious that "industrialized" medicine cannot rationally handle all the available information without the help of modern technology, notably of computers and microfilm devices. In view of the great variety of information needs – depending on the type of medical activity or medical speciality and on differences in personal background and education – at different localities in which identical activities are performed, there is an equally great variety in data collection and data processing procedures.
Thus, different procedures may effectively be employed within the same locality, comparison with any other locality being at the same time practically impossible /3/. Two approaches to the solution of this problem are possible: first, "official" institutionalization of all data from various medical fields and second, definition of a common minimum basic data set to be freely expanded and supplemented as various needs may require. The latter approach will be dealt with while utilizing local flexible processing facilities and keeping common data for comparison (e.g. application of local classifications).

2. ZAGREB HEALTH INFORMATION SYSTEM (ZHIS)

A programme for the development of a Common Information System of Health Insurance and Health Care of Zagreb, the so-called Zagreb Health Information System(ZHIS), was completed in 1978. Conceived of as an integral part of the health insurance system, the ZHIS was set the following general objectives:
1. Provide the necessary means for better and more comprehensive analysis of events and trends in health insurance and public health care as well as improve planning and programming in both fields,
2. Provide more complete information to support decision making in self-management, control, professional and operative activities,
3. Increase the efficacy, economy, efficiency and quality of health care and other forms of health insurance.

Unlike many other health information systems developed so far throughout the world, the ZHIS was designed to operate as an integral information system covering the fields of both health care and health insurance. While concetrating on individual patients needing medical care, it will at the same time collect, analyze and communicate relevant data about then as well as generate ordered aggregated information for the assessment of public health, control of health care activities, definition of user needs with respect to health care and health care planning /4/.

The ZHIS will thus provide assistance to medical personnel with their everyday professional tasks, support business and financial administration in health care and health insurance and facilitate control within the health care system.

2.1 Zagreb Health Information Subsystems

In order to provide for the basic functions of the public health care system in the city of Zagreb, the following subsystems were planned within ZHIS:
1. primary health (general practice) care subsystem,
2. outpatient health care subsystem,
3. hospital care subsystem,
4. health insurance subsystem,
5. health care institutes subsystem,
6. other subsystems.
Subsystems under 1-4 were designed each with a separate data bases whereas the remaining two were to make use of information generated within the data base of subsystem 4.

2.2 Entities and attributes

The principal entities (units on which data are collected) and attributes (features describing the properties of entities) within individual data bases include:
health care user (patient), health care renderer (hospital, department, physician), diagnosis, drug, medical service/procedure, visit/admission to hospital, right to sick-leave allowance, financial assistance and medical aids, name of company paying for health insurance, health insurance, decision/conclusion of health insurance companies, environment, sanitary-epidemiological factors.
The basic patient attributes include :
hospital identification, patient's number, name and surname, sex, date of birth, place of

birth(county),name of parents,marital status,basic occupation,present address,health insurance category,degree of disability,relevant medical data (blood group,allergies etc.)

Diagnoses are made in accordance with the International Classification of Diseases, Injuries and Causes of Death (ICD) which has been in use in our country since 1950. (6th revised version). In 1980 the 9th revised version of the ICD was put to use in Yugoslavia.The diagnosis and study of malignant diseases is covered by the TNM classification of malignant tumours.

The extended ICD-ZS classification containing a detailed presentation of a given disease is used in dental medicine and stomatology.

Also,there is in use a Classification of Ophthalmic Disorders containing a similar presentation of diseases on the basis of the 9th revised edition of the ICD.

Drugs : The use of drugs is regulated by the Yugoslav Classification of Drugs (JKL) where each drug is assigned a 7-digit code including information on dosage form,basic pharmacotherapeutic group (according to ICD),mechanisms and sites of action,subgroup and individual package number.

The principal attributes refer to the name of drug,JKL code,price and adverse effects. Drug consumption in a hospital is usually expressed as defined daily doses.

Medical services/procedures: A medical service is defined as any procedure described by the WHO International Classifications of Medical procedures and unequivocally defined by a 4-figure code provided by the classification. Occasionally, 5-figure codes may be used for coding specific procedures.

Environment: is defined as part of man's natural or man-made surroundings that may affect the quality of life and work if people are living in that environment. It may be urban,residential or occupational.

Sanitary-epidemiologicl factors are defined as determining the incidence and prevalence of disease within a given population or population group. They include environmental sanitary factors in a more general sense (atmosphere,water,soil),housing sanitation, working environment hygiene,food and household hygiene,sanitary-epidemiological care.

3. HOSPITAL INFORMATION SYSTEM (HIS) WITHIN A HOSPITAL

A HIS generally consists of 3 subsystems:
 PAS (Patient Administrative System)
 CLS (Clinical Laboratory System)
 CDS (Clinical Departmental Systems) /5/.
The most completely elaborated subsystem in our hospital is the Patient Administrative System used primarily for accounting and billing ipatient and outpatient treatment costs. Consequently,the requirements placed on the remaining two subsystems (CLS,CDS) will have to be such as to yield data needed for PAS operations.

3.1 Basic data set

The basic data set on inpatients are contained within the patient's case history. In addition to data required for accounting the costs of treatment,various additional parameters can be included to provide for medical and economic analyses.
The basic data set includes :
 - patient identification (number)

-surname and name
-date of birth
-sex
-insurance category (who pays treatment costs)
-date of admission
-source of admission
-diagnosis on admission
-department to wich the patient ia admitted
-date of discharge
-disscharge status
-main diagnosis (according to ICD-9 or local classification)
-other diagnoses
-residence
-complications
-treatment costs to be charged to

In addition to basic data collected for all patients alike, ther is also a set of others data or records concerning medical services rendered, examinations, drugs, surgical procedures, anesthesia if any, diet.

These records contain the following data:
-patient identification
-service, drug, surgical, obstetric or other procedure etc.
-date
-quantity
-department
-departmental period of stay
-miscellaneous

Patient identification and registration has so far been performed for each hospital separately so that at present there is no way of identifying the same patient in different hospitals. However, the problem will soon be solved by introducing national number for all Yugoslav citizens.

3.2 Local classifications

In order to improve the efficiency of local information systems in hospitals, local nomenclature codes and for some purposes even local classifications have been developed for the identification of most entities. There are two reasons for such an approach.
On the one hand, comprehensive general classifications (such as ICD-CM, SNOMED, Yugoslav Classifications of Drugs, etc.) have long codes which may unnecessarily complicate the identification procedure. On the other hand, less comprehensive classifications (ICD, Classification of Medical Procedures, etc.) are not sufficiently elaborated to allow the identification of a given entity in clinical practice /6/. In this case, the efficiency of local information systems and general applicability and comparability of data obtained at different locations can be reconciled by using local nomenclature codes and classifications, with general codes (e.g. ICD or Classification ofDrugs) contained as data within the basic entity record.

The practices have already yielded favourable results in terms of a common service, material and drug nomenclature (data needed for accounting treatment costs) where each record of the drug entity is assigned a code as provided by the JKL and each service a common health insurance code.

As regards diagnosis entities local diagnosis nomenclatures developed separately for various medical specialities are used, the record being assigned ICD codes. Each speciality group freely uses a 4-digit nomenclature code supplied with a control digit which allows easy coding, through diagnosis (up to 1000 within a speciality) an automatic conversion into ICD codes.

4. CONCLUSION

The definition of a minimum basic data set is a necessary step in bringing together data sets of different specialities from various hospital units. The use of local classifications and nomenclatures represents a further development in this respect. They allow a sufficiently detailed description of entities such as diagnosis, procedures and drugs at the level of hospital departments and at the same time the conversion of these data into generally accepted classifications (e.g. ICD codes, drug classifications codes in national and international terms).

5. REFERENCES

/1/ Roger, F.H., Opening address, MIE 84 Proceedings, Springer Verlag, 1984.

/2/ Madjarić, M., Development of Medical Information Systems: Possibilities and Restraints, Medical engineering JUREMA proceedings 26, Part 5, Zagreb 1981.

/3/ Common Information System of Health Insurance and Health Care of Zagreb – Conceptual Design Project, Associated Self-Management Interest Community of Health Care and Health Insurance, Zagreb, 1984, pp. 1035

/4/ Aurer, B., Gj. Deželić, B. Golec, S. Krajačić, T. Manhalter and M. Strnad, Common Information system of Health Insurance and Health Care of Zagreb – A Review of the Conceptual Design Project, Proceedings 6th Yugoslav Symposium "Social Systems of Informing '84", Zagreb, 1984.,

/5/ Lovrek, V., M. Madjarić, HIS Development under Conditions of Limited Hardware Resources, MIE 84 Proceedings, Springer Verlag, 1984.

/6/ Anderson, J. et al., Medical Informatics: Nomenclature and Classifications: SNOMED to ICD-10, Vol 8, No 1, London, 1983.

/7/ Roger, F.H., The minimum basic data set for hospital statistics in the EEC, Hospital Statistics in Europe, North-Holland, Brussels, 1982.

ADVANTAGES OF AN INFORMATION SYSTEM APPROACH CONNECTED WITH A THESAURUS FOR THE PROGRESSIVE, GLOBAL and COHERENT MICROCOMPUTERIZATION OF A CLINICAL DEPARTMENT.

+B. HUET, ++J.L. POURRIAT, +++C. ROLLAND

+Univ. PARIS-NORD, Fac. Médecine, Section Informatique médicale et Biostatistiques, 74 Av. M. Cachin, 93012 BOBIGNY Cedex, FRANCE

++Hop. AVICENNE, unité de réanimation, 125 route de Stalingrad, 93009 BOBIGNY, FRANCE

+++Univ. PARIS, Dépt Informatique, 12 Place du Panthéon, 75231 PARIS, FRANCE

ABSTRACT

Many microcomputers are everyday implemented in hospital clinical departments.COMMONLY there is only a little conceptual phase before implementation; the consequences of such an approach are : problems for semantical definitions, problems comming from redondance, problems for structure of data.
OUR approach is a conceptual study centred on the building of a semantical conceptual schema and of a thesaurus before any implementation in the department.
In our realization this conceptual study preceded the implementation of a real-time abstract medical record;two years later it was followed by evaluation of I.C.U. activity by Diagnosis Grouping Methods.
Today we are working about a consulting system.
Those various tasks progressively implemented in the department are coherent between them and will lead to a global microcomputerization in I.C.U. thanks to a semantical Information System and thesaurus approach.

I - INTRODUCTION

The aim of this paper is to present the concrete interest of an I.S. and thesaurus approach for the progressive, coherent and global implementation of several microcomputerized tasks in a clinical department.

We spent six months on the conceptual study (from February to August 1980) of the I.C.U. in the hospital Avicenne (located in the northern suburbs of PARIS - FRANCE) then implementation of a microcomputer has begun by one major objective: real-time (thesaurus based) abstract medical record; it was continued in 1983 by the evaluation of I.C.U. activity; today it is continued by research on a consulting system for I.C.U., in a few years we think to realize complete medical and administrative management of the unit on microcomputers.

This progressive microcomputerization in a medical ward is COHERENT because the first implementation was preceded by an important conceptual phase (chapter II) of which benefit is today perceptible.

The results are presented in chapter III; the interest of our methodology is highlighted in the discussion (chapter IV); conclusion is in chapter V.

II - METHOD

The functionning of an I.C.U. is complex, because analysis shows that there are many objects (medical records, patients files, analytical instruments, clinical examinations, doctors...) on which many operations are performed (sorting of medical record, validation of information...) in a manner that many interconnections exist along the dynamics of the unit; this necessitates to our sense an information oriented analysis before any implementation (1).

The conceptual phase of our realization was divided in two parallel researches:

* Representation of a static and dynamic view of the organization (I.C.U. department) to make sure coherence on data and between tasks.

In order to model any organization, ROLLAND proposed the diagrammatic representation of the perceived reality in terms of types, i.e. categories independent of any technical factor (2);this model is one among several ones: CHEN (3), FLORY (4), BRACCHI (5)....

Modelling in this way leads to a conceptual superschema, incorporating the methodolgy evolved in the ANSI/X3/SPARC workshop (6) and extending it to embrace the dynamic aspect (7).

For us a model may be defined as a set of concepts and the corresponding rules for their proper utilization.The superschema, dually comprising the static and dynamic, is a relational model (meaning of CODD E.F. (8)), theoretically defined by ROLLAND and his colleagues in 1978 and 1979; it is based on 3 concepts : object, operation, event.

An evaluation of the model proposed by ROLLAND was performed in several Information System (I.S.) design oriented I.F.I.P. workshops (1981, 1982, 1983); it is today the most complete I.S. design methodology (9).

In fact the importance of modelling before implementation of computers in organizations was underlined by our team since several years (10).

* Building of a thesaurus to get a semantical coherence between I.C.U. medical people :

The inventory of the specialized vocabulary (signs, syndroms, symptoms, medical therapy and surgical therapy) used by clinicians was followed by an analysis and a structuration; this led to a set of about 2700 wordings organized in two multilevel trees (T1 and T2) going from generalities to specialities.

The tree T1 regroups 2500 wordings on 9 levels, T2 is a general complementary tree for treatment, it regroups 210 wordings organized in 5 levels and can be called from any level of T1 (11).

These 2500 wordings come from the World Health Organization classification for 90 %,in 10% wordings are not in the W.H.O. classification.

Afterwards, we began the implementation of the first task on a current 8 bits microcomputer (32 kbytes core) equipped with a dual disk drive (170 kbytes each), a printer (90 car/s) and a current Basic.

III - RESULTS

The first target was reached in June 1981: from this period for each patient an abstract medical record is built during his (her) stay in reanimation by using the wordings of our thesaurus; at their outcome of the department the abstract is enclosed with a letter for the specialist or general practitioner (12).

Programs are built on an automaton which allows strictly the same application in an other speciality only by storing on disk an other thesaurus (13)without any modification of software.

Simultaneously to that task, we have built continuously a data bank constituted with (thesaurus based) abstract medical record.
The processing of this data bank was oriented towards evaluation of activity by diagnosis grouping.The first results were presented in M.I.E.84 (14), today groups are defined with a better precision because there are more abstracts.

we are searching today on a consulting system.

IV - DISCUSSION
----

* According FOUCAUT (15) the qualitative features of such a conceptual schema are

** Coherence :

A representation is coherent if there is no contradiction.

This coherence is provided by the method which is used to build the conceptual schema : relational approach, 3rd Normal Form, minimal cover (16).

In its final form this schema has no redundancy.

This coherence allows to implement progressively various autonomous tasks in a comprehensive project, it suppresses problems comming from redundancy and problems comming from dedicated structure of data of independent implementations.

** Completion :

The completion assigned to the conceptual schema does not mean exhaustivity, i.e. we do not want (and we cannot) to model all caracteristics of all phenomena of the organization in the conceptual schema, however the different points of view of users must be explained in the schema.

The conceptual schema will be complete if it assumes the various views (comming from the different users) useful for the organization.

This completion is the surety of a total view between the various independent computerized applications.

** Flexibility :

To integrate future evolutions of the organization the conceptual schema must be easy to modify; the relational approach provides this flexibility.

This flexibility allows a better evolution of the I.S. all along its life.

* The interest of a thesaurus in such an application is, to our sense, double :

** Suppression of a problem of semantical definition:

** More flexible processing of abstract medical record, especially for diagnosis grouping methods (GDM):

The regroupment of abstract medical records is very difficult to perform.

Many methods are used to constitute groups, they lead to various results going from a little number of groups (7) to a great number (10000) (17).

From the idea of Fetter (18) we assigned each case into one of the 383 groups defined by Fetter, then each of these groups was processed according to the same method.

This assignation is made easier by the thesaurus allowing to adjust groups, definition of new groups, subdivision in a group according the stage of illness.

There is a great flexibility for processing of medical records.

Today 80 groups are defined from the processing of 2500 abstract medical records.

V - CONCLUSION

The concrete advantages of such an approach are clear : suppression of problems of redundancy, suppression of problems of dedicated structure of data, suppression of problems of semantical definition, makes sure a global view between various independent applications, provides flexibility for the processing of medical records by diagnosis grouping methods.

Moreover, this approach can be used for a global, progressive and coherent microcomputerization in any hospital clinical department.

R E F E R E N C E S
----

1) - A conceptual approach of Hospital Information Systems
     HUET B., ROLLAND C., MARTIN J.
     Proc. MEDINFO 83, North Holland, 18-22, Aug 1983, Amsterdam, Holland

2) - Concepts for the design of an Information System conceptual schema and its utilization in the REMORA project
     ROLLAND C., FOUCAUT O.
     Proc. IVth Int. Conf. V.L.D.B., 342-350, 1978, Berlin, RFA

3) - Report on database management system
     ANSI/X3/SPARC
     Final Report, Washington, 1977

4) - The entity-relationship model toward a unified view of data
     CHEN P.
     A.C.M. Trans. Data Bases, 1 , 9-36, March (1976)

5) - Un modèle et une méthode pour la conception logique d' une B.D.
   FLORY A.
   Thèse ès -Sciences , Univ. LYON, 1977

6) - Binary logical associations in data modelling
   BRACCHI G.
   Proc. I.F.I.P. TC2, Freundenstat, R.F.A., 1976

7) - Tools for Information Systems Dynamics management
   ROLLAND C., LEIFERT S., RICHARD C.
   Proc. Vth Int. Conf. V.L.D.B., 251-261, 1979, Rio Janeiro, Brésil

8) - A relational model for large shared data banks.
   CODD E.F.
   Com. A.C.M., 13 , 6, 377-387, (1970)

9) - Information Systems design methodologies : a comparative review
   Proc. IFIP working conf., May 1982, Noordwijkerhout, Hollande

10) - Modelling and simulation of Information Systems:methodological advantages
   HUET B., MARTIN J.
   Med. Inform. 5 , n°3, 193-203, (1981)

11) - A semantical approach of microcomputerization in an I.C.U.
   HUET B., POURRIAT J.L., GABRY M.
   Proc. Int. Congress Anesthesia, Erasmus , 129, Sept 1983, Rotterdam;
Hollande

12) - Réalisation sur microordinateur d' un résumé d' observations en temps- réel
   POURRIAT J.L., HUET B., GABRY M., ROLLAND C., CUPA M.
   Revue de 1' Association Française d' Anesthésie - Réanimation, 1 ,
161-165, (1982)

13) - An automaton computer program for a microcomputerized real-time (thesaurus
based) abstract medical record
   HUET B., POURRIAT J.L., MARTIN J., CUPA M.
   Comp. Prog. in Biomed., 15 , 117-123, (1982)

14) - A microcomputerized evaluation of I.C.U. activity by diagnosis grouping
methods.
   HUET B., POURRIAT J.L., MARTIN J., BENHAMOU M.
   Proc. M.I.E. 84, Springer, 681-685, Sept. 84, Bruxelles, Belgique

15) - Modèle et outil pour la conception des Systèmes d' Information dans les
organisations
   FOUCAUT O.
   Thèse ès-Sciences, Univ. NANCY I, Juin 1982

16) - Contribution théorique à la conception et à 1' évaluation d' un système d'
information appliqué à la gestion
   DELOBEL C.
   THèse ès-Sciences, Univ. GRENOBLE, 1973

17) - Hospital case mix: its definition, measurement and use-Part II
   HORNBROOK M.C.
   Med. Care rev., 39 , 73-123, (1982)

18) - Case mix definition by diagnosis- related- groups
   FETTER R.B., SHIN J., FREEMAN J.L., AVERILL R.F., THOMPSON J.D.
   Med. Care (supplement), 18 , n°2, Feb. 1980

DML/3000 : A relational database retrieval language providing simultaneous access to a large number of clinical databases, full computational facilities and built-in interfaces with different statistical packages

M.A. de Rotrou, Y.N. La, N. Issakides and R. Gomeni
Laboratoires d'Etudes et de Recherches Synthelabo, Dept. of Clinical
Research, 58 rue de la Glacière, 75013 Paris, France.

1. Introduction

The large and ever increasing amounts of data involved in the management and analysis of clinical trials lead to the need for more efficient data processing techniques.

Conventional data storage, with unrelated files, causes users to be concerned with the physical layout in the computer. This storage usually generates file redundancy, as files have to be transformed for use by new applications. In addition, creating and deleting files endangers the clinical data integrity.

Database Management Systems (DBMS), have been since recent developments, recognized as the most efficient storage and management tool for data organisation. The relational database model, introduced by Codd in 1970 (1)and later extended (2), has acted as a foundation for many relational DBMS's.

But the use of these systems in medical research, was slowed down by the fact that these relational DBMS's lacked data integrity control, were not a friendly interface for the user and did not offer help facilities.

Because of the reliance on DBMS's, the need for query languages, using relational DBMS's, became necessary. CLINIC/3000 (3), developed on a HP3000 computer, is a clinical trial management and analysis system. It uses a relational DBMS system, RELATE/3000 (4). The query language, is named DML/3000, Data Manipulation Language. DML/3000 is a superstructure for RELATE/3000.

2. Data retrieval

a) Design

DML/3000 has been designed to access the clinical database. Medical doctors, statisticians as well as data processing personnel are meant to use it. Therefore, friendliness of use, security of transaction and built-in help facilities are some of the major advantages.

As an interface between the end users and the clinical data, DML/3000 may be used interactivly or by batch. Clinical data are organized in clinical studies, each study having a defined structure. The structure is modelled in a dictionary database. Therefore, DML/3000 maintains independence of the study structure and the language processor. The end user may acces one or several studies at the same time, depending on his requirements.

If one wishes to examine data for patients of a study (e.g. laboratory data), it is possible to retrieve a set of items from this study. This is a vertical examination of the items of a study structure. It is possible, by a horizontal exploration of an item extract all adverse reactions for patients in a set of studies.

As all items have a single name in a study, no confusion may occur, and if item names have been standardized in all studies, horizontal retrieval is even more facilitated.

b) Manipulation

The main feature of a query system, is the selection, possibility to select sets of items and to create views, by relating files together. Such relations in DML/3000 may involve an unlimited number of files and items of different studies. The most common key matches are made automatically and the user has just to type the special condition criteria.

Files and sets of items can be sorted on a temporary or permanent basis. All files may have permanent indexes as well as temporary, and it is possible to have up to nine permanent indexes on a file, involving as many items as necessary. Selected views may be copied to create new files of data, or merged to pre-existent files. Manipulation of data is very easy, and requires a minimum of typing from the user.

Each file is considered as a table and may be used for simple arithmetic computations (addition, substraction, multiplication,...). Items can be freely mixed up in such calculations. Totals are automatic and system variables (e.g. time or date) enhance presentation of data.

c) Display of the data

Data may be displayed in three ways :

- The most usual display is a row/colunm presentation, the rows represent patients and the colums represent items. This is the most used, as it allows immediate examination.

- The spreadsheet system puts the data into a spreadsheet form (the Visicalc type) for the users who are used to it.

- The most sophisticated display is the graphic : barcharts, histograms, piecharts or linegraphs, all use monochromic or colour graphic devices (terminals or paper plotters).

d) Printouts

The actual state of the study is shown by either standard reports or user reporting.

The standard reports can be generated giving information as patient I.D., item names and visit numbers, and produce listings ready for internal, statistical or official purposes.

- For a set of items and/or patients, this listing provides set of item values for the selected items and/or patients; one may need all the values of haemoglobin for patients who have sleeping problems and have never smoked.

- For a set of items, outside the normal limits; the purpose of this listing is the same as the former, except that only patients, whose items are outside predefined ranges, are printed.

- A summary of patients who have an item out of the predefined limits.

- A CHI-2, table of patients for an item, showing the difference of in-bounds, and out-of-bounds between two different visits.

User reporting consists of a few simple, but powerful commands that allow to lay-out the data in the desired format. With this system, very complex reports may be generated.

3. Statistical Analysis

One of the main aims of DML/3000 is to provide statistical computation facilities in order to analyse data, before or after transformation by user manipulation. The user generally selects subsets of data, based on logical criteria and then submits these subsets to statistical functions.

Simple statistics can be obtained by built-in functions, that give for example descriptive statistics, or even analysis of variance for a series of patients.
For example, to obtain descriptive statistics on laboratory data, the DML/3000 commands could be :

```
OPEN FILE BIOLOGY
SELECT BLOOD_PRES,HEAMOGLOB WHERE CIGAR_DAY<20
DESCRIPTIVE
```

DESCRIPTIVE is a built-in descriptive statistics generator function.

Data, in the CLINIC/3000 database, has a binary form. This data may be sent to standard ASCII character files; this ensures total compatibility with most existing software. These files can be submitted to BMDP, S.A.S or other full-fledged statistical packages.

4. Security restrictions.

The problems of security encountered have increased in line with the growing number of connected users at the same time. Data which have entered the study have been thoroughly checked during the Entry Phase of CLINIC/3000 and later by quality control. To ensure that integrity is maintained, every further access to the database must be controlled.

Security problems have two different levels of control :

- The first control concerns the users capability to access or not each study.

- The second security control concens the users capability to execute certain types of functions : reading, writting or updating data.Usually studies may only be accessed in read mode.

5. Network facilities

Total databases or only parts of the databases may be exchanged between two or more different computers and as no conversion is necessary, the integrity of the data is maintained.

Once CLINIC/3000 files have been transformed into ASCII character files, the later may be sent to remote computers for analysis using statistical packages (e.g. S.A.S. on IBM computer).
For example, to select some laboratory data, and send it to a remote IBM computer (assuming that a physical link has been established between the HP3000 and a mainframe IBM) :

```
OPEN FILE LABORATORY
SELECT BLOOD_PRES,SGOT,HEMATOCRIT WHERE AGE>21
CONVERT TO LABDATA
SEND LABDATA TO IBM
```

The CONVERT command will convert a CLINIC/3000 binary data file into a new ASCII file named LABDATA. SEND will transfer the file LABDATA to a remote IBM computer.

When a CLINIC/3000 file is transformed to an ASCII file, a second file may be created at the same time, containing the description of the data. This description file is very useful, when files are exchanged between computers, as data can not only be sent to a remote computer, but also used by the host relational database management system of this remote computer. In fact, the whole clinical study, including structure, can be sent to a remote computer, and utilisation is completely transparent for an end user. This has been done with DBASE II on a micro computer or INGRESS on a mainframe host, two relational DBMS's.

6. Conclusion

DML/3000 provides flexibility for retrieval, analysis and reporting of data within the CLINIC/3000 clinical database management system. It gives access to an increasing number of functions and enlarged statistical packages. Usable with a minimum qualification and knowledge of the computer, it has reached the objective : friendliness of use. DML/3000 has made the data structure transparent to end users and eliminated the boundaries between different tasks. Users have an edge : they can concentrate more on analysis and less on computation.

Due to development in "Distributed Informatics", integration in a Network System appears like the major future task for DML/3000.

References

(1) Codd E.F. : A relational model of data for large shared data banks
Comm. of A.C.M. 13, 1970, 377-387

(2) Codd E.F. : Extending the database relational model to capture more
meaning   Comm of A.C.M. TODS, 4, 1979, 397-434

(3) N. Issakides, M.A. de Rotrou and R. Gomeni : CLINIC/3000 a clinical trial management system. Lecture notes in Medical Informatics, MIE84, Springer Verlag, New York, 406-411, 1984

(4) RELATE/3000 : Reference manual, C.R.I., Santa Clara CA 95054 U.S.A., 1985

Rules for the Design of End User Languages

U. Engelmann, H.P. Meinzer
German Cancer Research Center
Institute of med. and biol. Informatics
Heidelberg, FRG

Introduction

Tools for the implementation of fourth generation languages are now available
(SCHA83). These tools facilitate the production of interactive systems. A language
is defined by a formal grammar in which the semantic actions are embedded (MEI83).

This process of implementation yields software systems for unexperienced users like,
in the medical field, doctors and nurses. The languages are problem oriented and
built to avoid hardware or software restrictions. A user expresses his demands in
his concepts and language and must not specify how a job is executed on the machine.
The systems are always specialized for the solution of defined tasks. It is assumed
that an increase of performance of 7:1 can be gained if compared to third generation
software.

The creation of good interactive systems can be supported by a careful design. The
authors develop systems for end users since ten years and won a lot of experience
which is presented here in the form of rules for the design of fourth generation
languages.

The design of a language

There are basically only three ways of man-machine communication, the sequential
dialog (question and answer), the menue technique (pick one of a set of commands)
and the command languages. The third alternative is the method of choice as it is
more powerful and flexible than the other methods of interaction (MEI83). The following ideas can support the design of command controlled systems.

- sets of commands

  Functionally correlated commands should be sampled as a well defined subset of the
  language. A collection of correlated commands in sets also supports the training
  of users. A user can concentrate on these subsets of his special interest and will
  not be confused by the others.

- active and parametric commands

  It is absolutely necessary that every command has only very few parameters, two is
  maximum, zero is best. This requires the possibility for the definition and update
  of defaults, which is done by the parametric commands. Active (or procedural)

commands initialize and execute a task under the conditions defined by defaults. Every set of commands should be split in a list of its procedural and the associated parametric commands.

- information commands

    There are two groups of information commands. The first includes answers to questions like

    - which file am I working with?
    - what is the actual value of a default?
    - how did I proceed to the actual state of my session?

    The commands can be named STATUS, DEFAULT or HISTORY. Other information commands answer the questions

    - which commands are available?
    - what are the possible parameters for a certain command?
    - what does a command do?

    These commands could be HELP (or simply ?) or EXPLAIN. Another category of commands support system management functions. These parts of a language have a more general character and should deal with the following features:

    - extension of a language by a user without changing the grammar.

    - creation of files or procedures that collect a set of commands for the solution of a given problem. It must be possible to include parameters and control structures.

    - definition of synonyms and abbreviations of commands under control of a user.

    - concatenation of commands to permit more than one function per line. Examples are 'AND', semicolon ';' and comma ','. This allows the use of basically simple commands to form longer and rather 'natural'looking input lines.

    - lines of comments usually make no sense in an interactive command language. They are very helpful if procedures or batch-jobs are developed.

    - conversational and batch mode must use the same commands. In special applications like e.g. image processing some routines are very time consuming. It should be possible to execute them in batch mode.

Features of a language

Close control of user yields useful hints on the quality of a system. Norman (NOR83) studied and classified user errors into five groups:

- mode error
- description error

- consistence error
- capture error
- activation error

From this classification the following design rules are derived.

1. Reduce the number of modes.

   Ideally there are no modes. Users get very easily confused, this requires a lot of complicated explanations.

2. Always clearly indicate the actual mode.

   As it is not possible to use no modes (at least you need WAITING and RUNNING) it must be made obvious where you are. Bad systems force a user to use trial and error methods where he tries to recognize a mode by its (different) error messages.

3. Avoid ambignity.

   An example can be the editor 'VI' (UNIX, Berkeley Release) where 'd' and 'D' and 'CTRL-d' have different meanings. More bad examples are to be found everywhere. Ambignity can be very harmful as unwanted but harmful decisions are possibly initialized.

4. Design a consistent language.

   Consistence errors occur if for example the sequence of parameters of a command is not obvious, or worse changing from command to command. A user is mislead by wrong analogies. If a new command is inserted into a language its consistence with the existing ones must be checked both in respect to its parameters and its name and function.

5. Support the users memory.

   A number of activation errors are based on people's short memory. An interupt of a session (e.g. by a telephone call) results in an unfinished process (out of sight is out of mind). Incomplete sequences of actions should be indicated, questions to missing answers should be repeated within a certain time.

6. Avoid prompting.

   Prompts are questions or remarks of the machine like
   - do you really want to erase this dataset?
   - this file already exists, select another name.

   These parts of a dialog are popular with users, especially with unexperienced ones. As the remarks are always the same the attention paid to them is reduced by the time and then they cause trouble again because users apply potentially dangerous standard answers to the standard questions. It is bad that the machine does not learn anything but constantly repeats the same message to the same error (MEI83). Especially disturbing are prompts if the language is used in a procedure

or batch job. As the answer to a question is missing, the next command line is
taken for the answer, of course not understandable to the machine. Worst case are
repeated prompts, the whole process ends up in a mess.

7. Permit an UNDO

Even the finest program design can not make failsave systems, it can happen that
a user applies a wrong command. In the case of a parametric command there is no
problem as a second input corrects the first. If an unwanted action was executed
real harm could have been initialized and in this case a function UNDO is very
helpful. In an editor e.g. DELETE commands are candidates for a reverse action. A
nice example is found in the LISA concept where a file is finally lost only at
the end of a session. No physical destruction is executed but some kind of logic
operation that can be reverted (LISA quotation).

8. Permit a software reset.

A common joke of computer people is the remark, if nothing else helps and you and
the system lost control of the interaction then use the 'hardware reset'. This
indicates a complete electric cut off of the power supply. This is not only not
elegant and time consuming for a new start but also dangerous as incomplete action
or open files can be the result. We found a command like RESET to be helpful. It
reinitialises the dialog, all defaults are set to their standard values. The
machine is put into a defined and well known state.

9. Use concepts of the end users.

The system must be as close to the concept and language of the users as possible.
Training and use is facilitated a lot.

10. Take special care of error messages.

Every programmer can tell stories of misleading or not understandable error messages. Tests have shown that improved error messages can increase the system performance by factor two (BRO82, BRO83, SHN80) not to speak of the subjective acceptance of a system. There are three main aspects:

- syntax errors

  In an interactive environment the syntax errors are identified by the parser.
  The location of the error in the input line can be indicated and a suggestion
  for correct continuation can be presented. A standard message like "unknown command" is less useful.

- semantic errors

  Actions usually depend on their semantic context, e.g. a certain command only
  makes sense if another action has been executed before. If the interactive system has been defined by its grammar and the correlated semantic actions special
  error checking routines can be inserted at the semantic level. These error
  actions should be given priority before executing the others. On this level very

sophisticated error detection can be implemented. An error and a possible solution can be described in much more detail as compared to the syntax errors.

- psychologic aspects

The negative image of computers to a great deal stems from the negative experience of user in the case of errors. As interactive systems lead users to an experimental approach ("let us try and see what happens"). "The user learns weather a system is a friend or a foe, when he makes errors" (BRO83).

Shneiderman described a few suggestions to message design (SHN82). He asks for readable and understandable error messages, the efficiency of which should be tested thoroughly by end users under control of a system designer. All messages that urge a user or scold him are bad. Good message are positive in form and action. Negative words like INVALID, ILLEGAL, ERROR or INCORRECT should be avoided. An error should be indicated, and a possible solution explained in detail, A message must be in clear text, don't use error codes that have to be analysed with the help of a reference manual. A user should feel that HE controls the system and not vice versa.

While developing and maintaining large end user systems we found an error documentation feature very helpful. The number and location of both syntactic and semantic errors can identify the two deficiencies in the concept of a system. It is then possible to update the system, the instruction manuals, the error messages and the education at the right point.

References

[ACS84] Archer, J.E. jr., Conway, R., Schneider, F.B.: User Recovery and Reversal in Interactive Systems. ACM Transactions on Programming Languages and Systems 6, No 1 (1984) 1-19.

[BRO82] Brown, P.J.: My system gives excellent error messages - or does it? Software Practice and Experience 12, No. 1 (1982) 91-94.

[BRO83] Brown, P.J.: Error Messages: The neglected area of the man/machine interface? Communications of the ACM 26, No. 4 (1983) 246-249.

[ENG85] Engelmann, U., Meinzer, H.P.: Bessere Mensch/Maschine Schnittstellen durch mehr Beachtung des Benutzerfehlers. Angewandte Informatik 1985 (in print).

[MEI83] Meinzer, H.P.: Der Dialog zwischen Mensch und Maschine in der biologisch-medizinischen Forschung. Dissertation, Fakultät für Theoretische Medizin, Universität Heidelberg (1983).

[NOR83] Norman, D.A.: Design Rules Based on Analyses of Human Error. Communications of the ACM 26, No. 4 (1983) 254-258.

[SHN80] Shneiderman, B.: System message design: Guidelines and experimental results. In Badre, A., Shneiderman, B. (eds.): Directions in Human-Computer Interactions. Norwood, N.J.: Ablex Publishing Co. (1982).

[SHN82] Shneiderman, B.: Designing Computer System Messages. Communications of the ACM 25, No. 9 (1982) 610-611.

[TEI75] Teitelman, W.: INTERLISP Reference Manual. Xerox PARC, Palo Alto, Calif., Dec. 1975.

[VER78] Verhofstad, J.S.M.: Recovery techniques for Database Systems. Comput. Surv. 10, No. 2 (1978) 167-195.

[WIL83] Williams, G.: The LISA Computer System. Byte 2 (1983).

USE OF U.S. VETERANS ADMINISTRATION SOFTWARE IN FINNISH HEALTH CARE

Jukka Koskimies
Department of Data Processing
Helsinki University Central Hospital
Helsinki, Finland

SUMMARY

The FileMan (File Manager) database management system and programming
tools and the Kernel utility software of the U.S. Veterans
Administration have been taken in use by Helsinki University Central
Hospital and several other health care institutions in Finland. In
system work the use of FileMan has created a standardized working
environment, facilitated technical communication and teamwork and
stimulated national and international co-operation. FileMan has been
extensively used and is well suited to end user database computing.
Problems of efficiency may arise if too complicated database
structures are defined. Other difficulties have been primarily
caused by the lack of detailed technical documentation of the systems.

INTRODUCTION

To take advantage of the rapidly increasing possibilities of
information technology health care institutions have two main lines to
pursue: installing traditional information systems and promoting end
user computing.

When installing information systems to clinical environments, many
institutions find it preferable to build their own systems instead of
using commercial packages, whereby the efficiency of working methods
and software tools becomes an issue of utmost importance. The same is
true of clinical end user computing: flexible and easy-to-use software
tools, especially database management systems, are needed.

Ideally, the same software should be usable for both application
development and end user computing. In this way unnecessary learning
overhead and maintenance of several software tools can be avoided. A
common tool for both systems people and end users also improves
possibilities for communication between end users and data processing
professionals.

A good application development tool should work in a friendly and
efficient programming environment and in its structure encourage
branches to user-written code to enhance the efficiency and
the functional properties of the resulting systems.

As a result of its search for efficient and flexible software tools
for both systems work and end user computing, Helsinki University
Central Hospital (HUCH) has committed itself to the use of the
database management system FileMan (also known as File Manager)
developed by George F. Timson of the Unites States Veterans
Administration (VA). In HUCH, FileMan has been the principal tool of
end user database computing since 1982 and of application system
development since 1983. Also several other health care institutions
and commercial enterprises in Finland have adopted FileMan for a
variety of purposes including large commercial system development
projects.

Within VA itself FileMan has developed into a standard tool upon which the development of all system utility and application programs for its hospital information system package is based. This package is presently being installed in about 170 VA hospitals ranging in size from 100 to 1200 beds (1). The VA hospital system programs will be used also by some other U.S. public domain health care organizations, e.g. the Indian Health Service hospitals.

In 1983, several health care organizations in Finland joined into a co-operative national effort (the MUSTI project) to develop a hospital information system package suitable for both small local hospitals and large university hospital complexes. After evaluating the existing possibilities the project selected FileMan as its principal tool. Obvious similarities between the working environments and the objectives of the VA project and the MUSTI project made it natural for the MUSTI developers to consider the possibility of taking advantage of VA hospital system software also beyond FileMan itself.

This paper reports experiences of using VA system software, especially the FileMan package, in Finnish health care institutions and in the MUSTI project.

FILEMAN (FILE MANAGER)

FileMan as such is a software package on some 140 ANSI Standard MUMPS programs (2). From the user's point of view it is:

- a stand-alone end user database management system
- an application development system and prototyping tool
- a set of programmer's tools.

As an end user database management system FileMan allows basic database applications to be created and run by end users after minimal training. Defining more complicated database structures and data relations and taking advantage of the more sophisticated functions of the system require experience and support from data processing professionals.

As an application development system and prototyping tool FileMan makes possible rapid definition of file structures and basic user functions, experimentation with system prototypes and easy modification of file structures and data relations. Depending on performance requirements the system may be run in production as such or may be modified by hand-coding. For enhancing the functionalities of a standard FileMan application the system provides numerous 'hooks' where strings of MUMPS code or calls to external MUMPS routines may be attached.

As a set of programmer's tools FileMan offers the possibility to use the individual routines of the package as building blocks of customized applications.

FileMan is a U.S. public domain program product and is available for a copying media and handling charge through international MUMPS Users' Groups. It is currently in use around the world in hundreds of organizations. Tutorials of basic and advanced FileMan techniques both for end users and for programmers are a standard part of international meetings of the users of the MUMPS programming system.

USE OF FILEMAN IN HELSINKI UNIVERSITY CENTRAL HOSPITAL

The first copy of FileMan was brought to HUCH in October, 1981. New versions have been obtained roughly once a year.

In system work the basic FileMan package is used to define and document database structures and to build prototype systems. Systems with low to medium performance requirements as well as relatively permanent auxiliary files in general, are left to be handled with standard FileMan functions (Enter/Edit, Print, Search, Inquire, Transfer), whereas parts of systems with high performance requirements are hard-coded. In many cases it has been found desirable to modify the standard FileMan user interface to fit the local standards or taste.

Two examples of FileMan-based application systems in HUCH are described is other papers presented in this meeting: an out-patient scheduling and administration system converted from a previous Costar-based system, by Hanna Kalpa, Tiina Pesonen and Sinikka Ripatti, and the MULTILAB system for clinical laboratories, by Esa Soini. Others to be mentioned are a regional statistical database of ca. 200 000 hospital in-patient encounters per year as well as numerous smaller systems for managerial statistics of the medical departments of the hospital. Also extract copies of the regional population census register, used by the out-patient scheduling systems of the departments of Gynaecology and Obstetrics (360 000 persons) and Pediatrics (155 000 persons) are standard FileMan databases.

Non-medical FileMan-based applications in HUCH include the personnel administration system of the hospital's 10 000 employees, a database of its 7000 medical instruments and their service costs, and a regional database of 1400 pieces of X-ray equipment. In addition, FileMan has become an everyday tool for a multitude of departmental and personal housekeeping functions within the data processing department. Examples are personnel and project administration, end user activity management, system maintenance, as well as documentation and maintenance of the terminal network.

The use of FileMan as an end user database management system for clinical applications in HUCH is described by Esa-Matti Tolppanen in another paper in this meeting. To facilitate the use of FileMan by end users a Finnish language User's Manual has been prepared.

USE OF FILEMAN ELSEWHERE IN THE HEALTH CARE IN FINLAND

At the moment MUSTI is the most extensive project in Finland relying on FileMan techniques. The participating three university hospitals, those of Helsinki, Kuopio and Turku as well as Kuopio University use FileMan in their system work. Kuopio University in particular, has used it since 1981 for a number of medical and non-medical systems.

Outside the MUSTI group the Department of Dentistry of Helsinki University is one of the established routine users of FileMan since several years. Commercial or semi-commercial FileMan systems run or are being developed in Finnish laboratories of surgical pathology and microbiology. The Finnish Cancer Registry and the Finnish Foundation for the Research of Alcoholic Diseases are among the health care institutions having adopted FileMan. In the non-medical area, a large commercial stock control project based on FileMan is underway.

OTHER VA SYSTEM SOFTWARE

The VA hospital information system consists of a set of FileMan-based application systems and a package of utility software, the Kernel, which provides an identical system enviroment for all the hospitals installing the system. The Kernel is an extension of the FileMan and includes, among others, a sign-on/security system, a menu management system, a background task monitor and an electronic mail system.

The first copy of the Kernel software was obtained to HUCH in June, 1984, and an update with a set of documentation of the system in October, 1984. Parts of the system were installed to HUCH and some other Finnish sites by the end of the year. A full set of Kernel programs is in production in one of HUCH PDP-11/44 machines at the time of writing of this report. It replaces earlier home-written systems of sign-on/security, electronic mail and, in part, menu management. The Kernel utilities will be used in the MUSTI system.

BENEFITS RESULTING FROM THE USE OF THE VA SYSTEM SOFTWARE

At first sight the most exciting features of FileMan are those of an application generator and end user database management system. Further acquaintance with the package leads one to appreciate it perhaps even more as a set of tools for defining standardized MUMPS database structures and for building standardized MUMPS application systems.

The technical advantages of using standardized file structures and application development tools are obvious. The use of FileMan has created a uniform working environment for system development, facilitated technical communication and teamwork and encouraged the development of further software tools for this environment. It has also encouraged to and facilitated exchange of experience and programs between institutions sharing the same system environment. The stimulation of co-operation, both national and international, and its effects upon information exchange and learning, have been among the major advantages experienced as a result of the use of FileMan.

The advantages brough about by co-operation and joint projects have been emphasized by the excellent portability of FileMan-based systems. Both FileMan itself and the Kernel employ special techniques to render the programs independent of the MUMPS operating system used. In fact, within VA the hospital system is to be run on at least four different operating systems, two of which (DSM-11 and M/11) are interpreters and two others (M/11+ and M/VX) are compilers. Within HUCH, all these except DSM-11 are used. Provided a system environment compatible with that of VA is adhered to, the VA programs have been found to run without difficulty in all of them. As a further experiment, the FileMan package and an application built with it were transported from our VAX-11/750 to an IBM PC with a Micronetics MUMPS system. Only one minor change in a device handler was necessary, and the system was in operation in the new enviroment within half an hour.

A utility is provided by FileMan to convert file definitions and (optionally) data into standard MUMPS routines which can be transported to any FileMan environment and run there to initialize an identical system. The Kernel provides further tools for transporting programs, files and data by means of its electronic mail system.

PROBLEMS ENCOUNTERED

Greatest difficulties have been encountered in cases, where the fact has been overlooked that although simple database systems can be built and run with FileMan with no problems, defining more complicated database structures and data relations requires experience and careful planning. The versatility of the system easily leads an inexperienced and over-enthusiastic user to define clumsy systems much too complicated to be utilized efficiently. This danger applies equally to end users and to data processing professionals

The technical documentation of the VA software, including FileMan, has not been very detailed. To improve the situation, about twenty people involved in the MUSTI development organized in the spring of 1983 a series of seminars to study the FileMan programs (which consist of, to put it mildly, extremely complicated code) and to write a technical manual of the FileMan system in Finnish language. Further technical advice was obtained during a three-day consultation seminar conducted by George Timson in Helsinki in October, 1984.

Some difficulty has been caused by the fact that to be usable in Finland, FileMan has to be translated, an effort that has been undertaken four times so far, as new versions of the package have been taken to use. On the basis of proper documentation of the previous cycles the work can easily be done during a weekend, but each time involves a further period of several weeks or even months before all errors have been tested out from the translation.

Although FileMan itself is independent of its environment and also the other Kernel programs as such are fully portable and can be installed in any standard MUMPS environment, their installation in an enviroment with a long-established culture of user interface and programming conventions may pose some difficulties. Of the Kernel programs only the sign-on program has caused problems in this respect. In our case we found it necessary to modify the VA sign-on program to behave identically with the old home-written one, to which the several hundred users had been accustomed.

Most difficulties encountered in applying VA software have basically resulted from the fact that these programs are primarily VA internal. Non-VA users, especially those as remote as in Finland, can not reasonably expect responsibilies of support or consultation from the VA or from the persons having developed the programs. Yet the willingness of the VA system specialists to spread knowledge about these tools has greatly alleviated the difficulties and contributed to the successful implementation of the VA system sofware into Finnish health care.

REFERENCES

(1)   Houser, Walter R.: End User Software Engineering: The Experience of the Veterans Administration Decentralized Hospital Computer Program. MUG Quarterly, 1984, 3/4:3-11.

(2)   Timson, George F. and Martin T. Ivers: Supporting End User Development of Complex Information Systems Through a Natural Language Applications Generator and a Library of Utilities. MUG Quarterly 1981, 2/3:43-45.

A METHODOLOGY TO INTEGRATE IN A DATA BASE:
Data-Items, Text, Graphics and Images.

M. J. de Matos Barbosa

Faculty of Medicine
University of Coimbra
PORTUGAL

1 - ABSTRACT

This paper is a solution to model documents at three levels: the logi
cal level, concerning the logical aspects of documents; the conceptual
level, relative to the notion of a structural model and the physical
level corresponding to the editing of documents. We propose, here, forms
to integrated in a Data Base: data-items, text, graphics and images.
We have defined this Data Base as INTEGRATED DATA BASE SYSTEM (IDBS).

2 - INTRODUCTION

An IDBS can be developed, based on the existing technology appli
ed to fields such as: Data Base, Image processing and Office automation. Therefore, with an IDBS is possible to manipulate information of
different kinds, structured according to a single model and accessible
through a language which should integrate compatible sub-languages such
as: SPLM-11 (1).

At conceptual level, the Schema is unique for various kinds of information, being it: data-items, text, graphics or images. Its manipula
tion can be done by the various commands built into language. Such com
mands can be used not only integrated in the host language, to build
complex applications, but also independently through interactive requests by the user.

The IDBS must guaranty the existence of principles such as: inte
grity, security, confidenciality and non-redundances. The information
models that it manipulate can be defined as: Data-items, Textual and
Pictorial Models.

3 - DATA-ITEMS MODEL

The data-model to be used can be derived from the following entity
and relationship classes:

a - <u>Entity-classes:</u> The entities of some kind are grouped into sets
called entity-classes. Each of these classes are
identified by a unique and significant name.

<u>Example:</u>

In a ward, the nurses are grouped in the same entity-class called
"NURSES", the patients into an entity-class called "PATIENTS" and the

terapeutics applied to the patients int an Entity-class called "TREAT MENTS".

Each entity of a class is described by a list of characteristics refered as "ATRIBUTES" and the values of the atributes are grouped into sets as "DOMAINS".

Example:

```
┌─────────────────────────┐
│ PATIENT                 │
├─────────────────────────┤
│ S.S.No                  │
│ Patient-name/Name       │
│ Clinical Hist.          │
│ etc....                 │
└─────────────────────────┘
```

Where:

PATINET in a class name;
S.S.No, is an attribute/
domain;Clinical History,
is an attribute.

b)- Relation-class: In these group, the entities of various classes can be associated. Associations of the same kind are grouped into classes called relations, and each relation is designated by a unique name.

A relation can be defined on two or more entity-classes. And inversely an entity-class can participate in the definition of several relations. Also one or more attributes can be associated to a relation.The type of a relation can be classified by the number of relationship existent. The classification of a relation (R) between two entity-classes (E_1) and (E_2) can be defined by:

K-L - Several entities of E_1 can be associated to E_2 and vice-versa;

1-K - One entity of E_1 can be associated to K entities of E_2;

1-1 - One entity of E_1 is associated to E_2 and vice-versa.

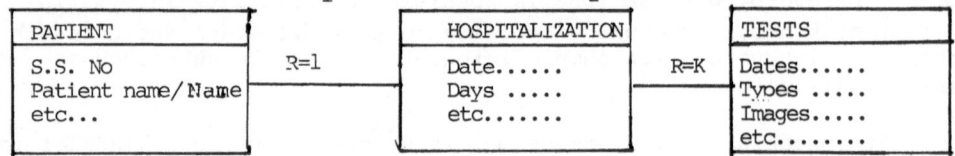

4 - TEXTUAL MODEL

A series of characteres with semantical meaning constitutes a Textual Unit. It is not restricted to the notion of a sentece or a paragraph. Commands might be inserted in a text to edit its contents in required way. A text can be for example: a summary of a clinical record of a patient or a curriculum vitae of a physician.

A text unit within a IDBS Schema, may be attributed to a class of entities. This attribute is different of data attribute refered early and it is possible to do some operations on its contents.

The lenght of a character string, at logical level, is not limited. The textual units may integrated into classes when their descriptive characteristics are identical.

Example:

```
┌─────────────────────────┐
│ PATIENT                 │
├─────────────────────────┤
│ S.S.No                  │
│ Patient-name            │
│ Address                 │
│ Clinical History        │
│ etc...                  │
└─────────────────────────┘
```

Where:

S.S. No, is a data attribute;
Patient-name, is a data attribute;
Address, is a data attribute;
Clinical History, is a text attribute

5 - PICTORIAL MODEL

Pictorial information covers, in general, all the visual represen tation of entities under different forms: simple graphics, static ima ges, dynamic images etc. However, for simplicity, dynamic images are not considered in this paper. But, whatever the type it can be proces sed at the same level by the system.

The different type of pictorial units which can be of more inter-est, in a clinical environment, can be defined as:

a)- <u>Simple graphics:</u> A simple graphic is composed of a series of: poin ts, circular arcs and straight segments in a plane. So, an entity such as: the trace of an ECG, a drawing of an element of the human body etc. can be represented. These graphics may be designed on a screen with the use of a light-pen, directly by a specific computer program or monito-red from some equipment such as an electrocardiograph. In any of the refered forms to represent a drawing a set of specific functions is used.

b)- <u>Images:</u> An image before being processed by the computer needs to be digitized. It is composed of a great number of elements called pix tels. The luminous intensity is represented by an associated digit.The simple way to digitalize a black and white static image consists in as sociate a 1 to o white point and a 0 to a black. Image size may vary from 128x128 to 4096x4096 pixels and the grayscale digitalization from 3 to 12 bits density resolution. Small dimentions, being typical for images of: CT, Digital Fluoroscopy, Ultrasound or Zooming on areas of interest, and large dimensions from chest quality images.

Typical operations which needs to be supported are for instance:

   i)- Simple direct access to name images or images sequences, to pro-vide flexibility viewing;

  ii)- Flexible spacial composition of images mosaics for side by side comparations of images of different resolutions;

 iii)- Fast and powerful images enhancements mecanisms;

  iv)- Quantitative analysis of simple images;

   v)- Ability to attach symbolic names to pictorial entities;

  vi)- Hierarchical access to images and sketch-like representations of images at various degress of resolution;

 Vii)- Support of flexible report generation and communication.

Regarding storage media for digitized images, mag. tapes and dis cs can be used but, the amount of space required is so high that such storage media for this use becomes too expensive. However, this prob-lem is partial solved by the utilization of optical discs, being the only problem the fact that the information cannot be errased.

The images can be viewed on the appropriated VDU or reported on a hard-copy, using electrostatic or laser printers.

c)- <u>Pictorial information structure:</u> In a similar way to the structu-re of a text a pictorial unit can be an attribute of an entitly-class or of a relation.

Example:

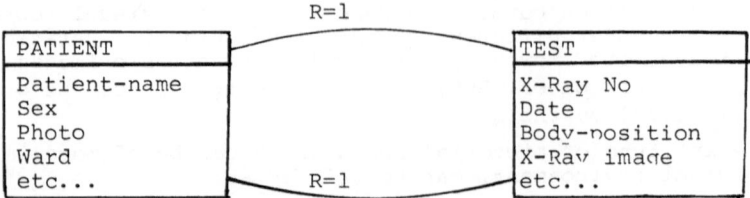

Therefore an attribute-list describes every identity, in the example refered as PATIENT, and every relationship to that identity. A code of two letters is associated to each attribute to indicate the type of in formation. So that a Data-attribute is identified by (DA), a Text-attri bute by (TA), and a Picture-attribute by (PA).

A relationship between entities and pictorial units can also be des cribed. In this kind of relationship a graphical representation of an identity is usually expressed. For example in an archive of images is possible to associate the description of every text made (entity) to its related images.

Example:

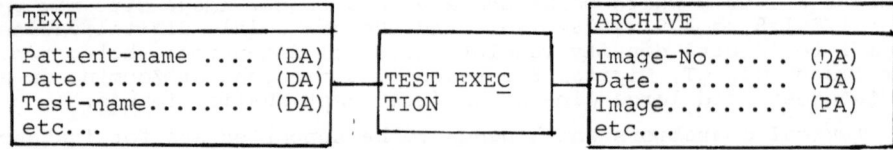

A pictorial entity is a general term which denotes either a pictorial unit or a more complex object generated from relationship between pic torial entities.

Example:

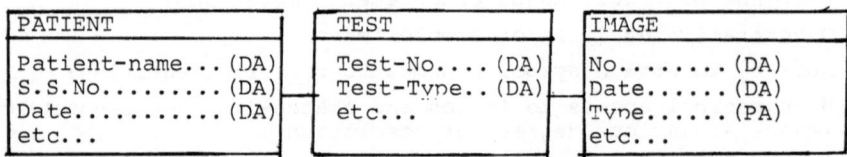

The class PATIENT contains the identification. The class TEST associa tes each test to the patient and the class IMAGE associates the Image- -type to the test.

6 - ELECTRONIC DOCUMENTS

Traditional most of the interchange of information in a hospital is done in paper, in document from. It is ussually composed of: text, graphics, data-items, tables etc., organized in logical sequence. Howe ver, paper documents as a communication system presents some problems such as: lack of security, slow transmition and difficult retrieving. Electronic systems documents minimize greatly the refered problems.

A document can be defined on the following two aspects:

  i) - Internal (logical or electronic), corresponding to the manner
           of which the document is recorded in a electronic system;

ii)- <u>External</u> (physical), which enphasizes the doment presentation on material from.

Documents are produced in four distint phases definition, edition pre sention and utilization. To describe an electronic document we have to describe at least the following two components: the logical structure and its contents.

To estabelish the structure of a document it can be decomposed in a se quence of parts called document units, which can be for instance: a ti tle, a chapter, a paragraph, a sentence etc. These document units can be of two types: simple and composed.

A simple document unit referes to homogeneous type of information, wich cannot be decomposed without losing its entirely meaning, being it a text class or an image class. For example: a date, an image, a paragraph etc. A composed document unit can be decomposed in a structu re of elementary units and sub-composed units.

7 - DOCUMENT PRODUCTION

During or after patient care, the various hospital services invol ved need to manage various technical documents related to the patients. These documents are used to provide adequate patient care or to help in research and development.

An IDBS permits integration of the following three levels of mani pulation of information, to produce a document:

a) - <u>Memory level</u>. At this level, the system mantains non-redundance as a consequence of the unique existence, in the data base, of textu al and pictorial units used in the various documents. Each docu- ment, at logical level, referes to that unit. Up-date is done only once, for all the the documents containing the same kind of infor- mation.

b)- <u>Process level</u>. At this level, the system uses a generalized program ming language to be possible to: retrieve automatically textual and pictorial units from the data base and to do manipulation of text and image together with the processing of normal data.

c)- <u>Pictorial level</u>. At this level the realization of different edi- tings of the same logical document is facilitated by the existing differences between logical and physical sqructure

8 - HARDWARE CONFIGURATION

To implement an IDBS is necessary to have, at least, the fo-lowing hardware configuration:

a)- <u>Word processing unit</u> for the manipulation of text;

b)- <u>Scanner unit</u> for digitalization of images;

c)- <u>Graphics unit</u> for CAD;

d)- <u>Secundary direct access storage unit(s)</u>, with large capacity, for storing the various types of data base;

e)- <u>Output unit</u>, Laser or electrostatic printer;

f)- <u>Central processor unit</u>, mini-computer.

9 - REFERENCES

Böhm M. and al. - Image management in the system CA/1 - SPIE,Vol.
318 - Picture archiving & Communications Systems for Medical Appli
cations(1982).

Cahuzac B. and al. - Information textuelle dans une base d'Informations Generalisee. Seminaire INFORSID, Toulouse (1982).

Chamberlin D.D. and al. JANUS: - An interactive system for document
composition. ACM SIGPLAN; SIGOA, Symposium on Manipulation Techniques. June (1981)

Chen P.P.S., - The Enttity-relation Model towards a unified view
of data. ACM, TODS, Vol. 1 (1976).

Gramps J. B. and al. - The BIG Project, second International Confe
rence on Data Bases, Cambridge (1983).

Thomas A. J. - Pictorial Information Systems and Arquitectures for
Diagnostic Imaging. SPIE, Vol. 318 - PACS (1982).

APPLICATION OF VIDEOTEX SYSTEMS TO MEDICINE

G. Pfaff[1], R. Süss[2] and M. Malter[2]

[1] Department of Paediatric Surgery,
University of Heidelberg
D-6900 Heidelberg
and
[2] Institute of Experimental Pathology,
German Cancer Research Center
D-6900 Heidelberg
Federal Republic of Germany

VIDEOTEX, the "New Medium" with the old ingredients (telephone, TV-set, post office computer) is being introduced in practically all Western European countries. Though still dominated by homebanking, electronic mail order and news services, the medical profession is just about to discover the possibilities of this new communication technology.

Published information is still scarce. We perfomed an experimental review of the existing medical programs. This survey is, however, limited: Cross country Videotex use is — to say the least — laborious; moreover, not in all cases did we find our way into closed user groups (CUG). We apologize therefore that we will dwell a little bit in some more details on our own two Videotex projects. Let us begin the commented list with the

United Kingdom

Great Britain has been the forerunner in Videotex technology and has introduced its PRESTEL system as early as in the early seventies. Besides this service of British Telecom there exist a variety of private viewdata systems.

MEDITEL is an information provider in PRESTEL. Its program aims mainly at general practitioners in the National Health Service and provides news related to managemental information and actual developments in the NHS as well as from medical societies. A daily news service reflects current articles on medical topics from the lay press. Growing attention is given to computer applications in medicine. MEDITEL serves within its CUG currently 2.200 terminals and estimates its users to number about 6.600 doctors.

TREATMENT VIEWDATA is the drug information service of a medical publisher [2] and is available via a private Videotex network. The main text of this database is derived from a loose-leaf handbook which is edited by Dr. Linda Beeley, The Queen Elizabeth Hospital, Edgbaston and Dr. V.W.M. Drury, Professor of General Practice at the University of Birmingham. The database corresponds thus to a conventionally printed book but can be updated practically any time new developments occur. The information available falls under the following categories: Therapeutic properties, contraindications, side-effects, interference with laboratory test results, recent reports of reactions and interactions, choice of drugs, comparative costs, administration, dose and preparations available.

The SCOTTISH POISONS INFORMATION BUREAU provides on a private Videotex system a database which allows authorized users (mainly hospitals but also general practitioners) to identify properties of a known toxicant, principles of its action and therapeutic countermeasures [5]. We rate this system among the best developments reviewed.

MEDILINK is a market research operation which maintains a weekly updated news service for general practitioners. This offer and a committment to pay back the telephone charges for connect time serve as an incentive for its currently 230 users to answer questions on a response frame. This serves to monitor rapidly the effect of marketing activities on the attitude of doctors towards new drugs.

The collection of data from field studies on new drugs has also been described [7].

PRESTEL has been tested for the collection of information on adverse drug reactions within the SUMIT-Project of the University of Surrey (personal communication: Professor Paul Grobb). This application is at present not further studied.

The Netherlands

The national Videotex system of the Netherlands, VIDITEL, uses PRESTEL standard. One of its information providers is the National Hospital Council ("Nationale Ziekenhuisraad"), a cooperation of hospitals. A publicly accessible set of information focusses on questions of public health care and hospital management, statistical data and the current state of health care legislation. Members of a CUG may access an actual noteboard ("NZR Prikbord") where information on forthcoming meetings, instruments and equipment to be sold or wanted and vacancies can be entered. To us, the most impressive feature is however a system used for the communication between the eight neonatal intensive care units of the country. As there is a permanent shortage of beds in these specialized treatment units, a Videotex table which is updated at least once daily lists the available beds in each unit. This facilitates the rapid organization of a transport for neonates in need of intensive paediatric care (personal communication: Dr. L.A.A. Kollee, Sint Radboutziekenhuis, Katholieke Universiteit Nijmegen).

Federal Republic of Germany

From 1980 until autumn 1984, the Deutsche Bundespost carried out a Bildschirmtext field trial based on PRESTEL in the cities of Düsseldorf and Berlin. Since autumn 1983 regular service in CEPT standard was gradually taken up and is now nationwide accessible.

Within the German Bildschirmtext (BTX) system, the MEDIZIN-BTX-POOL maintained by a medical publisher eases via an alphabetical index access to most information providers in the field of medicine. As in Great Britain, a number of pharmaceutical companies offer programs with a mixture of medicine-related news, convention calendars, new developments in drug therapy and advertisements. Only a few selected applications will be reviewed.

MEDICAL WEATHER SERVICE FOR DOCTORS: The Medical-Meteorological Research Unit of the German Weather Service (Medizin-Meteorologische Forschungsstelle des Deutschen Wetterdienstes) uses Bildschirmtext for a weather report on meteorotropic weather conditions which might influence diseases mainly of the cardiovascular and respiratory system.

Two examples from our own work. First, an effort in public medical education. In a "CANCER ENCYCLOPAEDIA" we try to compile reliable and responsible information. In a first edition some 1.000 pages described topics from risk factors to useful adresses for patients. The service has therefore attracted much attention and has found enthusiastic response in the notes left in our "mailbox".

Second, information on RARE DISEASES. The advances made in the prenatal diagnosis of fetal malformations raise the need for early and improved prognostic information on the possible outcome of pregnancy for both the expecting mother and the attending medical professionals, mainly the obstetrician and the family doctor. Due to the rare occurrence of certain malformations, the lack of experience outside specialized centers may lead in many cases to imprecise advices. In an attempt to create a source of information permanently accessible to medical professionals, an experimental database was compiled [4]. The information given refers to facts of general importance for the most common types of congenital malformations, especially prognosis and chances for therapy by planned pediatric surgery. This experiment aims at making a specialist's knowledge accessible to doctors outside specialized centres and at facilitating contacts.

The Institute of Medical Information at the University of Mainz is evaluating a private Videotex system for the collection of data on therapeutic regimens in PEDIATRIC CANCERS. To our knowledge, this application is still in a testing phase [3].

Switzerland

The Swiss PTT began in September 1984 with a nationwide Videotex field trial under CEPT. The SWISS HOSPITAL INSTITUTE (Schweizerisches Krankenhausinstitut – SKI) is one of the participants and offers access to its database via a Videotex gateway. Documents e.g. on questions of health care planning, socioeconomical topics, health status, preventive medicine and finance may be retrieved by a system combining descriptors and abstracts. The system tolerates typing errors by applying a soundex-code on free-term descriptors. Documents retrieved are available from the SKI library.

France

France follows a different approach from its neighbours both by its own national standard TELETEL and a network concept supporting many distributed databases instead of one central host. France has succeeded in overtaking Great Britain as Europe's number one in Videotex subscribers. About 4.7 percent of all French videotex applications are in the field of medicine [6] with almost 5.000 practitioners and 1.500 pharmacies already connected to TELETEL [1]. The most attractive applications combine Videotex terminals with an intelligent chip card. An experimental approach allows for example a user who identifies himself by a chip card to access background information about the medical history of a pacemaker patient. The card is kept by the patient who may hand it to his attending doctor anywhere in the country. To be mentioned are systems that allow the calculation of pensions using the central computer of the social security service (CUG) and of course public information about health care. Diagnostic and therapeutic pathways may also be checked via TELETEL. We regret that we will have most likely missed further applications of interest due to technical problems founded in the different protocols.

Other European Countries

As of January 31st, 1985, a review of the Austrian Bildschirmtext system did not yield applications to medicine. PRESTEL systems are either operational or in a testing phase in Finland, Norway, Sweden, Denmark, Spain and Italy. We could not obtain positive information about applications to medicine in the aforementioned countries. Unlike the systems described before which we accessed and searched over international telephone lines, the Videotex systems in these six countries were not reviewed by us. There are technical tests of a Videotex system in Belgium. No public Videotex systems exist in the Republic of Ireland, Luxemburg, Portugal and Greece.

Summary

Videotex is a new medium rapidly gaining acceptance as a tool for providing information in the field of medicine and health care. A variety of applications have already been developed: Health and drug information systems, note boards of medical societies, hospital associations and scientific journals, search facilities in databases, databases on registries and clinical trials and many more. Simplicity of use and a favourable cost/benefit relation invite its further development.

Acknowledgements

This review would not have been possible without the generous support of the Embassies of many states in the Federal Republic of Germany and their respective postal administrations. Most helpful was information received from: E. Davis, MEDITEL, West Bromwich; C. Ancliffe, Kluwer Publishing Ltd., Brentford; P. Barton, MEDILINK, London; Dr. A.T. Proudfoot and W.S.M. Davidson, Royal Infirmary, Edinburgh; V.G.M. Feldbrugge, Ziekenhuiscentrum, Utrecht; Mrs. R. Bäbler, SKI Aarau and H. Graf, Fa. Optima, Frankfurt. Our thanks to all of them.

References

1   Anonymous: Frankreich baut seinen Vorsprung bei Bildschirmtext zügig aus. Ärzte-Zeitung Nr. 202 (Nov. 13, 1984), 19.

2   Anonymous: TREATMENT VIEWDATA Drug Information Service. User Guide. Brentford, Middx: Kluwer Publishing Ltd. 1984.

3   Kaatsch P, Michaelis J, Rudolf S: Datenaustausch mit Hilfe von Bildschirmtext im Rahmen eines bundesweiten Registers für Malignome im Kindesalter. Proceedings, 29. Jahrestagung Deutsche Gesellschaft für Medizinische Dokumentation, Informatik und Statistik, Oktober 1984. In press: Berlin: Springer-Verlag.

4   Pfaff G, Schütze U, Schmidt H, Süss R: New ways in the counselling on prenatally diagnosed congenital malformations – an experimental application project using Bildschirmtext/Videotex. In press: Z Kinderchir 40 (1985).

5   Proudfoot AT, Davidson WSM: Acceptance of viewdata for poisons information. Br Med J 289 (1984), 1420-1421.

6   Texier AG: Teletel after two years of commercial service. In: VIDEOTEX International. Pinner, UK: Online Publications, 1984, 34-43.

7   Waldron HA, Cookson RF: Use of a viewdata system to collect data from a multicenter clinical trial in anaesthesia. Br Med J 289 (1984), 1059-1061.

"BILDSCHIRMTEXT" - THE GERMAN VIDEOTEX SYSTEM, ITS USE IN HEALTH CARE.
FUNCTIONS AND APPLICATIONS

K. Böhm
German Cancer Research Center
Central Data Processing
D-6900 Heidelberg, F.R.G.

1. Introduction

In the course of history man has developed ever new techniques for the purpose of
documentation of information and of communication. The hieroglyphs in Egypt, the
Greek alphabet, the use of paper as data carrier, the invention of the printing
press, the new media such as telephone, wireless, television, video films and, in
the area of electronics, computer storage and communication up to Videotex have been
milestones in this development. Characteristic for every new generation of data
documentation and of data carriers is the improvement of the presentation and
management by growing standardization, cheaper and faster production and reproduction
of data carriers, easier and faster transportation of information and finally - of
importance in our time - the possibility of a speedy actualization of the data.
Videotex, in German called "Bildschirmtext" or "Btx" for short, is one of the new
media also to be taken notice of in medical informatics on account of its use in
health care.

2. Function of Btx

The videotex system of the Deutsche Bundespost (DBP) is based on the information
system "Viewdata" developed in England in 1974/75 which also acted as prototype for
similar systems such as "Prestel", "Teletel" and "Videotex". The idea behind the
system is to grant every participant with minimum equipment access to an open
information network. The information network is fed by suppliers of information
who provide their data base in a computer of the DBP or in a computer of their own.
Any one can participate, e.g., a private household, in as far as it has the
following equipment:

A television set with 'decoder' (to transform the data into telepictures = Btx
pages), a remote control for the television set or a keyboard (for the interactive
dialog), a telephone (for the connection to the computer), a Btx connection box
(a modem for the transformation of data into sound frequencies on the line and vice
versa).

Thus, the investment costs for the Btx participant are in fact low. New television
sets are already equipped with a decoder (surcharge ca. DM 500,--); there is a
telephone in practically every household or every place of work; the charge for
using the Btx connection box amounts to DM 8.-- per month.

Pilot studies over several years were carried through in Düsseldorf and Berlin with 5,000 participants and 2,000 suppliers of information. In the second half of 1984 Btx was introduced nationwide. In 1985 any participant will be able to reach the Btx system at the cost of a local telephone call; in 1986 the DBP anticipates one million participants [1].

The use of the Btx system is very easy indeed. The number of the nearest Btx knot is dialled on the telephone to create a connection to the Btx central computer. The first Btx page appears on the television screen with the demand to type in a password known to the participant only. The knot computer checks the given password and uses it for accounting. Next, the participant receives a message if information from a supplier or another participant is available for him personally (comparable to the electronic mail). On the following page, there appears an overview of the Btx data bases which the participant can retrieve according to the search tree method in order to obtain a desired information. Movement within the search tree takes place by typing in a one-digit number by which the respective next page is called and appears on the television screen.

Already today the offer of information in the videotex system covers a wide range of information requirements. It is striking that this concerns long-lived information (e.g., a cancer lexicon) as well as short-lived information (e.g., the weather report). Btx is not only suitable for a passive supply of information, e.g., product information, information on timetables, events, but also for communication in dialog, e.g., for placing orders with suppliers, reservations and bank transfers.

Compared to the existing information media, the Btx system must be considered an important competition, especially for printed matter. Information like Btx pages can be quickly produced, constantly updated, distributed in seconds and is, to an increasing extent, available to anybody due to low investment costs; they meet the demand for fast, selective, brief information. In this respect, Btx is superior to printed matter.

Btx is superior to the telephone, the medium for short-lived information, by structuring and visualizing the information the quality of which remains constant. But this medium, too, is subject to essential limitations - the "cursoriness" of the information gathered. As long as there is no possibility to document the information shown on the colour screen, an essential gap remains - quite apart from the fact that the quantity of information offered is not yet sufficient - which continues to render the other media irreplaceable.

3. Applications in Health Care

Generally, it must be remarked that the expense for the installation and operation of a videotex system in a private household - as opposed to professional application - does not pay in the case of one sole application. Rather must the sum of a variety of applications form the basis for a cost-benefit calculation. The potential Btx applications in the medical field for the private household presented in the following are thus part of the entire spectrum of usage and in themselves would hardly release the procurement of a videotex equipment. The following is intended to show a variety of the possible uses of the new medium videotex in the medical field at present not yet available or merely available in rudimentary approaches. It will depend upon the publicly articulated demand and the readiness of state and private suppliers to engage themselves financially which of these applications will actually materialize.

The possibilities of medical information for the population by means of videotex can be classified into two groups:

- passive offer of information without feed-back, i.e. mere information retrieval by the user;
- offer of information with feed-back possibility, i.e. genuine communication between supplier of information and user.

3.1. Medical Information for the Public

3.1.1. General Medical Information

Today in most households general medical information is available in printed form. Even in households with but few books there is a 'home doctor' containing information on the human body, diseases and their cure. The benefit to be drawn from such a book and similar literature depends upon its traceability when actual demand arises, the frequency of use related to its costs, the intelligibility and presentation of the information, its specification and actuality.

It appears quite feasible that the demand for information regarding elementary anatomical and physiological functions of the human body may be covered by a supply per videotex. Since this demand for information occurs relatively rarely, its satisfaction by using Btx is less expensive than the purchase of a book. On the other hand, there is little need to update such information and the presentation in print is superior to Btx presentation so that materialization in videotex covering supplier's costs does not appear to be promising. Rather is the videofilm a serious competitor for the book, since its manner of presenting anatomical and physiological processes renders it superior.

3.1.2. Information about Prevention

In view of the wealth of information provided by the established media on the subject of prevention, the question must be raised whether the new medium videotex is to add a further offer in this direction. Since, in this field, there is little need of updating information, conventional media such as printed matter and television should be given preference on account of their better form of presentation. However, an offer in videotex provides unequivocal advantages in case of actual demand for particular information.

For example, the sporadic publications in the conventional media make it impossible to determine when, how often which inoculations are required for certain groups of persons (children, persons travelling overseas, occupational groups). Though the conventional media report on newly occurring health risks such as AIDS or certain drugs, obtaining such information is rather accidental for the individuum and cannot be repeated if the need arises. Thus, the benefit of videotex as a carrier of information in the field of medical prevention is based on the possibility of supplying a comprehensive offer of information, making relevant information accessible to the user at any time if the need arises.

3.1.3. Information on Early Detection

In the field of the early detection of diseases, information about screening methods with regard to cancer and cardiovascular diseases as well as with infants should be mentioned. In these instances, videotex information presenting the usefulness, the necessary frequency and the course of such a medical check-up would be to the purpose in order to reduce the fear of these measures and to attain a greater participation of the population. Moreover, benefits and techniques of self-diagnosis could be presented.

In the field of cancer, the German Cancer Research Center has since 1981 been offering a "cancer lexicon" in videotex at present comprising 1,000 Btx pages and also informing about prevention and early detection. Already at this time users show great interest in the "cancer lexicon" so that this can be assumed to be a purposeful application of videotex [2].

3.2. Btx for the Communication with Medical Institutions

Apart from the latent need of the population for medical information which will have to be updated to but a minor extent, there is another spectrum of information which will be required by private households under critical circumstances. What is meant is the use of information services.

3.2.1. Topical Information Services

In an acute situation, the medical emergency service can be immediately reached practically anywhere via telephone. Contrary to Btx, a telephone conversation permits direct communication about the steps to be taken and is thus superior to Btx application.

If, however, there is no emergency but merely a need for information about
- when which practice has consulting hours;
- whether and for how long a practice is closed, e.g., on account of holidays;
- which practices act as substitutes;
- which pharmacies are on night duty,

the satisfaction of this need for information, particularly outside office hours, is often hardly possible. It is true that this information is largely printed in the local newspapers. However, when needed, it is frequently not traceable. Finding out about a substitute and his/her consulting hours outside office hours may also be tedious or even impossible.

A corresponding offer in videotex, which has today been partially realized, is apt to close this gap and to provide the topical information at any time.

3.2.2. Poison Center

A similar situation exists in case of actual need for information about the address of the nearest poison center. In order to compare the effectivity of the Btx system with conventional retrieval of information via telephone, an experiment was carried through in Heidelberg. Dialling the Btx computer of the DBP, browsing through the key-word index and selecting the relevant supplier with the correct address of the nearest poison center required 11 Btx pages. The entire process took exactly two minutes.

The same search using the telephone directory at once showed that a relevant entry for "poisoning" or a similar term was missing in the telephone directory. Telephone calls with the Heidelberg university hospitals yielded different results. Apart from time-consuming cross-references to other hospitals, correct information was also given; however, each process took at least two minutes.

A comparison of the results shows that already today the Btx service is as effective as the existing sources of information and even superior to them as far as the constancy of the quality of information is concerned.

3.2.3. Drug Information

Information about side effects of drugs, cosmetics and cleaners used in the household turns up within creasing frequency. This information is spread by the media; it is, however, sporadic, reaches the individual user rather by chance and cannot be retrieved in toto and selectively if need arises. Here a full updated offer of information in videotex, e.g., in connection with tips for the equipment and upkeep of a medicine chest, should be basically useful. In particular, this applies to the announcement of side effects with drugs as they are given on the packet insert which are frequently not traceable when needed.

3.2.4. Fixing Dates

Every Btx participant automatically receives "electronic mail" where other Btx participants may leave personal messages. Sending such a Btx page costs 40 Pfennige, that is less than the postage for a postcard.

Communications of private households with the above named medical institutions refer essentially to fixing dates with practices and ordering ambulance services. Fixing the first date via telephone is definitely to be preferred to doing so per videotex on account of the direct communication of the two partners; if, however, one of the two partners cannot be reached via telephone - the practice out of office hours, the private person not at home during the daytime -, the Btx message, especially for scheduling consultations, e.g., for a follow-up examination, and postponing consultations, can be a useful complement, less expensive and faster than normal mail.

3.2.5. Financial Transactions with Physicians and Insurances

The business transactions of private patients with medical institutions are more complex than those of patients with obligatory health insurance. The private patient receives a bill directly from the physician. The amount in question is then transferred in the conventional manner by filling in a transfer form which is forwarded to a bank.

Videotex offers the possibility of "home banking" already today; the transfer is then arranged from the patient's home. For this purpose, the Btx participant dials the computer of his bank, is informed about the last bookings and the actual balance and can fill in and send off a preformated page for the transfer. He thus saves the way to the bank or the postage, and the payment is made more quickly.

This also applies in a similar manner to the reimbursement of costs of medical treatment to the patient by private health insurances.

3.2.6. Btx Communication for Disabled Persons

A group of the population, whose communication with their environment and with social institutions is severely restricted due to physical disablement, is formed by persons who are deaf, blind, non-vocal or motorically handicapped. Their living space is mostly limited to the domestic sphere, and an optimal communication with the outside world is, therefore, of particular importance.

Deaf and/or non-vocal individuals cannot use the most important means of communication, the telephone.

In the living space of the disabled, which is restricted to their own domestic sphere, Btx grants access to sources of information, education, games, tele-shopping, business transactions and communication. If two participants are logged onto the Btx system at the same time, they will be able to exchange personal messages interactively, i.e. to communicate almost as using the telephone.

Contrary to persons who cannot hear or speak, but can use videotex without restrictions, motorically handicapped persons may, according to the type of their disability, encounter difficulties when operating the input keyboard. For this reason, special input devices have been developed, particularly in North America, enabling, for instance, a control and operation of the keyboard by mouth [3].

The use of videotex does not present any problems today for motorically handicapped persons able to operate an input keyboard. For them and, to an increased extent, for persons suffering from an impairment of hearing and/or speech Btx opens up new possibilities of enlarging their living space by additional access to information and communication and thus to become active members of society.

References

[1] Bundesministerium für das Post- und Fernmeldewesen (Hrsg.):
     Die Post informiert über Bildschirmtext.
     Bundesministerium für das Post- und Fernmeldewesen 1983

[2] Goerttler, K.
     Aufbau eines aktuellen Krebslexikons.
     In: Geschäftsbericht für das Jahr 1981.
     Hrsg.: Krebsverband Bad.Württ. e.V. Stuttgart (1982)

[3] Staisey, N.L., Tombaugh, J.W., Dillon, R.F.
     Videotex and the disabled.
     Int.J.Man-Machine Studies 17, 35-50 (1982)

REPORT OF A PILOT STUDY TO EXAMINE THE USE OF INTERACTIVE VIDEODISC CARDIOPULMONARY RESUSCITATION INSTRUCTION

Margaret Edwards
Associate Professor
The University of Calgary
2500 University Drive N.W.
CALGARY, Alberta
Canada   T2N 1N4

The linkage of computer technology with interactive video has allowed for the development of innovative health education delivery methods. The American Heart Association has developed a self-training system for cardiopulmonary resuscitation (CPR) that utilizes both technologies. Development of the CPR learning system began in 1980[1] with production models becoming available in late 1983.[2] Components of the CPR learning system are a Sony VDP-1000 laser optical videodisc player, two monitors, an Apple II computer, a random access audio machine and a light pen. Also included is a sensorized Laerdal manikin (adult and infant) which provides input to the computer concerning performance skills. The CPR learning system exemplifies the zenith of the new hybrid technologies. One of the remarkable features of the system is the capability of stopping the videodisc at a certain address, and while keeping the disc stopped, providing voice over instruction via the random access audio machine. This capability allows for over four hours of instruction to be provided through the use of only one thirty-minute videodisc. A second feature of interest is that the CPR learning system has segments that are voice activated. For example, in performing two-rescuer CPR, the learning system functions as the second rescuer. When a student is performing compressions and the learning system is providing ventilations in response to the compression rate, the student can shout "change" and the learning system will begin to provide compressions while the student commences ventilations. The CPR learning system provides an excellent example of very high interactivity. The CPR learning system is a menu-driven program. This facility allows the student to be in complete control of the learning sequence. The student can stop the instruction at any time, or he/she can choose the section to be viewed. Other menu selections include review of sections, manikin practice, vocabulary check and frame stepping. The third feature of interest is the sensorized manikin.

Traditional CPR manikins produce, at the end of practice, a paper tape scribed in response to compressions and ventilations. The sensors in the CPR learning system manikin sense all the steps in a CPR assessment.

The sensors include: a mercury switch that responds to a 10° change in position, allowing assessment of shaking a victim to establish unresponsiveness; a light sensor in the manikin's chin, sensing the checking for respirations by looking, listening and feeling; a voice sensor which registers a call for help; and a carotid pulse generator and sensor that records the checking of the pulse. The input of the sensors is shown on the monitor as a computer graphic within one-thirtieth of a second of the stimulating performance. The immediate feedback to the student in terms of skills performance allows the student to very quickly make the changes necessary to meet performance criteria.

All of these technological considerations that explain the CPR learning system lay the ground work for examining the learner benefits[3] of the system. Because the CPR learning system can so quickly evaluate a student's performance, far more precise and immediate coaching about the student's sequence and depth and rhythm of compressions and ventilations can be provided by the system than by a traditional human instructor. Adult learning principles indicate that learning is more effective when the learner is in charge of the learning situation, as in the use of the CPR learning system. Individual needs of each student are further met through the provision of different levels of explanation, implementing a "mosaic" concept of learning. In addition to the benefit given to the individual, use of the mosaic approach allows for the satisfaction of several different levels of learning needs or programs by one system using the same videodisc. Standardized information, presentation, coaching and testing would also seem to contribute to a more consistent learner output as well as addressing the problem of lack of standardization among human instructors.

Theoretically, the use of the CPR learning system has many positive features providing learner benefits. However, during the system verification only one small study of nursing students without CPR experience was conducted by the developer. As the study was for internal component testing purposes only and not to establish the efficacy of this delivery method as a teaching strategy, there are no plans for publication of these results.

After viewing a prototype of the CPR learning system in 1982 and desiring to investigate this novel delivery method, a system was obtained in January 1984 through a Canadian Heart Foundation grant. The

Canadian Heart Foundation also supported the pilot study of the CPR learning system that will now be reported.[4]

A pilot study to begin to examine the validity and reliability of the CPR learning system as a teaching method was conducted by researchers in the Faculty of Nursing at the University of Calgary commencing in January 1984. Specifically, information was sought to address the following questions: what is the nature of the relationship between group membership (control=traditional instruction, experimental=CPR learning system instruction) and initial cognitive knowledge score, initial skills performance, gain score (pre-test to post-test), three month and twelve month cognitive knowledge retention and three month and twelve month skills retention; and what are the notable relationships that appear to exist between the above measures and variables such as age, gender, education and computer experience.

The population for the pilot study included sixty-five employees of a major oil company that routinely offers CPR training. The design for the pilot study was quasi-experimental utilizing control and experimental groups measured along two dimensions - skills and cognitive knowledge at three times-immediate post-training, three months post-training and twelve months post-training. In addition, a demographic data sheet and a cognitive knowledge pre-test were completed prior to the instruction in either group. As was previously mentioned the control group was taught by traditional methods including lectures, slides and skills practice while the experimental group was taught solely by the CPR learning system.

The statistical results of the pilot study can be summarized very succinctly. Using Crosstabulations with Yates' corrected Chi-square statistic or Fisher's exact test statistic and Students' T-test[5] for matched pairs, there were no significant differences noted between the control group and the experimental group along the dimensions of initial cognitive knowledge, initial skill performance, gain score, three month cognitive knowledge retention, three month skills retention, twelve month cognitive knowledge retention and twelve month skills retention.

These results are summarized in Table 1.0.

Table 1.0 - Summary of Crosstabulations[*]/T-tests[t] of Group by
        Seven Dimensions

Dimension	df	probability
initial cognitive knowledge	5	0.2697[*]
initial skills performance	1	1.0[*]
gain score	60	0.68[t]
3 month cognitive knowledge	32	0.786[t]
3 month skills performance	1	0.4895[*]
12 month cognitive knowledge	24	0.1696[*]
12 month skills performance	1	1.0[*]

Two entries in Table 1.0 require explanation. Both traditional
instruction and the CPR learning system coach to mastery in skills performance; therefore, there were no failures. The twelve month skills
retention reflects the dismal fact that no person in either the control
or the experimental group demonstrated a passing performance when re-
tested.

The interpretation of the results requires firstly a reminder that
as this was a pilot study with an "n" of sixty-five, statements of
universal prediction cannot be made based on the results. The statement that can be made is that these results begin to demonstrate that
the CPR learning system is able to provide instruction to students that
enables them to do as well on standardized cognitive and skills tests
as students taught by traditional instructions. The pilot study design
is currently being replicated using a sample of four hundred people.

A major supplementary finding of the pilot study was the determination of the amount of time utilized by a student in completing a
course through the CPR learning system. Prior to the inception of the
pilot study many combinations of numbers of people and hours were tried.
The optimum condition seems to be three people working with the system,
at the same time, for eight hours to complete a CPR course for the
first time. Traditional courses require sixteen hours to complete and
are taught by one instructor to eight people at a time. One of the
greatest potentials of this technology is the time saving incurred.
The shortened learning time resulting from the interactivity, remedi-
ation and reinforcement of the CPR learning system translates into less
lost productivity and greater monetary advantage to companies providing
such instruction to their employees.[6] For the individual student the

shortened learning time seems to translate into less decreases in motivation and concentration due to fatigue, as well as decreasing the number of days one must be away from his own job responsibilities.

The CPR learning system can be viewed as the standard-bearer for interactive videodisc instruction. The learning advantages seen to result from use of the system can be predicted to occur in other applications of this hybrid technology, provided that the same degree or greater degrees of interactivity are achieved. Within the nursing and medical communities there exists many skills that could be taught by similar technologies. Additionally, where vast geographical areas must be serviced with continuing education, for example, interactive videodisc technology is particularly appropriate as well as being a very efficient and convenient delivery method. As the technology of interactive videodisc instruction becomes increasingly more popularized, nursing and medicine will want to carefully examine this alternative delivery method.

References Cited

1. Hon, D. Interactive training in cardiopulmonary resuscitation. <u>Byte</u>: 108
June, 1982.

2. Cassidy, D. Chairman, Interact Inc., Oklahoma City, Oklahoma, U.S.A.
personal communication, June 29, 1982, August 9, 1982.

3. Edwards, MJA & Hannah, KJ. An examination of interactive videodisc CPR
instruction for the lay community. In <u>Proceedings of C.O.A.C.H. Conference VIII,</u>
Halifax, Nova Scotia, Canada, May 13 - 16, 1984.

4. Edwards, MJA & Hannah, KJ. An examination of the use of interactive videodisc
cardiopulmonary resuscitation instruction for the lay community. In <u>Proceedings</u>
<u>of First Annual Nursing Conference on Computer-Assisted Interactive Video Instruction</u>,
Sacremento, California, U.S.A., February 27 - March 1, 1985.

5. Nie, NH, et al. <u>Statistical Package for the Social Sciences (2nd edition)</u>,
Toronto, Ontario, Canada: McGraw-Hill Book Company, 1975.

6. Edwards, MJA. A cost analysis comparison of traditional and interactive videodisc CPR instruction. In <u>Proceedings of International Symposium on Nursing Use</u>
<u>of Computers and Information Sciences</u>, Calgary, Alberta, Canada, May 1 - 3, 1985.

TELEMEDICINE: NEW APPLICATIONS AND DEVELOPMENTS

A.ROBERTO, G.VALENTINI
SIP-DIREZIONE GENERALE
ROME-ITALY

- INTRODUCTION

Research and experiments over the past twenty years have shown that the joint resources of informatics and telecommunications are capable not only of providing medical care to patients far from health centres (telediagnosis systems), but make other advantageous innovations in the health system possible, in particular with regard to first-aid services, hospital management, keeping medical personnel up to date and training paramedical personnel (tele-health).

The human and social advantages of telemedicine can be resumed, briefly:
- better utilization of the various skills and structures of the health system;
- more effective and timely diagnosis in case of emergency treatment (first aid);
- assistance to patients while being moved (ambulances);
- constant availability to small hospitals of the skills and knowledge of specialists;
- more health care for outlying communities and greater access to the National Health Care Service;
- possibility of checking patients in their homes (monitoring);
- provision of guidance to paramedical personnel;
- less need to move patients and shorter hospitalization periods;
- wider possibilities of teaching, medical up-dating, training of paramedical personnel and health education;
- availability of already organized emergency services in case of disasters (calamities);
- propagation of health education.

Telemedicine also permits considerable economies to be made in costs. There is no doubt, in fact, that a substantial share of human and social costs of the Italian health care service are due, on the one hand, to the length of hospitalization periods, to moving of patients and, on the other hand, to the irrational proliferation of analyses, to waste of medicaments, to lack of hygiene and of preventive care: in other words, to factors which can, to a great extent, be remedied by telemedicine.

It's a matter of course that such benefits cannot be achieved unless there is a constant and firm commitment to experimenting the resources offered by informatic and telecommunication technologies. There is a need, in fact, for research, both in hardware and software, and for extensive field testing, in other to evaluate, step by step, the various needs of the national health care system and the relevant possible solution .

This is the way in which SIP, the italian company for the domestic communications, has been and is working, in collaboration with hospitals, universities and industries, proposing apparatus and telemedicine systems for different branches of medicine, both to assist in medical diagnosis and to contribute to the renewal of the health services, all this without neglecting research for new solutions in the field of biomedical technologies. Following it's described what has been done and what we hope will be possible to do in the closest future.

- CARDIOLOGY
- Cardiotelephone

A transceiver apparatus used for transmission of electrocardiograms, complete with 12 leads.

It permits collection and transmission from outlying points (for instance, consulting rooms, first aid station, sport centers, civilian emergency units, ships at sea, patients being monitored at home etc.) to a center equipped with receiving units supervised by cardiologists.

The receiving unit permits to display simultaneously, on a monitor, the signals transmitted and, on a paper recorder, the related tracing.

The portability and the easy usability of the transceiver, as well as the great precision on the signals recorded by the receiver, are the main characteristics of the cardiotelephone, which is indispensale in emergencies in order to have a correct diagnosis and a subsequent appropriate treatment.

The cardiotelephone is at present on the SIP list.

- Cardio-bip

A portable apparatus used to record, memorise and transmit a standard ECG branch.

It allows hearth patients suffering from arhythmia to record an attack as soon as it starts and subsequently to transmit the signal, by means of a simple acoustic connection with a normal telephone, to a center equipped with receiving apparatus and supervised by specialized medical personnel.

The small dimensions of the transmitting unit, the high level of technology and the tremendous assistance which it can give to health patients are the main characteristics of the Cardio-bip.

The Cardio-bip is on the market from 1/1/85 on.

- Automatic processing system for electrocardiograms.

The system consist of three parts:
- a central processing and memorization unit based on a HP series 1000 computer (the possibility of the latter to be placed into a SIP exchange is being studied);
- one or more consoles to be installed in highly specialized coronary units, both at regional and national level, where the ECG tracings processed will be displayed and the diagnoses checked by experts;
- portable terminals (to be distributed to outlying places, small hospitals, various specialized departments, first-aid station, schools, industries, etc.) which make it possible to:
-    take the electrocardiograms and print them on the spot on millimetre paper;
-    memorize up to a maximum of twenty tracing, with the possibility of reprinting them;
-    transmit the information to the processing center, where the results are printed and checked by an expert.

The system also permits all the tracings to be filed in a magnetic memory for subsequent comparison and for statistical purposes.

This system is at present in an axperimental phase.

- NEUROLOGY
- Tele-electroencephalograph

A transceiver apparatus used for the transmission of complete electroencephalograms from a hospital or outlying consulting room to a center presided by neurologists or neurosurgeons.

The apparatus has a particularly wide application in emergencies where it is necessary to evaluate, in the shortest possible time, serious pathologies, such as the conditions of an injured person, a state of coma, an epileptic fit and any neurological disturbances.

The apparatus is being experimented in the Neurological Clinic of the Umberto 1 polyclinic in Rome.

- HAEMATOLOGY
- Tele-analysis

Apparatus used for the complete transission of blood and urine tests.

It consists of a transmitter, situated in a remote locality and used by unspecialized personnel, linked to a central analysis laboratory.

The receiving apparatus is capable of controlling the transmitter by means of a computer which can evaluate the validity of the tests and subsequently produces a document giving the patient's name and listing the results of the tests, pointing out those with pathological characteristics.

Tele-analysis avoids to bring far away patients to laboratories, effects the analyses promptly and,moreover, supply surgeons, in hospitals that have no laboratories, with data essential for an emergency operation.

The system is being experimented in Emilia Romagna between the hospitals of Alfonsine and Lugo di Romagna.

- RADIOLOGY
- Teleconsultation system

The system allows consultations between medical centers, distant from each other, with the same or different specializations. It can be used as part of the normal routine of a hospital department or, in emergencies, in a first aid center whenever it's necessary to have a "consultation" with teams in other departments of the same hospital or in other hospitals.

Any center can, therefore, avail itself of the advice of experts in the sector present in the principal institutions, universities or others. Successively, depending on the result of the consultation and on the needs of the situation, the patient may be cared entirely in the original center or transferred to another more suited to his case, or, if necessary, treated partly in one and partly in the other.

In this way, unnecessary moves and stays in hospital are reduced, the regional health structures are more evenly distributed and, furthermore, the knowledge of medical techniques and technologies, that now is the prerogative of only a few specialized centers, will be made more widely available.

The system permits:
- the transmission of picture (x-ray, tracings, documents, hospital files, picture of patients, etc.);
- the transmission of text, tabulations and drawnings;
- the transmission of voice in full-duplex;
- access to data banks.

Trasmission and reception of pictures is done by means of a telecamera, of a monitor and of a high definition "still picture video" apparatus. The latter takes the picture from the telecamera or from other biomedical instruments, and subdivides into 256X256 basic picture elements (pixels) each with 256 level of grey. The pixels are then transmitted sequentially to the receiving station where the picture is recomposed and displayed on the monitor. Transmission time is about 40 seconds.

Transmission of text is done by means of the fac-simile terminal which permits any type of written information to be reproduced at a distance: typescript, manuscript, drawings, printed matter, etc. (the model used permits the reproduced of 8 levels of grey).

In this way the teleconsultation centers can:
- book, or in first aid centers request, a teconsultation session by sending a standard form (these types of terminal are equipped with automatic answering and identification of the caller);
- transfer the documentation related to patients, such as anamnesis, hospital files, results of lab tests, plans for treatment, prescriptions, tracings, etc.;
- confirm a diagnosis or treatment by sending the signature of the doctor in charge of the case;
- use it for administrative and management purposes or, simply, as an electronic mail system.

The audio connection between the two centers is done by means of "direct voice" apparatuses which, having microphones and laudspeakers separate from the telephone receiver, ensure autonomy of work and of consultation. It's possible, in fact, not only to work with "free-hands", but also permits simultaneous communication between the members of the two teams present in the respective rooms.

Connection with data-banks is made by a TTY terminal, asynchronous, suitable for remote-job entry operations. Furthermore, the use of the public switched network gives access to:

- national and foreign data bases, for bibliographical up-dating;
- calculation centers for programs and data of general or statistical type (indispensable for processing the data of patients of the participating centers, for checking the quality of the treatment plans, etc.);
- and, in the future, Expert Systems and Computer Conference networks.

Use at present consists of a network of centers for oncologic radio-diagnosis. The experimental phase was completed on 30/6/84 and the system is now on the SIP list.

- High resolution tele-consultation system

Although the tele-consultation meets the present requirements, it is not, and is not intended to be, in it's final form. Experiments carried out have, in fact, shown what innovations should be introduced and what types of apparatus should be used.

For this purpose a new system of tele-consultation is in the experimental phase, consistong of:
- high resolution still-picture video apparatous capable of memorizing and transmitting picture of 512X512 basic picture elements;
- very high definition and sensitivity telecamera, with an ultricon type tube, with more than 700 lines at the center of the picture;
- a high persistance and definition monitor with large bandwidth;
- possibility of analogue registration (on audio band) of the picture to be transmitted or of those received.

The system will be assembled in a rack, fitted with wheels for easy movability, and will include the previously described apparatuses, as well as:
- the diaphonoscope, mounted, for the operator's convenience, on the work table and fitted with a light intensity regulator for a better picture lighting;
- the telecamera, mounted on a joined head to enable the patient, or part of him, to be filmed (an auxiliary video entry permits the telecamera also to be mounted on a tripod with wheels);
- the control panel and the interface to any other biomedical instruments.
The first prototypes of the system are expected to be ready in May 85.

- Transmission of digital diagnostic images.

Current radiographic systems utilise for the data acquisition and display a film screen area detector, chemical processor, illuminated display and film archiving.

This systems are characterised by excellent resolution but have relatively poor contrast, sensitivity and dynamic range. They are also inefficient in storage, retrieval and transmission of image data. A considerable amount of radiography involves the use of contrast media to opacify vessels and organs of interest. On the contrary, current approches to digital imaging improve dynamic range and contrast sensitivity and add capability for image manipulation, interactive analysis and quantitative informations. Moreover, data storage and retrieval is easy and economical being based on magnetic tape or disc and advances await developments in optical disc technology.

Digital diagnostic system allow, at real time frame rates, the selection of optimum reading curve, windowing, contrast enhacement and frame averaging. Moreover, digital equipment may olso be used for post image analysis and forprocessing functions such as image arithmetic such as smoothing, edge detection and for quantitative analysis of spatial density disytribution and statistics required in different analysis.

Tipical digital diagnostic systems are the digital radiography, the X-ray computerized tomography, ultrasound with the sonographic imaging, the doppler imaging and the transmission reconstruction imaging, the nuclear magnetic resonance and others with less diffusion.

In this field, in response to numerous request from users, a system capable of taking, transmitting and memorizing TAC pictures is being studied.

The study aims at a communication protocol suitable for transmission of this particular type of information and the realization of interfaces which can be connected with the principal manufacturers presently on the italian market.

The system also provides for the use of personal computers which, among other things, will allow the use of programs suited for the handling of a pictures file and of a whole X-ray department. Local processing of the pictures to be transmitted and/or received will be possible, such as:
- contrasts enhacement;
- edge detection;
- compression and decompression;
- enlargements;
- high-pass, low-pass numerical filtering;
- equalization of distribution of greys;
- calculation of distances, perimeters and areas;
- transformation by rotation and/or specularity;
- extraction of isolevel curves;
- definition of single or multiple interest curves;
- calculation of statistical parameter;
- comparison of values taken from previous picture, etc.

- NEPHROLOGY
- Home dialisis
A preliminary agreements is being negotiated with CSELT concerning the industrialization of a system in the field af dialysis at home.
The system envisages a control center capable of collecting data on the working of the dialysis machines whether in operation in homes or in consulting rooms.

- OBSTETRICS
- Perinatal medicine
Within the framework of the National Programme for Research in Telemedicine, instituted by the Ministry for Scientific and Technological Research, SIP is partecipating, in agreement with the University of Perugia, Mistel S.p.A. and Biotronix s.r.l., in the experimentation and the putting into operation of a system of home monitoring for care of expectant mothers at risk, by means of the transmittion of fetal heart frequency signals and uterine pressure.
The system consist of a transmission apparatus which is given to the patient and of an apparatus installed in a maternity hospital, supervisited by specialists round the clock.
The expectant mother, at intervals established by the doctor or in case of suspected alarm, can connect herself with the control center, transmit the signals of the fetal heart frequency and TOCO signals and receive, through the normal domestic telephone receiver, the instructions and advice of the specialist.
The system, for what concerne the positioning of the transducer is such that the apparatus can be safely used by any patient after a short practice period.
Furthermore, the instrumentation uses doppler type ultrasonic techniques and makes a double correlation of the signals, using both the information on power and on short and long term speed. This guarantees an accurate evaluation of the signals and enables their transmission by telephone line with absolutely no distortion, even when the lines are very disturbed.
A prototype of the transmission apparatus has already been made and is under experimentation at the University of Perugia. Manufacture and commercialization of the system is expected to start this year.
The research programme also includes:
- a system for the prevention of apnea in premature babies and of cot deaths of newborn babies at home;
- a mobile unit equipped with apparatus for maternal-fetal tele-monitoring and assistance and rianimation of the expectant mother, of the fetus and of the newborn child at risk.

CANADA'S NEW MANAGEMENT INFORMATION SYSTEM GUIDELINES

by: Betty Lowry, M.I.S. Project Director

In Canada, the longstanding concern for the development of standards
and maintenance of solid management tools in the health care field
has, until recently, mainly concentrated on accounting standards as
provided in the various editions of the Canadian Hospital Accounting
Manual. In the last decade, the "Information Revolution" has focused
attention on the problems and possibilities of national cooperation on
health care issues, particularly good management of resources. The
time came to find, develop, and document tools that would go beyond
accounting standards and that would, therefore, help any size or type
of health care facility manage its resources more effectively and make
useful contributions to the ongoing national dialogue on health care.

Over one million dollars was provided by the Federal and Provincial
Governments to fund the initial three year Management Information
System Project and close to two million dollars is being funded by
Governments and Provincial Hospital Associations to support the M.I.S.
Project Team for implementation and maintenance of the Guidelines
during the next three year period commencing in 1985.

The M.I.S. Guidelines provide departmental managers with tools for
effective resource management. They also provide executives, trustees, and physicians with sound information on which to base resource
allocation decisions, and with which to assess the impact on resource
utilization of various kinds and methods of treatment and services.

Effective management depends on comprehensive information. The Guidelines describe the information that must be recorded, relate the information to its source in a functional centre, and suggest an organization for the collection and reporting process.

The Guidelines are not a substitute for thoughtful decision-making;
they only provide input (information) to the decision-making process.
The Guidelines also do not address the question of quality assurance.
They measure only what is utilized and what is produced in the operation of the facility; they do not measure what is "best" or "right" in

the relationship between resource utilization and services provided. Finally, the Guidelines are not, in themselves, a management information system. They do not obviate the necessity for detailed system specifications in the system's planning process. Rather, the Guidelines give health care facilities a common ground for recording and comparing information. Where, how, and when the information is collected is the choice of the individual facility.

The complete set of Guidelines comprises these features:

° A structure consisting of three frameworks, or views of the information being collected by a facility; the departmental/ global dimension framework, the management information systems framework, and an underlying functional grouping referred to as the functional centre framework.

The departmental and global dimension framework of the Guidelines will assist facilities in determining what they need to know in order to manage resources effectively. To this end, the departmental/global dimension framework identifies the resource utilization and cost reporting structure within which all other aspects of the Guidelines have been developed. It also answers the following questions:

° What resources are required to produce a specific product within a specific department? (departmental dimension)

° How many and what kinds of resources are required to provide a specific kind of care or to treat a specific patient or patient group? (global dimension)

Each dimension has its own set of inputs and outputs:

TABLE A
Departmental/Global Dimension Inputs and Outputs

Departmental Dimension		Global Dimension	
Inputs	Outputs	Inputs	Outputs
Earned hours Supplies Equipment Purchased services etc. Allocated Overheads	Units of service identified by Workload measurement systems	Units of service	Numbers and kinds of patients treated

The departmental dimension enables administrators to manage resources effectively by treating the department as a business, and by relating, in a standard manner, the resources utilized to products produced, thus determining the costs of specific services.

In the global dimension, the units of service produced in each department are assigned to specific inpatient, ambulatory care, research, education and ancilliary services. As a result, independent or collective analysis of resource utilization and costs, by specific patients, or patient groups, or other services can be performed.

The management information systems framework proposes what information should be collected what processing performed, and what reports produced. Well-planned information systems, whether manual or automated, will not only fulfill their functions as individuals systems (i.e. central registry, payables, order entry, etc.) but are designed to work in support of the information structure laid out in the Guidelines.

The M.I.S. Project studied current health care systems for their usefulness in a variety of areas, particularly the production of useful information for department managers. The reporting requirements of the agencies which regulate health care in Canada were also checked, and a list of possible system applications for health care facilities was drawn up.

The discussion of each system covers the purpose of the application, the objectives and functions and identifies the data elements and reports to be generated by the system.

The functional centre framework is a lavered breakdown of all the functions that can possibly be carried out in a health care facility. Other features of the Guidelines are based on this functional centre framework.

The functional centre framework makes logical and practical divisions by function. These divisions are standard, but the individual facility decides what level of detail to adopt in its record-keeping. In the example, facilities which separate their high-risk antepartum mothers from the general post/antepartum population may keep detailed "level 5" records. Other, smaller facilities, which do not treat any high-risk mothers, may keep records only at the third or fourth level of detail. It is up to the management to decide how much information is needed.

When it comes to reporting the information, facilities can indicate the level from which the data is drawn. Statistical comparison among facilities, therefore, becomes simpler and more valid. Comparisons can either be drawn between facilities that report on the same level of detail, or the data can be "rolled up" until all facilities can be compared at a less detailed level. (It should be noted, though, that the higher the level of comparison, the less reliable the conclusions.)

For each function at each level, the functional centre framework also gives a description of the function, and a specification of what the function includes/excludes.

Within the three major frameworks just described, the M.I.S. Guidelines provide definitions, accounting and workload measurement systems, statistics and indicators, and also provide managers with guidance and how to apply the information in management functions.

° In any information-gathering effort, everyone involved must have a clear idea of what is being recorded. Whenever two people use the same term to signify different things, or whenever two or more terms are used interchangeably for the same idea, statistical comparisons become questionable. Definitions are therefore an integral part of the Guidelines. All terms used within the context of the Guidelines are defined, and all information items that are, or might be, recorded by a health care facility are listed.

° The M.I.S. Accounting Guidelines provide a new chart of accounts, a chart of statistics, and expanded discussions of current accounting issues. Items of particular interest in the new Accounting Guidelines include:

° a <u>modular chart of accounts</u> with variable length coding
   structure, which supports financial statements on the integrated basis and the funded basis;

° a <u>chart of statistics</u> that defines the non-financial component of the indicators;

° <u>updated procedures</u> to account for revenues, compensation expense, purchased services, equipment operation expense,
   acquisition and renewal of capital assets, and a <u>revised</u>
   <u>format</u> for general purpose financial statements;

° <u>cost accounting methodologies</u> for the allocation of Administrative and Support Service expense in order to determine
   the full cost of operating departments and providing patient
   care and other services, and for the development of unit
   costs as a departmental management tool and a link to program and patient costing.

° The M.I.S. Project has adopted existing workload measures in a
variety of diagnostic and therapeutic services (developed under
the aegis of the Sub-Committee on Productivity Improvement,
Health and Welfare Canada) as an integral part of the Guidelines. Workload measures in other diagnostic and therapeutic
services, which are now under development, will be adopted when
complete.

In the nursing and ambulatory care services, existing workload
measurement systems were reviewed. Using these as a basis, the
M.I.S. Project developed criteria for workload measurement in
nursing that will help to standardize the collection and reporting of workload information.

Wherever workload measures have not been available, and are not
likely to be for some time, the M.I.S. Project has defined interim workload measures for current use.

Workload measurement data is one component of the statistics
generated on the **departmental dimension** in order to determine how well each service is functioning, whether in comparison
to its own past performance or to the performance of the same

service in another facility. This method of getting a grasp on
the performance of departmental services is central to the
Guidelines. However, for those who wish it, measurements made
at the departmental dimension can also be tied to individual
patients in order to obtain a **global view** of resource utilization. For example, given the same diagnosis, it becomes possible to contrast the resource utilization resulting from one
course of patient treatment with that resulting from a different
course of treatment in the same facility, or among facilities.
The possibilities for health care research as well as effective
management of resources are tremendous.

° The statistics that should be used in health care management
  have been divided into the following categories: financial,
  workload, activity, staffing, and profile.

  The Guidelines identify the statistics that may be collected
  within specific functional centres. Those statistics used in
  resource utilization and costing reports are included in the
  chart of statistics.

° Indicators are carefully defined in the Guidelines. Basically,
  indicators are those calculations and "roll-ups" that assist in
  analysis and decision-making. The Guidelines also suggest which
  indicators are most useful to department managers, to executives, and in comparisons with other facilities in a peer group.

It appears a daunting task to make the shift in focus recommended by
the Guidelines. For this reason, every effort has been made to make
the Guidelines complete and comprehensive. At the same time, flexibility has been an important component. For the most part, it is
possible to select and implement portions of the Guidelines according
to the will and resources available to the individual institution.

Before closing, we wish to leave you with some food for thought and
discussion regarding some of the areas of impact of the M.I.S. Guidelines.

° Strengthened Departmental Accountability - As a result of the
  greater precision and definition of financial and statistical

measures provided in the Guidelines, there will likely be a downward shift in delegation of authority, as well as strengthened departmental accountability. These changes should free senior management to concentrate more heavily on evaluation of results, rather than on continual reviews of management processes.

° Improvement in Usefulness of Data - Standard indicators and definitions will increase the accuracy, consistency, and comparability of data used by managers.

° Increased Ability to Assess Impact of Treatment Methods - For those health care facilities that implement the global dimension framework, accurate impact analyses concerning the treatment of specific numbers and kinds of patients will finally be possible. For the first time, physicians will be able to assess the impact of differing treatment methods on resource utilization. By matching this knowledge with the productivity and financial information on the departmental dimension, it will be possible to allocate resources to the best advantage of the patient community.

° Creation of Standard Performance Indicators - In reporting to external agencies, health care facilities will be assured that assessments will use identical performance indicators.

° Improvement in Program Planning - Trustees, physicians, and health care executives will be able to apply the information available through the global dimension framework to accurately plan the introduction of new programs, or the expansion or deletion of existing programs. The degree of managerial confidence in predicting the impact of such actions will be greatly increased.

° Increased Ability to Use Resource-Based Reimbursement Schemes - Full implementation of the global dimension framework will permit consideration of reimbursement schemes that are based on the actual resources required to treat groups of patients with unique care needs. However, such consideration must be approached cautiously and should only be entertained after the global dimension framework has been fully implemented.

The M.I.S. Guidelines, which consist of eighteen manuals, are registered for copyright under the name of the M.I.S. Steering Committee and have been published in English and French.

THE INFORMATION SYSTEM OF LAZIO REGION
FOR THE DEATH CAUSE DECLARATION

Arca' M.[1],Lagorio S.[1],Perucci C.A.[1],Ricci F.L.[2],Tasco C.[1]

[1] O.E.R.-S.I.S.,Regione Lazio, Via Rosa Raimondi Garibaldi 7,00145 Roma,Italy
[2] I.S.R.D.S.-C.N.R.,Via Cesare De Lollis 12,00185 Roma,Italy

The Lazio Region information system for the death cause declaration is described.It is conceived to harmonize the data use at local level,where data are collected,with a different use of the same data at regional level.

Introduction

The organization of National Health Service (SSN) in Italy is based on three organizing and decision-making levels;each level has its own independent duties regarding administration supervision and planning: central (State), intermediate (Regions) and peripheral (USL= local health authority). Each level uses the same data to satisfy their tasks, even though the objectives are different.

A same fenomenon can be observed from different views;if we consider,as example,the hospitalization of a person,we can extract useful information for: a) planning health services in the area where the hospital is located; b) epidemiological analysis regarding the health status of the resident population. Since the citizen can receive health assistance by SSN structures in any part of Italy,indipendently of his residence,the services at the same organizational level may analyze the same data from different views. Therefore the specific information thought collected only once (and generally by the periferic level that use it at first for its ordinary administration tasks) it's later trasmitted not only to the immediately upper level at the point of data collection, but also to all interested structures wherever located.

The SSN is trying to adapt the information system on mortality (SIM) to the new needs caused by the health reform; in other words the objectives are: a) to rationalize the procedures to verify of the cause of death; b) to unify different forms concerning a single case; c) to keep a "cause of death register" in the USL. The cause-specific mortality rates lost sensivity as measure of intervention efficacy,for the incidence decreasing of the infective diseases and the increasing of the chronic degenerative diseases. In spite of that,they remain the most objective and reproducible indicators of the population's health status. It's not to be understimated that a nomenative file of death causes allows retrospective and prospective epidemiological surveys. [1]

In this paper the Lazio Region SIM is described;the description of the system concerning central structures is omitted. [2]

Method

The SSN set up a strong co-ordination among the structures, hierarchically subordinate but with the decision capability. Therefore a design methodology of information and organization system,was need,suitable for the integration of the total view of system with the local self-government: the Superposed Automata Nets (SAN). The SAN are a methodology fit to describe the whole system and its sub-systems by decomposable structure. In this way,we model different connected processes (USLs and Region) and show up the parallelism and the interaction between them. Besides the SAN are a sub-class of Petri nets and use the condition-event couple concept;thus we can analyze all the system function conditions and garantee data diffusion between different sub-systems. The SAN start with the task formal definition,the old system description and the analysis of all the function situations to arrive at the new organization and information system. [3]

For an USL there are three functional cases: 1) an its own citizen dies in its territory; 2) an its own citizen dies in the different USL; 3) a citizen from another USL dies in its own territory . Every USL is interested to know both the trend of mortality by cause occurred in its territory and the causes about all the death only for citizens registered in its territory,because some causes are linked to the environmental factors. It is clear that the information about death must be avalaible to every interested USL. Then it is necessary not only to propagate the information,but to inform about the available information;in this way the different sub-systems of SSN know the confidence degree of their data.

The new information system is shown in picture in a semplified way (only the stations and the files).

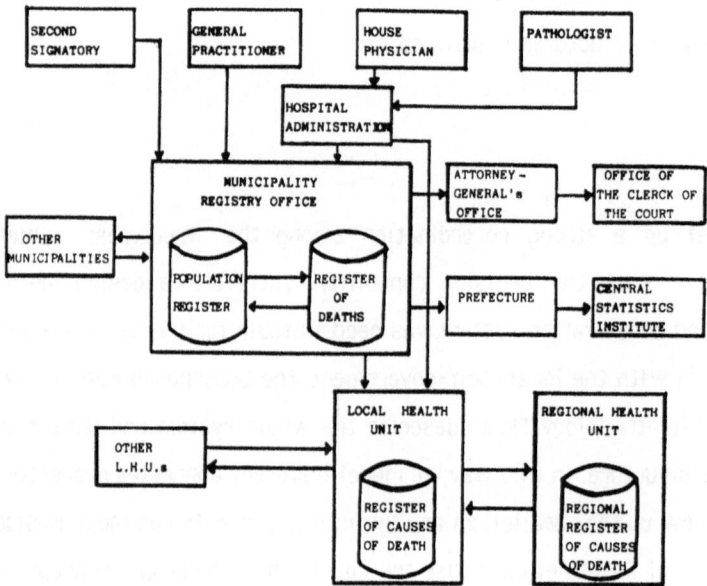

Comparison

It is up to the USL to compute periodically the mortality rates and to check whether or not the observed mortality agrees with the expected values,obtained on the basis of time and geographic trends. It is up to the Region to collect the ULS's mortality rates and compare them in order to provide information about regional mortality trends,particulary with regard to low incidence diseases. The periodic data recording would allow to identify at the proper moment the occurrence of potential health problems,using epidemiological methods. In order to allow the USLs to perform such a surveillance program some simple procedures must be implemented: a) to set up and update a case-register; b) to select and list cases according to different criteria; c) to compute a few selected statistics (confidence intervals and simple hypothesis tests).[4] The data that such a system has to process cannot be prefixed; the system must be flexible enough to be used in many different situations as the various USLs present.

At regional level the system must : a) set up and manage files of both individual and aggregated data; b) select and list cases according with different criteria; c) apply a number of even advanced statistical techniques.

In both cases therefore the matter is to sequence a data base management system with a statistical package.

Because the different sizes of processed files,the system works on a personal computer at the local level and on a main frame at the regional level. Here the problem of interface between data base management system and statistical package comes up,because the latter may change according with the requested processing.

Discussion

Different uses of the same piece of information at different levels of SSN are due to the different tasks to be performed as well as to the different degrees of knowledge and skill of the operators involved. On one hand you cannot carry out a refined analysis using poor or badly collected data,on the other the quality of such a data analysis strongly depends not only on the operator's skill in using tools and techniques,but also on his consciousness of social and medical problems pertaining to the area where he works. Therefore,going on with the SIM implementation and gaining more and more experience,it will be possible to increase the number of individual data to be recorded and to develop more refined analysis techniques.

To provide good quality of data an important point is the cause of death codification. In the Latium Region the death certificates are now undergoing three different and indipendent (blind) codifications at three different level (USL,Region,Istat). The aim is to estimate advantages and disavantages,in term of information validity and reproducibility af a peripherical codification system. Such a codification would be of course "rather close" to the death and thus likely to provide more accurate information (even thougt certainly less reproducible) than a centralized procedure,far from the event. In order to secure a codification procedure with sufficient pledge of reliability even when applied at USL level an ongoing research (by CNR,Ministery of Health and Latium Epidemiological Regional Unit) will provide a codification aid system. The aid of such system is to avoid that the different local operators willcodify in different ways a single succession of causes as written on the death certificate.

Conclusion

We described the Latium SIM and emphasized the different use of same data at USL and Region level,because the aim of these levels is different as the operator's skill in using the statistical techiques.

The crucial point of SIM is to codify the death certificates and then an codification aid system is under consideration.

References

1. Arca' M.,Forastiere F.,Perucci C.A.,Tasco C.,Valesini S. **Riorganizzazione del sistema informativo per la rilevazione della mortalità.** Progetto Salute,vol. 1,n° 1,1982

2. Verdecchia A.,Capocaccia R.,Mariotti S. **An interactive inquiry system for mortality data.** Proceedings of MIE'84,Springer-Verlag,1984

3. De Cindio F.,De Michelis G.,Pomello L.Simone C. **Superposed automata nets: application and theory of Petri Nets.** Informatik Fachberichte,52,Springer-Verlag,1982

4. De Rosis F., Franich A.,Pizzutilo S.,Ricci F.L. **Handling and analyzing epidemiological data by microcomputer.** Proceedings of MIE'84,Springer-Verlag,1984

TERTIKA-DATABASE AS A PLANNING INSTRUMENT FOR MUNICIPAL HEALTH AUTHORITIES

I. Parvinen
Chief Health Officer
Health Office
City of Turku, Finland

General

The health status of the population should administratively be controlled and examined in the same way as the health status of an individual. This could be made by doing and interpreting "laboratory examinations" and controlling "the patient's" welfare continually.

From the standpoint of the health administration, this kind of control involves a medium, by which necessary "samples and examinations" can be done.

Converted to the data processing language this means an effort to set up a system, where the database is always up to date. From this database it is possible to obtain necessary information for planning and decisions.

It is easier to create a database like this in those countries, where the local planning and providing of health care is fixed by law. In Finland the communes have this kind of an obligation, which particularly concerns primary health care. These same communes must, however, organize and finance most of the remaining health care, too, including f.ex. health services in the university central hospitals. In Finland this is carried out by setting up federations of communes, which maintain f.ex. the central hospitals mentioned above.

To control the total situation it is necessary to develop a database, which to a sufficient extent includes basic data on resources used to maintain the health status of the population and on the allocation of these resources.

A prototype of a database like this is presented to you during the lecture by some practical examples.

TERTIKA-database

TERTIKA is the health centre's management information system based on direct operations.

With TERTIKA a user can:
- form a general view how health services are used in the communes or the federations of communes.
- follow up the development of operation in the health centre and compare it to other health centres.
- clarify how customers are directed.
- clarify the services supply for all age-groups.
- improve continuation of health care.
- get a good basis for the comparison of costs and economy.
- plan the personal's purposeful use.
- clarify the development need for all health care methods.

TERTIKA has been started to build up on the basis of the primary health care and it includes a data set which by APL-programmed menu solution can quickly be taken into operation. All data for TERTIKA is collected by TEHO-system which is an information system for health centres' administrative data processing. The inauguration of TERTIKA cuts out the most paper-printing of TEHO-system, because all information on visits, customers, laboratory and x-ray examinations are available whenever grouped as decided from TERTIKA. Naturally exact numeral paper-printings are also available.

TERTIKA consists at present of the following subsystems.

Table 1

TERTIKA SUBSYSTEMS

- primary health care services
- dental health services
- laboratory
- x-ray

Information can be obtained according both to visits and patients, which makes it possible to select the following variables.

Table 2

LIST OF VARIABLES

- related/absolute numbers
- federation of communes/commune
- providers of health services (physician, nurse etc.)
- place of provision (health centre, home, institution etc.)
- contents (preventive health care, consultations by physicians etc.)
- age groups
- examinations (laboratory, x-ray)

The extension of the system towards hospital statistics is just going on. The data describing the economics of health care will also be put in the database in the near future.

The Finnish State Computer Centre has carried out ADP-systems for planning and controlling the whole state's health care. These systems are used by the Ministry of Social Affairs and Health, and the National Board of Medical Service. The systems between local stages and ones of the state have been integrated together so that health centres can get information from the total system of health care via the data communications network, as well transmit data collected from TERTIKA in the machine readable form to the total system of health care.

The database includes a special output program for the information of annual reports necessary for the governmental authorities. This information can automatically be transferred for the use of the provincial health administration. Test runs will most likely be done this year.

To use TERTIKA requires that the health centre purchases a microcomputer provided with data communications software including a display terminal, printer and graphic multicolored plotter as peripheral devices. The microcomputer is connected via the telephone network to the mainframes of the State Computer Centre. The equipment also can be used for many other purposes besides TERTIKA, e.g. for TEHO-data storing, word processing and personal table-accounting. TERTIKA is an interactive and user-friendly system. The Finnish State Computer Centre organizes TERTIKA training. A customer learns to use TERTIKA independently already after one day's training and some hours' practising.

TERTIKA is a part of ATLAS, the whole health centre's computational total system.

ATLAS contains:

TEHO - information system for health centres' administrative data processing

TERTIKA - management information system

TAVA - appointment system

KULAUS - accounting system

SAPLA - system of salaries calculation, and

systems for accounting of property, stock and pharmacy meant for the material administration's data processing.

Connections to other databases

It seems that the data gathered by the Finnish Social Insurance Institute will also form a separate database in Finland. Thus we are in practice coming to the stage where planners, managers and decision makers have data base management tools at their disposal (a terminal equipment & dataprocessing programs). By this equipment they can combine,transform and process the available administrative information of health status of the population (the administrative information of health care) by using different databases.

Fig 1

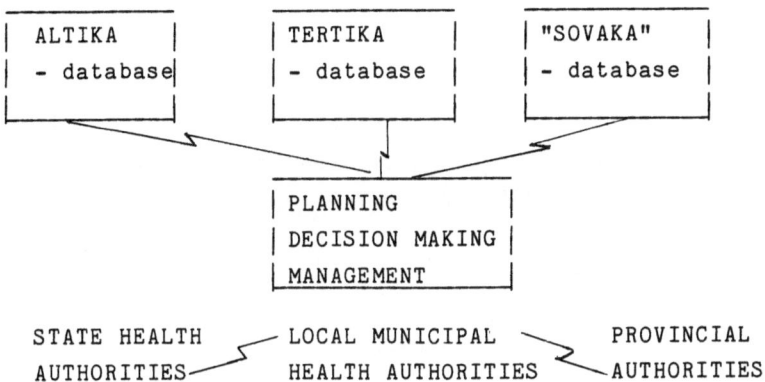

The ALTIKA-database consists of f.ex. demographic file of the population grouped municipally and provincially and covering the whole country. The database is produced by the Finnish State Computer Centre which also maintains the TERTIKA-database.

DEVELOPMENT OF A DATA MODEL OF THE NORWEGIAN HEALTH CARE SYSTEM

Petter Hurlen

Directorate of Organization and Management

P.O.Box 8115 Dep, 0032 Oslo, Norway

Summary

The development of a data model of the Norwegian health care system with the SYSDOC and SYSTEMATOR products is described. The design and possible practical use of the model is discussed.

Introduction

The use of modern information technology in the health care system in Norway is increasing rapidly today. Unfortunately, the development of information systems has been, and is, taking place almost without colla- boration or co-ordination of any kind. This has resulted in a variety of health care information systems running on different computers, program- med in different languages and based on different understanding and defi- nition of even major technical terms in the health care system.

Variety in understanding and definition of the technical terms the infor- mation systems are based upon, creates a major problem whith regard to computer communication and information exchange. It also complicates the data collection for the Health Authorities. This author believes that a common understanding and definition of the technical terms is necessary and essential in the further development of the health care information systems. One possible ground for the discussion of such common terms, is a data model of the Health Care System. This paper will deal with certain aspects of such a data model, developed by the author.

Material and method

For the manifestation of the model, the SYSDOC® and SYSTEMATOR® products
were chosen (1). SYSDOC is an information system design methodology while
SYSTEMATOR is a software tool which may give computer aid for the information system development process. The SYSDOC methodology is primarily
data-oriented. A SYSDOC conceptual datamodel contains three main types of
concepts: Entity types, relationship types and data element types. These
concepts can, however, be elementary, derived, generalized or grouped.
Each occurrence of any of the three concept types is given a unique
identifier.

An __entity type__ description is a description of the general rules that may
apply and the properties the entities of that type may have. An entity
may be a physical object, an abstract object or an event. The generalized
entity type is used to express that a given entity occurrence may be
considered as being of different types in different contexts. In the
examples elementary entities are drawn as squares, generalized entities
as squares enclosing squares.

A __relationship type__ description is a description of one particular type
of relationship that may exist between the entity occurrences. A relationship type may be of one of the following degrees: One to one, one to
many or many to many. The relationship type description contains information regarding what entity types the relationship may involve and other
essential information. However, a relationship in SYSDOC may __not__ be given
any attributes, as opposed to for instance the ERA model (3). The "inverse" of a relationship is handled in SYSDOC by giving context dependent
names to a relationship where the context is given by the starting point
of a relation (an entity). In fig. 1 relationships are drawn as lines. A
line containing an arrow at one end indicates the degree of one to many.

A __data element type__ description contains a definition of its type and
description of length etc. A data element type normally describes an
attribute of one entity type, but may apply to several. A group of individual data element types may be given a name.

Information about the health care system was obtained by participation
in, and observation of, the health care system, and by communication with
health care personnel. Some of the information obtained have previously
formed the basis for the Norwegian Medical Information System - NOMIS.
NOMIS is a hospital information system developed for Norwegian hospitals.

A list of data elements was produced based on the combination of the
NOMIS system description (2) and a data dictionary made by the SYSTEMATOR
data base schema scanner. Simultaneously a graphic representation was
made describing the health care system as accurately as possible in terms
of entities and relationships. The graphic representation was developed
in collaboration with the former leader of the SYSTEMATOR project, Bernt
M. Mostue.

Results

The data model developed in this way, consists of 32 entities, 55 relationships and 490 data elements. The most detailed level of SYSDOC data
model documentation contains 670 pages, and is thus impossible to present
in this paper. However, the complete model will be demonstrated at the
congress.

The model is meant to portray a selected set of the properties of the
Norwegian health care system, and all the terms originally used were Norwegian. In the figures and the model to be presented at the congress,
English terms are used to make the model comprehensible to English-
speaking readers, even though it was not always possible to find
completely corresponding terms for the translation. Fig. 1 shows an
important subset of the graphic representation of the model. It portrays
certain administrative aspects of a patient's stay at a hospital, the
persons involved, the hospital owners, the departments of a hospital and
so on. The data elements belonging to one of the entities are shown in
fig. 2.

Discussion

Many questions may arise from the development of a data model. Whether
the model is correct and complete, given the modelling tools, will be
considered elsewhere (4), since a discussion of this topic presumes
detailed knowledge of the Norwegian health care system. In this paper, I
will raise the question of whether a model developed using SYSDOC may
portray the Norwegian health care system in a satisfactory way.

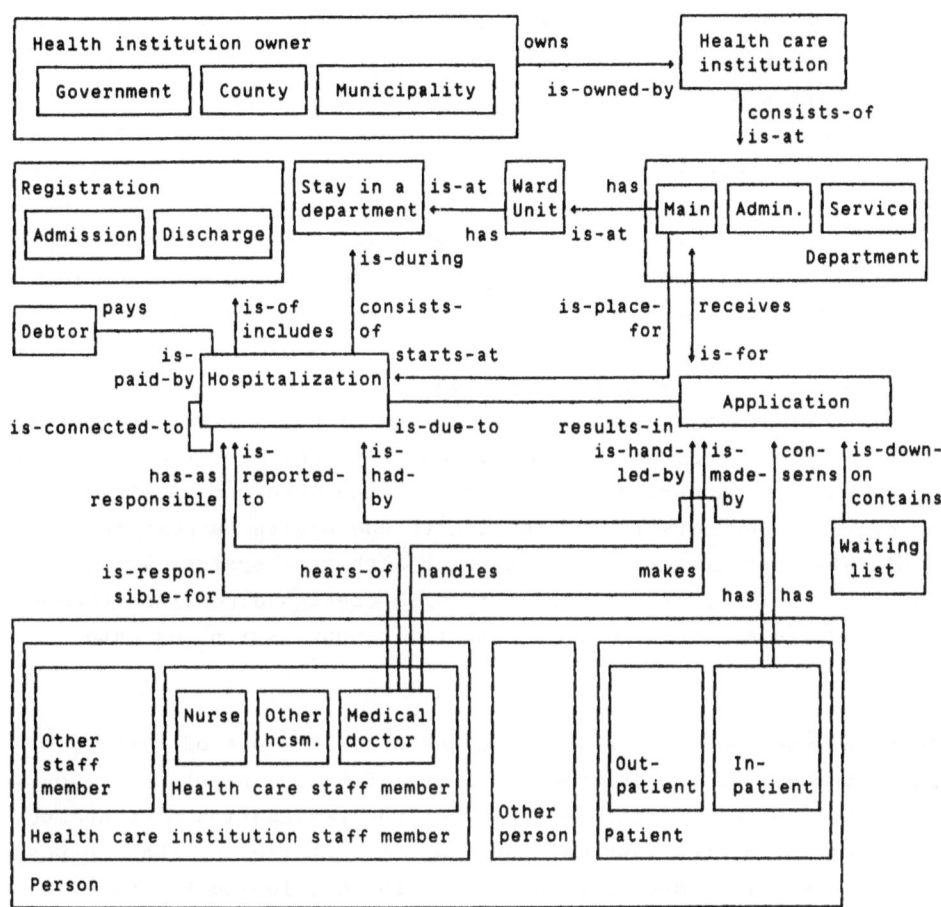

FIG. 1. A SUBSET OF THE GRAPHIC REPRESENTATION OF THE MODEL.

ADMISSION:

Data element Name	Data element Type	Maximum Length	Definition/ Remarks
DATE	N	6	DDMMYY
TIME	N	4	Hours & minutes
DIAGNOSIS	N	5	ICD-8
PLACE	N	4	Institution or other place
WAY	N	1	The way of admission

N= Numeric

FIG. 2. THE DATA ELEMENTS OF THE ADMISSION ENTITY.

The SYSDOC methodology facilitates the description of objects and events, and their properties and relationships. This permits all major parts of the health care system to be included in the model. The graphic representation of the model only contains objects and events familiar to health care personnel. There is no extra sybols with special meanings complicating the model. It is thus rather easy to comprehend, even without much previous knowledge in information system design. This makes the model a useful means of communication when completing and correcting the information collected in collaboration with health care personnel.

Another majore advantage is the detailed description of data elements which may be produced from the SYSDOC data dictionary. This may serve as a ground for clarification and definition of technical terms, and is a valuable source of accurate information for the development of information systems. Furthermore, it reveals to the health authorities which kinds of data that are collected in the health care system, and thus may be reported regularly or on demand. It also creates a possible common ground for defining standards for computer communication and data exchange.

In addition, the model may serve as a basis for the use of "4th. generation languages" in the information system development process. However, the model presented was not developed for the realisation of a health care information system, and may thus not be suitable for that purpose. As stated in the introduction, the reason for developing the model was the lack of common comprehension and definition of technical terms in the health care system, and the subsequent difficulties concerning computer communication and information exchange. A model developed for the realisation of an information system would possibly be different. In addition, one would have to consider the special difficulties involved in the design of very large databases.

However, there is also some aspects of the health care system that is not so easily described by the use of the modelling tools. First and foremost, there is no easy way to describe constraints with the SYSDOC methodology. For instance, in Norway an application which must be written by a physician, may result in immidiate action or be deferred to a waiting list. This could be described in a more detailed data model documentation, but it could not be revealed in the graphic representation, wich is a disadvantage. However, a description of constraints would probably also complicate the model, and require a greater ammount of knowledge of the modelling methodology from helth care personnel.

There is a general concensus that some matters, for instance a patient's problems, are not satisfactorily described by the use of data elements only. Free text description also appears necessary (5). It is, however, not possible to use the tools for modelling matters that only can be satisfactorily discribed by the use of free text. In addition, parts of the health care system can be regarded as time-consuming actions. For instance, a patient is admitted to a hospital, stays in one or more departments, undergoes examination and treatment, and is finally discharged. It is difficult to describe this as time-consuming, partly concurrent and partly successive actions with the modelling tools used.

However, these objections have appeard to be of minor importance as far as this model is concerned, and thus the model developed seems to portray the health care system in a satisfactory way.

References

1) Aschim, F. and Mostue, B.M.: IFIP WG 8.1 case solved using SYSDOC and SYSTEMATOR. Information systems design methodologies: A comparative Rewiev (editors Olle & al.) North-Holland Publishing Company 1982

2) Buvig, H. & al.:NOMIS BHB/SPES 1-9, Statens Rasjonaliserings- direktorat.

3) Chen, P.: The Entity-Relationship Model Toward a unified View of Data. ACM Transactions on Database Systems, Volume 2, No.2, June 1977.

4) Hurlen, P.: Informasjonsutveksling i helsevesenet (In preparation).

5) Østbye, T.: Free text retrieval of medical information. To be presented at MIE 85.

ACTUAL UTILIZATION OF THE COMPUTERIZED NATIONAL DANISH DEATH REGISTER.

K. Juel
The Danish Institute for Clinical Epidemiology (DICE)
25, Svanemøllevej
DK - 2100 Copenhagen Ø, Denmark

Introduction

The National Danish Death Register contains information on 1.88 million deaths during the period 1943-83. The information in the register is derived from the death certificates and is filed on magnetic tape. The organization of the register and its content will be described in the following. Furthermore, examples of applications of the register will be shown.

Organization and content of the register.

The National Board of Health uses the statutory death certificates as basis for the official, annual statistics of causes of death. For this reason the information in the death certificates was transferred to punched cards for automatic reading. The cards were stored after use. The punched cards conserning the period 1943-60 were handed over to DICE in the beginning of the 1960's, and in 1973 DICE received the similar punched cards for the period 1961-70, altogether 1.2 million cards. From 1971 and onward DICE has received a magnetic tape covering all deaths, after the National Board of Health had made use of the material for the annual statistics of causes of death.

At the time, when the organization of the register was initiated, some of the cards were more than 30 years old and reading them was a time-consuming task even though the cards were in a fairly good condition. Another problem consisted in the lack of continuity of information during the period, and this was further complicated by insufficient documentation of the information on the cards in some years. Since 1976, the register has been ready for EDP-use and a number of control tabulations have shown that there is a high degree of accordance with the official statistics of causes of death.

A total of 1.88 million deaths during the period 1943-83 have been filed on the magnetic tape. All the information is derived from death certificates. There are both demographic and medical informations. The demographic information includes sex, age, marital status, occupation,

residence, dates of birth and death. The medical information concerning
the death includes the underlying cause of death and one or two contributory causes, and information from autopsy.

There are two problems involved in the application of this information. Firstly, not all information is available each year, e.g. occupation
is stated for only a few years, and information from autopsy is available for only a part of the period. Secondly, some of the variables have
different meanings in different periods. Thus, four different classifications of causes of death have been used. From 1943 to 1950 a special
Scandinavian classification was used, from 1951 to 1957 the 6th revised
ICD was used, from 1958 to 1968 the 7th revised and subsequently the
8th revised ICD has been applied. In addition, a number of different
ways to classify residence have been applied.

Examples of application

The register has been applied for a number of different tasks, and in
the following three main types will be described: Studies of regional
and temporal variations, Elucidations, and Occupational health investigations.

Regional and temporal variations.
The regional variation in death from all causes in Denmark during the
period 1971-80 was the subject of a descriptive analysis (Juel 1984).
Denmark was divided into either 16 or 275 regions. Men and women were
analysed separately during two periods 1971-75 and 1976-80. The different age distributions in the regions was taken into account. In the
capital two municipalities Copenhagen and Frederiksberg had a unique
pattern of mortality with a distinctive, high mortality in the age
group from 30 to 60 years. The remaining 14 counties in Denmark showed
only minor differences. The difference in mortality in the county with
the highest mortality and the county with the lowest mortality was approximately 10%. When the analysis was carried out at the municipality
level the estimates were more imprecise, and the mortality in the municipality with the highest mortality was twice as large as in the municipality with the lowest mortality.

The significance of frequency of autopsy for the statistics of causes
of death has been analysed based solely on the register (Juel 1981). For
this reason all municipalities in Denmark which satisfied the following
3 criteria were selected. Firstly, they should lie outside the capital
region, secondly, the municipality should have between 25000 and 80000

inhabitants, and thirdly, there should be a hospital in the municipality.
26 municipalities satisfied these criteria. These municipalities were divided into three groups according to frequency of autopsy, and the pattern of mortality was analyzed in the three groups.

In the period 1943-78 the mortality from cancer in Denmark was analyzed with regard to residence, birth-cohort, and age (Juel 1983). The
mortality was studied separately for men and women and for 14 different
kinds of cancer. The applied mathematical model allowed tests for differences in mortality between birth-cohorts and between the capital and
the provinces.

Currently, a project under EC's program for research and development
applies the register in an analysis of avoidable deaths; that is, death
from diseases which according to medical experts should not lead to death,
or mortality should at least be very low. The period 1970-83 is in this
study divided into three periods, and Denmark is divided into 16 counties. It is thus possible to evaluate temporal and regional effects. The
calculated regional mortalities will at a later stage be related to social indicators and different indexes of the health services in the region.
A preliminary report for the period 1971-80 has been published (Kamper-
Jørgensen and Juel 1982).

Elucidations.
In the last decade several examples can be found in Denmark where local
residents have observed clusterings of certain diseases or deaths - mostly cancer - within a geographically limited area, often close to a factory. These observations are often extensively commented in the media.
The health authorities are for this reason under pressure for fast reactions. The register has on several occasions been applied where different environmental factors' influence on health status should be evaluated.

The conditions near Cheminova, the chemical plant in Thyborøn-Harboør
municipality represents such an example. The issue started in 1982 as a
result of a parliamentary inquiry. A report published in 1984 compared
the mortality in Thyborøn-Harboør municipality with a control region in
the period 1956-80 (Juel and Jacobsen 1984). The period was divided into
5 five year periods, and the deaths were divided into 4 large categories
of disease. Firstly, it was of interest to investigate whether there was
a difference in mortality between Thyborøn-Harboør and the control region. If there was a difference, it was considered of interest to establish
whether this difference had been constant during the whole period. The
plant was founded in 1953 and taking a latency period of 10 to 30 years

into consideration, one would expect an increase in excess mortality
during the period if the plant had a major effect on mortality.

Occupational health investigations

Much epidemiological research is concerned with the study of groups of
persons who have been subject to a certain influence: Employees at a certain factory or a group of persons who in other ways have had the same
experience. The data are often rather old making follow-up difficult. A
central population register (CPR) was introduced in Denmark in 1968.
Every person was assigned a unique number comprising birthdate and a serial number . Knowing the CPR no. it is possible through the CPR to establish whether a person is alive or not, if the person was alive on January 1. 1968. If the person is dead, the cause of death can be found in the
death register.

Persons who are not found in the CPR are either dead before 1968 or
data are erroneous. In these instances the death register will be of value. By matching date of birth and name it is possible to get a list of
all persons with the same date of birth and name, and thus possibly establish whether the person died before 1968. A copy of the death certificate can then be obtained from the National Board of Health. The remaining group can be obtained through the local offices of the National Register. The follow-up of 1582 persons who had been in KZ-camps during the
2nd World War is an example. It was possible to establish the status of
all persons (Nielsen 1983).
When the follow-up is finished it is possible from the death register to
calculate the expected number of deaths in the group under study if the
mortality is equal to the mortality of the whole population. The studies
of mortality among brewery workers (Jensen 1980) and cryolite miners are
examples (Grandjean et al. 1985).

Conclusion

The above mentioned examples show that the National Danish Death Register
has been applied in a number of different contexts. Analyses covering a
long period of time currently 41 years are possible. Classifications
which cannot be found in the official statistics are made possible, for
instance different regions, other groups of diseases or other age groups.
Analyses are made possible which could not have been carried out if the
National Danish Death Register did not exist. The register has greatly
facilitated in tracing causes of death in different groups of patients

and in occupational health investigations. A copy of the death certificate is not always needed, thereby significantly reducing the number of
inquiries to local offices of the National Register. It is evident that
use of the register greatly reduces time.

The register of causes of death which is accessible through EDP has until now been used frequently and is a valuable tool in research, evaluation, and health planning.

References

Grandjean P, Juel K, Jensen OM (1983) Mortality and cancer morbidity after occupational fluoride exposure. AM J Epidemiol, 121 (to appear).
Jensen OM (1980) Cancer morbidity and causes of death among Danish brewery workers. Lyon: JARC.
Juel K (1981) Autopsihyppighedens betydning for dødsårsagsstatistikken
(The significance of the frequency of autopsy for statistics of the
causes of death). Ugeskrift for Læger, 143: 2669-74.
Juel K (1983) Demographic factors and cancer mortality: a mathematical
model for cancer mortality in Denmark 1943-78. Int J Epidemiol, 12:
419-25.
Juel K (1984) Dødelighedsindeks for kommuner og amter 1971-80 (agestan-
dardised mortality index for Danish municapalities and counties 1971-
80). Dansk Institut for Klinisk Epidemiologi og Sundhedsstyrelsen.
Vitalstatistik I:7. København.
Juel K, Jacobsen P (1984) Dødeligheden 1956-80 i Thyborøn-Harboør og i
et kontrol område (The mortality 1956-80 in Thyborøn-Harboør and in a
control region). Dansk Institut for Klinisk Epidemiologi og Sundhedsstyrelsen. Hygiejnemeddelser: 4. København.
Kamper-Jørgensen F, Juel K (1982) Aspects of preventable deaths in Denmark (Preliminary report). Presented at EC-Workshop: Health status
Assessment Paris, 1-3 december.
Nielsen H (1983) Dødelighed 1943-79 blandt danske modstandsfolk deporte-
ret til tyske koncentrationslejre (The mortality in the period 1943-
79 among members of the Danish resistance movement who were deported
to German concentration camp). Ugeskrift for Læger, 145: 345-50.

THE SYSTEM OF MEDICAL STATISTICS IN THE GDR AND TARGETS UP TO 1990

Bernd Schirmer and Doris Panzer
Ministry of Health, Berlin, GDR
Institute of Medical Statistics and Data Processing, Berlin, GDR

During the 36 years of its existence, in the GDR a high level of health protection of the population has been achieved and an efficient health service has been built up in keeping with the social development. In this way the stipulations of the Constitution of the GDR to guarantee the protection and promotion of the health of all citizens are realized. During the past 15 years there has been, above all, a very rapid development of the human, material and financial prerequisites for the health and social care of the population.

Since 1970 the number of employees in the health service has been rising by more than 150.000. At present, more tan 520.000 persons are working in the health and social services devoting themselves to the life and health of their fellow-citizens (5). They make up more than 6% of the working population of our country. In many places new hospitals, policlinics and other health and social care facilities were established during the past years. 70 % of the eligible children from 0 to 3 years are devotedly cared for and educated in crèches in close contact with their parents. The care for the elderly in their communities has been further improved and new homes for adolescents and adults needing care were built. On the basis of these developments physicians, nurses and other personnel in the health and social sector were able to substantially expand the scope of their services. The modern and effective structure of health care provides primarily a qualified primary medical care based upon the family physician concept. Everybody can choose the physician of his confidence. The high number of medical and dental consultations is a reflection of the presence of a developed and effective network of health facilities. These developments provided the basis for the steady improvement of the health status of the GDR population which is shown by a careful morbidity and mortality analysis (6). Indices such as the infant mortality rate and the mean life expectancy are an illustration of the dynamics of this process.

New tasks to be solved in the years to come also arise from what we
have stated above. Extensive projects aimed at further improving health
and social care of the population will be carried out in the period up
to 1990. Entirely new demands will be made on the management and planning sectors of the health service. To meet these demands a distinctly
better collection, processing and utilization of information at the
various levels will be needed, especially since our health service is
territorially run. One important health political principle is, however,
not to allow unjustified territorial differences and to gradually overcome existing differences. It is necessary, therefore, to establish a
uniform information system for the health and social services which
requires an effective mechanism for accounting and statistics. Already
in 1966 there began the creation of a uniform national system for accounting and statistics under the responsibility of the Central Statistical Office of the GDR (1).

The following general principles are necessary for the information
system of the health service:
1. The Ministry of Health is responsible for formulating the indices
   on the basis of the National Socioeconomic Plans. The uniformly
   designed records are passed on through specific channels of information.
2. Facilities are legally required to report data. Their managers are
   also responsible for informing the working people in order to involve them widely in the management and planning processes of the
   facilities thus fulfilling the principles of democratic centralism.
3. The Health Statistical Service is an integral part of the Public
   Health Service while maintaining a relative independence and guaranteeing the collaboration with the Central Statistical Office (4).

At the present stage of our long-term plan the health information
system has the task of
- reflecting the health status of the population as completely as
  possible by using data about care provided in preventive, out-patient,
  in-patient and rehabilitation services,
- contributing to the improvement of the quality and efficiency of
  medical and social care,
- achieving an optimum relationship between cost and benefit with regard to the resources made available,
- achieving meaningful integration between the organization of health

care and the information system,
- utilizing the data derived from the information system for the competent planning of the facilities and of their location, for the long-
  term and annual planning as well as for the measuring of the execution
  of the plan and for the target-oriented operational control by all
  levels of management,
- developing into a decision-oriented information system, especially
  for the county and ministry levels.

Here we fully agree with proposals of WHO as they were expressed at the
Fourth European Conference on Health Statistics, Copenhagen, 1981 (7)
and other international events (8).

The German Democratic Republic has created the basis for gradually at-
taining the goal of a suitable countrywide linkage of information and
data. The information system is increasingly better incorporating the
principles of a socialist health policy such as
- treatment of patients as whole persons;
- implementation of the unity of prevention, diagnosis, therapy, and
  after-care in medical and social care;
- replacement of old patterns of care by new forms of care and the
  central position of the family physicians;
- creation of health facilities of a rational size and implementation of
  optimum forms of cooperation, coordination, and communication (4).

In our country the information system of the health and social services
is until 1990 being constructed and extended on such a basis, namely
according to three meaningfully integrated columns:
(a) information related to persons and patients, i.e. to those to be
    cared for;
(b) information related to health facilities, i.e. to facilities and
    services provided as well as costs;
(c) information on persons employed in the health service (3).

Early in 1985 the Institute of Medical Statistics and Data Processing
of the Ministry of Health was founded in Berlin which serves as a guiding centre for the information system for management, planning, accounting and statistics and is responsible for stimulating scientific progress in this field. The new Institute is involved in solving problems
concerning the health status of the population, computerbased information projects and the computer strategy for the information system.
Among the tasks of this Institute is the provision of the total in-

patient morbidity statistics which has been conducted as a computer project since 1969. Another task is the health facility report which is to gradually replace a great number of isolated reportings. The target is to link the projects developed as partial reports by means of a register of the facilities into a uniform entity (2).

The results achieved so far and the before-mentioned tasks for the next years provide a good basis for implementing in the GDR an effective information system for the health and social services. It is prerequisite for the more efficient funktioning of the health service, for the assessment of its activities and for setting out the next important steps. In this way the health service of the GDR will increasingly better comply with its responsibility to make an important contribution towards fulfilling our main task - to do everything for the well-being of the people.

References

1. Donda, A.; u.a.:   Statistik
                                       5. Auflage, Verlag die Wirtschaft, Berlin 1981

2. Kleinecke, R.; Voß, G.; Wolf, K. und H. Ziesemer
   Das Einrichtungsregister als Mittel und Voraussetzung für die Rationalisierung des Berichtswesens im Gesundheits- und Sozialwesen
   Z.ges.Hygiene 25(1979)8, S.618

3. Otto, J. u. W. Schneider
   Die Weiterentwicklung des Informationssystems für die Leitung und Planung, Rechnungsführung und Statistik im Gesundheits- und Sozialwesen
   Z. ärztl. Fortbild. 72(1978)18, S.878-884

4. Panzer, D.; Schneider, W. u. N. Fichtner
   The System of Medical Statistics in the GDR and the Tasks of Postgraduate Training of Physicians and other Personnel. Lecture at the European Symposion on Biostatistics/Medical Statistics, Berlin, October 22-26,1984

5. Schirmer, B.:
   Auf dem Weg zum XI. Parteitag - unser Plan 1985
   Humanitas 25(1985)1, S.1

6. Seidel, K. u. B. Schirmer
   Effektives sozialistisches Gesundheitswesen - Garantie für hohe Qualität der medizinischen Betreuung
   Einheit 38(1983)2, S.180-186

7. Regional Office for Europe, WHO, Copenhagen 1981
   Health Statistics, Report on the Fourth European Conference

8. Fourth World Congress on Medical Informatics
   The Netherlands, Amsterdam, August 1983

MANAGEMENT EVALUATION OF THE HOSPITAL INFORMATION SYSTEM
AT THE LEUVEN UNIVERSITY HOSPITALS (BELGIUM)

ir. R. Vanderstappen
Associate Director
Leuven University Hospitals - Belgium

ABSTRACT

The paper presents a management view of the computer phenomenon at the
Leuven University Hospitals. It traces the decision making process as
to the development of the hospital information system (H.I.S.) -
focussing particularly on the cost-benefit analysis and implementation
strategy aspects - its impact on the hospital organization and the
implementation of the information system as a management tool.

INTRODUCTION

The Leuven Hospital Information System is operational in three acute
hospitals totalling 1877 beds (Gasthuisberg, St. Rafaël-St.Pieter,
Pellenberg) and one psychiatric institute of 425 beds, all geographically separated, with one central management.

In 1984, acute care has been given to 50.000 inpatients and 380.000
outpatients, representing approximately 500.000 inpatient days and
6.500.000 medical acts; this comprises a.o. 4.850.000 laboratory tests,
280.000 radiology procedures and 23.000 surgical interventions.
Over the same period, the pharmacy carried out 1.550.000 prescriptions,
utilizing 2.000 different drugs.
The personnel employed counts 5.100 people, including 600 M.D.'s
(staff and residents) and 2.250 nurses.

A network of computer systems has been elaborated based on one central
IBM 3033 main frame with 390 terminals,mainly for hospital and patient
management applications, and 16 dedicated Hewlett Packard mini-computers
(thirteen 21 MX, two 2100 and one HP 3000) with 180 terminals, mainly
for laboratory automation and other specific medical applications.

DECISION MAKING PROCESS

1. From the beginning, every decision for a major hard- or software
   investment was to be justified to the Board of Directors on the
   basis of a financial benefit,generated by the considered applications.
   The benefit resulted either from a production increase with positive
   marginal economic effect, or from an efficiency increase with
   demonstrable cost savings.

   From a management point of view, this financial approach is to prevail, keeping in mind however that an information system has non-
   negligible intangible advantages. A computer and its subsequent
   major extensions should not be considered as an unavoidable
   "production" machine or as similar auxiliary equipment (such as
   telephone exchange system),resulting from other primary policy
   decisions.
   The operational disadvantages experienced with this kind of approach
   are that a major system change had to take place roughly every two
   years, each time whenever for a longer period the existing equipment
   found itself overloaded.
   Meanwhile, at any such occasion, all the applications were re-
   examined critically and the tuning of the computer operating system
   was necessarily improved.

   It is also clear that the approach of financial justification is a
   method easily understood by the Board of Directors, who usually
   have had little, if any, computer exposure.

2. The central management decided on an implementation strategy, which
   aimed at an integrated hospital information system by linking
   centralized processing on the IBM main frame(s) and decentralized
   processing on the HP mini-computers, each system being supported by an
   independently operating group of experts, reporting respectively
   for the IBM system to a manager with an engineering background and
   for the HP system to a manager with a medical background.

   An integrated system was expected to be an information system,
   wherein every relevant part of new information is recorded once and
   only once near the source and transferred automatically to different
   applications and authorized users. This option was successfully

implemented , taking into account the technical linking problems
of non-compatible hardware.

As can easily be understood, this "dual" organization causes coordination problems, but, because of the desirability of the two
before-mentioned professional backgrounds in hospital data processing, it has furthermore the advantage that developments in the
administrative and the medical fields were progressing at the same
time in a self-correcting counterbalanced way, while increasing the
probability of a better user acceptance in both areas of applications.

A dilemma has been created by giving up in 1982 the highly reliable
concept of dual (IBM) main frames operating under DOS-VM software,
in favour of a single larger system, operating under MVS, completed
with a no-break power supply, supplying more teleprocessing facilities, but requiring a higher computer availability.
This situation may call for a re-examination of the degree of centralized processing, excluding however data definition and maintenance.

IMPACT ON THE HOSPITAL ORGANIZATION

1. Introducing a central management for the afore-mentioned group of
   four hospitals has been the all-pervasive change since 1973.
   Fundamental organizational development , aiming at standardization
   of departmental administrative and logistical procedures and
   overall data communication has been part of the scene continuously.

   A major positive factor in this effort has been the gradual pene-
   tration of the H.I.S., whereby the introduction of a specific
   computer application resulted automatically in the desired standardization and data collection.

   In a university hospital with its strong centrifugal tendencies,
   obtaining user acceptance for this is finding the delicate
   psychological balance between giving up part of the user's autonomy
   and the substantial advantage he finds with the application for
   fulfilling his own goals.

2. Impact of the H.I.S. has been fundamental, as well quantity- as
   qualitywise, on the central and departmental administration (i.e.
   the systematic collecting, processing and supplying of information
   for management purposes) by the mass introduction of terminals in
   the working environment of all administrative personnel.

   The functioning of the patient administration department (including
   admission, discharge and transfer of clinical patients and central
   billing of all medical procedures) has been influenced most dramatically so far. Automation enabled to cope with the processing of
   approximately 100% more data with an increase of personnel of 28%
   for the period 1973 te 1984. Proper training could for most clerical
   personnel lend the necessary skills for terminal work, while
   overcoming the psychological resistance to change.
   More difficulties were encountered with the older supervisory
   personnel, whose organizational constraints changed dramatically :
   direct hierarchical influence on a rather isolated administrative
   process found itself replaced by technical bargaining with younger
   e.d.p. specialists about one subsystem interlocked in an integrated
   H.I.S.
   The experience in the patient administration department provides
   us with a useful outlook for future developments in the entire
   administrative sector.

3. It is nearly impossible to discern the actual influence of the
   introduction of automatic analyzers and computerization on the
   chemistry laboratories, including haematology and coagulation.
   The combined result was an output increase of 84% from 1973 to 1984
   with 43% more lab analysts.

IMPLEMENTATION OF THE H.I.S. AS A MANAGEMENT TOOL

Information   is needed on the central and the departmental level for
running a complex hospital organization, more specifically for preparing
management decisions and for controlling their execution afterwards.

From a central viewpoint, most day-to-day management decisions are
related to the allocation of resources (personnel, equipment, space)
between competing medical departments within the long-term objectives

of the hospital. Important criteria influencing these decisions are, besides the existing resources per department, the output and the financial result, emphasizing direct costs and income.

The <u>output</u> of the <u>medical departments</u> are all diagnostic and therapeutic procedures,daily about 21.000, out of a variety of approximately 2.000 different activities, originating in 180 different production centers.

In the past, this basic information was gathered
- by requesting it periodically from the written - more or less detailed records of the departments, based on local data definition (with the exception of the labs with real time data acquisition) and,
- by analyzing the cumulative billing records, based on reimbursement rules of the national health insurance system and captured incompletely after a certain lapse of time.

Therefore, a centralized subsystem has been set up with a user-friendly data base of medical procedures, inclusive of an automatic conversion to reimbursement units (for billing purposes) and statistical processing of the data. Organizational development is in progress with the aim of immediate data collection at the source.
User acceptance is assured as soon as the local department head takes interest in fast and complete production data, which can be used for justifying his share of resources.

It is obvious that this is only a first step in the development of a full-fledged computer-based management information system.
Another step will be the transfer into the above system of basic data, resulting from existing <u>departmental</u> management sub-systems, such as the accounting system, the personnel management system, the pharmacy and materials management system, the catering and laundry system, the patient classification system and the technical department system.

REFERENCE

Boel, A., Willems, J.L. : Building a hospital computer network at the University of Leuven. In "Communication Networks in Health Care" (Eds. H. Peterson and A.I. Isaksson), North Holland Publ. Amsterdam, 1982, pp. 145-153.

THE CANADIAN WORKLOAD MEASUREMENT SYSTEM- A NATIONAL HOSPITAL PRODUCTIVITY IMPROVEMENT PROGRAM

H.H. Rubarth, Ph.D.
Health Services Directorate
Department of National Health and Welfare
Ottawa, Canada K1A 1B4

INTRODUCTION

Productivity Improvement is a key issue which confronts us all in every economic sector of society and particularly those working in the health sector. Conceptually, productivity is a simple notion: it is the relationship between the physical output (workload in units) of an organization and the input (paid or worked personnel hours) utilized to produce the output. Productivity can be quantified by dividing the output by the input. And productivity can be increased by improving this output/input ratio.

Productivity applies to all the factors of production, labour, capital, and material that a hospital organization utilizes in producing an output. However, in the context of Canadian Hospital Workload Measurement Systems, productivity will only be applied to human resources, which consume as much as 80% of a hospital's operating budget, and thus make workload measurement a prerequisite to labour performance evaluation and productivity improvement. Workload Measurement Systems (WMS) are now considered essential proven tools for the effective management of Canadian Health Care Facilities, their departments and services. They provide a nationally uniform basis for the measurement of workload according to standardized units of production and thus provide the means for evaluation and management of personnel productivity.

This uniform approach to the quantification of workload permits various statistical comparisons within individual hospitals, or between peer groups on a regional or national scale. The information and comparative productivity indicators derived from such systems can be used in the planning, programming, budgeting, control and monitoring functions of the manager.

While each of the departmental WMS have been designed as stand-alone systems, they represent the key building blocks of an integrated total Hospital Management Information System(M.I.S.).

HISTORY OF CANADIAN WMS

In the 1940's the Nuffield Foundation in the United Kingdom devised a system for measuring workload in laboratory departments based on the total time expended by all personnel involved in each individual test and expressed in ten-minute time units. Canadian hospital laboratories adopted this system of workload measurement and in 1954 the Dominion Bureau of Statistics (now Statistics Canada) commenced collection of hospital laboratory statistics in units of time.

In 1965, the Canadian Association of Pathologists received a grant from the Department of National Health and Welfare to develop new units for procedures based on standard time studies. As a result of this project, the unit was restructured to represent one minute instead of ten and the concept of productive time was introduced and defined. Statistics Canada published the first unit values derived from actual timed measurements in 1969.

CURRENT STATUS OF WMS

The National Hospital Productivity Improvement Program is a joint, cost-shared Federal/Provincial Program directed by the Federal/ Provincial Sub-Committee on Productivity Improvement under the aegis of the Federal/Provincial Advisory Committee on Institutional and Medical Services.

Its mandate includes the development, promotion, evaluation, approval and funding of Workload Measurement Systems and Staffing Methodologies in collaboration with representatives from the Department of National Health and Welfare, provincial health authorities, national professional associations, the Canadian Hospital Association/M.I.S. and Statistics Canada.

The Health Services Directorate of the Department of National Health and Welfare has the responsibility for overall program coordination and administration, while Statistics Canada is responsible for the provision of national health statistics.

To date, National Workload Measurement Systems have been implemented in the following five specialty areas: Clinical Laboratory, Diagnostic Radiology, Occupational Therapy, Physiotherapy and Respiratory

Technology/Pulmonary Function. Twelve new WMS are currently in various stages of development: Audiology and Speech Pathology, Social Work, Pharmacy, Health Records, Radiation Oncology, Nuclear Medicine, Materiel Management, Operating Room, Recovery Room, Emergency, Obstetrical Suite, and Physical Plant - Operation and Maintenance.

WORKLOAD DATA REPORTING MECHANISM

Figure (1) indicates the direction of flow of workload data from the worker, through the internal reporting system to the external reporting system. A limited amount of aggregate data is required at the federal government level, while more data is required successively by provincial governments, the hospital administration and the department's manager. The figure is triangular in shape to denote the quantity of information required at each reporting level.

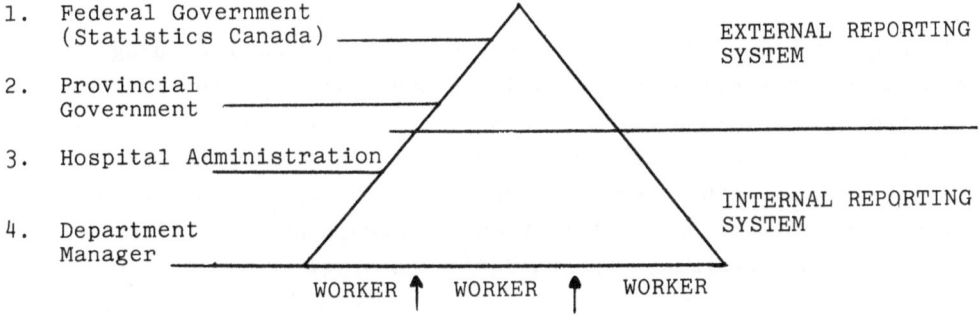

Figure 1

The data collected through WMS is reported on an annual basis both federally and provincially by all Canadian hospitals. A voluntary QUARTERLY HOSPITAL INFORMATION SYSTEM was also instituted by the federal government to provide over 700 participating Canadian hospitals quarterly with comparative operating statistics, which enables administrators and departmental managers to compare their hospital's performance with other hospitals of similar type and configuration.

STRUCTURE OF WORKLOAD MEASUREMENT SYSTEMS

Canadian WMS represent measures of production which are based on the application of methodologies which provide for the nationally uniform

measuring and recording of personnel time expended in the performance
of specified and defined patient care and non-patient care activities.

The cornerstone of the Workload Measurement System is the UNIT.
For uniform national reporting purposes, work output is expressed
in standard units, where

> **ONE UNIT** equals **ONE MINUTE** of personnel time
> spent in the provision of patient care activities.

In all national Workload Measurement Systems, the unit is used as
the standard measure to express output.
Due to the diversity and complexity of the work within departments,
two different methodologies have been employed in the development
of Canadian Workload Measurement Systems:

1. The Average Time Recording Methodology
2. The Actual Time Recording Methodology

The Average Time Recording Methodology consists of the recording of
predetermined **unit values** for activities/procedures/examinations based
on average time values derived from a series of time studies, which
were carried out across the country in hospitals of varying size and
complexity. This methodology was applied to the W.M.S. in Laboratory,
Diagnostic Radiology, Respiratory Technology/Pulmonary Function,
Nuclear Medicine, Pharmacy, and Radiation Oncology WMS.

The Unit Value is defined as the average number of units (minutes)
of professional*, technical and support personnel time required to
perform all activities to complete a specific procedure or examination.
  * (non-medical)

The Unit Value consists of the recording of actual time spent by
personnel in the performance of unit producing activities. This
methodology was selected for the Occupational Therapy, Physiotherapy,
Social Work, and Audiology/Speech Pathology WMS.

W.M.S. Design Features give recognition to the diverse aspects of
the delivery of health services and patient care, while providing
a link through the uniform use of components which are common to

Workload Measurement Systems:

(1) Classification and definition of patient care activities
(2) Categorization of patient care activities
(3) Classification of non-patient care activities:
   - Support Functions
   - Service to Hospital/Community/Profession
   - Education
   - Quality Assurance
   - Research
(4) Methodology for measuring and recording workload
(5) Methodology for calculating workload
(6) Options for system expansion
(7) Managers Guide
   - Reporting of Workload Data
   - Comparative Performance Indicators

An example of the conceptual framework of the Occupational Therapy W.M.S. is given in figure (2).

MANAGEMENT USE OF WORKLOAD MEASUREMENT SYSTEMS

W.M.S. are considered improved management tools which are needed by managers to assess departmental performance and labour productivity. Workload data from the W.M.S. can be used, in combination with other hospital statistics, to derive numerous indicators for such purposes as evaluation, planning, budgeting, control and peer group comparison. Examples of key indicators are presented in figure (3) to demonstrate their construction and utility. The number of key indicators usually included in W.M.S. manuals varies between ten and twenty.

324

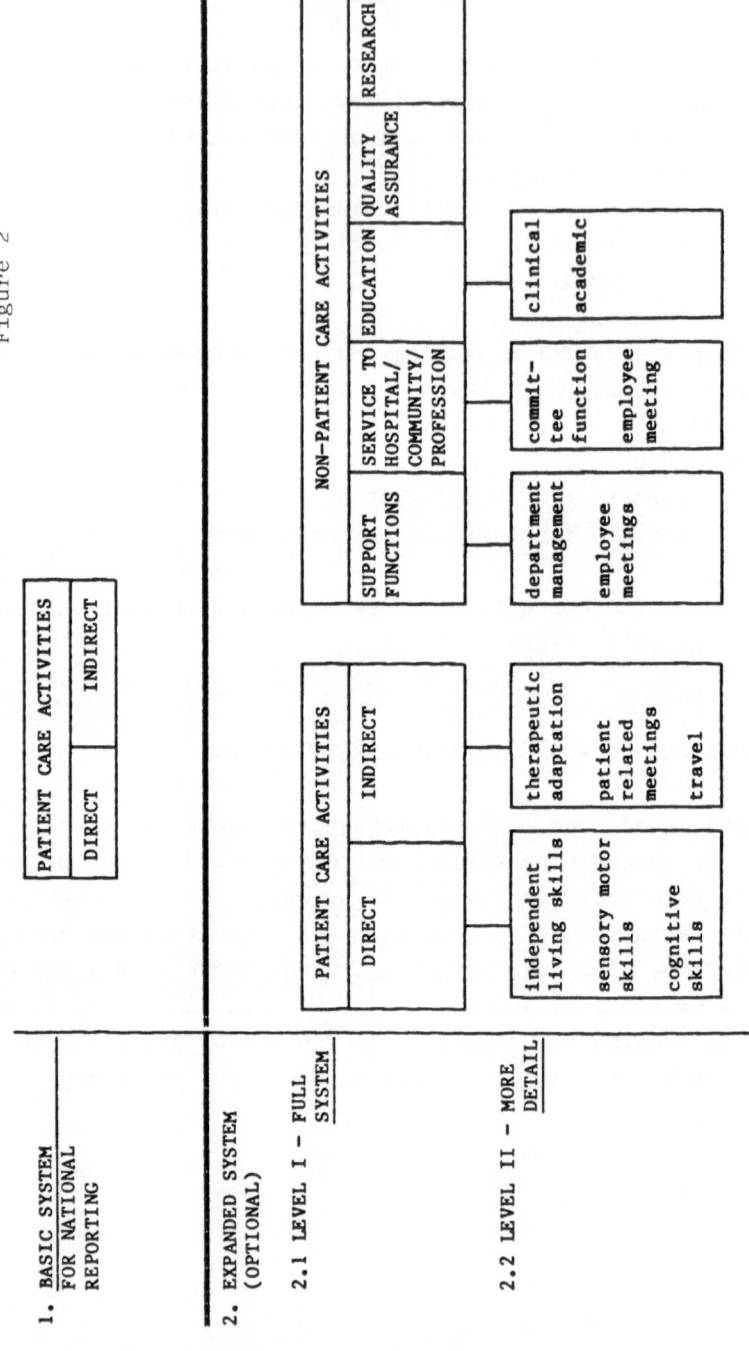

Figure 2

Figure 3

EXAMPLES OF PERFORMANCE INDICATORS

INDICATOR	CALCULATION	DEFINITION	KEY PURPOSE
PRODUCTIVITY INDICATORS: Unit-producing personnel worked productivity index	Patient care units in period x 100 / Unit-producing personnel worked hours in period x 60	The percentage of all unit-producing personnel worked hours spent in the provision of patient care	Control evaluation planning
Units per unit-producing F.T.E.	Patient care units in period / Unit-producing personnel F.T.E. in period	The average number of patient care units generated by each unit-producing personnel full-time equivalent	Control evaluation planning
UTILIZATION INDICATOR: Inpatient new referral rate	Inpatient new referrals to department in period x 100 / Total hospital inpatient admissions in period	The percentage of total hospital inpatient admissions during the period referred to the department or service	Evaluation planning
STAFFING INDICATOR: Total full-time equivalent (F.T.E.)	Non-medical paid hours in period / Normal hours in period per F.T.E.	The total number of full-time equivalents in the period	Control budgeting planning

USING DRGS TO SEPARATE CASE MIX IN THE UK FROM TRENDS IN LENGTH OF STAY

L.M. JENKINS, M.J. BARDSLEY,
CASPE Research, 14 Palace Court,
London W2 4HS.

Abstract

Patient records from acute hospitals in four health districts in the UK, altogether serving a population of one million, have been assigned to diagnosis related groups (DRGs). The workload over the period 1979-83 was examined for changes in complexity of case and in treatment practices. Using a statistical technique of separation into components, marked reductions in DRG-specific lengths of stay were identified in combination with small changes in overall case complexity . The analysis was repeated after excluding cases with extremely long stay lengths or chronic illness to examine the effect of these cases on the stability of the results.

Introduction

Much interest has been generated by the development of diagnosis related groups [1] and other patient classification schemes [2] as an attempt to measure hospital output. Since the adoption of DRGs in setting reimbursement rates for a large section of the US population whose health care is federally funded, many other countries are looking at the potential of DRGs in their health care setting. Some early analyses suggest that the US groupings with only small adaptation are applicable elsewhere, in the areas of planning services, monitoring performance and building budgets [3,4,5,6].

In the UK a government funded research project was set up to investigate changes in case mix during an experiment in clinical budgeting. The study described here formed a part of that project and investigated the changes in lengths of stay (LOS), and the extent to which the observed fall in LOS was due to a simpler case mix or to real reductions in LOS by case type.

The approach used DRGs to define case types. They were chosen because they represent one of the most widely tested, comprehensive in-patient classification schemes available and because they are based on routinely recorded abstract information. It was hoped that by assigning cases to DRGs it would be possible to identify both qualitative changes in case mix, as well as the quantitative implications of these changes on resource utilisation (which in this case is estimated using LOS as a proxy). In this way it would be possible to identify the extent to which changes in case mix, as reflected in the mix of DRGs treated, were responsible for changes in the overall average LOS.

By using a technique first described by Kitagawa [7] and later employed by Fetter [1], it is possible to quantify three specific components responsible for differences in LOS.

1. Differences due to case mix - one sample may have proportionally more or less complex or resource intensive types of patient.

2. Differences due to LOS - the average LOS for each type of patient may have changed.

3. Interaction - the effects due to combinations of changes in case mix and LOS.

Mathematically the relationship between these three can be described as follows. For two samples with average LOS a and A, the proportion of cases in the ith DRG being p_i and P_i and LOS a_i and A_i.

$$a-A = \Sigma\ P_i\ (a_i - A_i) + \Sigma\ A_i\ (p_i - P_i) + \Sigma\ (a_i - A_i)(p_i - P_i)$$

Avg.LOS =Difference due to + Difference due + Difference due to
difference   LOS   to case mix   to interaction

Method

Within the context of the clinical budgeting research programme four non-teaching districts provided data on inpatients over the five year period 1979-1983. Annually this totalled 90,000 deaths or discharges from a catchment population of just over a million persons. Cases were assigned to DRGs using a computer program developed to handle diagnosis and procedure codes used in the UK and incoporating minor adaptations to Yale's DRGs to match UK practices.[8] A small percentage of cases was "lost" because a DRG could not be assigned. This was due to incomplete or missing data in the patient record or to lack of specificity in ICD9 diagnosis codes, but left 97% of cases successfully assigned.

The analysis was based on the interpretation of the components of case mix and length of stay changes. Each district was considered separately and successive years compared to the base year. In this way any fundamental differences in the mix of patients and the patterns of treatment between districts was not considered, only the changes each experienced over five years. A form of null hypothesis was proposed that there was no overall change in average LOS, and that each component was also zero. In practice the interaction was examined first; if it was large in relation to the other components the effects of LOS and case mix complexity could not be separated. If the interaction was non-significant we looked for significantly large components as indicators of change. Finally the sum of these values may produce an important overall difference although the effect of individual components is small.

A criticism of DRGs is that there is considerable heterogeneity within groups, often seen in excessively long staying patients. Our data was no exception, and omitting a small proportion of cases from some DRGs had a dramatic effect on average length of stay. This gave rise to concern about the stability of results based on all the data, and the extent to which observed changes in the overall population might simply be due to the relatively few, but influential cases with extremely long LOS. Therefore the analysis was repeated using a smaller sample which excluded cases which fell outside the limits of ± 2 standard deviations from the mean of the logged data. In addition all cases in the 'geriatric' specialty on discharge were excluded on the grounds that they may contain patients not receiving typical acute care.

Results

The results for all districts studied are given in the table, and show a clear fall in average LOS. This fall was broadly consistent with published statistics at regional and national level [9], despite inter-district differences in overall provision of services, case mix and the possible efficiency with which the available resources were used. The data presented was the end-point of a trend of falling LOS which can be seen , with minor fluctuations, in the intervening years.

Changes in average LOS split into components

District	LOS (Final Year)	Change in LOS	Components of change		
			Case mix	LOS	Interaction
Untrimmed					
1	8.4	-0.74*	0.54*	-1.11*	-0.16
2	8.6	-1.83*	-0.09	-1.93*	0.19
3	12.9	-1.55*	-0.16	-0.85*	-0.54
4	11.0	-1.93*	0.23	-2.14*	-0.02
Trimmed					
1	5.4	-0.85*	0.08	-0.84*	-0.09
2	6.1	-1.02*	-0.27*	-0.76*	0.01
3	8.1	-1.44*	0.40*	-1.45*	-0.40*
4	7.3	-0.49*	0.38*	-0.93*	0.06

* Significant, using 95% confidence limits.

The interesting feature of these results is the separation of overall change into its component parts. The most consistently significant change in all districts was the reduction in DRG-specific LOS of 1 to 2 days. In contrast, only district 1 untrimmed could demonstrate a significant change in case mix. This was a shift toward more complex cases causing an increase of 0.54 days on the average LOS. The interactions between complexity and stay length were small, apart from district 3, and not significant for the untrimmed cases.

The construction of both the DRG classification scheme and the component analysis technique employed, allowed observed changes to be traced back to a particular major diagnostic category (MDC) or even specific DRGs. For example the large interaction in district 3 could be attributed to mental disorders (MDC 19), where an increased number of cases had been accompanied by a large reduction in the average stay.

It is possible that effects observed in the whole workload may be due to changes in only a few cases which have a very long LOS. Removing these cases by trimming, left 80-90% of cases which used 50-60% of the occupied beds. These were regarded as roughly corresponding to the "routine" acute caseload.

Results for the trimmed data also demonstrated a clear reduction in average LOS, within which the most important component was the fall in DRG-specific LOS. Unlike before, significant changes in case mix were seen in three districts, with only district 1 showing no changes in complexity when outliers were removed. The complexity of cases seen had increased in two districts (although district 3 also had a significant interaction which could swamp the case mix effect), and decreased for the other district. Tracing these effects back to major disease categories showed orthopaedic cases to have major but conflicting contributions to districts 2 and 4, and district 3 was most affected by the mental illness cases as explained before. These results, dealing more specifically with the "routine" acute case load, therefore provided a refinement to those observations on the whole data set.

Further analysis on the "routine" cases in the trimmed data and the excluded cases can be carried out. The same component analysis can be used to study the relative contributions of these two groups to changes in district LOS. Though not presented here results of this further analysis suggested that the the effects due to outliers varied in their impact on overall stay length. Reducing LOS in districts 1 and 3 was largely explained by the changes in normal acute (trimmed) cases. In districts 2 and 4 the picture was more complex as both the proportion of outliers had increased and their LOS fallen, the net effect being that these cases made a larger contribution to the changes observed in the distrct average.

Discussion

This study offers an explanation of the falling LOS in the UK, namely that changes were due to a reduction in DRG specific LOS rather than case mix differences. In fact there was evidence to suggest that in some districts the case mix complexity was actually increasing which would, other things being equal, tend to increase average LOS.

Comparing trimmed and untrimmed samples there were both similarities and major differences. To explain overall changes in the district averages it is obviously necessary to include all cases, yet to produce more stable values representing the normal case load within the district, the trimmed study would seem most appropriate.

One feature of the results which made the interpretation easy was the predominantly low value for the interaction component. This was because the changes in case mix for successive years were relatively small within the same district, reflecting a general stability in the DRG profile.

Acceptance of such conclusions about case mix complexity relies on the assumption that DRGs distinguish "medically acceptable" and statistically homogeneous patient groups. Whilst it is true to say that in the UK we are still in the process of validating this assumption, for the types of analysis performed in this study there are no suitable alternatives to DRGs.

Having produced the empirical observation that DRG-specific LOS was falling it is tempting to speculate on the possible explanations. At the district level it is difficult to make generalisations about either changes in the forms of treatment, or the increasing efficiency with which care is provided. However, it is possible to exploit what commentators have described as the "construct validity" of the DRG classification, to identify those areas most responsible for changes in the aggregate figures. In conjunction with the component analysis technique, observed changes in resource consumption (or as near as can be approximated using LOS) can be equated to the patient care services provided, and so suggest appropriate explanations for specific changes. The development of the aggregated, district-wide summary statistics presented in this study, is only a small part of the possible practical applications of these techniques.

References

[1]   Fetter R.B., Shin Y., Freeman J.L., Averill R.F. and Thompson
      J.D.   Case mix definition by diagnosis related groups.
      Medical Care Supplement to February 1980, 18, 2, 1-53

[2]   Hornbrook M.C. Hospital Case Mix definition, measurement and
      use. Part I The conceptual framework. Part II Review
      of alternative measures. Medical Care Review 1982, 30,
      2, 1-123.

[3]   Rodrigues J.M., Girardier M., Fetter R.B., Freeman J.L.,
      Mullin R., & Valois J. Evaluating productivity of
      hospitals using US DRGs as a case mix measure on a
      French database. Ed. F.H. Roger et al - Lecture Notes
      in Medical Informatics, 1984, 24, 479-484. Springer-
      Verlag, Berlin.

[4]   Hofdijk W.J. and de Jager K. The DRGs going dutch.   Ed.
      F.H. Roger et al - Lecture Notes in Medical Informatics,
      1984, 24, 485-491. Springer-Verlag, Berlin.

[5]   Jenkins L.M. and Coles J.M.   Information tools for the
      future. Health and Social Service Journal, 9 August
      1984, 948-9

[6]   Palmer G. and Wood T.   DRGs: recent developments and their
      adaption and application in Australia. Australian Health
      Review, 1984, 7,2,67-80

[7]   Kitagawa E.M. Components of a difference between two rates.
      Journal of the Americal Statisical Association, 1955,
      50, 1168-1194.

[8]   Sanderson H. and Andrews V. Monitoring hospital services.
      Report from the London School of Hygiene and Tropical
      Medicine, Keppel Street, London, 1984.

[9]   DHSS.   Hospital in-patient enquiry, 1979.   HMSO, London,
      1982.

Confidentiality Problems in the Federal Republic of Germany

G. Wagner
Cancer Research Center
Heidelberg, F.R.G.

In almost all western democracies the idea has gained more and more
ground during the last twenty years that the citizen's personal data
are in need of increased protection in view of the practically
unlimited possibilities offered by the computer in setting up and
working with the most extensive databases. This development also has
considerable impact on research inasmuch as the latter depends upon
work with personal data. The fact that the understanding of jurists
of the scope and necessity of data protection frequently differs
greatly from the requirements of the medical researcher (e.g., the
epidemiologist) has in the past led to innumerable discussions, reflected in unpleasant articles in the press which, among other things,
spoke about "giant data collections at the cost of the patient", about
"ferocious epidemiologists" and of "cancer patients whose data was to
be turned into cash" (13). One of the rare examples to the contrary is
the article in the New Statesman of 3 March 1967 with the caustic
title "To Hell with Medical Secrecy".

It goes without saying that no manner of dealing with this problem can
claim to be generally valid for "law, unlike medicine, knows national
borders" (3). I will, therefore, restrict myself to conditions in the
F.R.G. as they now present themselves to the epidemiologist.

The discussion on the execution of data protection has, in the Federal
Republic of Germany, been determined by uncertainty as to the legal
conditions and by an increasing criticism of research. This conflict
situation follows from the fact that two so-called fundamental values
of our constitution are touched by this legislation: first the personal
right laid down in article 2, par. 1 warranting the protection of the
individuum and his right to alone dispose of his personal data;
secondly, the freedom of research declared in article 5, par. 3, making
it a duty of the state to see to it that scientific research can work
freely, protected against outside aggression (14). Thus, we have two
partly contradictory fundamental values which are, however, equally
legitimized, and whose mutual harmonization has, unfortunately, not
yet been satisfactorily achieved (12).

The Federal law on data protection and the subsequent laws on data protection of the Länder were conceived as protective laws in favour of the individuum against the intervention of public authorities and private agencies with the informational right of self-determination. It is evident and appears plausible that the authorities set up to control the observation of these laws (the so-called "Landesdaten-schutzbeauftragten")are inclined to prove their competence by offensive interpretation of these laws. The fact that conflict situations between data protection and research had not been anticipated when these laws were conceived proves the lack of a so-called research paragraph in the Federal Privacy Act (2).

Present Legal Situation

Principally, data protection is nothing new. Personal data have been protected in the Federal Republic of Germany by other, partly older regulations, too (e.g., the medical professional regulations, the Federal Law on Statistics, the social legislation and the Funeral Laws of the Länder).

Competence concerning legislation is divided between the Federal and the Länder governments. Apart from the Federal Law, there are eleven Privacy Laws on a Länder level. Thus, the Federal Privacy Act, as far as medical research is concerned, applies to all private hospitals, to hospitals belonging to the churches and the welfare agencies. On the other hand, the respective privacy acts of the Länder are valid for the universities and university hospitals (4).

Only four of the eleven privacy acts of the Länder do contain a "research clause", namely those of Baden-Württemberg, Hesse, North-rhine-Westphalia and Rhineland-Palatinate. Largely coinciding as to their contents, if not phrased identically, these clauses roughly contain the following:
Universities and other public institutions engaged in independent scientific research may, within the framework of their tasks for certain research projects, store or change personal data, ...if the person concerned has agreed to this or if his interests to be protected are not impaired (due to the nature of the data, their notoriousness or the way in which they are used).....

Just as vaguely phrased and accessible to controversial interpretation are the regulations about medical secrecy, frequently of prime impor-tance for medical research. While the representatives of the medical professional organizations admit that medical research as a basis of progress in medicine serves the interests of the individual patient as well as those of society and is partly dependent on the acquisition of personal data (1), they argue at the same time that safeguarding medical secrecy must, in every instance, be the supreme principle of any medical action and that § 203 of the Criminal Code threatens with punishment anyone laying open medical secrets without the knowledge or against the will of the patient concerned.

What is to be understood by "laying open medical secrets" depends upon the professional law laid down in the medical regulations of the Länder. This is being rigidly interpreted to an increasing extent. While earlier passing on patient data to research institutions was considered unobjectionable if these were medically directed, today any physician passing on personal data for the purpose of medical research makes himself liable to punishment according to the opinion of most representatives of the profession. This opinion feigns blindness with regard to the fact that undermining medical secrecy within the framework of public health insurance is a social reality and a necessary manifestation of our public service society (9). It is hard to understand that in this situation it is the scientist, and apparently only he alone, who is being classified as potential "abuser of data", against whom patient data must be protected by any means.

The Problem of Epidemiological Research

In the field of medicine, one may differentiate between treatment-related and not treatment-related research (6). The former includes research at the patient's bedside, the entire therapy research as well as research on drug safety. The second group includes fields of research such as epidemiology, genetics, certain projects of hygiene, setting up disease registries as well as health systems research. In the following, I want to restrict myself to the example of epidemiological research and its obstruction by the present legislation on data protection.

As opposed to the clinical researcher, the epidemiologist is not entitled to personal data on the basis of an agreement about treatment with the patient. Therefore, he is, to an increasing extent, refused access to primary and secondary data required for the solution of his tasks.

Not all epidemiological projects are equally affected by the restrictions of today's legislation on data protection. With prospective studies it will frequently be possible to obtain the so-called "informed consent" of the probands envisaged; with retrospective investigations, however, this will generally not be possible.

If, for example, an epidemiologist wants to investigate the late sequelae of certain occupational activities, it will be necessary to follow up the fate of those workers who had been engaged in these particular activities. There is, however, no legal basis for covering and subsequently following up the fates of such cases. How is the epidemiologist to obtain the consent of a proband whose present address is not known to him and of whom he does not even know whether he is still alive? If, after more or less tedious inquiries with residents' registration offices, he has at long last succeeded in finding out his last place of residence, it then turns out that the patient or proband has meanwhile died. The public health offices and residents' registration offices refuse to an increasing extent to give information on causes of death.

It goes for many fields of epidemiological research that they simply cannot do without personal data, but that such data are only needed for an interim period. The epidemiologist is not interested in the individuum; for him the individuum is but a statistical counting unit which, however, must be correctly identifiable in order to make an exact record linkage possible, i.e. in order to correctly coordinate data from different sources (11).

On the basis of an inquiry among German members of the faculty initiated a few years ago, I was able to establish an increasing resignation with a view to the chances of epidemiological research in the F.R.G. By the way, this frustration is not specific to our country; it can be seen in other countries, too. Thus, the US-American epide-miologist A.Z. Smith, author of a famous study on food additives and cancer, wrote some years ago: "One year of my career was invested in contacting hospitals, completing redundant forms about informed consent and privacy, assuring skeptical clinicians of the value of epidemiologic research such as mine, and writing letters repeatedly awakening slumbering administrators to the urgency of my request. It shocks me now to realize that I spent roughly 3 per cent of my scientific career trying to get permission to conduct a single study, which in itself took only three years" (8).

Hoping for an Improvement of the Situation

The fact that certain fields of medical research - in particular epidemiology - are being obstructed to an extent almost exceeding what
is tolerable by too "offensive" a handling of privacy acts and ever
more restrictive regulations of the medical profession is recognized
even by sensible and farsighted representatives of the "opposition".
Attempts are, therefore, made on the part of the legislators, the
data protectors and professional representatives as well as the
researchers to arrive at a compromise acceptable for both parties.
Technical solutions (such as, e.g., improved methods of anonymization)
are under discussion as well as legal solutions (such as, e.g.,
setting up data trustees and more specific legal regulations). Patent
solutions are not to be expected in any of these fields; a legal
regulation offering a tolerable compromise would appear to be most
promising.

Data positivism on the one hand and data neurosis on the other hand
are the two diametrally opposed poles between which the work with
data, in particular social data, takes place today (10). It will
certainly not be easy to find a golden mean.

References

1. Bundesärztekammer: Thesenpapier - Empfehlung zur Beachtung der
   ärztlichen Schweigepflicht bei der Verarbeitung personenbezogener
   Daten in der ärztlichen Berufsausübung. (Als Manuskript gedruckt).

2. Deutsche Forschungsgemeinschaft: (Unterkommission Datenschutz der
   Senatskommission für empirische Sozialforschung): Vorschlag zur
   Novellierung des Bundesdatenschutzgesetzes (BDSG) vom 1. Sept.
   1982. (Als Manuskript gedruckt).

3. Glazebrook, P.R.: Medical Confidences, Research and the Law.
   In E.D. Acheson (Edit.): Record Linkage in Medicine, pp. 323-332.
   Edinburgh and London: Livingstone 1968.

4. Kilian, W.: Rechtsfragen der medizinischen Forschung mit Patienten-
   daten. Datenschutz und Forschungsfreiheit im Konflikt.
   Beiträge zur juristischen Informatik, Band 9. Darmstadt: S. Toeche-
   Mittler Verlag 1983.

5. Kilian, W., Porth, A.J. (Hrsg.): Juristische Probleme der Datenverarbeitung in der Medizin. Med. Informatik und Statistik,
   Band 12. Berlin-Heidelberg-New York: Springer 1979.

6. Reichertz, P.L.: Kontextabhängigkeit medizinischer Informationen. In P.L. Reichertz, W. Kilian(7), S. 204-210.

7. Reichertz, P.L., Kilian, W. (Hrsg.): Arztgeheimnis-Datenbanken-Datenschutz. Med. Informatik und Statistik, Band 38. Berlin-Heidelberg-New York: Springer 1982.

8. Smith, A.Z.: Memoirs of an epidemiologist. New York: Augur Press 2002.

9. Steinmüller, W.: Der Schutz "medizinischer" Daten: Terminologische, rechtliche und organisatorische Aspekte; sowie ein Vorschlag zur gesetzlichen Regelung des Datenschutzes bei Forschung und Planung. In W. Kilian und A.J. Porth(5), S. 135-148.

10. Überla, K., Zeiler, J. (Hrsg.): Datenschutz und Wissenschafts-administration im Gesundheitsbereich. bga-Schriften Nr. 5/83. München: MMW Medizin Verlag 1983.

11. Wagner, G.: Krebsregister und Datenschutz. In W. Kilian und A.J. Porth(5), S. 71-77.

12. Wagner, G.: Datenschutz und Onkologie. In P.L. Reichertz und W. Kilian(7), S. 117-126.

13. Wagner, G.: Krebsregister: notwendig, wenn auch nicht unproblematisch. Klinikarzt 13 (1984), S. 753-762.

14. Wissenschaftsrat: Stellungnahme zu Forschung und Datenschutz vom 5. Nov. 1982 (Typescript).

GUIDELINES FOR PRIVACY PROTECTION IN DUTCH HEALTH CARE

O.F.C. van der Leer

Advisory Board for Automation in Health Care
P.O. Box 439, 2260 AK Leidschendam
The Netherlands

1. Introduction

At the time of writing this paper, in the Netherlands a data protection (privacy) act is still in preparation. It is to be expected that the introduction will take some more time and that such an act will not provide for specific measures in health care concerning acquisition, handling and retrieval of medical (patient related) data.

Therefore the Dutch Advisory Board for Automation in Health Care (BAG)[*] was asked by the Ministry for Welfare, Health and Cultural Affairs to frame the necessary guidelines for privacy protection in health care. 'Privacy' means in this context: safeguarding the patients' claim to confidentiality of his medical data.

The Board framed two pattern regulations: one for health care institutions (hospitals, public health services, etc.) and one for individual medical professionals, such as medical doctors, pharmacists, dentists, therapeutists. A distinction between these categories has to be made in terms of organisation and working methods. However the tendency of both regulations is identical.

2. Purpose of these regulations

- Steering and co-ordinating 'self-regulating' and preventing simular studies (and costs) by individual institutions.
- To improve quality of existing guidelines.
- To reach more uniformity in rules.

---

[*] This is an independent advisory board for the Dutch government, in which representatives of ministries, health care institutions, health care insurers and medical profession groups participate.

- To offer more legal security (to the patient).
- Stimulating and structuring discussions at issue.
- To speed up the process of privacy (health care) legislation.

3. Status of these regulations

The Board will probably advise the Minister for Welfare, Health and Cultural Affairs to give these regulations a legal status what means, that the regulations have to be adopted by existing health care legislation and/or have to be part of agreements between Sick Funds and individual health care professionals and health care institutions.

4. Contents of regulations

The regulations consist each of the following sections:

a. general rules	art. 1 + 2
b. characteristics of the registration (patient files)	art. 3 - 5
c. patients' rights	art. 6 - 11
d. keeping terms and use of patient related data	art. 12 - 14
e. Visitation Committee	art. 15
f. temporary and final provisions.	art. 16 - 18

An explanatory memorandum discusses the regulation in general and then clause by clause.

ad a.: This section treats definition and consideration of terms.

ad b.: This section treats purpose and procedures concerning the registration and the data recorded.

It is provided that the keeper has to add an appendix to the issued regulation, in which he describes the purpose(s) and procedures and data recorded in the registration (f.e. categories of data which exclusively can be found in patient files). No other personal data may be recorded than those which are in accordance with the purpose of the registration. The recorded data may not be used for another purpose than described in the appendix to the rules.

Besides this provision attention has been paid to the relation between keeper, manager of the registration and originator.

ad c.: Patients' rights provided in this section can be summarized as follows:

1. The patient has to be informed explicitly and individually when his identifiable personal medical data will be used for another purpose than concerning his medical treatment and/or described by the keeper or a purpose of which the patient is not aware. It is generally assumed that patients are aware or can be aware of the fact that their personal data have to be registered in aid of their medical treatment. Apart from that the advise must be given that keepers draw the patients' attention to this fact in general, f.e. in waiting rooms or by means of brochures, and make known that regulations on guaranteeing the patients' privacy do exist.

2. The patient may inspect his personal data recorded in the registration (his personal file).

3. The patient can request that (some of) his personal medical data will not be recorded in the registration.

4. The patient can request that (some of) his personal data recorded in the registration will be corrected.

5. The patient can request that (some of) his personal medical data will be removed from the registration or will be made anonymous for further use.

6. In principle the patient can block disclosure of his personal file in case of intended external use (see below ad d and 6).

In cases of 3, 4 and 5 the keeper (or medical attendant, who should not necessarily be the keeper) can reject the patients' request, after which appeal can be made to an independent committee (see below). The findings of this committee are absolute. The keeper has to point out to the patient that his request can cause consequences for medical treatment or as costs or charges.

ad d.: The keeper has to add an appendix to the privacy regulation, in which he describes how long the data recorded in the registration will be kept. Of course it would be well advised to pursue similar terms per category of health care institutions or medical profession group.

This section does also provide for rules concerning access to the registration and data retrieval. Generally spoken, only authorized users of the registration have access to the recorded data. Also an originator has access, but the keeper doesn't necessarily.

Concerning data distribution and external use a principle rule emphasizes the patients' claim to confidentiality of sensitive personal data: the patients' written consent has necessarily to be obtained before his data, if directly related to his identified person, are distributed or used for external purposes.

Some exceptions to this principle rule are possible, particularly related to medical research (see below).

Besides, this section provides that the patient can table a complaint against a keeper, who does not obey the rules; the complaint can be lodged with the Visitation Committee, which will make inquiries into that complaint and will possibly give judgement.

ad e.: This section provides that there is a Visitation Committee.
It has been advised to set up such a committee with the following terms of reference:
- superintending the proceeding of keepers
- to accede to certain alterations of the regulations
- complaint-address
- to arange possible disputes.
In order to carry this advise into effect it is evident that such a committee must dispose the necessary competence and authority. If more visitation committees will be set up it is recommendable that their proceedings will be attuned to each other.

ad f.: The temporary and final provisions concern the regulations' term, transitional (arrangements) and conveyance, alteration and coming into force.

5. Data linking

No explicit rule provides against data linking. It was considered that provisions particularly concerning competence of keepers and users, purpose of the registration, access and data retrieval must be sufficient in order to protect the privacy of the patient. These provisions must prevent inadmissible linking personal files and make possible significant (legal) linking.

6. Medical research

As stated before, the patients' written consent has necessarily to be obtained before his data, if directly identifiable to his person, are distributed or used for external purposes. Two exceptions on this rule are important when distribution of medical data seems to be necessary for the sake of medical research: one exception effects distribution of medical data if the receiver (research-worker) is not able to relate those data to an individual. Otherwise it is in principle possible to make medical research part of the purpose of the registration (think of university hospitals f.e.). In this case the research-worker can have access to the registration as an authorized user and if the patient has been pointed out to that fact (assumed or informed consent). These provisions have been developped for the time being; it was advised to set up a specific committee for studying this complicated and important subject in order to build a bridge between patients' individual interests and common interests.

CONSIDERATIONS ON THE EFFECTIVENESS OF PROTECTION BY PASSWORDS

A.R.Bakker and C.P.Louwerse
BAZIS, Leiden University Hospital
Leiden, Netherlands

Introduction

In health information systems in general a significant part of the stored data is of a confidential nature. An adequate protection is thus of vital importance.

In most terminal based information systems the access protection is based on a password that the authorized user has to offer to the system when he tries to access it. In general there is a password for each individual user; two strategies can be distinguished :

A. The system generates the passwords periodically.

B. The user can choose his own password and can be forced to change it periodically.

The first approach has as disadvantage that the password will be difficult to remember, with as a consequence that users will tend to write it down in a place easily accessible to themselves (e.g. their diary).

The second approach involves the risk that users will choose as a password a string of characters they are familiar with (e.g. a first name, a telephone number, a car number etc.). There is an enlarged risk that such passwords might be guessed by an intruder who knows the user personally.

Guessing passwords is a time-consuming activity when done by human beings, so up till now the risk in general was considered to be limited. However, with the arrival on the scene of personal computers, equiped with data communication facilities, the risk for passwords being guessed deserves our attention.

In this article the use of passwords in two terminal based systems in the Netherlands (a large hospital information system (I) and a university research/education system (II)) is considered. Apart from characteristics of the use of passwords, also possible strategies for the reduction of the risks are considered.

Passwords and probability

At first sight the password system where each user individually chooses a string of characters as his password seems to be a rather secure system. When the password consists of N characters and the characters are chosen from a characterset with C different characters the probability of guessing a password is $C^{**}-N$.

Usual values for C and N are 64 and 6 respectively, which leads, when the characters are choosen at random, to a risk to guess the password of $1.5*10^{**}-11$. This figure is definitely too optimistic, since users will not always choose N characters as a password, but take less characters, e.g. to save time when logging on. In figure 1 the distribution of the length of the passwords in two systems is given.

Figure 1.

Distribution of
length of passwords

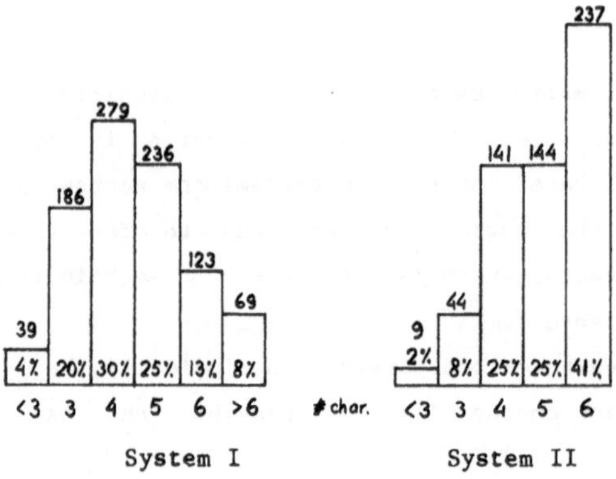

System I   System II

In well-organized systems there should be a lower limit to the length of the passwords in number of characters. At least in system I a check is made on such a limit when entering new passwords. The limited number of passwords with less than 3 characters have a historical background; changing these passwords will automatically solve the problem. Recently the keeper of the information system concerned decided that passwords should be changed at least every 3 months, which will be checked by software. So for further considerations we can neglect the very short password (that of course is in itself a large security risk).

For a length distribution as given in figure 1 we find as the risk to guess a password by random selection of a number of characters the values $8*10^{**}-7$ and $3*10^{**}-7$ respectively. The values are already about a factor 1000 larger than those mentioned earlier. If passwords consisting of only 3 characters were forbidden, risk values would drop to $3*10^{**}-8$ and $6*10^{**}-9$ respectively, which implies a reduction of the risk by about a factor 30.

The characters in a password are in general not choosen at random, which might lead to a higher risk for guessing a password, if some pattern of behaviour in choosing passwords can be detected. The following assumptions on the use of passwords were suggested :

- the passwords might be equal to the telephonenumber of the user or some other number he often is using (e.g. his bank account number)
- passwords will often be pronouncable words without digits or other special characters
- within the class of pronouncable words some words like first names may have high probability.

On letters and digits

Within the two systems considered here, it was checked which percentage of the passwords consisted of letters only. The results are shown in figure 2. Moreover, it was checked which percentage of the passwords consisted of digits only, this turning out to be 3% and 1% respectively.

The probability of guessing a password when the distribution of the length of the password is known is given by

$$\sum_i p(i) / c^i \qquad (1),$$

with p(i) being the probability of finding a password with length i. Taking into account that a certain fraction f(i) of the passwords with length i consists of letters only we find the probability by

$$\sum_i \left\{ \frac{f(i)\,p(i)}{26^i} + \frac{(1 - f(i))\,p(i)}{c^i} \right\} \qquad (2).$$

Substitution of the values from figure 2 in (2) yields as result the probabilities $1*10**-5$ and $4*10**-6$. Taking into account the passwords that consist of digits only will have a moderate increasing effect on these figures.

Figure 2.

Percentages of passwords consisting of letters only

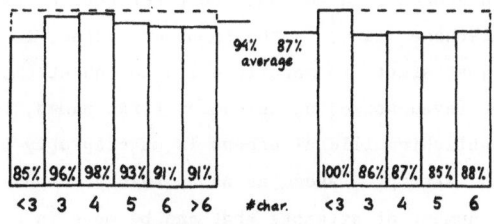

85% 96% 98% 93% 91% 91%   94% 87% average   100% 86% 87% 85% 88%

<3 3 4 5 6 >6   #char.   <3 3 4 5 6

System I   System II

The use of first names

For the two systems the passwords used were considered in more detail. It was found that a significant percentage of the passwords consisted of first names being in use in the Netherlands. In figure 3 the percentage of the passwords consisting of a first name is given for the various lengths of passwords.

The percentage of passwords corresponding to a first name, as given in figure 3 indicates that the guess risk is even higher than calculated till now. Assuming the number of candidatenames per length class to be NC(i) we can calculate the risk by means of

$$\sum_i \left\{ \frac{f(i)\,p(i)\,g(i)}{NC(i)} + \frac{f(i)\,p(i)\,(1-g(i))}{26^i} + \frac{(1-f(i))\,p(i)}{c^i} \right\} \quad (3).$$

Taking for NC(i) the values 100, 300, 500 and 500 we find an increase of the guess risk by a factor 10.

The estimation of the guess risk might be made more accurate by taking into account the frequency of occurence of certain first names. This will lead to an even higher outcome of the risk estimate.

Figure 3.

Percentages of passwords that are equal to a first name

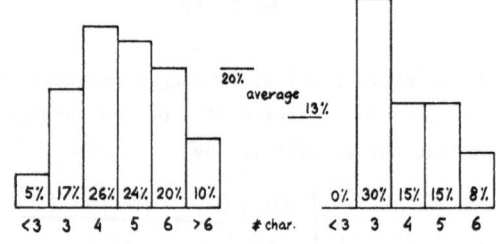

System I   System II

Defence strategies

The results found in the previous section demonstrate clearly that a possible intruder, who disposes of a personal computer that he can connect (e.g. by means of a dial-up telephone line) to the computer system, is a serious security risk. If this intruder just starts to make repeated log-on attempts, using at random strings of letters, or (even worse) using common first names, the probability that he will succeed in establishing illegal access is unacceptably high. Let us assume that a failing log-on attempt takes as an average t seconds (typical values of t being 2-10) then the number of attempts that can be made in one hour amounts to 3600:t.

Confrontation of this figure with the risk estimation found in the previous chapter makes clear that measures must be taken.

Measures to be implemented may be aiming at two different effects :
* reduction of the guess risk
* reduction of the possible number of log-on attempts in a certain period of time.
As to the first approach, one might reconsider the possibility to let the system issue the passwords. As mentioned in the introduction this principle has as a disadvantage that such passwords are difficult to remember and users will write them down somewhere, thereby increasing the risk that usernumbers will be misused within the organization. For an outside intruder (with his personal computer) however, this approach would be rather effective since the guess-risk is reduced by at least a factor 10**6.
Even if the principle is maintained that users choose their own password the guess-risk can be reduced in a number of ways. As a first step short passwords e.g. with only three or four characters could be forbidden.
According to (2) this would lead, in case of random choice of letters, to a reduction of the risk by a factor 30 if the three-character passwords are forbidden and a factor of 1000 when also the four-character passwords are forbidden. However, we should bear in mind that in practice passwords are not chosen at random and if the percentage of passwords corresponding to first names remains the same, the effect is limited. If the total number of candidate first names amounts to NT and pc percent of the passwords are first names, then the risk is equal to pc:NT.
As a defence strategy one might forbid certain passwords, e.g. christian names and other common words. Such a strategy might be implemented by adding all passwords being ever used in the system to a blacklist and refusing new passwords when they are on that list. By forcing users to change their passwords every W weeks, easy passwords will be filtered out rapidly. A serious disadvantage is, that it might become time-consuming for users to find passwords that are not on the blacklist.
A possible way out is to let the system offer to the user a number of suggestions for passwords and to leave the choice to the user. This might be a good compromise between user selection and system generation of passwords. The guess probability would be low if passwords of six characters length are used. The probability will be higher than the figure of 10**-11 found earlier, since users will prefer passwords that can easily be remembered which implies in practice a reduction of the characterset to 36 possibilities (letters and digits) and moreover a preference for readable passwords.

In chosing a strategy to limit the number of log-on attempts we should strike a balance between the restricting effect on a possible intruder and the burden for a normal user.
Sometimes the simple strategy is implemented where after more than a predefined

number of consecutive failing log-on attempts, the usernumber or terminal is blocked. This might be an effective strategy to reduce the risk, however, the burden for normal users will become unacceptable if an intruder has the possibility to try via a dial-up telephone line a large number of usernumbers, which would lead to blocking a significant part of the user community. For fixed telephone lines however, this approach seems to be attractive and acceptable.

For dial-up lines a strategy might be implemented with as basic characteristic a system-generated waiting time, that depends on the log-on history for the terminal connection (telephone line) and user number concerned. For a normal attempt this waiting time should be virtually zero, but in case the attempt was preceeded by unsuccesful attempts the waiting-time should increase, e.g. exponentially. The size of the effect that can be obtained in this way is indicated by the following example.

Let us assume that a log-on action takes normally 3 seconds. This implies that the possible number of attempts without any special measures amounts to 1200 per hour. If the waiting time is increased exponentially ($2**i-1$ seconds) for the i-th unsuccesful attempt, then the number of possible attempts per hour is reduced to 12. However, the waiting time will be unacceptable for a normal user who tries to log-on later on via the connection (or terminal) concerned. Strategies that combine user friendliness with high effectiveness deserve more attention.

Concluding remarks

This study demonstrates clearly that the password protection system based on user selected passwords implies a much higher guess-risk than often is assumed.

Use of personal computers as a tool for an intruder increases his potential to generate log-on attempts.

Defence strategies should be aiming at two effects :

- Reduction of the guess-risk by implementing some form of control on the use of passwords; requirement of a certain number of characters and exclusion of passwords that can easily be guessed.
- Reduction of the number of log-on attempts that can be generated by an intruder in a certain period of time.

A HAND-HELD SYSTEM USABLE BY RURAL HEALTH WORKERS FOR MEDICAL DECISION-MAKING.

B. Auvert, V. Gilbos (*), Ph. Aegerter, Le Thi Huong Du, Ph. Boutin,
JL. Monier and X. Emmanuelli (*).

INSERM U88 91 Bd de l'Hôpital 75013 PARIS-FRANCE
* MEDECINS SANS FRONTIERES 68 Bd St Marcel 75013 PARIS-FRANCE

A great part of the world's population is cured by rural health
workers who also collect data for epidemiological studies; these
workers have a low level of medical training and work in a poor
technical environment. At the request of an international
humanitarian organization (Médecins Sans Frontières), we have
developed an integrated system (TROPICAID) based on a hand-held
computer, designed to increase rural health workers' effectiveness.
The software is easy to use, allowing access to an internal data base
on 60 drugs. The decision making module analyzes the patient's
parameters and indicates possible diagnoses and relevant treatments.
The system knows 240 diagnoses. In addition, individual medical data
can be collected for elementary statistical analysis. The computer,
sturdy and compact, runs on battery power rechargeable by a solar
panel. Program and data are stored in high capacity EPROMs (320 K
bytes). This system is currently being evaluated in several places in
Chad. The first results show that this system is intensively used and
gives valuable information to the user.

1 INTRODUCTION

Our main goal is to improve the technical level of curative care
dispensed in developing countries, essentially by offering a kind of
help which is immediate and applicable to a wide variety of likely
situations with only minor adjustments.

In most developing countries, the local health center plays a
major role in the health network. In the health centers, medical
care is given by a para-medical, equipped with little material for
surgery and few beds for hospitalization. The pharmacy of the health
centers contains about one hundred drugs. The personnel is trained
for a period of about two years.

Recently, hand-held computers (HHC) were proposed to produce a
diagnostic system, for workers having rudimentary medical knowledge
to ensure more appropriate diagnoses (2). Together with "MEDECINS

SANS FRONTIERES" (MSF), we have worked out an entire system TROPICAID capable of helping medical personnel to make diagnoses and to prescribe therapy. The system also allows for the collection and analysis of medical activity data.

2 HARDWARE

Because no available HHC had a memory capacity large enough to contain our software, we have developed one (BLAISE) especially for this task. It has been partly described previously (3).

The prototype is the size of a book (29x20x5 cm), having a 8x40 character liquid crystal display. The keyboard contains 51 characters and five functionkeys. It is waterproof and shockproof. There is a standard serial interface connection plug. To get electrical autonomy, we have chosen the CMOS technology. The processor is a NSC 800 (National Semiconductor). The RAM capacity is 128 K bytes. ROM used are 16 K bytes NMOS EPROM which are disconnected once a program segment has been loaded into the RAM memory. The ROM is considered by the software as a secondary memory storage for programs. Actually we use 320 K bytes including a P-code interpreter. Cd-Ni batteries can be recharged by a solar panel. The autonomy of the system is 2 weeks of constant use.

3 SOFTWARE

We have chosen Softech P-system as an operating system and Pascal UCSD as a language. Thus the application software has been developed on a micro-computer using P-system (VICTOR S1) and then transferred to the ROM of the HHC by means of an EPROM programming system. Program and files are stocked in ROM. During operation, only index files and needed segments are present in RAM (64 K-bytes for P-system). All the data-files are packed. By using indexed files, response time is independent of the quantity of data.The software allows four main functions:

1) Informations on drugs: We created a data-base of 64 drugs used by MSF in health centers and appearing in the list of "essential drugs of the World Health Organization (WHO)" (4). For each drug we collected the following data into coded thesauri: commercial name, international name, contra-indications, side-effects and the way to control them, interactions and the way to prevent them, posology (dose, duration of the treatment and the route of administration), pharmacological class and properties, follow-up measures,

presentation, signs of toxicity, overdose or reaction and the way to treat it. The posology is calculated according to the patient's medical profile including weight.

2) Information on disease treatments: A therapeutic data-base for the 240 diseases most frequently occurring in developing countries includes, for each disease, the following information: a) clinical description and therapy management. It indicates, for instance, whether the patient should be transferred to a hospital; b) therapeutics: the name of the drug(s) is indicated in order of preference and with the posology as above; c) general remarks: for instance, management of the patient, and the advice to give him or her. Treatment may depend on certain parameters: clinical appearance (high fever); patient type (child or pregnant); epidemiological conditions (epidemic); type of treatment (curative or preventive). The data-base contains appropriate treatment for each possible set of parameters. All this information is codified using thesauri, except for the clinical description and remarks which appear as text, limited to the size of two screens (640 characters).

3) Diagnostic decision aid: We used diagnostic pathways, derived directly from those described by J.B.Essex (5), by which one can obtain possible diagnoses through successive questions and answers. These pathways were progammed to avoid repetition of a question. A chosen path will be completed but, it is possible to jump to another one before returning to the preceding one. This can be done in a recursive way. These pathways are represented as a set of nodes. Each node contains the code of the question to ask and, for each possible answer, the code of the next node or the code of a diagnosis. The text of the questions is located in a file together with their possible answers. For certain questions, the "Help" key allows the display of an explanatory text. The network contains 460 questions and 120 messages. At the end of the process, the diagnoses are listed and the user can then have access to their specific therapies.

4) Medical data collection: It is possible to store in non-volatile memory for each patient and up to a maximum of 2000 patients, the following characteristics: age-group, sex, month of the year, geographical origin, symptoms, diagnosis and medical action. A module permits the user to define for each of these items the number of possibilities (up to 14) and their labels (up to 17). A statistical program may give numbers according to selected criteria, as well as the total number of registered patients.

4 FIELD EXPERIMENTATION

In the spring of 1984, the prototype was tested in Chad by about 50 people (doctors from MSF and Chadian doctors and nurses). All those interviewed stated that the system was simple to use, fast to answer and full of information. A Chadian nurse succeeded in using TROPICAID for his clinic after just 30 minutes of initiation. The MSF doctor, who assisted the clinic, agreed with the system's therapy recommendations. The short instructional period for using the system (about 15 minutes) can be provided by the systematic use of the selection frame (6). There are 3 operational keys: START, HELP, and PAGE. The START key returns the program to the beginning. The PAGE key allow to pass to the next step. The test has also proven the resistance of the system. It did, in fact, resist dust, heat and the many voyages (about 1000 Km of hard road). Recharging the batteries on solar panels was no problem.

5 DISCUSSION

A system like TROPICAID seems really advantageous and useful only for someone with sufficient basic medical knowledge. Of course, the system asks, as well, a minimum of goodwill and interest.

The parts of TROPICAID concerning the drugs and therapeutics needed only small additions: direct access to the drugs through their international denominations, follow-up or after-treatment suggestion.

Some major faults appeared in the diagnostic part, leaving open to question the technique used: a) once elaborated for a certain situation, the pathways are fixed and not adaptable either to seasonal or geographic variations, or to epidemiological influences, or to differences in the training level of potential users; b) because of the separation of the diagnostic and therapeutic modules, the diagnostic path could lead to a diagnosis not within the realm of the therapeutic possibilities of the user; c) the technique of diagnostic pathways does not really correspond to the medical approach (7) and cannot perform an explanation of a diagnostic decision, so they do not contribute to a true diagnostic teaching approach.

The data-collecting module appears to be of precious help. Its main interest is the possibility of surveillance of disease patterns at basic curative levels.

TROPICAID is an aid in making a medical decision, but it can be used as a teaching instrument as well, which seems really necessary for someone who got only two years of training. This would also be very useful for foreigners working in the medical field and having only limited experience.

We are convinced of the potential interest in the use of hand-held systems in the medical field. The cost is continuously decreasing (around US$ 1000 in 1984). In the future, even if such a system is still more expensive than paper, the low cost and the small dimensions will permit large distribution. The possibility of continuous teaching and the harmonization of medical practice will simplify the organization of medical care.

1-ATMA-ALTA PRIMARY HEALTH CARE Health for All Series (Number 1). World Heath Organisation, 1978

2-GOLDBERGER H., SWCHENN P., "Man-Machine Symbiosis in the Assistance and Training of Rural Health Workers: A Proposal" in "Meeting the Challenge: Informatics and Medical Education" (J.C. Pages, A.H. Levy, F.Gremy and J. Anderson, eds) Elsevier Science Publishers B.V (North Holland) IFIP-IMIA, 1983

3-TAVERNIER H., AUVERT B. and LE BEUX P., "BLAISE: A PORTABLE CMOS Bio-Terminal Programmable in Pascal" In The Best of Computer Fairs, Vol VII, 1982, 250-253

4-SELECTION OF ESSENTIAL DRUGS. Technical Report Number 641. World Health Organisation, 1980

5-ESSEX B.J.,"Diagnostic Pathways in Clinical Medicine" Churchill Livingstone, 1980

6-LE BEUX P. "Frame selection system and language" PhD Thesis, University of San Francisco Medical Center, 1974

7-POPLE H.E.,"Heuristic Methods for Imposing Structure on Ill Structured Problems: The Structuring of Medical Diagnostics" in "Artificial Intelligence in Medicine" (Szolovits ed) Westview 1982

NUCLEOTIDE SEQUENCE ANALYSIS SYSTEM ON MINICOMPUTER

M. Kataja and M. Sarvas
National Public Health Institute
Mannerheimintie 166
SF-00280 HELSINKI, Finland

Summary

A program package to analyse nucleotide sequences of DNA and RNA on a
minicomputer is described. The package 'DNAW' is designed for rapid
analysis of strictly known data to support the well known programmes
of Rodger Staden for the analysis of partially known DNA-sequences.

The package 'DNAW' is written using standard FORTRAN IV for PDP-11
series but it runs also on smaller PDP:s and even on CP/M based microcomputers provided that a FORTRAN compiler exists. The package is very
fast in execution since the sequences are supposed to be known exactly.

1 Introduction

Important methodology aids for recombinant DNA work are computer programmes for the analysis of nucleotide sequences of stretches of DNA
and RNA. Many versatile and comprehensive programmes have already been
published and are available (1,2,3,4). Methods of recombinant DNA-
technology are, however, applied in increasing number of laboratories
which use only basic cloning techniques and do only a limited amount
of the DNA-sequencing analysis.

In such laboratories there is need for a fast, compact program for
analysing the basic DNA-sequence data, while more comprehensive programmes would seem either too tedious to install or too demanding for
the computers available.

Our laboratory has now for a few years used recombinant DNA-technology
for studying protein secretion of bacteria and its possible application for biotechnology. The main part of work has consisted of cloning

and subcloning of pieces of DNA into various vectors, trimming the pieces with exonucleases, and sequencing short "critical" stretches of DNA.

In planning our system we already knew that in due course we would get access to the program package of Rodger Staden (1,2,3,4) and we there- fore decided to limit the package to our specific needs, to find:

- cleavage sites for restriction endonucleases,
- homologies between short DNA-sequences, and
- to deduce the amino acid sequence encoded by a stretch of DNA.

It took about six weeks time of the authors to write and test the DNAW package. It was operational in August 1981 and was used two years with only a few minor improvements. In November 1984 it was transferred to a VAX-11/750 and a routine for combining new sequences was added.

2 Purpose of the system

The goal of DNAW-system is to help to find out all possible or some special cleavage sites for restriction endonucleases in DNA-sequences. Technically an analogous task is to find longer parts of the DNA- sequence of some protein, or some stretch of DNA sequenced.

The DNAW-package performs all those tasks specified before the devel- opment and some others included later:

- Processing a restriction endonuclease list to internal mode; vali- dity, consistency and symmetry are checked.

- Processing a given DNA or RNA sequence to internal mode; validity is checked and reported for corrections, which are made by a text editor to the primary text file.

- Combining a new DNA sequence from parts of sequences already stored in the system.

- Finding the cleavage sites for a given set of restriction endonuc- leases. There are three alternatives to report the sites:

- a short list giving only the codon numbers,
- graphical presentation horizontally with the enzyme names on appropriate places, and
- a vertical list, three codons and three amino acid translations per line, with the enzyme names if fitting.

- Reporting the amino acid translation or all three translations of a given sequence.

- Finding various homologies, either exact or with given percentage of fit. Included are:

  - homologies with a sequence given by the operator (repetitive),
  - homologies within the sequence itself,
  - homologies in two given sequences,
  - homologies with the sequence inverted,
  - homologies with the sequence inverted and completed,
  - homologies on the amino acid level meaning that three codons (64 alternatives) are coded to an amino acid (21 alternatives).

3 GENERAL SOLUTION

3.1 The data

The DNAW-system utilizes two kinds of files, one type for data entry by a terminal and another, processed form, for the analysis. This simplifies the maintaining of primary files in allowing the use of normal text editors. The high speed of the program package is achieved by using the data in processed form where, for example, all conversions and nearly all consistency checks are omitted.

There are two types of primary data, one for the restriction enzymes and another for the DNA-sequences. At the moment we have seven different sets of enzymes adopted from various published sources. For example one set gives those enzymes whose key sequence is six elements long, another gives all those with four elements. Emphasis has been laid on the enzymes available commercially. As the sudy data we have all DNA-chains sequenced in our laboratory and also some known useful sequences from the literature, such as penicillinase of Bacillus richeniformis or Semliki Forest Virus 26S RNA.

3.2 The Structure of DNA-data

Nucleotide sequences are coded in a kind of tertiary based system with A, C, G, and T (or U in RNA) as basic elements. Since in our system only exactly known sequences are handled, we can take a real tertiary algebra in use and code the sequences according to this without redundancy.

The use of this compact coding helps also to form the code of the cleavage sites of the restriction enzymes in a short way. When the key lenght is limited to six elements we have exactly 4096 possible keys. One key with five elements 'masks' four locations in key table and one with five elements occupies 16 locations in the table.

We thus have a very straightforward means to describe the properties of the enzymes by a table of 4096 elements giving the identifications of the restriction enzymes. An element is empty if the combination of the address is not fit by any enzyme.

The DNA-data are coded similarly in pieces of three codons in a computer byte (six leftmost bits used) allowing the use of normal arithmetics. Otherwise we would have the problem with negative integers.

The structure of DNA-data makes it quite easy to write simple and efficient program code to compare two stretches of DNA sequence, which is the only initial goal of the system. The code array of the cleavage site of a restriction enzyme is also a sequence although a short one.

3.3 Technical solution

The DNA-data are coded so that the basic elements have binary values:

```
A      00    Adenine
C      01    Cytocine
G      10    Guanine
T, U   11    Thymine, Uracile
```

By this selection the symmetry in DNA-data is returned to simple arithmetics in the computer. For example the complement code of AACGTT <000001101111> is gained by the operation 4095 - code resulting in <111110010000> giving decoded TTGCAA.

The comparison of two sequences is thus returned to arithmetic comparisons of two six bit wide elements. This is made floating so that the other sequence is shifted in two bits increments. Thus the program logic to compare the sequences need only some few lines of code.

3.4 Input, operation and output

The programmes are used in conversational mode. The primary selection is made by choosing the appropriate program from a list of eight routines (DNA#, where # = B, D, J, H, Q, R, S or W). Most of the tasks are included in the routine DNAW to keep the operation simple. The others are to prepare the data, to compare a sequence with full complement of the same sequence or with the sequence itself to find internal homologies. The newest routine DNAJ combines a new sequence of pieces specified by the operator. The output of DNAJ is produced in the source form to allow the use of a text editor for adding titles and comments.

The programmes give only short messages to the operator's terminal and write the output to a file which can be edited if needed and further printed to a hardcopy device.

The DNAW-package is capable to handle restriction enzymes given six codons or less. The lenght of a sequence is limited to 12000, which value is hardly ever exceeded. A sequence of amino acid residues for the homology comparison may not exceed 166 amino acid residues (498 codons). These limitations are far beyond the practical sizes of sequences.

The main program DNAW has two operation modes, interpretation and homologue recognition. Interpretation is used for translating the sequence to one or all three possible chains of amino acids. It is also used for marking possible cleavage sites if a set of restriction enzymes is defined.

The homologue recognition may be done on a specified level of accuracy (100 % for the exact fit). The sequence of godons is given by the operator. The character '*' is allowed to describe "any character" at that specific location.

The recognition may also be done on the amino acid level which is no
more an exact comparison in the original sense. We have found this
very useful in attempts to locate the coding sequences of specific
small oligopeptides.

5 EXPERIENCES and AVAILABILITY

The program package has markedly shortened the time needed in the
analysis of DNA data and in planning of the subcloning and sequencing
strategy. It has also given us a neat tool to document our results.
The time invested in the development of the system was gained back in
the first runs. Especially the program package has been very useful to
look for possible restriction sites for optimal subcloning and trimming strategy.

After completing the system the excellent volume 10 of Nuclear Acids
Research (5) devoted to the computer research on nucleic acids was
published. We still do not have the feeling of being invented a wheel
once more. Our solution is unique and serves us well. The volume 10 of
NAR shows clearly that there are many ways to solve DNA sequence analysing problems with mini- or microcomputers.

The program package may be delivered on magnetic tape (1600 bpi, ASCII
or EBCDIC, readable for most computers) by sending an empty 600 feet
reel to our address. DNAW compiles by every FORTRAN compiler on PDP
and VAX machines.

REFERENCES

(1) Staden, R. Nucleic Acids Research 4, 4033-4051 (1977).
(2) Staden, R. NAR 5, 1013-1015 (1978).
(3) Staden, R. NAR 6, 2601-2610 (1979).
(4) Staden, R. NAR 8, 817-825 (1980).
(5) Nucleic Acids Reseach 10, (1982).

REGISTRATION OF TOTAL HIP REOPERATIONS ON HOSPITAL AND COUNTRY LEVEL BY AID OF ROUTINE SURGERY STATISTICS

T. Niinimäki
Oulu University Central Hospital, Department of Surgery, Oulu, Finland

The total endoprosthesis operation of big joints has become a mass product of the hospitals during the last 10 years. In Finland about 2500
such operations per year are done. The patients are aged and have often
other diseases. Ability to move is essential to them since daily living
manageability at home is absolutely the best. Less pains produce a better standard of living whereas continuous languishing does not prohibit
walking and sleeping. This is why the endoprosthesis operations are generally accepted as one of the most helpful procedures of aged people,
although they are expensive and sometimes complicated, too. The problem
is to join the living organism to a technological product. Despite 20
years of intensive development work, the prostheses tend to loosen and
cause reoperations. The loosening happens years after the application,
the frequency is about 0.5-1 % every year. Collecting a sufficient
amount of patient loosenings to prove some prostheses weakness takes
much time. That is why almost all studies concerning these operations
are multicentric. How do we have this continuous follow-up multicentric-
ally ? In Finland we have a particular register for endoprostheses, it
collects data immediately after the operation and a year later. In Sweden a reoperation register is in use in some parts of the country.

The aim of this study is to examine whether a routine surgical statistics could give enough information from this particular operation method
and could it help in making decisions of care policy. In Finland we
have a wide spread system of routine surgical statistics. It uses a
Finnish modification of the list of the operations. This list was planned and developed during the years 1976-80 and also had two test versions. During that work endoprosthesis reoperations were thought particularly profoundly.They were separated into their own group, and the purpose of the procedure was also pointed out. The joint and the component
received their own codes, too. This code is somewhat complex and needs
a registration system, which takes two or three numbers in.

The amount of reoperations, infections, loosenings, luxations and which
component is probably dissatisfied are all seen in the computer report.
This is quite descriptive in own hospital where all details of

operations are well known, for instance which model and version of the prosthesis is usually used.

Is it necessary to know the model and version of the prosthesis ? The general registration of the reoperations means that their number is a reference to all units concerned with these problems. The aim is to have the standard of care above the mean, that is the minimum level. If one uses such a method, which does not reach this standard, it is a reason to choose another prosthesis and check the process in the operation theatre thoroughly. The need to know the model is thus essential in a hospital, but not in the country.

Other data which is also worth discussion are the repeated reoperations. If we inspect the number of reoperations as an indicator of the quality in primary operations, we are then interested in,which patients come for a reoperation. The interval between two operations can be even 10 years and to solve this problem by searching for the old data is rather irksome. A simple solution to this problem is to develope the list of the operations to such a direction that the first reoperation can be identified. Then we use the first reoperation as a measure to the primary operations and the follow-up reoperations concern the possible quality of the former one, not the primary.

When the data processing has become easier, need to compite special registers for some diseases or methods is evident. When planning these systems, it is always necessary to consider how the existing other systems can serve us and give nearly the same information. If it is possible, it makes the data collecting much easier in working places. Data systems in Finland are able to collect routine surgical statistics into one central register. It is possible with the same procedure as the diagnosis collecting.

By developing the list of the operations into a suggested direction, it is possible to obtain such information which is necessary for hospitals to control their own standard of care and to make decisions, which lead to better results in these operations.

The systematics of codes for total hip joint operations:
1. Primary operations
    the method
    - cemented
    - non cemented

2. The first reoperations
   the cause of reoperation
   - infection
   - loosening etc

   the component involved
   - femur
   - acetabulum

   what is done
   - change
   - reapplication

3. The later reoperations
   cause
   component
   what is done

References

Total Hip Joint Replacement, National Institutes Health Consensus
Developement Conference. Summary, vol. 4, 4, 1982, Maryland.

The list of operations (Finnish). Sairaalaliitto, 1983, Finland.

DIAGNOSTIC CLASSIFICATION OF MUSCLE BIOPSIES BY A MICRO COMPUTER

Vesa Kuusela
Rehabilitation Research Centre of the Social Insurance Institution
SF-20720 Turku, Finland

Leo Paljärvi
Department of Pathology
University of Turku
SF-20520 Turku, Finland

Introduction

In diagnostic histopathology the diagnosis is often made on the basis of a
visual pattern which may be difficult to define precisely and yet is fully
diagnostic in the eyes of an experienced observer. Muscle pathology, however, is to a large extent analytical in nature: muscle disorders manifest
themselves as a limited number of histological features, which are likely
to be fairly easily agreed upon by different pathologists, but none of
which alone is usually diagnostic as such. To make a histological diagnosis, one has to recognize the quantitative association of features characteristic of disease in question. To do this successfully, one needs to
memorize a large amount of data on the occurrence of histological features
in various diseases as well as to have a command of heuristic rules for
diagnostic classification.

Muscle diseases being rare, such knowledge accumulates slowly, and particularly a beginning histopathologist is in need of algorithms to help
him in this complicated task. However, no algorithms based on statistical
methods has been available although a practical algorithm - a decision
tree in bud - is given in the Appendix of a leading handbook (Dubowitz and
Brooke 1973). Computers and multivariate statistical analysis provide for
means to take into account a great number a simultaneous changes in order

to construct a formalized diagnosis system. In the present paper a description of a quantitative diagnostic classification system of muscle biopsies is given.

Training set

Training set consisted of 124 patients examined by the muscle diagnostic team of the University of Turku Hospital in 1977-1983. Those patients were included, in whom a definite diagnosis was reached by a panel of neurologists, neurophysiologists, neuropathologists and geneticists. Muscle biopsies taken with the "semi-open" method (Henriksson 1979) were frozen-sectioned and stained with HE and Gomori trichrome; enzyme histochemical reactions included NADH-TR and myofibrillar ATPase after preincubation in pH 9.4 (or 10.4), 4.6 and 4.3. The numbers of cases in the diagnostic classes are given in figure 1.

Feature analysis

The biopsies were analyzed for the presence or absence of 25 histological features (some features were analyzed semiquantitatively in scale 0-3). The features covered changes in fiber size (seven variables), type differentiation and distribution (three), nuclear pathology (two), internal structure (nine), necrosis and regeneration (two), inflammation, fibrosis and fatty infiltration.

The predictors were selected by the logistic regression analysis (see Anderson 1974) of the BMDP statistical library (estimation was done by the maximum likelihood method). The logistic analysis seemed to be the only appropriate one because of the small number of cases in the training set and many different diagnoses, and it has been reported to be at least as reliable as the linear discriminant analysis (see Schmitz et al. 1983).

Diagnostic model

In the logistic regression analysis the probability that a (multidimensional) observation $\underline{X}$ is from a population D is given by

$$prob(D|\underline{X}) = 1/\left[1+exp\left[-(b_o+\underline{B}'\underline{X})\right]\right]$$

The observation vector $\underline{X}$ is composed of the predictive feature set of the diagnosis class D ($\underline{B}$ is a vector of regression coefficients).

365

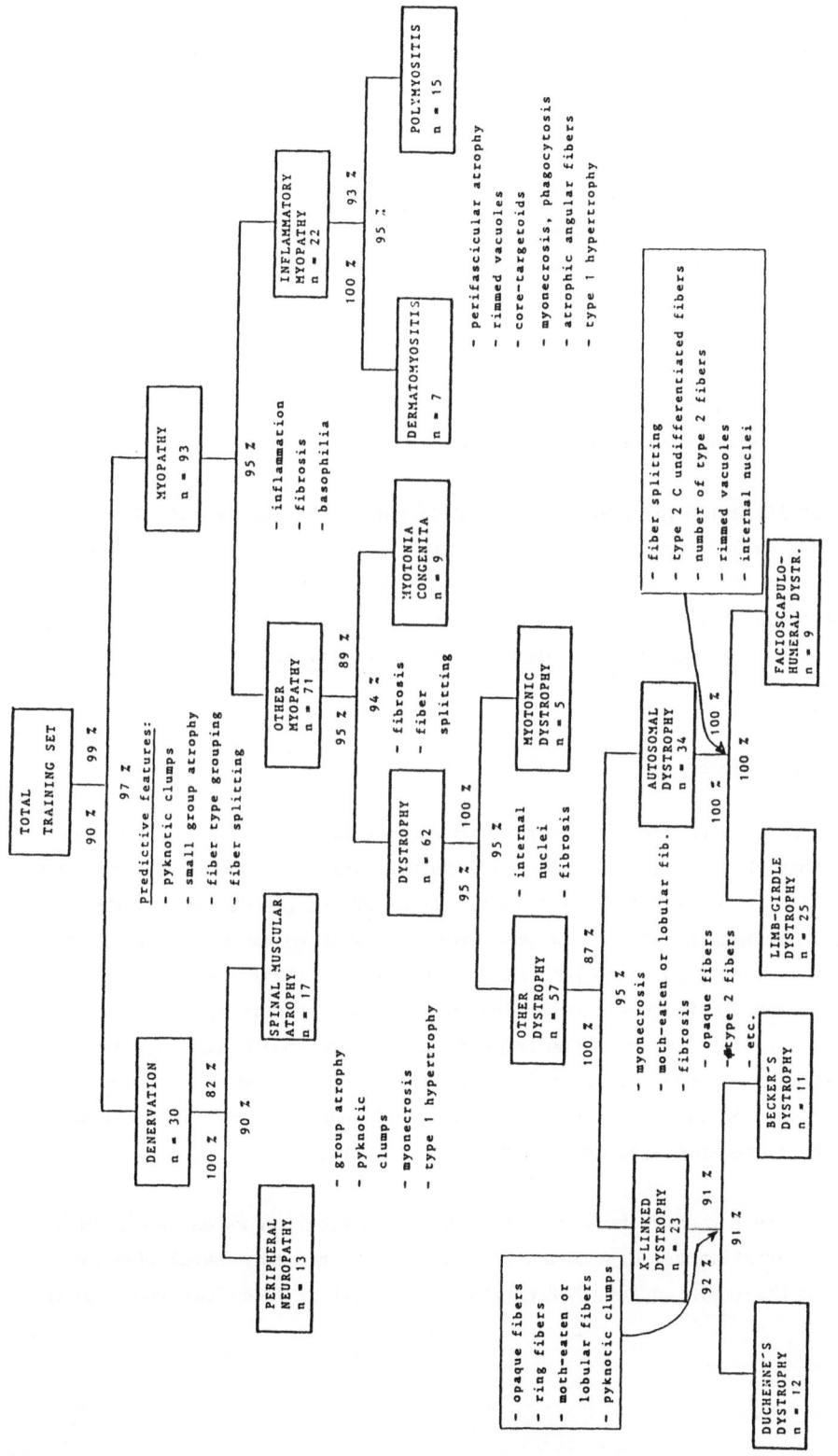

Figure 1. The hierarchy of diseases, predictive features and classification rates (%).

Logistic regression deals with a dichotomous criterion variable. That is why a hierarchy of diagnoses was employed (see figure 1) where in each node a classification into a more specific disorder is accomplished. The hierarchical structure has six levels and the discrimination in each level is specific to the node. Parameters of the diagnostic model and the classification rates are displayed in figure 1. The rates are theoretical and obviously overestimates. Actual misclassification rate could not be estimated reliably due to small amount of new cases.

Computer program

The program is made in a standard BASIC by an IBM PC compatible micro computer. Hardware and memory requirements are minor.

The classification program has two modes: interactive and batch. In the batch mode all 25 predictive features are given at the same time and the result is a tentative classification accompanied with all available and relevant classification data. In the interactive mode the hierarchy of the diseases is followed and features will be asked for in the order they are needed.

Concluding remarks

The diagnostic accuracy of our program was encouraging (Fig. 1), and suggests that the system could be useful in practice. The misclassified cases were all more or less "obscure" in the light of the predictor set, which is an indication of absence of some relevant features or of the fact that the panel classified these patients principally on the basis of clinical and laboratory data. When the system will be further developed, clinical variables will be added to the regression function and/or the Bayesian classification (see e.g. David 1976) will be incorporated by allowing the user to give a priori probabilities to some diagnoses. There is no doubt that the diagnostic accuracy could be still increased.

It should be stressed, however, that the classification rates shown (Fig. 1) are overestimates: discrimination tends to be too successful when applied to the training set. A fresh validation set is therefore required to

obtain a realistic estimate of the performance of the system. The inter-
observer reliability of feature analysis is also necessary before the
practical value of the system can be assessed.

Apart from the true diagnostic value of the system, it should have educational applications: particularly a beginner in the field is likely to
improve his diagnostic acumen, when he has to face the logical consequences of his primary observations.

References

1 Anderson JA. Diagnosis by logistic discriminant function: further practical problems and results. Appl Statist 1974:23;3:397-404.

2 David AA. Diagnostic data distributions. Biometrics 1976:36:1-37.

3 Dubowitz V, Brooke M. Muscle biopsy: a modern approach. WB Saunders,
   London 1973.

4. Henriksson KG. "Semi-open" muscle biopsy technique. A simple outpatient
   procedure. Acta Neurol Scand 1979:59:317-323

5 Schmitz PIM, Habbema JDF, Hermans J. The performance of logistic discrimination on myocardial infarctation data, in comparison with some
   other discriminant analysis methods. Statistics in Medicine
   1983:2:199-205.

COMPARATIVE RESEARCH, PREVENTION AND AUDIT IN GENERAL PRACTICE
USING THE SYSTEM ORIENTED REGISTRATION METHOD.

Roland Billiet M.D. (*)   Luc De Norre Drs. Sc. (**)

INTRODUCTION

Although a detailed description of the System Oriented Registration (S.O.R.)
has yet been published in the Proceedings of the M.I.E. 84 (1) some of its most
important principles are repeated here, for reasons of better understanding the
research possibilities offered by the program-package. New features of a
steadily expanding and improving program are also added.

The S.O.R. method is automated and contains now four main sections :

1. Patient registration and supervision of all patient files.
2. Complete secretarial work.
3. Total accountability.
4. Audit : Prevention and research programs.

As items 2. and 3. can be different from one country to another they will not
be discussed here. Nevertheless these items offer valuable information for
further research. Also they can be used in the prevention and audit schemes.

METHOD

In the S.O.R. there are 36 subdivisions that correspond mainly to organ
systems, specialisms or subspecialisms. Each system is represented by a
condensed mnemonic code of 3 characters.

e.g.: 1. ALL   ALLERGY + IMMUNOLOGY   : ...
      2. COL   COLLAGENOUS DISEASES   : 35. TRO   TROPICAL DISEASES
      ...   : 36. VEN   VENEREAL DISEASES

The patient's medical file consists of 8 different items :

First a brief description of the different items will be given, then followed
by a discussion of the research possibilities they offer.

A. GENERAL DATA :

  A patient's file is always opened at first contact by entering all different
  general data.

- Patient identification : the first 4 letters of the family name, followed
  by the first 2 letters of the Christian name. In case 2 or more patients have
  the same identification code a number is added :
  e.g. Smith Albert ---- SMITAL   Smith Allan ---- SMITAL2

- Card number : the two first numbers are the year in which the new file is
  opened, then followed by the number under which all the documents concerning
  the patient are classified.

- Date of first contact is noted.

- Matrimonial state : noted in codified form.

- Family relation : to make family related search possible the relationship is noted using the identification code of all the family-members in a zig-zag structure : e.g. the family of Mr. Allan Smith, his wife Jenny Jones and their 2 children Bryan and Cindy.

For each of them we mention the previous and the following member:

SMITAL2	Previous :	AAAAAA-	Following :	JONEJE-
JONEJE-	Prev. :	SMITAL2	Foll. :	SMITBR-
SMITBR-	Prev. :	JONEJE-	Foll :	SMITCI-
SMITCI-	Prev. :	SMITBR-	Foll. :	ZZZZZZ-

In this way the whole family is enclosed between AAAAAA- and ZZZZZZ-.

- The previous professional state as well as the actual one is noted, so that it can offer supplemental information on professional diseases.
- The activity code is noted as follows : the professional actives are coded in capitals whereas the pensioners are coded in small letters. Different letters are used to define various professions, giving an idea of the social classes.
- People living in a community can be grouped under the heading of an institution, such as elderly people in homes, children in boarding schools etc.

B. and C. PERSONALIA and VACCINATIONS :

- In this item the allergies, risc factors, intolerances and habits can be noted and coded. As a reminder this code will appear on each of the following items in a specific color.
- The vaccination state can be updated at any time by entering the given vaccin and the repeat date. Up to six different vaccinations can be noted at a time. A global idea of the state of vaccination in a practice can be obtained and using the planification a preventive program can be started.

D. and E. ANTECEDENTS and JOURNAL :

The S.O.R.-method is applied in the antecedents as well as in the journal.

A problem is registered in the journal as Active (A). When the problem is no longer active, the code A is changed into Passive (P), and the problem at hand is automatically transferred into the antecedents survey, classified per date. Once a contact is localised in one of the 36 SYSTEMS, which is useful to situate a main problem, a further discription is necessary for an efficient registration.

Therefore SUBPROBLEMS are used, represented by a mnemonic code of at most 4 characters. Introduced in condensed form they appear in full on the screen or on the outprint. Using a combination of different subproblems a more clear description of the problem is obtained. By giving a specific meaning to each subproblem, a given complaint gets an even better circumscription :

e.g. 1 : the organ, 2 : the lesion, 3 : further specification.

In this way the subproblems can be used to register syndromes as well as diseases, organs, signs and symptoms and even impressions. Each G.P. can make his own unlimited list of subproblems. The subproblems can be linked to any other classification such as the I.C.D. or the R.C.G.P.(2), which can be of great help in the analysis of the collected clinical material.

In the Survey of the Journal or the Antecedents the date of the consecutive contacts is displayed followed by the code of the System and full circumscription of the Subproblems. With the dates that have been collected so far the M.B.D.S. i.e. the Minimum Basic Data Set can be realised in G.P. (3)

ITEM F : LONG TERM MEDICATION :

The repeat medicine is entered in this screen. The date of the last prescription is memorized, allowing control on the patient's compliance.

ITEM G : BIOMETRICS :

All the biometric values such as bloodpressure, pulse rate, length, weight and any of 4 free chosen other measurements can be noted at the same time and can be displayed in a synoptic scheme. If a specific medecine is prescribed for any of these parameters this can be noted in this scheme.

ITEM H : GRAPHICS :

All the biometric measurements as well as the lab-results can be represented in graphical form. The corresponding medecine is also displayed.

ITEM J : PREVENTION :

In a spread-sheet way any kind of anamnestic- or examination-charts can easily be drafted. They are usefull for specific examininations, such as geriatric procedures or gravidity follow-up. These charts can be of great value in prospective morbidity studies.

COMPARATIVE RESEARCH AND AUDIT

A. AUTOMATED FORM OF PRACTICE DENOMINATOR.

In countries with no compulsory registration with a G.P. the total number of listed patients will not be a good parameter to compare results between different practices, nor does it give a real idea of the practice size.

It has been prooved that the total number of first contacts with patients in one year (Y.A.G : Yearly Attending Group) is a more relialable parameter.(4) However it has also been prooved that registrating all first contacts during a period of 12 weeks provides a practical way of calculating the practice size: within this period nearly 42% of the total patient number (T.N.P.) has been seen. The Y.A.G. approximates 70% of the total number of patients i.e. the practice size.(5)

In the automated registration this 12 week first contact group can be measured day by day, providing daily the practice size denominator.

These first contacts can be found in the journals. A correcting factor can be introduced for example to eliminate all acute respiratory or gastrointestinal infections due to season influence.(4)

In the item accountability the total number of contacts is known as well as the kind of contact, so the average number and place of contacts per patient (surgery or at home) can be given.

B. AGE DISTRIBUTION AND SEX RATIO.

As the date of birth and the sex have been systematically noted in the general data, an Age/Sex register can be updated on a daily base. Since supplemental information can be obtained by testing the activity-state code and by consulting the code of the actual profession, it becomes possible to have an idea of the distribution in social classes.

By testing the actual and previous profession, valuable information on occupational pathology can be obtained.

As mentioned above, the family relation was noted and so family related search can be done.

Information about people living in an institution can be selected.

For the standardized specification of a practice 4 well defined parameters have been proposed (5) :

1. The practice size denominator
2. The sex ratio and the age distribution
3. The average number of contacts per patient
4. The distribution in social classes

Using the S.O.R.-program package these parameters can be produced in an automated form. To make comparability even more accurate all the further results can be expressed in terms of thousand patients.

C. STATISTICAL POSSIBILITIES.

In the following an enumeration of the possible data on which can be tested simultaneously is given below :

1. General Data :
     11 : Date of first contact/ 12 : Post code / 13 : Sex/ 14 : Date of birth/
     15 : Matrimonial state/ 16 : Activity code/ 17 : Profession code/
     18 : Institution
2. Personalia
     21 : Allergies/ 22 : Risc factors/ 24 : Intolerances/ 25 : Habits/
     26 : Vaccinations
3. Antecedents and Journal
     31 : System/ 33 : Subproblem(s)/ 34 : Active/Passive/ 35 : Consulted Doctor
          and place : ambulatory or hospital/ 36 : Medecine(s) options : 1-5
4. Long term medication : 41 : Medecine(s) options : 1-14

5. Biometrics :

   51 : Bloodpressure : R. or/and L.; Standing/Sitting/Lying

   52 : Pulse : At rest/After 10 knee flexing/1 minut later

   53 : Weight/ 54 : Length/ 55,56,57,58 : Option 1-4 :e.g. neckcircumference,

                                       angulation, temperature, etc.

6. Laboratory results : 61 : Combination of all different tests : free choise

7. X-Ray: 71 : Combination of all kinds of X.R. : free choise

Each of these data "N" can be selected one after another, and for each of them a criterion "X Y Z" can be given. This criterion can be:

- data "N" must be equal to criterion "X Y Z"

- data "N" must be different from criterion "X Y Z"

- data "N" must be greater than criterion "X Y Z"

- data "N" must be smaller than criterion "X Y Z"

- data "N" must contain criterion "X Y Z"

By using an age/sex register, a wide range of possibilities in practice survey, practice audit and statistical work is opened in an automated form to the G.P. Examples of these possibilities do not fit within the restricted space of this communication but could be demonstrated during the congress.

SUMMARY

An automated practice size denominator is presented. Research and audit is possible not only within one practice but also between different practices. Of all the previous mentioned parameters the statistical results of the search can be presented in graphics and synoptic print-outs.

The Minimum Basic Data Set can be realized on the general practice level.

Some of the possibilities using an automated medical record system are emphfasized. The program-package is called Medipraxis and runs on I.B.M. Personal computer XT. with a hard disk station of 10 MB and a color screen.

LITERATURE
(1) R. Billiet : System Oriented Registration in General Practice: a global
      computerized method as a variant of the problem oriented medical
      record system. Medical Informatics Europe 84, Proceedings, Brussels,
      Belgium 1984 p. 546-551.
(2) K. Hodgkin : Towards earlier diagnosis in primary care. Translated in Dutch
      by J.B.M. Vismans : Vroege diagnostiek in de eerste lijn. 1984 De Tijd-
      stroom.
(3) F.H. Roger : Le résumé du dossier medical, indicateur informatisé de
      performance et de qualité des soins. 1982. Thèse d'Aggrégé de
      l'Enseignement Superieur. Centre d'Informatique Médicale de l'U.C.L.
      Avenue Hippocrate, 10 B - 1200 BRUXELLES.
(4) J. De Loof : Practice Size. A fraction of the yearly attending group as
      practice size indicator. Allgemeinmedizin. International. General
      Practice: A.M.I. 3-1983, p.127-128.
(5) J. De Loof : Analyse der praxisstruktur. A.M.I. 1-1981, p.19-23.

(*) Roland Billiet M.D. General Practitioner. Elslo 24, B-9050 Evergem Belgium.
(**) Luc De Norre Drs. Sc. Kortrijkse steenweg 321, B 8730 Harelbeke Belgium

COMPUTERISING FAMILY PRACTITIONER SERVICES

John G Handby FBCS
NHS Information Technology Branch
Department of Health and Social Security
Market Towers
1 Nine Elms Lane
London SW8 5NQ

'Nobody is healthy in London, nobody can be.'

Emma by Jane Austen

New management arrangements for family practitioner services (FPS) in England are
being introduced from 1 April 1985 which offer opportunities to improve the use of
information technology in the administration of these services. From this date the
Family Practitioner Committees (FPCs) that look after the registration of patients
with general medical practitioners and are responsible for the payment of all
practitioners (doctors, dentists, opticians and pharmacists) will be directly
responsible to the Department of Health and Social Security (DHSS).

In preparation for this change a study was commissioned from a firm of management
consultants (Arthur Andersen & Co) to advise on the future development of computer
systems and their report was produced last year.[1] Decisions have now been reached
to go ahead with the proposals contained in the report and the first steps taken
along the road advocated. This paper outlines the proposals and our plans for
implementing them.

BACKGROUND

There are ninety FPCs in England of which the majority hold their records on an
entirely manual basis. Standard software has already been developed to undertake
registration and other tasks by the FPS Computer Unit at Exeter, which is directly
managed by the Department. This operates on DEC PDP equipment and has ensured the
introduction of a common system by most of those FPCs that have computerised. The
NHS Central Register (NHS CR) run by the Office of Population Censuses and Surveys
(OPCS) supports the FPCs by maintaining an manual central index showing the FPC in
which each patient is registered. The Dental Estimates Board (DEB) is responsible for
processing all claims for dental treatment and informing FPCs what payments to make to dentists.
This work is already partly computerised. The prescription Pricing Authority (PPA)
is responsible for calculating the amount due to pharmacists for each prescription
item dispensed and informing the appropriate FPC. Its operations are currently
being computerised.

STRATEGIC APPROACH

The view was reached that greater use could be made of information technology in the administration of these services and that there would be particular advantages in adopting a coordinated approach to development. A number of principles were identified on which the strategy should be based, viz:

- Administrative systems should be integrated so that they support a complete process and recognise the interconnections between the various organisations within the FPS;

- Data should be captured as close to its source as possible;

- Data should wherever possible be captured as a by-product of routine tasks;

- The systems developed should support good professional practice by helping to improve the quality of service provided to the patient eg through assistance for practice registers, call/recall programmes;

- Confidentiality of patient and practitioner data should be preserved, and in particular clinical data should only be accessible with the practitioner's knowledge and consent;

- The systems should aim to improve patient access to health care;

- Multiple potential uses of data held in the various administrative systems should be recognised and, subject to confidentiality safeguards, exploited.

FPS administration is seen as being based in the future around five major systems, These systems will be linked together but do not all need to be developed at the same time. A brief description of each one follows.

Registration The registration system will take the form of a computerised registration database for each FPC, linked and cross-referenced through a similarly computerised national central index operated by the NHSCR. These individual systems will be linked together into a network which will greatly speed up the process of initial registration and registering with a new doctor. In time it is expected that the majority of practices will have their own computers so that registration details can be input electronically to the FPC; so offering further advantages in terms of speed and convenience. Quite apart from these operational improvements the provisions of a computerised central index will strengthen the ability of the NHSCR to support medical and statistical surveys.

Doctor Payment This system will be operated by FPCs and linked to the registration system. It will calculate capitation and item of service payments to be made each quarter, add practice allowances and any other amounts due and make payment to each practice.

Prescription Processing and Pharmacist Payment The proposals for handling prescriptions take advantage of the high usage of microcomputers in pharmacies and will ensure the capture of data as early as possible. On presentation of prescription to the dispensing pharmacist details will be recorded on the pharmacy computer and the necessary labels produced, stock records updated etc. Details of items dispensed will then be periodically transmitted electronically to the PPA so that they may be priced. The PPA will then inform the relevant FPC of the payment of be made to the pharmacist.

Dental Claims Approval and Payment The strategy will support expansion of the current experiment to pay capitation fees in respect of dental treatment for children as well as the continuation of the present item of service payments for other patients. Claims will continue to be sent to the DEB for assessment, who will then authorise payment by the appropriate FPC. The way in which they are handled will however differ considerably. Some claims will continue to be submitted on paper but as computers are installed into dental practices direct electronic transmission of claims to the Board's computer will grow. Even those on paper will be fed in on arrival and the Board's staff will use computer terminals to call up claims to review them.

Optician Payment Arrangements for payment of sight tests and NHS prescribing will continue as at present, opticians forwarding details to the FPC for payment. It is expected that FPCs will use small computer systems to support the authorisation and payment of claims.

TECHNICAL ISSUES

A number of technical issues arise in seeking a more coordinated approach to the use of IT within the FPS. Firstly there is the question of the extent of standardisation to be sought in the equipment and software used. There is already a variety of equipment in use and our view is that it would be unrealistic to look for total uniformity in the future. But standard software is already being used in the current

FPS: Main Agencies and information flows

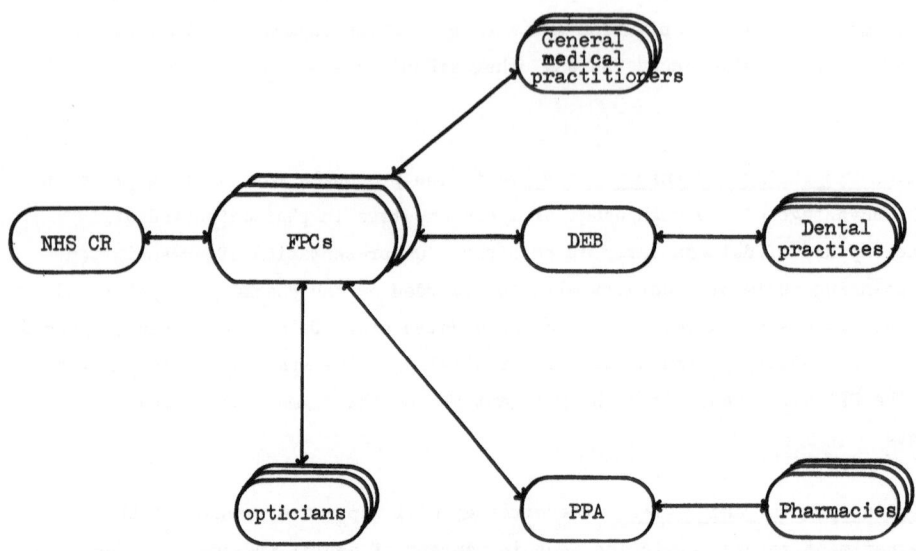

generation of FPC systems and there are strong arguments for standardising on one range of equipment and/or a computer operating system. This is particularly so as the FPC network will form the basis of the new technological infrastructure for the FPS.

Beyond this it is necessary to ensure compatibility between the various systems and this will be achieved by the adoption of a number of common technical standards; principally in the areas of data management and communications. In the case of the former data modelling techniques have already been used to structure the data used within the FPS and its relationships. This work will be extended and agreed data definitions drawn up. It will continue to be undertaken in conjunction with similar work being carried out in respect of data used in the hospital and community services so as to ensure links with computer systems operating in these areas.[2]

For communications the ISO open systems interconnection (OSI) standards offer the obvious basis to facilitate the exchange of data between systems and these will be adopted. These will be used not only to link the various administrative systems but also to determine the specification of the interface protocols that practice computers will have to meet in order to communicate with these administrative systems. By

making this known at an early stage we hope to encourage suppliers of such systems
to turn their attention to meeting this requirement in equipment they market.

A good deal of thought has been given to the nature of the FPC network leading to the
conclusion that each FPC should have its own computer. Other possibilities were
considered including the centralisation of computing facilities or the sharing of
them by consortia of FPCs at a number of regional sites. The cost differences are
not great and there is a natural reluctance on the part of FPCs to share equipment.
A highly distributed option of the kind planned seems to be well in line with the
expected trend in technology.

IMPLEMENTING THE STRATEGY

Three stages in implementation are envisaged:

- Stage one to be principally concerned with the development of a new generation of administrative systems; introduction of a comprehensive computerised
  registration system for all FPCs and the NHSCR, new financial systems in
  each FPC, completion of the PPA computerisation programme and replacement
  of the DEB machine.

- Stage two to involve the widespread introduction of practice computers,
  following earlier trials, so that the majority of administrative data can
  be collected at source.

- Stage three to provide further developments of benefit to patients and
  practitioners based on the results of the earlier work. Computer readable
  medical cards and diagnostic support for doctors are two of the possibilities.

This sequence of implementation reflects both management's priorities and the inter-
dependancies between related systems. The key management priority for FPS administration is to improve efficiency and effectiveness by reducing costs and at the
same time raising the quality of administration through such things as:

- the provision of services to patients or practitioners more quickly;

- making available additional services or supporting practitioners in doing so;

- simplifying the way in which services are made available to patients.

It will also be clear that once the administrative systems proposed for stage one are in place they will form a natural basis for the later developments planned.

The strategy I have outlined is significant in terms of cost and the technological skills required. To be successful firm management is essential. We have established a three tier management structure to this end consisting of:

- a strategy steering committee (SSC) representing the various interests involved to have overall direction of the implementation of the strategy and its regular review;

- a central management unit (CMU) to be responsible for the planning and control of the strategy, identifying and defining projects and securing their implementation;

Advanced tools and techniques will also be important. A common design methodology (SSADM) will be used and appraisals are under way of various developments tools (fourth generation languages, designer and programmer workbenches, application generators etc) to reduce the level of effort required as well as improving the standard of systems produced. Each project will be making use of the PROMPT progress control methodology in planning its work and ensuring the production of outputs to time. In addition the CMU will be monitoring the progress of each of the projects using a computer based progress control package. This will allow a regular review of progress and the reporting of problems in achieving particular milestones to the strategy steering committee.

CONCLUSION

I have tried to give a broad picture of the strategy recently developed to improve the use of information technology in the FPS in England. It is ambitious and will take some 10-15 years to implement in its entirety, although significant benefits should be secured much earlier than this. Decisions have been taken to go ahead and work is underway to define projects, establish the various teams and set appropriate control mechanisms in place. We expect the next few years to witness considerable gains in improved efficiency and effectiveness of the various administrative systems involved.

REFERENCES

1.   Arthur Andersen & Co

Report of a study of family practitioner services administration and the use of computers. Department of Health and Social Security, London, 1984.

2.   Handby J G

Harnessing Technology to health care - the challenge for the future. Springer-Verlag, MIE 84 proceedings, pps 616-621.

AN OUTPATIENT SYSTEM ESPECIALLY DEVELOPED FOR FINNISH
STUDENT HEALTH SERVICE'S DATA PROCESSING

H. Taberman
Finnish Student Health Service
Töölönkatu 37 A, Helsinki/Finland

1. Finnish Student Health Service

Finnish Student Health Service (FSHS) is a primary health care organization for the
primary health care of all university and some college students - at this moment
about 80.000 students.
To this end, FSHS runs health centres in every university or college town, 16 towns
in all. The central administration is in Helsinki.
As a special service, every "first year student" is invited to a comprehensive
health examination. About 80-85 % of freshmen attend for the health examination.

In addition, the organization provides all the usual primary health care services:
medical care (physician and nurse consultations, vaccinations, physiotherapy,
laboratory and X-ray), dental care and mental health care. The medical care includes
almost all the specialist services such as gynecological, otorhinolaryngological,
dermatological and internal medical.
The running costs of FSHS activities are covered partly by the students themselves
(37 %), partly by the Social Insurance Institution (49 %) and partly by the
state (12 %).
The student pays an annual health service fee - a sort of insurance premium
which entitles him/her to utilize the services of FSHS.

2. The outpatient information system of FSHS

At the beginning of 1980, the minicomputer-based, real-time system for patient
information processing was implemented in two of the 16 FSHS health centres.
Since then, the system has been implemented in other two big health centres
of FSHS. The databases of the system now include the records of about 55,000
university student (Figure 1). FSHS has planned, developed and built this outpatient
system for its own use. The system's activities correspond to those of FSHS.

The user-oriented system comprises:
- recording and updating of patients'personal data
- recording and updating of consultants' timetables
- time scheduling
- recording and updating of patients' medical data
- recording and updating of all the statistical information

All the data are organized in three databases: time scheduling, patient information and parameter databases, of which the patient information database is the most comprehensive.

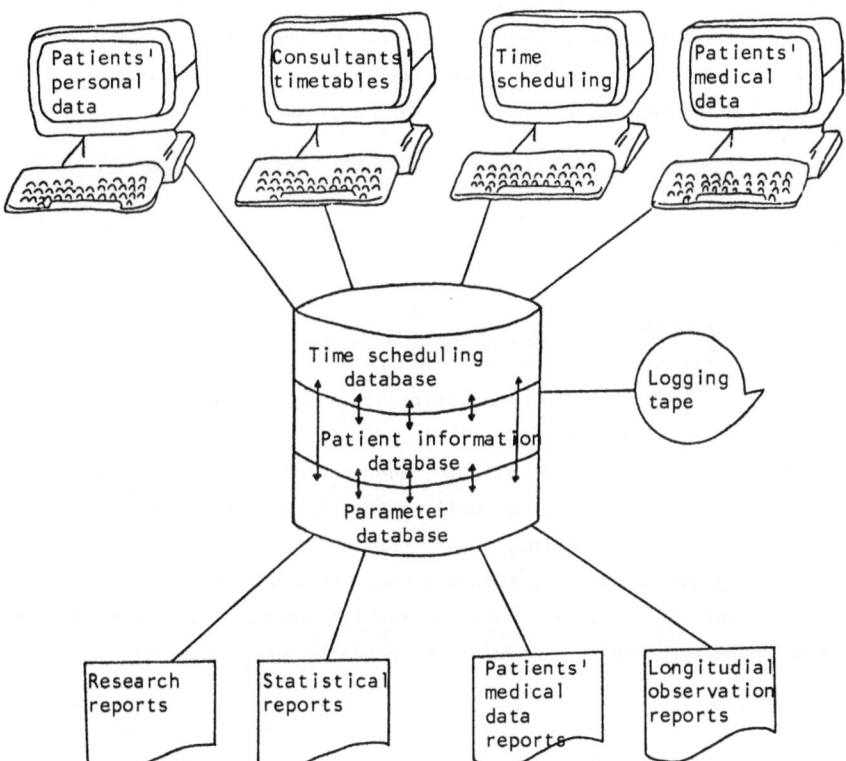

Figure 1. Patient information system

2.1. Patients' personal data

Patients' personal data are either updated directly by data from the universities' databases or recorded during the patients first visit to the health centre of FSHS. They are available to every user at the display terminals. The student's social security number is used for patient indentification.

2.2. Consultants' timetables

A personal timetable of consultations is prepared for each consultant (physician, dentist, psychiatrist, etc.). The schedule can be seen at the display nine weeks ahead in one- or two-week periods. The timetable can always be changed if necessary. The timetables are the basis for appointments.

2.3. Time scheduling

Appointments are made for:
- medical consultations
- dental consultations
- psychiatric and psychological consultations, and other services, such as
- physiotherapy and dental hygiene

The terminal user can make appointments, query, cancel or change appointments. He can see all the appointments as well as the first three free hours of consultation for each consultant.

Time scheduling automatically produces a computer-generated output of the appointments for the consultants and the archive and collects the daily numbers in the database for long-term reports for planning and management.

2.3. Patients' medical data

Limited medical history data are collected acoording to the services (medical care, dental care, mental health care) used by the patients. Limited data are also collected at every visit and according to the type of the visit: health examinations, medical consultations, dental services, mental health services, laboratory examinations, X-ray examinations.

Work to develop unlimited patients' medical information continues. The unlimited medical patient data will be keyed-in with the wordprocessing application as a part of the patient information system.

2.4. Statistical information

All the patients' personal and visit data records include some fields with required statistical information.

3. Utilization of the system

The most important use of the system is the daily interactive data processing between the large databases and the terminal users. In addition, there are numerous reports and listings which can be printed out. Some examples are given in the following.

3.1. Some daily listings

The scheduling listings contain information on consultations, for example the number of patients' visits, unreserved consultation time, uncancelled non-attendances by patients. All the laboratory tests and their results are printed for each patient before he sees the physician.

3.2. Use in planning activities

The system is also used for planning and developing activities. The following is an example of health examinations:
One purpose of health examinations for "first year university student" is to detect risk behaviour and to provide health education and counselling with the public health nurse.
All the data obtained from the health examinations, including the health behaviour items and symptoms are recorded in the system.
The system produces the numbers of students who have participated in health check-ups, the numbers of students referred to physicians for further examination and treatment, the listings of the behaviour items according to the different background variables, etc.

In addition, the behaviour risk points are computed for each student on the basis of the behaviour items. It is then possible to produce figures concerning the students' behaviour risks automatically. This kind of information can be utilized in planning future health education activities, such as activities for obese students, smokers, etc.

3.3. Use for research

The opportunities for research given by the system can be illustrated by examining the multitude of information collected from each patient. The first visit is usually the health examination at which, as already mentioned, the information on health behaviour, the symtoms and the results of somatic tests are entered in the system. Data on consultations with the physician, dentist, mental health specialist and nurse, physiotherapy, laboratory tests and X-ray examinations are added over a 3-7 year period to this basic information. The system also enables longitudinal observation of one specific patient or patient group.

3.4. Statistical reports on activities

The system provides access to all reliable and up-to-date statistical reports needed by Finnish Student Health Service's own decision makers and the local and state authorities. The number of patients and the number of visits are needed separately for the three main activities (medical care, dental care, mental health care) once a year.

MICRO COMPUTER APPLICATION

IN A MEDICAL SOCIAL WORK DEPARTMENT

Tony Carroll
Administrative Officer
Rotunda Hospital, Dublin 1.

The Medical Social Work Department of the Rotunda Hospital interviews almost *8,000 patients each year and processes numerous telephone and indirect enquiries each day relating to a broad spectrum of problems. Because the Rotunda is a Maternity Hospital most patients have to be followed-up during the course of their pregnancy and also for quite some time after delivery. The problems which are encountered in the Department are wide-ranging and often very complex. In many instances their final solution can only come about through the interaction of Community Care Services and other agencies which the Department works with in close co-operation. The Department has a staff of three Social Workers and two Secretaries.

Manual System:

In the past, when a patient first presented, a record card was created by the Medical Social Worker. This card was held in an "active file", until such time as the patient's problems were satisfactorily resolved. At the end of each year the cards were reviewed and edited and the information transferred to a "social register", which was really a quantitive summary of all attendances at the Department. Obviously, some patients at this stage would still be "active", in which case they continued on to the next year's register. This system of record keeping was time consuming, often inaccurate and served no real purpose other than to provide a means of collecting annual statistics.

<u>Illegimate Pregnancy</u>: Home situation, placement of mother during pregnancy, outcome of pregnancy, placement of baby, details of putative father. (Age, civil status, occupation and relationship with the patient).

<u>General Counselling</u>: This includes legal, psycho-sexual, bereavement, infertility, general supportive information, termination of pregnancy, marital breakdown, and in-depth counselling.

DATA ENTRY

The information from the forms are put on the Micro by the Department's Secretarial Staff during a three hour session once a week. As the problem identification section of the form is quite comprehensive, a coding system is used for convenience.

CONFIDENTIALITY

The patient's record can only be identified by a reference number while entry to the system is via a password.

VALIDATION

By specifing as many parameters as possible in each field, transcription and other errors can be minimised.

HARDWARE

Rank Xerox 820-11 Micro Computer (operating CP/M) double sided disk drive utilising eight inch floppy disks giving formated byte storage of 490 K per drive. Xerox 630 daisy wheel printer.

Computer System:

In January 1983 with the aid of the Hospital's Micro Computer facility,
a computer based system was introduced with the following objectives in
mind.

1. To develop a computerised Social Record that would meet the needs
of the Department and the Community Care Service in the Hospital's
catchment area.

2. To establish a comprehensive social register for research and follow up.

3. To compile quantitive statistics.

The description of the system in detail is as follows.

METHODOLOGY

A data collection form is completed for each new patient attending the
Department. The form is divided into two sections, section 1 being
used to record standard social and identification details while section
2 consists of a comprehensive list of pre-printed social factors under
a number of major headings, which are ticked off by the Medical Social
Worker in respect of the patient's visit to the Department. The divisions and the contents in this section of the form are;

Housing: Shared, inadequate, homeless, traveller.

Financial: Unemployed, long term illness, off work to care for children,
1 parent family, other.

Personal Problems: Physical , terminal, psychosomatic or psychiatric
illnesses. Physical or mental handicap, immaturity, isolation.
Alcoholism, gambling, drugs, crime, illiteracy, relationships.

Birth: Miscarriage, stillbirth, neo-natal death. Physical or mental
handicap, poor parenting skills, other.

SOFTWARE

Data Management System (DMS) Package.

The information is grouped at present on one floppy disk for each year.

ADVANTAGES

The advantages of the system may be enumerated as follows.
1. The data base provides a speedy method of identifying high risk follow up cases and is invaluable for social research.

2. The compilation of statistics for management and the social services is less tedious and more accurate.

3. The Social Workers have fewer administrative chores to do and thus can concentrate more on patient care.

4. This system is extremely cheap.

ACKNOWLEDGEMENTS

Professor G.R. Henry, Eleanor Holmes, Margaret Horner, Angela Long, Alison Colclough, Geraldine O'Sullivan, Mary Powell and Roisin Marrey.

*Rotunda Hospital Clinical Report 1983.

COMPUTERISATION OF THE MEDICAL ADMINISTRATION IN A GROUP PRACTICE OF OCCUPATIONAL HEALTH SERVICE (GOHS)

J.J. Weijers; F. Burgmans
Occupational Health Service
Oostelijk Gelderland
7000 GE DOETINCHEM
The Netherlands

Summary

For advicing individuals, groups of employees and companies about the connection between health on the one hand and work and workenvironment on the other, we need a regular medical examination of the individual and investigation of the workplace.

The tremendous amount of medical data, obtained by appointment examination, periodical examination and consulting hours has to be arranged and transformed in relevant information. Computerisation is indispensable.

oooooooooo

In the Netherlands companies and institutions, which are too small to maintain their own Occupational Health Service (OHS), have the opportunity to become a member of a Group Practice of Occupational Health Service (= GOHS).

At the end of 1984, there were 46 services of this kind and they provided this possibility for the whole country. This means that within a reasonable distance (approx. 15-20 km) each company can be supplied with occupational health service. The number of employees in such a GOHS, that has to be taken care of, ranges from about 3.000 to 40.000, the number of pnysicians from about 2 to 15.

The GOHS Oostelijk Gelderland in Doetinchem, situated in the eastern part of the Netherlands, takes care of about 37.000 employees, in an area of 30 by 40 kilometers; besides a central department, this GOHS also has four sub-departments in other small cities in the region.

Nineteen thousand of the total number of employees are working in a variety of industries such as the metallurgical and machine industry, paper-mills, wood processing industry, food industry; ten thousand in the building industry; one thousand in road-transport and passenger transport; one thousand in the printing trade; five thousand in service industries, mainly in government services.

One of the most important tasks of an OHS is to advice individuals, groups
of employees and companies, about the connection between health on the one
hand and work and -environment on the other. This requires a regular medical examination of the individual and investigation of the workplace.
One of the most important conditions therefore is that the data collected
are registered uniformly and in a standardized way. These methods of investigation are focused on:
- identification of occupational hazards,
- identification of employees who are liable to risks,
- prevention of occupational hazard and exposure to risks.
The medical data of the employees are mainly obtained by means of an appointment examination, periodical examinations, and from the doctor's consulting hours, the latter often as a consequence of long term absenteeism
for health reasons.
Anamnesis, physical examination and laboratorical analyses are the main
parts which have to provide us with a picture of the people examined.
Each day 45 examinations are carried out and each examination consists of
400 items. This tremendous amount of data has to be arranged and transformed into relevant information. For this purpose our GOHS and the computer manufacturor Sperry have developed the so-called MAO-system (MAO =
Medical Administration Occupational Health Services), a soft-ware system
for supplying information of OHS's.
Starting-points of MAO are:
- the data-collections are based on so-called standard forms,
  which are being used by a large number of GOHS's since 1981;
- the system answers questions concerning:
        - the individual,
        - occupational groups,
        - company/department/type of work,
        - management of the GOHS;
- the answering of additional questions;
- different types of accessibility.

Execution of data-collecting in practice

Eighty percent of the GOHS's collect and record their data uniformly,
which means: they use the so-called standard forms which are introduced in
1981. Each examination consists of the following standard data:
- name, date of birth; name of the company; date of examination;
  file number; native country; civil status; kind of shift;

kind of examination; name physician, medical assistant and
clerical assistant; nature of the company and type of work;
- former schooling and jobs.
All these data are added to the computer in coded form, if possible natio-
nal-coding-systems are used.
The main part of the health questionnaire of the AE (appointment examination) and PE (periodical examination) are identical.
Also during the PE-examination, a questionnaire concerning work has to
be filled out, containing 41 questions on work-experience. All the questions can be answered with a "yes" or a "no".
Generally, "yes" means that further attention needs to be paid and the
doctor concerned will ask further questions during a further anamnesis-
inquiry.
The questions concerning health are devided into twelve groups which contain 30 primary questions, i.e. questions which at all times have to be
answered with either a "yes" or a "no", and furthermore 19 secundary
questions which only have to be answered when the patient has answered
the primary questions with a "yes"; next, previous diseases, treatments
and operations, use of drugs/medicine, family diseases, smoking and alcohol, physical activities, health-complaints due to profession.
During the medical examination, the occurence of certain defects or indications pointing to affection of the tracts are recorded on another list.
This is considered as a hint for a certain pathology.
During the anamnesis as well as during the medical examination the physician can make additional notes separately.
The biometry-form offers the possibility to make a note of frequently
occuring items, such as length, weight, audiometrics, visus examination,
lungfunction test, bloodpressure, ECG, urine-examination, blood-examina-
tion (BSE, Hb, cholesterol, glucose, creatinine, ALAT, γ-GT, HDL).
In this way relevant data can be recorded for each individual. The main
data as well as all indications resulting from the questionnaire, the
medical examination and the biometry are - after having been coded -
added to the computer.
The PE takes place every four years, is meant for all ages and is carried
out in a period as short as possible. This means that in the course of
1985 the periodical examination will be held for the second time with the
same procedure and the same contents as in 1981. The data of both examinations can be compared longitudinally.
The computer gives a profile of every person examined, by which the physician is immediately informed about any pathology. By way of this profile the person examined can be informed about the outcome and given

advice. The relation between work and this record is important in this. These individual-data can also be arranged into group-data. Of each company the results from all items on the questionnaire and from all items of the biometry and physical examination are recorded. In this way groups of people, of whatever composition, can be compared.

The contents of MAO is as follows:
- soft-ware for the build-up, dating, reproduction and securing of:
    - NAD-file (name, address, domicile),
    - individual-file derived from data of the standard form,
    - historical individual-files,
    - files on prolonged absenteeism;
- support-files;
- charts for purposes of comparison;
- soft-ware for the re-call of data:
    - fixed: - individual risk-profile consisting of:
                       - personal data,
                       - data on work,
                       - signals resulting from questionnaires,
                       - biometry marked with 1-4 stars according
                         to their degree of abnormality;
                     - individual summary of schooling and occupa-
                       tional history;
                     - name, address, domicile data;
                     - group data:
                       - department, company,
                       - department-data compared,
                       - age categories,
                       - occupational groups,
                       - sex,
                       - Dutch/foreign,
                       - shift work;
    - additional: "Escort": a program-generator which is used for
                   counts, selections, comparisons, statistical
                   processing, surveys.

The use of information inside this GOHS relates to:
- individual employee: a review of recent examination data and data
  from the past, to detect trends in the development of the state of
  health;
- groups of employees with deviations from certain standards;
- workplace, department or concern: data about occupational hazards;

- connecting individual persons or a group of persons with the workplace to find out whether there is a relation between the state of
  health of the employee and the working-conditions;
- management: assesment of efficient functioning of the GOHS;
- medical audit: functioning of (para)-medical employees of the GOHS.

Examples of the use of data

1. Two departments of a metallurgical concern:
   - department A has a high score in physical working-conditions
     (noise, changes of temperature), but scores favourably concerning
     the head of the department (social support, cooperation, organi-
     sation).
   - department B scores favourably concerning physical working-
     conditions, but there are many complaints about the head of the
     department.
   In cooperation with the company, a plan was made to pay attention to
   the physical circumstances at the workplace in department A and to
   the leading of department B.
2. In a company with a work force of over 500 employees, there are many
   health complaints of persons older than 55 years, but hardly any objective pathology. A plan was set up in cooperation with the company,
   for reorganising the tasks, in order to prevent people older than 55
   years doing any strenuous work.
3. 9.000 ECG's spread over different categories of age did not show under
   40 years any abnormalities which needed any treatment.
   Conclusion: ECG's under 40 years only when complaints have been noticed.
4. There are great differences in anamnesis at appointment-examination
   (AE) and at the periodical examination (PE), taking place only $1\frac{1}{2}$ to
   2 years later.
   The scores of the same questions were sometimes 5 times as high at
   the PE as at the AE. It is very unlikely that these differences have
   been caused by the work and workenvironment.
   So this shows the relative value of the anamnesis for the prognosis
   at the AE.

DEVELOPMENT OF A SYSTEM OF COMMUNICATION TO COLLECT MEDICAL DATA AT A REGIONAL LEVEL.

*F. A. ALLAERT, **P. DUSSERRE, ***H. BASTIEN, *L. DUSSERRE, ****F. KOHLER.
* Service d'Informatique Médicale. Bd Mal de Lattre de Tassigny
21034 DIJON CEDEX - FRANCE -
** Laboratoire de Pathologie Humaine et Expérimentale. Rue Sainte Anne
21000 DIJON - FRANCE -
*** Laboratoire d'Anatomie Pathologique. Centre Leclerc, rue du Profes-
seur Marion 21034 DIJON CEDEX - FRANCE -
**** Service d'Informatique Médicale, Faculté de Médecine 54500 VANDOEU-
VRE LES NANCY - FRANCE -

INTRODUCTION

The computerization of private medical offices is presently developing in several countries (1, 2) and particularly in France (3). However, in several more cases the technical solutions proposed to doctors do not take into consideration one of the essential objectives of this process : the possibility of gathering together medical data in the framework of a regional epidemiology.

As a reaction against this evolution, the "A.I.M" (Association for the Development of Medical Informatics) is promoting for the last 3 years, in Burgundy, a project entitled "computerization of private medical offices in a compatible and coherent way in order to establish a gathering together of data at a regional level". The first part of this work made up by a survey on the computer needs of medical practitioners was presented at the last M.I.E Congress (Brussels, september 1984).

We are presenting now, the second part of this study : realisation and evaluation of computer systems.

OBJECTIVES

This computerization of the private medical offices must respond to 5 needs that were expressed in the survey of january 1982 :
- to computerize the medical record of the patient.
- to assure the statistical analysis of this information.
- to permit the connection of the computer system of the private medical office to the different available data banks.
- to make possible a direct communication of information between doctors themselves and also with a regional computer center.
- the house calls still being inseparable in France from the private medical practice, the system must easily permit the consulta-

tion and the completion of the patient's medical record at his bedside.

REALISATION

At first, the creation of this computer systems was envisaged in the framework of an hospital university laboratory or another public institution. However, if the above could take over the technical production of such a system, they do not have sufficient personnel to guaranty the optimal conditions of maintenance necessary for commercialisation.

From this fact, a commercial offer was proposed to the computer supply companies under the aegis of A.I.M.

After selection of different competitive companies, 3 of them were taken in, due to their technical competence and their experience in the medical profession :
- MEDICAL COMPUTER FRANCE COMPANY
- MEDISOFT COMPANY
- SOPRA COMPANY

The 3 companies committed themselves to realize or to modify their existing programmes (MEDIGEST, MEDIS) in such a way as to be conformed to the functionnal needs described by the medical profession.

FIRST CHARACTERISTICS OF THE SYSTEMS

We present here, the first technical solutions that were chosen to respond to the different objectives of the project.

- To computerize the medical record of the patient, the solution that appears to be the most satisfactory is that of "preprogrammed" forms. The system gives the possibility to the pratitioners to create by himself, without having to program them, the forms corresponding to the different aspects of the pathology. The only thing to be defined is the heading of the column and the size of their content. These forms are then called upon according to the needs to make up the medical record of the patient.

- The statistical analysis of the information of the medical office is realized by a multicriteria research programme taking into account both administrative and medical data.

- The transfer of the information to the patient's bedside is accomplished by a "pocket" computer HP 71B. The latter is connected to the general system before the doctor leaves indicating the names of patients whose clinical forms he wishes to make with him. This information is automatically introduced in the memory of the portable system and could therefore be consulted and then completed from a medical and financial view-point at the patient's bedside. When he comes back, the new data is automatically integrated into the system.

- Access to the data banks is realized by the connection of the system to the french network videotex : "TELETEL" .

- The transfer of information between doctors or to an epidemiological study center is also accomplished through the intermediary of this videotex system . However, the system cannot be directly questionned by this network because no matter what the complexity of the access code certain people could find it out and thus violate the medical records. In order to guaranty this confidentiality the exchange of information will be made by the intermediary of a "computerized post office box" whereby the doctor will be able to receive messages and to leave the records that he whishes to take with the knowledge of his collegues. In no case will a medical file be able to be consulted without the doctor himself having put it as his collegues' disposition in this message bank.

THE EVALUATION PHASE

The different proposed methods are presently in experimentation amongst practicing doctors in 3 french cities : DIJON, NANCY, MONPELLIER. After a three months trial period, thes practitioners will provide to "A.I.M" a report on the conformity of the programmes to their functional needs. If succesfull , the A.I.M will give the companies a quality label justifying the adaptation of their products to the needs of the medical profession.

THE CREATION OF A MEDICAL NETWORK

In our region, different groups of specialists already use a computer in their practice. The first were the pathologists. As far back as 1975 these practitioners were interrested in this new technologie and tried to create a product especially adapted to their needs. Their attempt was succesfull and now we can use a general register of tumors. Then the gastro-enterologists and the gynaecologists understood the value of the computer for the development of epidemiological research and organized their specific register of tumors.

But all the information was still coming from the public domain . Our work will permit the necessary participation of the private sector to the medical network and thus will allow the establishment of a regional Health policy. (scheme 1)

CONCLUSION

The interest of this study essentially rests in the straight collaboration between Health and Computer professionals to create a product adapted to the needs of the medical office. It shows the wish of the medical corps, to possess computer methods that would allow it to create a computerized medical network of communication in the private sector. This is the condition necessary for the development of an epidemiology of ambulatory diseases in the regional framework. (4,5,6)

REFERENCES

1- Cerutti S, Perez De Talens F, Nizzari D. Medical record system for the general practitioner. Health information systems: The italian approach. Ed Fernandez Peréz De Talens.1983.

2- Manacorda PM. Computer in general practice : an european survey. Fourth World Congress on Medical Informatics. MEDINFO 1983 AMSTER DAM .

3- Allaert FA, Bastien H, Guisiano B, Dusserre L. Survey of computer needs by medical practitioners in an administrative division of FRANCE (cote-d'or). V European Congress on Medical Informatics MIE 1984 BRUSSELS.

4- Speck P.K. Computerized methods for ambulatory care. Fourth World Conference on Medical Informatics. MEDINFO 1983 AMSTERDAM.

5- Lion J., Malbon A. Data base development: public health policy and ambulatory case mix . Fourth World Conference on Medical Informatics. MEDINFO 1983 AMSTERDAM.

6- De Moel J. General practitioners information system. Fourth World Conference on Medical Informatics. MEDINFO 1983 AMSTERDAM.

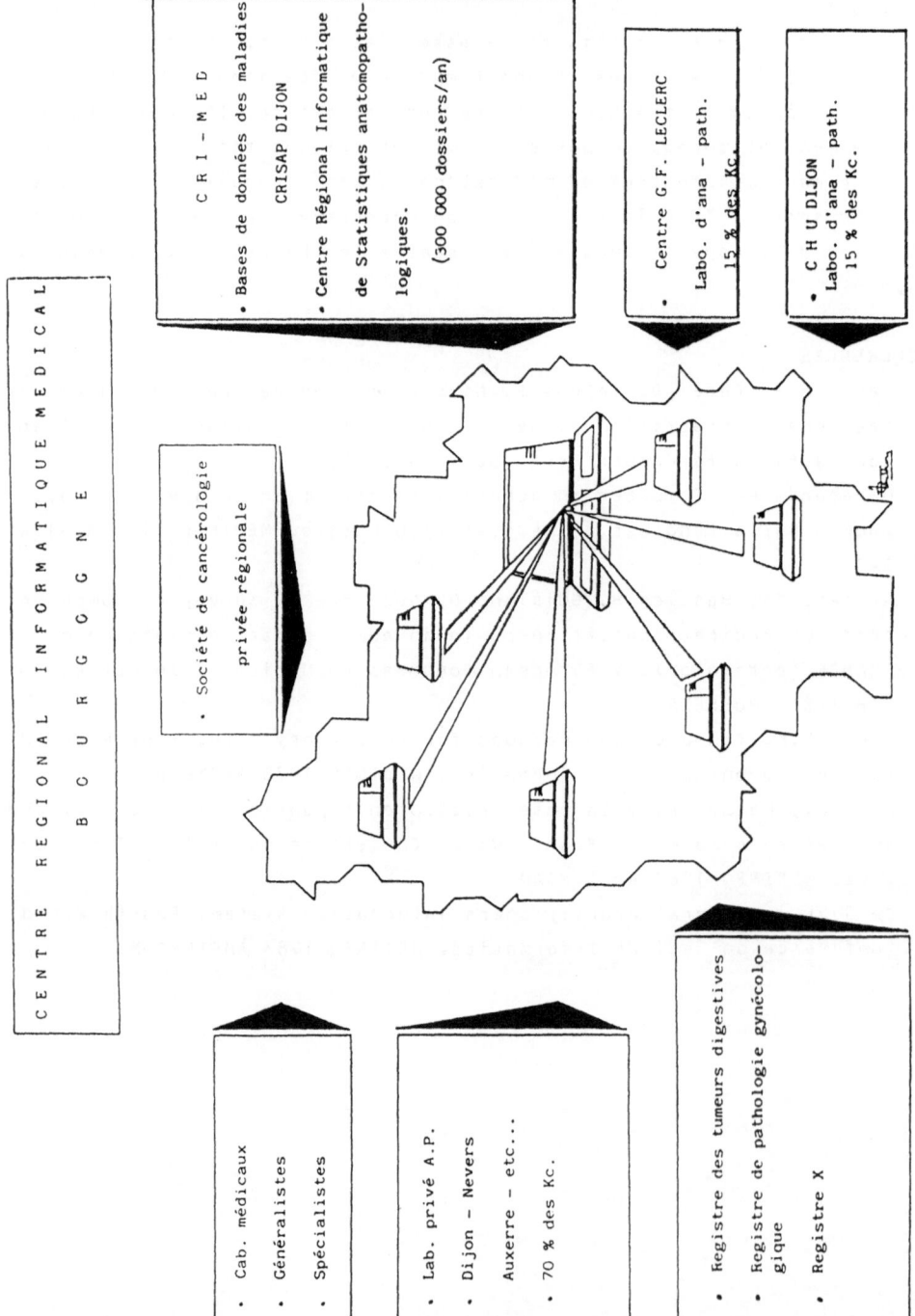

CENTRE REGIONAL INFORMATIQUE MEDICAL
BOURGOGNE

C R I - M E D
- Bases de données des maladies
  CRISAP DIJON
- Centre Régional Informatique
  de Statistiques anatomopatho-
  logiques.
  (300 000 dossiers/an)

- Centre G.F. LECLERC
  Labo. d'ana - path.
  15 % des Kc.

- C H U DIJON
  Labo. d'ana - path.
  15 % des Kc.

- Société de cancérologie
  privée régionale

- Cab. médicaux
- Généralistes
- Spécialistes

- Lab. privé A.P.
- Dijon - Nevers
  Auxerre - etc...
- 70 % des Kc.

- Registre des tumeurs digestives
- Registre de pathologie gynécolo-
  gique
- Registre X

MEASUREMENT OF PRODUCTIVITY IN PRIMARY CARE

Ilkka Vohlonen
Health Services Research unit
National Board of Health
Kalliolinnantie 4
00140 Helsinki 14
Finland

Introduction

In most developed countries there is a system of social and health insurance.
These systems are partly or totally subsidized by the state. With the decreasing
gross national products the development of health care has also become strongly
dependent on the limited public funds. In order to develop the health care system
it is necessary to monitor the implementation of the health services more carefully
than before. The relationships between planning, implementation and evaluation of
the nationwide supply of services are the prerequisites for a balanced allocation
of the health resources. The relationship between the supply and the demand of
health services can be thought of as a chain of costs (resources)-services
(operations)-effects (outcomes). The relationship between costs and services is
referred to as productivity. The relationship between services and effects is
referred to as effectiveness, and the relatioships between costs and effects is
referred to as efficiency. The health services consist of preventive and curative
services, which can further be classified as primary, secondary and tertiary care.
The aim of this paper is to present some results from a study measuring the
productivity in primary curative care, and to suggest some recommendations for
nationwide monitoring of primary care services.

METHODS

In order to study and develop a nationwide monitoring system of primary curative
services (medical care), data has been gathered from several municipal health
centers in the years 1981-84 in various parts of Finland. The data have been
computerized centrally and they have been stored as individual outpatient visits.
The date of the visit, the social security number of the patient and the licence
of the medical officer have been processed. In the town of Jyväskylä the data was
stored during three consecutive years. The town has about 60 000 inhabitants and
most of the health services are provided by the municipal health center. In addition,
data were gathered from the four large cities of Finland, Helsinki, Lahti, Tampere
and Turku during the spring and the fall of 1984. The proportions of primary medical
care supplied by the public and the private sectors vary between the four cities.

The data consist of the information gathered only in the municipal health centers, which provide a relatively equal supply of services in the four cities. The operations of the primary medical services were described by three different indeces. The first was the coverage of services, which was defined as the proportion of people who had utilized the health services during the follow-up period. The second index was the reuse of services, which was defined as the number of visits per patient during the follow-up period. The third index was the continuity of services, which was defined as the proportion of patients who repeatedly had been seen by the same physician. The continuity of services was computed as Kappa-coefficients, which take into account continuity of services due to chance (e.g. the effects of the number of patient visits and the physicians).

Results

The data on the utilization of primary medical services were gathered from the information collected for local administrative purposes. Therefore, no additional registration was performed for the study. On the basis of the data, it oould be estimated that, with a density of about 2700 inhabitants per general practitioner, about 70+/- 5 percent of the population annually sought help from primary care. Each person visited the primary care physician approximately 3 times per year. It could be calculated that a population of 100 000 would generate a need of approximately 230 000+/- 10 000 physician visits annually. The variation of coverage, reuse and continuity of primary health services most strongly depended on the amount of resources. There appeared no statistically significant variation between the three consecutive years in the age and sex standardized rates. The seasonal variation was only slight and it was consistent from one year to another. Children of under 3 years of age and the elderly of over 64 years utilized the services about 1.5 times more per inhabitant than the rest of the population. The continuity of services was low. About 15-20 percent of the patients had been treated repeatedly by the same physician. The variations of coverage, reuse and continuity of services were also examined with respect to the age and sex of the patients, the number of patients observed, and the length of the follow-up period. There appeared a consistency with the earlier mentioned results regardless of the chatacteristics of the patients or the size of the group of patients being followed. However, the lenght of the follow-up period seemed to determine the value of the three indices. The relationships between the length of the follow-up period and the values of the three different indices were quite linear (Figures 1, 2 and 3).

Figure 1.

The coverage (%) of primary medical services (2700 inhabitants per doctor) by the length of follow-up periods (mths).

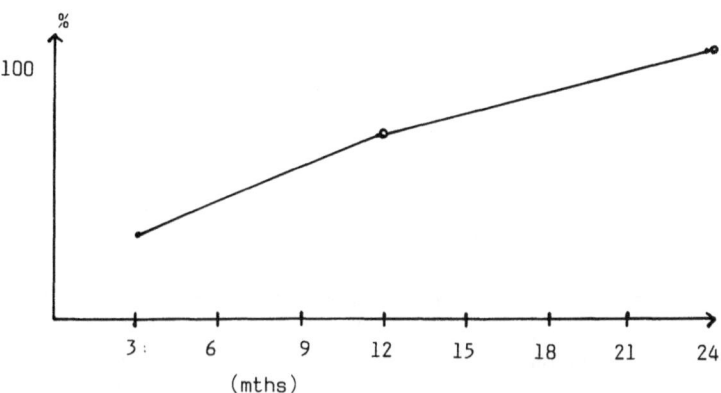

Figure 2.

The reuse (number of visits) of primary medical services by a patient (2700 inhabitants per doctor) by the length of follow-up period (mths).

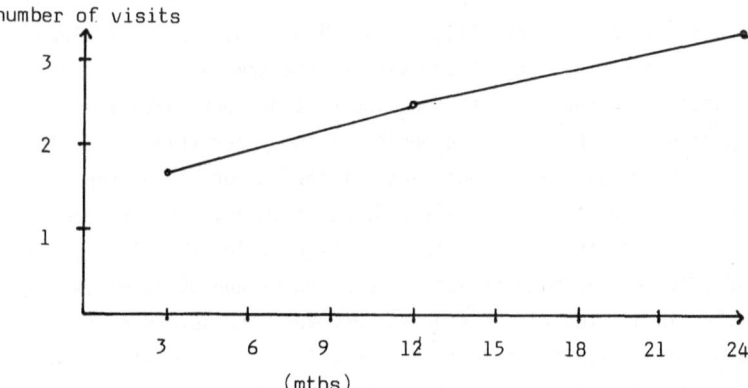

Figure 3.

The continuity (%) of primary medical services among patients (2700 inhabitants per doctor) by the length of follow-up period (mths).

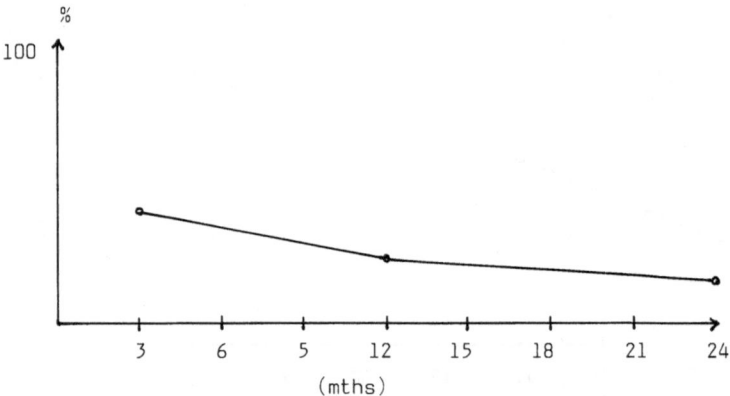

According to the curve of figure 1, in one year about 65 percent of the inhabitants of the population being served had utilized at least once the primary medical care services, and in two years the respective rate was about 95 percent. The reuse of services within one year was 2.5 times per patient, and within two years the rate of reuse was about 3.2 visits per patient (figure 2). Within one year of follow-up, about 20 percent of the patients had repeatedly visited the same physician, while reoccuring visits by chance had been counted for. The rate of continuity (Kappa coefficient) was 15 percent for the follow-up period of two years (figure 3). The curves of the three figures were similar regardless of the age or sex of the patients, although the levels of the rates differed. For example, the coverage was highest for the young children, the reuse of services highest for the elderly women and the continuity of services was highest among the women of age 34 to 64 years. The results were similar in all the cities studied. However, the levels of the curves varied and it was conceived to reflect the variation of the supply of the primary care services and, more so, the variation of the productivity of the primary care services. For example, between the two extreme cases there was a two-fold difference in the rates of coverage, yet, the resources for primary care were approximately the same in size and content. Again, the differences between the cities were consistent regardless of the sex or age of the population group or the patients being treated by their primary care systems.

Conclusions

The measurement of the productivity in primary care was done without a special information. The data consisted of the information collected along with the local administration of primary care services. The coverage, reuse and continuity of primary medical services could be described on the basis of three items of information about each patient visit. There was no annual variation in the examined rates, and their relationships with the length of the follow-up period were quite linear. On the basis of the results it could be concluded that the monitoring of primary care productivity is sufficiently done by respresentative sampling of patient visits. However, close attention should be paid to obtaining information about the health resources and the costs of the supply of primary care. For the comparison of various clinics or chronological follow-up of the same clinic, it is quite necessary to age and sex standardize the rates of observations. At present, more research is required to develop the methods of measuring the morbidity of the population or the patients serviced. On the basis of the preliminary findings, it seems possible to measure the prevalence and attack rates of the causes generating the need for primary medical care. If so, the effectivenes of the primary health services can be measured and the efficiency of the services estimated.

References

Armitage P. Statistical methods in medical research. Blackwell Scientific Publications. Oxford 1971.

Fleiss J. Statistical methods for rates and proportions. John Wiley & Sons. New York 1973.

Kohn R., White K. (ed). Health Care: An international study. Oxford University Press. Norwich 1976.

Purola T. A systems approach to health and health policy. Med Care 10:1972:373-379.

WONCA. International classification of health problems in primary care. Oxford University Press. Oxford 1984.

INTERACTIVE PATIENT RECORD

Peter Dvergsdal
General Practice
Drammensveien 327, N 1324 Lysaker, Norway

Summary

A computerized medical record system. Each patient's record is integrated with a menu system comprising about 500 standard medical texts. Using these it is possible to achieve semi-automatic writing of medical records and communications to be sent or handed to the patient.

Basis

The system is based on the INFODOC patient record but it is hoped that this work will also assume more general importance and that it may contribute to the process of standarization of automatic computerized medical records and automatic medical communication.

Functions

1. Standard texts from text register to record.
2. Standard texts from text register to forms.
3. Combination of a variety of standard texts.
4. Editing of standard texts before use.
5. Adjustment of the system to NS 4060 (Norwegian Standard for health service forms. Cf. Bruusgaard/Dvergsdal, article in Journal of the Norwegian Medical Association 10 May 1984).

Objects

1. Quicker and better printouts.
2. Ensure that actions carried out are always automatically entered in the patient record.
3. Standard note in the patient record.
4. Build up a diagnosis register with numerical code.
5. Build up a register of standard expressions for records.

6. Prepare proposals for later standardization.
7. Make it possible to use statistics at all levels in the record.
8. Arrange for automatic editing of the patient record.
9. Standardize the patient record to such extent that it can be transmitted to other systems (hospitals).

Programming

A preliminary specification for a program of this kind was drawn up in the autumn of 1981. It turned out that this work had to be done more or less from scratch. After thorough specification, the whole system was programmed by Informasjonssystemer in Bergen. It was tested in parallel by me.

PRESCRIPTION AND TEXT REGISTER

In the course of 1983 I completed a system which was capable of getting from the register and printing out texts for prescriptions, various requisitions and other communications. At the same time, the system made a note in the patient record of actions carried out.

The registers comprise about 1000 basic texts for prescriptions, and several hundred modules for various form texts (laboratory requisitions, references, medical certificates, letters to patients).

These are arranged in several menu trees, an expert system which assists the doctor in selecting what he requires. The menu tree for prescriptions is arranged in accordance with the Anatomical Therapeutic Chemical Classification System (ATC).

DIAGNOSIS REGISTER

Structure

ICD9. All diagnoses are numbered according to ICD9. Most have 4-digit numbers, but some are at 2 and 3-digit levels. All diagnoses that may be expected in general practice are included. Efforts have been made to maintain a relatively high level of precision, but unprecise diagnoses and symptom diagnoses have not been neglected. This is an expert system which demands a certain degree of precision on the part of the user, yet still allows less precise work if desired.

My register now comprises between 1500 and 2000 diagnoses. Since ICD9 has not yet been introduced in Norway, I have used a Norwegian list, ØMI ICD8, for writing; this is in Latin.

ICPC (International classification of primary care, final revision April 1984). The structure of this list differs from ICD8 and ICD9.

The structure of ICD9 is partly organ-oriented, with special classifications for infectious, neoplasm, injuries and intoxication, and with a register of symptoms and ill-defined etiologies. Users find ICD9 difficult to use.

ICPC is structured on a more consistent organ system pattern. At the next level there is a list of the various diagnoses and complaints.

I have divided up my diagnosis groups according to ICPC, using letter codes to build them up into a menu system. In this way the desired organ system can be entered simply by pressing one letter key.

In addition to ICPC I have set up a second level in the register. This level is etiological (see example). I have included ICD's special register at this level (infectious, neoplasm, injuries, intoxication, iatrogen, treatment without sickness). In this way it is possible by simply pressing two keys to scan about 300 options, largely without reading the menus.

At the next level the various diagnosis alternatives are listed. Where there are more than 20 diagnoses there is also a fourth level. On average, the time taken to find a diagnosis in this register is about the same as it takes to write a diagnosis manually. What is achieved is a somewhat more detailed diagnosis than usual. Moreover, the diagnosis is coded according to ICD9, and it is always written in the same way.

With a little practice, it is easier to find a diagnosis in this way than to write one by hand.

SYMPTOM REGISTER

I have also prepared a symptom register.

Purpose - To make the patient record <u>unambiguous</u>.
   - To impose certain <u>minimum requirements</u> as regards case history.
   - To carry out an experiment in <u>standard syntax</u>.

UNAMBIGUOUS: Few standard words are used, the intention being that in time the system shall recognize all important words used in the text. It is also conceivable to let the computer search for certain standard words, e.g. "pain".

MINIMUM REQUIREMENTS: The system is so designed that certain requirements are imposed in addition to the naming of the symptom. Details of characteristics of the symptom, duration, influential factors, improvement or aggravation, and possible previous occurrences are required by the system. In addition, arrangements have been made for registration of supplementary symptoms.

STANDARD SYNTAX: Each sentence is of hierarchical structure. First comes the organ system with possible sub-grouping and (:), next comes the key word of the symptom and (,), then characteristics (,), duration (,), possible aggravation (,), and previous occurrence. Punctuation is (;) before new key words in the same organic system and (.) at the end of the anamnesis for an organic system. Example: Respiratory: throat: pain, moderate, 3 days, improvement, previous occurrence 3 times 1 year; Secretion, yellow, copious etc. General: fever, moderate etc.

Future advantages are obvious. First and foremost it will be possible to develop a system which is able to recognize and sort the contents

of the records.   The system will be capable of editing and re-
editing the records as required.   In principle, it will also be
possible to extract a range of statistics without the need for
special registration.   Standard syntax will also simplify the transmission of records to systems of other makes.   The records will be
completely universal as regards hardware and software.

FINDINGS REGISTER

This register has much in common with the other registers.   Here
too, efforts have been made to develop standard texts for organ
systems, and standard works.   We differentiate here between normal
and abnormal findings so that the system can easily sort between
important and unimportant findings.

FINAL REMARKS

None of the registers are as complete as perhaps they should be in
the future.

It should be possible to proceed with the building up of a standard
text system for medical use.

It would seem sensible to set up a Norwegian or Nordic working group
to assume responsibility for this work.   At present the use of
interactive medical records seems to be a peculiarly Norwegian
phenomenon.   In this country the concept has been adopted with
enthusiasm by doctors and computer enterprises.

Developments have now reached a stage where one should proceed to the
production of a computer and a program-independent medical record.
This would also pave the way to problem-free communication.

Bibliography:

Journal of Norwegian Medical Association, 10 May 1984:   Dag
Bruusgaard - Peter Dvergsdal: "Skjema i helsevesenet".

EXAMPLES

1st LEVEL BASIC MENU

1   Sickreport
2   Prescription/Advice
3   Laboratory
4   Regiograms
5   Anamnesis
6   Findings
D   Diagnosis
F   Physiotherapy
H   Referral

2nd LEVEL DIAGNOSIS MENU

A   AbdDigest
B   Blood(Bloodforming)
C   Cardiovasc.
D   Dermatology
E   EndocrinImmun
G   General
H   HearingEar
M   Muscleskelet.
N   Neurological
O   Ocular
P   Psychological
R   Respiratory
U   Urological
E   ReproductEtc
X   Female
Y   Male
Z   Social
1   Perinatal

3rd LEVEL DIAGNOSIS MENUS A, B, C, D
E, G, H, M, N, O, R, V, X, Y
Etiological lists of diagnoses

4th LEVEL DIAGNOSIS MENU 3
Selected list of diagnoses

2nd LEVEL PRESCRIPTION MENU

A   AbdomMetab
B   Blood(Bloodforming)
C   Cariovasc
D   Dermatology
G   GenitoHormUr
H   Hormones
J   Infection
M   Muscleskelet.
N   Nervous syst.
P   Parasites
R   Respiration
S   Sensoryorgans
V   Varia

3rd LEVEL PRESCRIPTION MENU C

1   Hearttherapy
2   Hypertension
3   Diuretics
4   Vasodilators
5   Vasoprotectors
7   Beta blockers

4th LEVEL PRESCRIPTION MENU C
Selected list of beta
blockers

FREE TEXT RETRIEVAL OF MEDICAL INFORMATION

Truls Østbye
Directorate of Organization and Management
P.O.Box 8115 Dep.0032 OSLO 1

SIFT (Searching In Free Text), a retrieval system developed by the Norwegian public sector is described. Its general relevance and applications in medicine are discussed, followed by a description and analysis of a specific example - a test of SIFT using "Felleskatalogen", a
catalogue of all proprietary drugs in Norway.

The amount of printed information is growing exponentially, both in
general and within medicine. Therefore, it is increasingly important to
find relevant information about a topic quickly, without being over-
whelmed by unnecessary, marginally interesting information. Information-
Retrieval systems (IR-systems), where one can store information, change
it and freely search for single concepts or concept combinations that
appear in the text, are EDP-tools that are becoming more and more useful
in this context.

The Norwegian Directorate of Organization and Management, in collaboration with several other institutions, has developed a general IR-
system, SIFT, for use by state and other public institutions (1).

SIFT is a part of a larger whole, intended to be the foundation in
several future information systems. In addition, SIFT is to be used in
conjunction with several existing information systems.

SIFT

SIFT is an acronym for Searching In Free Text (Norwegian: Søking I Fri
Tekst). Furthermore, The Universal English Dictionary states (2):

> Sift, verb .... 3. To examine carefully and critically so as to
> separate the true from the false, the useful
> from the worthless etc.

And this is exactly what the SIFT system does; it goes through large
amounts of text and picks out the information of interest according to
specified criteria.

PROPERTIES OF SIFT:

Searching in the whole text

Most existing retrieval systems allow searching in a resume or index-
word-list. An advantage of SIFT, is that it allows retrieval from the
whole text. Therefore the system is also referred to as a fulltext
retrieval system.

Fields

It is possible to delineate sections of the text as fields (e.g. title-
field, author-field, introductory field etc.). By defining fields in
this manner, it is possible to carry out a more precise search.

The system allows freetext retrieval from the whole text, from the unstructured text and from the defined fields. Numerical fields (incl.
data fields), can be retrieved also by specifying intervals (e.g. "find
documents written between 15.12.1954 and 1.12.1958").

Query language

The query language in SIFT is easy to use, while simultanously being very general and powerful. There are no practical limits to the complexities of the questions. The query language allows ordinary Boolean operations ("and", "or", "not" and combinations of these) at a document level, as well as at the level of paragraphs and sentences.

Relative word positions may also be specified (i.e. the maximum or minimum distance between words).

Complex queries that are often repeated, can be defined and stored for later use.

Masking

Masking of parts of words enables retrieval of all words starting with a specified letter combination (e.g. ast* for asthma, astenia, asthmatic etc).

Thesaurus

Plans for further development of SIFT include designing a system for words which are related to each other. The development of such a _thesaurus_ will enable the system to "know" which words/concepts have the same or approximately the same meaning. Furthermore, the system will be able to compare if certain concepts are "wider" or "narrower" than a given concept, for instance if the given concept is "psychosis", "mental disease" is a wider concept while "schizophrenia" is narrower. This adds a further possibility for nuanced search.

Formats

In order to get a better overview, it is possible to present long documents by defining special formats. For example, the information presented on the screen can be limited to a document's title, author and an introduction.

Focusing

Quick retrieval of wanted information is improved by "highlighting", where the words/concepts which are of interest light up on the screen brighter than the rest of the text.

Access control

A secret password controls access to the documents. In addition, access can be limited by storing the information on different levels, i.e. some users have access to everything in all documents, while others only have access to certain documents or certain parts of the documents .

Machine independence

During the development of SIFT, machine independence was emphasized strongly, so that the system can, in principle, run on any type of machine over a certain size. The system has a clear-cut bounderyline which makes it easy to adapt to new computer types. Today the system runs on equipment from Norsk Data, Digital, Cromemco and Univac.

Storage method

In principle, text is stored _twice_. First, the ordinary text is stored in a "document file". However, before searching in this document file, an "inversion" of the text is carried out. A programme goes through the documents, makes a word list called a "search file", where the words and their corresponding addresses (page, line, position) are stored. This is done so that instead of searching through the whole text (i.e. the document-file) to find a given word, the actual word is accessed directly in the search file. If the word is found in the search file, the document that contains it, may be found directly.

Updating

The updating function is critical. Direct on-line updating of the system can be carried out while the system is being used for ordinary purposes. The search file is built up around B-trees (3).

General Medical applications

IR has many useful applications in various fields, ranging from library-science to law, to medicine. IR-systems have been used in medical research for several years. These earlier systems have been relatively difficult to master, and have only limited search capacities (usually search only by certain index terms such as title, author and date of publication).

With SIFT, it is possible to search the entire text if it is stored in the computer. Today books, articles and other publications are stored on a computer in the print-stop to make the graphical process easier. However, the potential for increasing the level of acessibility of these publications to the professional community has yet to been taken advantage of.

If free-text-search is going to be a useful tool in everyday clinical life, it is a precondition that the lay-out of the display that is presented as an answer to a question, must strike a delicate balance between being succinct and comprehensive.

In a patient oriented situation the information that is displayed must be structured in a clear "overview" format so that only the useful amount of information that can be assimilated quickly to aid diagnosis, is displayed. Merck's Manual is a medical text-book whose structure would be suitable for this purpose. (4)

Ideally, it is possible to computerize reference manuals/text- books which give an overview of problem areas at different levels of detail. For example, if the query is:

> FIND DIABETES

The answer could be an overview of the disease, which covers a few pages. However, if the question is:

> FIND (DIABETES AND VON HIPPEL LINDAU SYNDROME)

the answer would provide more specialised information concerning the relationship between these two diseases, possibly with litterature citations. One could also consider several intermediate levels with varying coverage between these two extremes.

Medical records

In many hospitals the medical records are already contained in text processing equipment. These records are well suited for use with SIFT. Using SIFT, these data can be used as "raw material" for further processing and analysis. For instance one can imagine queries like the following: "find all documents (records) which contains the concept "meningitis", searching in patients born in the period "1969-1978" and with place of residence "London".

"Felleskatalogen"

Felleskatalogen is a catalogue of all proprietary drugs in Norway (about 2000). Each drug is described by a text of 100-2000 words. The description has two parts; a structured part (drug name, ATC-number, producer etc.) and a semistructured, detailed, free text with paragraphs covering topics such as indications, contraindications, side effects etc. The data are the property of Felleskatalogen Ltd.

In the SIFT-context one drug definition is treated as one document. Each paragraph was defined as a field, to enable greater detail in the queries.

Some "Formats" were also defined for a better screen presentation of the drug descriptions. For example, the negative aspects of a drug are displayed through the format ANTI (consisting of the fields title, ATC-number, contraindications and side-effects).

Typical queries are shown. The first ones in table 2 are included to show the use of the Boolean operators "and", "or" and "not". The lower ones illustrate the flexibility of the query language and examples of queries that could be of interest, but which are difficult to answer using the printed form which Felleskatalogen has today.

Table 2 Examples of SIFT-commands used with "Felleskatalogen"

Problem	SIFT-command
Give an overview of all databases connected to the system	> LIST DATABASES
Find all documents (drug descriptions) containing the word "klorofyll"	> FIND KLOROFYLL (abbreviated:) > F KLOROFYLL)
Show these drug descriptions on the screen, first drug's first page first	> SHOW
Find all drug descriptions containing the word "antidot" or the word "vaksine"	> F ANTIDOT OR VAKSINE
Find all drug descriptions containing both the word "antidot" and the word "vaksine"	> F ANTIDOT AND VAKSINE
Find all drugs used against herpes zoster(ie. containing the word "zoster" in the indication field	> F ZOSTER IN INDIK
Find all drugs used against hypertension that may be given to patients with asthma	> F HYPERTENSION IN INDIK AND NOT ASTMA IN KONTRA
The patient had a narcosis yesterday, today she hallucinates. Her record is lost. Which drug did she get?	> F NARKOSE IN INDIK AND (HALLUCIN* OR HALLUSIN*) IN BIVIRK
Which tranquillizers exist as injection drugs? (In the field "pris" the drug types are mentioned)	> F TRANQ* IN TITTEL AND INJ* IN PRIS
Finish the search	> EXIT

Use:

The system in this context can be mastered in about 2 hours by anyone who has access to a terminal.

The system serves as a tool to find the raw-material. The final decisions about which drugs to use of course remain the responsibility of the one who uses the information.

Future prospects concerning "Felleskatalogen"

The aspects that could be improved could be more standardized presentation concerning drugs and their prices, so that comparison of similar
drugs will be even easier.

If an information-system like this is to be developed further, the
presentation of information must be emphasized, taking the screen
terminal's advantages and limitations into consideration.

In its written form the total amount of information presented appears
reasonable to the user. With an "electronic Felleskatalogen" it will be
possible to include even more information on each drug. Then, one could
define different levels of details in the drug descriptions. The
simplest would be a list of drug names in connection with one indication. One window could equate the "Felleskatalogen"as it exists today.
Furthermore, it would be possible to have an extensive drug information
bank with references to original journal articles to which the articles
themselves could be connected.

Today the Felleskatalogen on EDP could be used by Felleskatalogen's
editors to design an improved edition. It could be used by pharmacies,
drug control authorities and in drug research. It may also have applications in clinical practice.

In the future, instead of distributing "Felleskatalogen" as a thick
volume to all physicians and pharmacies, updated diskettes could be
distributed and put into the pharmacies', the hospitals' or the primary
health care physicians' own computers. With the new video-disc technology that is now being introduced, the problem of mass storage seems to
be solved.

Furthermore, later editions with general medical information structured
in somewhat the same way as the drug descriptions in Felleskatalogen
could be a further step on the way to having "all medical knowledge on
the screen".

Conclusion

Searching many different kinds of documents by means of systems like
SIFT is possible within medicine: routine correspondence, epicrises,
medical records, text books and reference works, drug information and
journal articles.

The EDB-tools exist already; what remains now is to synthesize the
"materia medica" and EDP technology so that the field of medicine can
gain maximum benefits from EDP for retrieval of information in every
relevant situation.

REFERENCES

1. SIFT. Design specifications.
    Directorate of Organization and Management, Oslo 1980.

2. The Universal English Dictionary.
    London: Routledge and Kegan Paul Ltd., 1982

3. Comer, D. The Ubiquitous B-tree.
    Computing Surveys 1979, II-2: 121-137.

4. The Merck Manual of Diagnosis and Therapy.
    14th Ed., Ralway, New Jersey: Merck, Sharp and co., 1982.

5. Felleskatalog over farmasøytiske spesialpreparater
    registrert i Norge 1984. 26 edition, Fabritius forlag, 1983.

INTEGRATED BUREAUTICS AND MEDICAL CARE UNITS

Dujols P. *,   Aubas P. **, Godard P. **, Romero M. ***,
Geoffroy F. ***, Gremy F. *, Michel FB. **
*   Departement de l'Information Medicale
**   Service des Maladies Respiratoires
*** Centre Regional d'Informatique Hospitaliere
555 route de Ganges, 34059 MONTPELLIER Cedex, FRANCE

   Hospital medical records meet four main requirements :
patient follow-up, communication between physicians whether
inside or outside the hospital, medical research and analysis of
the medical activity of departments [19].
   Based on a formalized thinking and precise protocole of
data-gathering, clinical research and activity analysis have been
successfully improved with computer [15]. On the same level,
computer based patient follow-up systems have been approached in
medical specialities [12][13], and some are still active in daily
medical practice [2][4][22]. In this field, all relevant cases
share a precise   investigation field (speciality,   ponctual
technique), a well defined aim, a deep knowledge of   the
interesting clinical data and, mostly, a perfect adequation to
praticians needs.
   But, those realizations correspond only to a part of
the requirement. This perfect adaptation to a precise medical
field involves at the same time a difficult extension to
polypathological records or to a wider investigation field.
Medical   improvements   imply   an   increasing   medical
multidisciplinarity, and a certain number of patients who, up to
then, belong to a monopathological status,   now turn out to a
polypathological status. Medical records, therefore, must fulfill
both synthesis and communication necessities [17][19].
   General computer based clinical data processings have
already been created [5][8][9][10], or analysed [1][6][12][13]
[22]. However, their preferential aim was to pick up patient
groups on a common set of data. Therefore, they respond better to
administrators [15] and medical committee [16] designs than to
communication within the hospital staff.
   A survey on information systems has been carried out to
reveal user's attitude to computer based medical record system.
The questionary was sent to 1,300 physicians and 1,000 responses
(data not published) have been collected. One of the conclusions
is that the first need is dealt with quality and disponibility of
medical records. 99 % of the praticians believe in the necessity
of a communicaiton network. This confirms the analysis of Young
[21] and Cerutti [1].
   A medical record may be considered to be made up of two
parts of different interest. The first of them arises from the
compiling of clinical examination and laboratory results carried

out when the patient was in. This part represents most of the writings, but they are only a writing-pad and of immediate interest. On the opposite, the second part consists in the lot of type-writings (discharge letters, condensed reports,...). A first attitude consists in reading only this part in a yet treated patient record [7], for it contains its main important elements [9].

So as to show first that this second part of the clinical record, typed-writted by the secretary, was the key to a general care computer based system and to any communication between praticians teams, an integrated bureautic experiment has been carried out in a medical department. The second aim was to show that a minimum record based upon the type-writings and opened to medical practice 24 hours a day was worth of interest.

MATERIAL AND METHOD

The experimental site is the Respiratory Diseases Department. It includes 5 clinical units (two casual hospitalizations, an out-patient unit, a daily hospitalization and a clinical allergology unit) to which are connected 3 exploratory units (respiratory function test, bronchial motricity, bronchialendoscopy). The medical team consists in 6 full-time physicians, 4 part-time physicians and 4 residents.

For the experiment, the 4 secretarial offices have been equiped with bureautic microcomputers. These autonomous machines have been linked to the hospital network already equiped with an IBM 3083 computer working in a CICS environment. The kind of connection desired was an interactive emulation BSC 3270 or SNA SDLC. The choice was made on the CORAIL B4000 (BULL company), for its connecting abilities. The operating system, CTOS, enables to consider the emulation primitive programs as functions to be called by any of the applications. Moreover, with a core memory of 256 KO, a Winchester 5 MO fixed disk and a Diablo printer, this machine is not to be challenged by any similar equipment.

Programs using the very own connection functionnalities of this machine have been implemented and enable a chronological recording of the medical texts in a both administrative and medical database already implemented in a DL1 environment in the central computer. The access to that database allows not to be obliged to seaze again a great number of data (identity for instance) and to secure the mailing of the medical data.

A typology of the writings has been created after a study of the records and has revealed the essential role of the discharge letter in the communication needs as a faithful summary of the patient stay.

The experiment held in two times. The first one lasted one month and dealt with the setting of microcomputers in a self governing manner only. It has shown the necessity of a period of probation for both medical and secretarial teams. The second time begun with the connection of the computers and involved a complementary management for fully mastering the problems and methods of communication.

A cost-advantage study was to be carried out to evaluate the system. It would consist in examination of frequence and facility of the access to records, the gain in secretarial productivity, the improvements on the compounds of medical texts and on the communication.

RESULTS

After a constant working during one year and a half 9,600 texts have been created, corresponding to 5,200 patients. They average to 2,210 characters (+/- 660). The number of characters of each letter is not significantly different before and after the experiment. The typology used gives us the following results :

	DL	OL	LR	DH	EX	BRON
CONSULTANTS	32	4,922	640	/	16	23
HOSPITALIZED	2,782	66	116	881	8	114

DL = discharge letter   DH = daily hosp. discharge letter
OL = out-patient letter   EX = expertise report
LR = lab. examination report   BRON = bronchialendoscopy report
                                         (since Dec 1984)

A two times ergonomic study (before the experiment and after six months) has shown that the secretarial type-writing activity which represented 30% of its work, has decreased, relatively, of 30%. This point seems due to the introduction of bureautics. At the same time, the filling and managing of the paper recordings, 40% of the secretarial work, has decreased of 30%, this saving being due to a systematic access to the magnetic record instead of the paper record. The amont of the savings has allowed to cope with the rising of the daily hospitalizations (plus 300% in three years) and that of the out-patient consultations, all this with the same number of secretaries.

If two full-time praticians have invested about 10% of their time during the first year of the experiment, a Delphi analysis has shown that the average relative gain is about 10% of the total medical charge of the department.

On the two points of text compounds improvement and communication, an acurate study has not been led until now and must be part of a research program. However, the overall feeling of the users is a real gain on those points. For instance, it takes now 20 minutes to prepare a consultation instead of 90 before. By an access to the information out of any station of the network, the physician, called outside his department, can be informed about data of the patient he has been called for.

DISCUSSION

Even if the evaluation of the system is still a little bit inconsistent and has to precise all medical and secretarial advantages, this experiment shows the real interest of the magnetic housing and restitution of the whole medical text during daily and emergency practice [21]. This point is not opposite to the experiments based upon standardized records which have their major place in patient specialized follow-up [3].

It is true that, if communication needs are fulfilled, with the options on the worknet now in place, it is not the same as for as the documentary function and its outlets (epidemiology, DRG's...)[15][17][19]. But an index module, close to that foreseen by Gleser [6] or Cerutti [1], is about to be written in the database. The gain, already aquired on the quality of the elements of medical texts, should lead to a similar gain on the accuracy of the indexation of patient hospitalization and, therefore, on the coming studies (documentation, activity analysis).

At last, introducing bureautic procedures in daily medical life, this system answers questions already solved in an industrial environnement [14]. It also resolves some of the reasons set by Young about the non-acceptability of computer systems by clinicians [18][20][21] (computer systems inflexibility, medical time-consuming use of these systems, patient care not significantly improved by the use of them...). As Reichertz notices [17], this kind of solution, based upon both micro-computers and central ones, connected in an adapted network, allows a better information disponibility and larger possibilities than independant approaches. In a period of inflation and technical evolutions [11], such an approach can be considered as one of the elements of medical problem solving, as far as the information cost represents 30% of the total hospital cost and as the number of physicians concerned with the health of one patient is increasing.

BIBLIOGRAPHY

[1] Cerutti S,Longhini E, Pinciroli F. A computer-oriented
approach to the comprehensive organisation of information in
hand-compiled medical records. Meth.Inform.Med 18(1979) 138-145
[2] Degoulet P, Hu HA, Chatelier G, Devries C, Plouin PF,Menard J
Hypertension management: the role of computer in improving
patient compliance. Med.Inform. 7(1982) 49-55
[3] Degoulet P, Chantalou JP,Chatelier G, Devries C, Goupy F,
Zweigenbaum P. Structured and standardized medical records.
MEDINFO (1983) 1164-1168
[4] Fabre A, Bouhanna A. Un systeme d'archivage de dossier
medical en pediatrie. AWAMI (1982) 283
[5] Frutiger P. Analyse de la demache medicale à l'occasion de la
redaction des comptes rendus d'observations cliniques:
proposition d'un langage clair exploitable par ordinateur. (These
bio. humaine PARIS 1983)
[6] Gleser M. The medical event vector. Meth.Inform.Med 18(1979)
127-131
[7] Gleser M,Young G, Woods D. A database built upon the medical
event vector. Meth.Inform.Med. 18(1979) 131-137
[8] Heaulme M, Mery C. Remede: an artificial language for medical
reports on computer. MEDINFO (1974) 935-941
[9] Heaulme M, Anderson J. Exploitation of medical records.
Med.Inform. 3(1978) 333-334
[10] Hernicot P, Deyres C, Dequatre A. Le systeme Dostam.
Gestions hospitalieres (1976) 417-426
[11] Jenkin MA. Clinical informatics: a strategy for the use of
information in the clinical setting. Med.Inform. 9(1984) 225-232
[12] Koens ML, De Vroome H, Op Het Veld W. The checking and
registration of radiotherapy treatments. AWAMI (1981) 271-276
[13] Krone RJ, Igielnik S, Miller JP. A computerized report
generating/data management system for a cardiology division.
AWAMI (1982) 277-282
[14] Nauges L. Cinq ans pour reussir la bureautique dans les
entreprises. Datafrance (1983) 21-26
[15] Omenn GS, Conrad DA. Implications of DRGs for clinicians.
N.Engl.J.Med. 311(1984) 1314-1317
[16] Price HC. The medical record. The key to the computerized
hospital information system. AWAMI (1982) 355-360
[17] Reichertz PL. The challenge of medical informatics:
delusions or newperspectives? Med.Inform. 7(1982) 57-66
[18] Shortliffe EH. The computer as a consultant. Arch.Int.Med.
140(1980) 313-314
[19] Van Bemmel JH. The structure of medical informatics.
Med.Inform. 9(1984) 175-180
[20] Young DW. A problem-orientated information system.
Med.Inform 3(1978) 105-111
[21] Young DW. Doctor's attitude to a computer-based clinical
information system. Meth.Inform.Med 20(1981) 196-199
[22] Yamamoto K, Ogura H, Furutani H, Kitazoe Y, Takeda Y. System
design of summary records compiled by clinicians in hospital
information system. Med.Inform. 9(1984) 103-109

COMPUTER-AIDED PRESCRIPTION FOR GENERAL PRACTITIONERS USING A HAND-HELD COMPUTER

B. Auvert *, Ph. Aegerter *,B. Diquet **, E. Benillouche *,
Ph. Boutin *, J-L. Monier *, Ph. Gerard * and P. Le Beux ***.

* INSERM U 88   91 Bd de l'Hôpital 75013 PARIS
** Department of Pharmacology   91 Bd de l'Hôpital 75013 PARIS
*** University of Technology of Compiègne

Until now, personal computer software designed for general
practitioners has allowed only file management, word processing or
drug interaction advice. But no information system permits the user
to get other relevant information on drugs or to determine a
therapeutic strategy.

We have designed an integrated, autonomous and portable system
for prescription aid. This system called PHARMAID includes a powerful
hand-held computer designed for such bio-medical applications and
specifically written programs. This software has been written in
PASCAL and includes a therapeutic knowledge data base which is easy
to use.

Then, we discuss the future of such hand-held systems in
medicine. We show that it is probable that these systems will have a
very wide usage in the next ten years, and that they are
complementary with telematic information networks.

KEYWORDS: Computer-aided decision-making, drug information, hand-
held computer, knowledge base.

1- INTRODUCTION

The general problem of information in medicine is crucial,
especially for the general practitioner and the specialist out of his
own field. This problem is connected with the very large amount of
medical information which doubles every ten years. It is quite
difficult for a physician to have simple and practical access to
specific and relevant information about a specific medical problem at
a specific moment (papers, reviews and books do not solve this
problem). Such information will allow the practitioner to have in
mind all the basic elements (and only those) necessary in making the

best decision.

Our particular problem is the choice of which treatment the practitioner should prescribe. The concern is mostly with the patients. Errors in this field are quite frequent and expensive for the patient and for society; therefore, the physician needs an information system which allows him or her: 1- the choose the most appropriate treatment for the patient. Criteria should take into account for example: the patient physiological condition and diseases; the drug protocols with possible interactions or contra-indications; the ease of administration. 2- access at any time the pharmacological data about a given drug. 3- use the system in different circumstances including home visits or consultations in a very quick and easy way.

In this paper, we present PHARMAID which is the hand-held computer with specific software we designed to solve these problems.

2- SOFTWARE

The software is composed of the operating system, the language and the application programs. We have chosen P-System for the operating system. The system is based on PASCAL. Which is a powerful language which allows structured programming so one can write modular programs which are easy to maintain and to extend. It is available on almost all microcomputers, thus guaranteeing the compatibility of the application software. This also allows us to develop the software on desktop computers. The application software is composed of four parts:

1. The therapeutic knowledge base: This base is composed of the characteristics of the 500 main molecules used in human therapeutics. These characteristics are the following: name, composition, pharmacological class and action, indications, contra-indications, side-effects, interactions, pharmacokinetics, toxicity, recommendations for use, forms, posologies and treatments. This information, except posology and treatment, is recorded drug by drug in order to compile dictionaries. Posology includes, notably, duration of administration, minimum and maximum doses and when to administer. A treatment chapter includes an indication code number, the patient's characteristics (new-born, renal failure, ..), a code for the form and for the posology and messages to the physician. Thus, a drug record contains only references to the previous

dictionaries. This structuring saves room in memory; each drug occupies 100 bytes. Furthermore, all the files are packed. The user can access directly the whole record of a drug through several functionkeys: brand name, composition and pharmacological class. The remaining data is then available through frame selections.

2. Selection of treatment: The selection of the treatment is made by moving in a graph formed by successive frames. These frames allow the user to select more and more narrow fields in medicine, for instance: cardiology, then coronary disease, then angina pectoris and so on. Finally, all the drugs corresponding to the patient's disease are displayed. In this last selection, one can choose a particular drug according to one or more of the following items: drug which can be given by mouth with a low frequency per day; drug with the least number of side effects; drug with no interactions with previously selected drugs; drug which can be given to a pregnant woman, child or patient with renal failure.

3. The user-machine interface: The software uses frame selection because it appears to be easier and faster to use by untrained people (1). The one exception is when one must introduce a string variable. This happens only when searching characteristics of a given drug. The user types the first three letters of the drug's name. The system proposes a list of drugs beginning with these letters. Then the user selects the desired drug in this list. A "MESSAGE" function key allows the user, at certain steps in the program, to be informed of the medical background of choices. These explanatory messages are not mandatory, so a trained user can get the information very fast.

4. The "prescription" function The "prescription" function enables the system to store a selected list of drugs. One can check in the list for pharmacological interactions or drugs with similar effects. The user can print the prescription, including brand name, posology and advice for the patient.

3- THE HARDWARE ARCHITECTURE

Such a system must be available not only at a doctor's office but also for home visits. Commercially available hand-held computers, however, were not sufficient to support this software. Indeed they do not have a convenient memory size and their operating system cannot

manage data base in ROM using a high level language. Therefore we
developed our own model of a powerful hand-held computer for such biomedical applications (4).

Our system is 21x29x3 cm large and weighs 1.8 kg. It is sturdy
and dustproof. The system runs on rechargeable Cd-Ni accumulators. It
includes an 8x40 liquid crystal display, a full alphanumeric keyboard
plus a set of function keys for ergonomic purposes: START, CONTINUE,
MESSAGE. On one side are three connectors: one is a standard RS232C
serial interface; the second is a regular phone plug; and the third
allows the user to recharge the batteries.

To get a low power consumption and increase the autonomy, we
have chosen the CMOS technology. The processor is a NSC 800 which is
software compatible with the Z 80. The RAM capacity is 64 K bytes.
ROM used are 16 K byte NMOS EPROM. They are disconnected once a
program segment has been loaded into the RAM memory. The ROM is
considered by the software as mass storage for files and program
which are stored in two ROM pseudo-disks of 272 and 256 K bytes. The
integrated modem allows fast and easy connection to central data
bases. The autonomy of our system is about 20 hours in constant use
and four weeks in stand-by.

4- HARDWARE-SOFTWARE COMPATIBILITY

Software was developed on a micro-computer running P-System
(Victor S1) and then transferred to the ROM of the HHC by means of an
EPROM programming system. During use, only index files and needed
segments are loaded into RAM. Due to structuring, the software does
not need to scan through the whole file. So the response time is
independent of the number of drugs and treatments. It is usually
about one or two seconds; this makes the system acceptable to and
convenient for the user. In addition, the software (programs and
data) can be updated by changing the ROM packages where they are
stored. The portable system is compatible with central
pharmacological data bases such as BIAM (3): the integrated modem
allows access to the central base, but this will be necessary only if
the portable base is insufficient.

5- CONCLUSION

A prototype of PHARMAID is already operational and is currently
being tested among GPs. The drug data base has been limited to the

500 most used drugs in general practice. A second phase of this project includes enlargement of the base to 2000 drugs and adaptation of an expert system to treatment selection.

We have surveyed a sample population of about 2000 French physicians to determine their impressions of portable information systems in medicine. This study showed great interest in such systems especially if they are easy to use, autonomous, powerful and, of course, not expensive.

The constant decrease in the cost and size of electronic components (decrease by a factor of ten is usually expected in the next ten years), and the progress in structuring and management of knowledge will probably ensure an increase in the number of users of intelligent portable information systems. Medicine appears to have numerous and various application fields: decision making, pharmacological or therapeutic knowledge bases, and analogical signal analysis. Consequently, the physician could save time and make better decisions. The expected benefits are an increase in efficiency and a decrease in unnecessary or harmful prescriptions.

(1) B. AUVERT, E. CHARPENTIER, B. DIQUET and al. THERAP-HELP: A hand-held computer using a therapeutic knowledge-base. MEDINFO 83 (Abstract), North-Holland.

(2) M. FIESCHI Intelligence artificielle en medecine. MASSON editor 1984.

(3) M. GOLBERG, C. SANTINI, B. LOYON and al. A drug data bank: specific problem in connection with the nature of information and operation methodology. MEDINFO 1974, North-Holland, pp 869-874.

(4) H. TAVERNIER, B. AUVERT and P. LE BEUX. BLAISE: A portable C-Mos Bio-Terminal Programmable in Pascal. The Best of Computer Fairs, Vol VII, 1982, p 250,253

HAND HELD COMPUTERS IN MEDICINE

B. Auvert, Ph. Boutin, Ph. Aegerter, P. LeBeux (*), Ph. Gerard,
E. Benillouche, Le Thi Huong Du, R. Allouche and JL. Monier

INSERM U 88, 91 Bd de l'Hôpital 75013 PARIS
* University of Technology of Compiègne

INTRODUCTION

Mainly because of technological progress and the reduction in
cost, computers are available to many people: in hospitals and in
general practitioners' offices; to nurses and even to patients.

Mainframe and mini computers are mainly used for management, for
handling large statistical or epidemiological studies and for patient
data recording in hospitals, while micro-computers are specially
designed for personal utilization, including file management, small
statistical study calculations and control of analogical devices.

A new type of computer is gaining in use. Portable computers
or hand-held computers (HHCs) are of the same size as a calculator
yet have the power of a micro-computer. Taking into account the
development of artificial intelligence, one is led to ask what is
(and will be) the use of such portable computers in the medical field.

HARDWARE

The main feature of the hardware of portable computers is
the necessity of using C-MOS technology, allowing these
computers to be operated on rechargeable batteries. Most of the
CPUs of 8, 16 or 32 bits have or will have a CMOS version. CMOS
static RAM has a maximum capacity of 8 K bytes allowing about
256 K bytes on a circuit board 16x20 cm. Many types of mass
storage are used. Some HHCs use ROM. These memories are
available in CMOS version but their capacities are small (8 K
bytes) compared to the capacity of NMOS version (64 K bytes). It
is possible to use NMOS ROM in HHC, but these memories have to
be disconnected between readings (1). Using these ROM, one can
make a 1 Mega byte memory circuit board on a surface 16x20 cm.
HHCs tend now to use the new 3.5 inch mini-floppy disk of high
memory capacity (about 400 K bytes). Bubble memories allow
storage about 200 K bytes in a small volume. The screen
currently used is a 8x40 character liquid crystal display. A
25x80 character LCD is already available. Generally, HHCs have a

standard RS232C and some have an integrated modem for connection
to the regular telephone network.

SOFTWARE

Available operating systems on HHCs are mostly CPM, MS-DOS and P-
System. At the present time none runs Unix. Programming languages
are Basic, Forth, C and Pascal. General application software has been
implemented on HHCs for word processing, statistics, data management,
accounting and spreadsheets. But general application medical software
is still under development, certainly because of the large size of
these programs, which have to be easy to use but also have to
contribute to improving the health worker's effectiveness or allow
him or her to spend less time in routine work. Potential medical
applications of HHCs are mainly: 1) decision-making for health
workers and for patients; 2) collection of medical data; 3)
intelligent analogical instruments.

1.1 DECISION-MAKING IN HOSPITALS

Recently (2) a hand-held programmable calculator has been used
by emergency-room physicians to identify potential heart attack
victims. In hospitals, computers can be used to manage patient data.
Intensive care units where the amount of data is rather great, a
computer terminal has been placed at each bed. Soon a HHC will
probably replace this terminal. Each HHC will manage each patient's
data independently but will be connected to the hospital network in
order to transfer data from other departments. It will be able to
monitor physiological parameters by means of captors. It will also
keep in memory the physician's prescription and help the nurses to
follow it.

1.2 DECISION-MAKING FOR GENERAL PRACTITIONERS

One of the main medical decisions of a physician is the
prescription. A team has already written a drug prescription-aid
software (PHARMAID) for HHCs (3) which includes 1) a drug data base
on about 300 drugs; 2) a module to help to choose the 'best'
treatment taking into account the patient's profile; 3) a module to
analyze the correctness of a prescription and to print the
prescription. With increased storage capacity, such a tool will
contain all the main information needed to make a good prescription;
then it will become widely used, leading to a decrease in the number
of prescription errors.

1.3 DECISION-MAKING FOR PATIENTS

HHCs are autonomous computers and can also be an element of a
complex medical information network. An example is the recently
developed HHC (named DIABAID) which is specifically dedicated to
diabetes mellitus therapy (4). It has been designed to be used by the
patient to correctly dose them daily insulin therapy using an
automatic glycemia analyzer. It also stores data for later monitoring
by the physician and from the physician and then to a larger data
base devoted to epidemiological research.

1.4 DECISION-MAKING IN DEVELOPING COUNTRIES

At the request of an international medical organization
(Médecins sans Frontières), a hand-held system (TROPICAID) usable by
rural health workers for medical decision making has been developed
(5). The software is easy to use allowing access to an internal data
base on 60 drugs. A decision making module analyzes the patient's
parameters and indicates possible diagnosis and relevant treatments.
The system knows 240 diagnoses. In addition, individual medical data
can be collected for elementary statistical analysis. This computer,
sturdy and compact, runs on battery power rechargeable by a solar
panel.

2 COLLECTION OF MEDICAL DATA

In epidemiology, the collection of disease patterns must be
provided by medical practitioners. Classic systems with record sheets
are time consuming and allow all kinds of biases. HHCs, when running
a special purpose program, can check diagnoses to limit biases due to
inter-person variation; can collect data without time lapse or errors
due to manual transfer to a record sheet and data from different
areas can be directly transferred to a central unit. The benefit of
such a system is quite obvious for developing countries where the
main problem of data collecting is the lack of validation and
comparability of records, and the absence of reliability of medical
figures (6).

3 INTELLIGENT ANALOGICAL INSTRUMENTS

The pacemaker was one of the first medical instruments to use a
micro-processor. New types can be programmed using a computer
connected to electrodes on the patient's chest, so the medical team
can adapt the program of the implanted pacemaker to the cardiac
status of the patient and data memorized by the pacemaker can be

transferred to the external computer for analysis. Computer analysis of electrocardiograms is a very advanced project, but largely accepted by GPs and cardiologists (7), although the price is still high. Today, one can transfer the complex evaluation of ECGs programs into HHCs which are powerful enough and available for a reasonable price, thus improving: 1) quality of data; 2) arythmia detection and analysis; 3) diagnostic strategy; 4) comparison of serial ECGs. For such analyses, one might use an HHC containing an appropriate analogical interface and printer. Artificial intelligence modules might be necessary for the data interpretation.

CONCLUSION

Because of both the small size of HHCs and their large capacities, a large amount of medical knowledge can be easily available. For each patient, a physician has to make the "best" medical decision and because of the complexity of the parameters to be taken into account, a computer can be of help in medical decision-making.

A new concept in medical information science, Intelligent Medical Books (IMB), is now appearing. IMBs will have a structured knowledge base and their software will be adapted to the users' problems. IMBs will largely use artificial intelligence techniques; a general expert system for medical applications which runs on a HHC has already been developed (8). IMBs will be used in decision-making, but also in training and reinforcement. These two possibilities (decision-making and training) will probably increase their use in developing countries as well, especially with a decrease in the cost of HHCs.

HHC are already beginning to be used extensively in the medical field by doctors, nurses and patients in both developed and developing countries. In the near future, HHCs will be thoroughly into the medical information system network. Because of the possibility of using such a powerful information system, some aspects of medical education will be changed. It will become more important to manage medical information than to keep all this information in mind. Despite all the advantages and contributions of HHCs, however, they will never replace the actions which have traditionally characterized the practice of medicine: human contact with the patient, appraisal of signs and assumption of responsability for medical decisions.

(1) H. TAVERNIER, B. AUVERT & P. LEBEUX
    BLAISE: A portable C-MOS Bio-Terminal Programmable in Pascal.
    The Best of computer Fairs, Vol VII, 1982, p 250-253

(2) M.W.POZEN, R.B.D'AGOSTINO, H.P.SELKER, P.A.SYTKOWSKI,
    W.B.HOOD.
    A predictive instrument to improve coronary-care-unit admission
    practice in acute ischemic heart disease: A prospective
    multicenter clinical trial.
    The New England Journal of medicine. 1984,310,1273-1278.

(3) B.AUVERT, B.DIQUET, Ph.GERARD, Ph.AEGERTER, E.BENILLOUCHE,
    Ph.BOUTIN, J.L.MONIER, P.LE BEUX.
    Computer aided prescrition for general practionners using a
    hand-held computer.
    Micro-computer applications in medicine and bio-engineering.
    Oct 22-24 1984. New-York.

(4) R.A.ALLOUCHE, A.AURENGO, B.AUVERT et al.
    A specific portable micro-computer dedicated to diabetes
    mellitus therapy.
    MEDINFO 83, North-Holland. pp 804-807.

(5) B.AUVERT, Ph.BOUTIN, Ph.,D.GERARD, LE THI HUONG DU, Ph.AEGERTER,
    J.L.MONIER, F.VAN LOOK, J.M.DARIOSECQ, B.HAP, X.EMMANUELLI.
    A hand-held computer usable by rural health workers for medical
    decision making.
    Micro-computer applications in medicine and bio-engineering.
    Oct 22-24 1984. New-York.

(6) Notification of medical information by non-medical personal.
    WHO publications. 1978.

(7) J.L.TALMON.
    Pattern recognition of the ECG. A structured analysis.
    Vrije universiteit te amsterdam. 1983.

(8) D.FONTAINE, J.F. BOSSEAU, P.LEBEUX, B.AUVERT, Ph AEGERTER,
    Ph.CAZENEUVE, H.MAURY, J.Ch.TALABAR,M. CAILLAT.
    SUPER: An expert system for medical applications.
    Micro-computer applications in medicine and bio-engineering.
    Oct 22-24 1984. New-York.

A PATIENT DIRECTED INFORMATION AND MANAGEMENT SYSTEM FOR NEUROLOGISTS

Arends J.B.A.M.(1), Puts C.M.(2), Smits M.G.(2) and Vos A.J.M.(2)

1) Department of Neurology, Catholic University of Nijmegen, Reinier Postlaan 4, 6525 GC Nijmegen, The Netherlands.

2) Department of Neurology, Juliana Hospital Ede, Stationsweg 86, 6711 PV Ede, The Netherlands.

SUMMARY

A program that contains actual information on the status of neurological patients is described. It includes a medical diagnosis system and automatic printing of the invoices. Additionally the program generates information for the consulting hours, and reminders for control measurements. Instant surveys, both medical and financial, help in managing the practice.

1. INTRODUCTION

Running a practice highly burdens the medical practitioner. Computer programs can facilitate data management for diagnostic, therapeutic and financial purposes. General medical packages most often do not combine these aspects. We developed a program for neurologists that facilitates medical accuracy, improves management of the out- and inpatient clinic, and automatically composes the invoices. It can be run on any CP/M microcomputer with 64 kB internal memory and one hard disk.

2. DESIGN

The program was based on an a system analysis by neurologists and written by a professional programmer. The total investment for hardware, software and first year programming support amounted $ 12.000. Since a professional programmer should maintain the program, a yearly additional cost of $ 2.000 was scheduled.

Since a good data structure is essential for optimal performance (Wirth, 1984) and a changing environment asks for versatility of the data, we used the DBASE II package, a registered trademark of ASHTON-TATE, which allows changes in data structures, without the need of profound alteration of program structure. Passwords limit unauthorized use of the data.

Each record (one for every diagnosis in a patient) includes the identification, the dates of first and last visit or admission, referring person and diagnosis at referral, recent investigations, and a final diagnosis (ICD-9-CM). The list of diagnoses forms a separate file. Other databases include the names and adresses of referring practitioners, insurance companies. These files can easily be modified by the secretary. All current investigations are coded twofold. The first code determines, whether or not a certain investigation is carried out, if the results are present, and which result is found. This enables us to give messages at subsequent visits. All messages, such as ' the patient has had an EEG and the results are known' are given only once. The second code is manually given for the invoice constructing program. When the visit or investigation has been invoiced, this is registrated in an 'invisible' part of the record. The invoices are generated automatically by a series of procedures that scan all available records, extract the data and store them into a separate database. Additional modules enable the operator to make changes in each invoice proposal and independently edit and print the bills. These procedures save much time and money.

The diagnosis is classified (ICD-9-CM) both at the time of referral and at the end of the investigations. Since each diagnosis belongs to one major class, like cerebrovascular diseases, two positions were added to the four number code of the ICD-9-CM. This enables the practitioner to use each major or minor class for the diagnostic follow-up or therapy control, to be carried out by the assistant during a visit. We, for example, advice the recording of the blood pressure for each patient with cerebrovascular disease, or testing the motor abilities of a patient with Parkinson's disease. In this way the program manages the medical part of the daily out-patient consulting hours. Furthermore all types of surveys can be generated, for example to create a population for studying drug effects.

Of course, rigorous procedures are necessary to ensure a correct data input. Along with the development of the programs, we instructed all assistants working in the practice, and designed two main logbooks for data input. The first included patient identification and current investigations, the second all medical data to be filled in by the practioner. The secretary was asked to care for proper collection of the data at the end of each week. Even with this simple system, correct data input required continuous attention from the neurologists.

3. DISCUSSION

The continuous attention of the neurologists for proper data input improved their diagnostic accuracy and only temporary increased their workload. Saving money and time is often the reason of existence of programs like these. The medical applications, however, are

the most interesting features and are combined with automatic generation of invoices. The current data structure enables us to find
recent information on the patients, to select diagnoses and screening measurements. Furthermore the connection with a word processor
enables the development of standard letters.

One should also be aware of the limitations of this type of
patient records. A most important restriction is formed by the fact,
that this data structure only contains the most recent data about
the patient's diagnosis. Longitudinal historical data acquisition
requires data structures that are not equal for different diseases
and must be very carefully constructed. Now we are planning such
longitudinal disease records.

A second problem is the communication of individual data banks
from practitioners with general hospital information systems. One
should consult the person in charge of the hospital records before
building one's own system.

REFERENCE

Wirth N., Data structures and algorithms, Scientific American 251-3,
48-57, 1984.

EVALUATING THE SCHIZOPHRENIA PROJECT

A. Hakkarainen
The National Board of Health
Siltasaarenkatu 18 A, 00530 Helsinki, Finland

2. INTRODUCTION

Before the change of the Mental Health Act in 1978 the population of long-stay (L-S) mental hospital patients had been in a stationary state. The size of the population, the influx of new L-S patients and the flow of those separated (discharges and deaths) from the L-S population had been constant since the stabilization of the number of hospital beds in 1963 (abt 18 000 or 4 per 1 000). The size of the L-S population of schizophrenic patients was abt 7 500 persons and expected length of stay of a new L-S patient was 8 years in 1978 (1).

Immediately after the change of the Act which put the emphasis on voluntary treatment and the development of outpatient services the equilibrium of the L-S patient population was disturbed. In 1979 the flow of new schizophrenic L-S patients sank from 800 patients/year to over 600/year and the whole patient population started to decrease.

The national plan to develop the diagnosis, treatment and rehabilitation of schizophrenic patients, in other words the Schizophrenia Project was started in 1981. In the next 10 years it will have two main targets: First, to decrease the number of new schizophrenic L-S patients from the former level of 800 to 400 patients/year and secondly, to rehabilitate every year 400 schizophrenic L-S patients out of the hospital into ambulatory care. When the Project was started the rapid decrease of the L-S patients had begun to slow up.

2. METHODS

The "new" L-S patient is defined as a patient whose hospital age (HA) or the time after admission on a certain census day varies from 365 to 729 days when the day of admission is excluded. The average HA is 1.5 years. Since all the mental hospitals have a yearly census on Dec. 31 the group of patients present at their second census is defined as the cohort of new L-S patients, which is abt 5 per cent of all admissions. In operational terms the first target of the Project means that the cohort of schizophrenic patients at their second census should be decreased into 400/year.

Other researchers have also defined the status of the new L-S patient on the basis of census data (2,3). The method of measurements is not exact but it is practical and has been proved to work. The whole patient population can be cut in two: the short-stay and the long-stay patient population. In Finland these populations have developed in quite different ways (4).

The population of L-S patients includes all patients whose HA is at least one year. It thus includes the cohort of new L-S patients (1 year $\leq$ HA < 2 years). The purpose of the Project is to rehabilitate 400 "old" L-S patients out of the hospital. This group is called the patient population whose HA is at least 2 years (PP whose HA $\geq$ 2 years).

The cohorts of new L-S patients in the 21 Mental Health Districts were measured in 1980- 1982. The yearly random variation of these cohorts is largely due to their small size. Therefore three-year averages are used in regional comparisons. The incidence of long-term hospitalization is computed by dividing the cohorts by the number of inhabitants. The regional incidence figures are indirectly standardized by sex and age so that they can be compared to the national index which has the value 100. The yearly prevalence of PP whose HA $\geq$ 2 years is also computed for each District in 1980 and 1982.

In order to evaluate how a certain District has managed to control the flow of new L-S patients one has to compare its development to the target. In 1980 and before the start of the Project, the national cohort was 649 new L-S patients while the target is 400, i.e. 38 % lower. If the District can diminish its cohort by 38 % it has achieved the set target.

The rehabilitation programme will increase the number of separations from the patient population and the separation rates at different HA:s (separations/patient population). It will also change the hazard function (q_x) of the hospital population life table. q_x is the probability of a patient to be separated in the next year after having achieved a certain hospital age x. In the era of stability before 1978, these indicators did not change but they have changed thereafter.

The success of the Project cannot be evaluated without knowledge of the "normal" and the "successful" development of the patient population which means the achievement of the Project targets. The available information is not quite sufficient for this evaluation. The q_x-function should be known at the start of the Project as well as the change of the function at different HA:s if 400 extra patients were separated each year. The Project has not given any statement whether the rehabilitation programme is aimed at a patient cohort of a certain HA of e.g. 2 or 20 years or at all cohorts beyond the HA-limit of 2 years.

Table 1 is based on the approximate separation rates from 1977 (5) and the projective life table of 1978 (1). Projection A shows how the schizophrenic L-S population would have developed in the whole country in 1980-1982 if the Project had already been active then. Projection B follows the normal course of development.

The separation rates of 1977 have been applied on the row I. They were .0877 for patients whose HA $\geq$ 2 years and .0850 at the HA $\geq$ 3 years. The values of q_x applied to the cohorts on the rows II and III are as follows: $q_{1.5}$= .27 and $q_{2.5}$= .25. In this calculation it has been assumed that the rehabilitation programme has been aimed only at the patients admitted before 1979.

3. EVALUATION

Table 2 compares the observations in 1982 to the projections. According to projection A the PP whose HA $\geq$ 2 years is 18 % smaller than in 1980. The observed number is 8 % and projection B 3 % smaller than in 1980. The new cohort of L-S patients is 4 % smaller than in 1980. Projection A would have meant a decrease of 38 % and projection B zero decrease.

One District has managed to surpass the Project target (18 %) in diminishing its PP whose HA $\geq$ 2 years. Five Districts have better results than the whole country (8 %).

The District indices representing the standardized incidence of long-term hospitalization vary widely. The lowest one is 39 and the highest 171 (the whole country = 100). The random yearly variation of cohorts hides the 3-year trends. However, in some Districts the downward trend is so clear that it cannot be missed. It is often associated with a small L-S patient population but not necessarily. A big population with long average length of stay has a weak flow of patients to and from the population.

The studies on the incidence and the prevalence of schizophrenia show that the incidence does not vary regionally very widely whereas the prevalence does (6, 7). High prevalence of the disease seems to be attached to high incidence of long-term hospitalization.

The evaluation system could be improved by using life table methodology. A life table should be made for the year 1981 as well as for the end of the Project period. They would indicate how the Project will change the hazard function and the expected length of stay in the Districts.

REFERENCES

(1) Hakkarainen A. Psykiatrinen laitosväestö Suomessa 1960- ja 1970-luvuilla (The Finnish mental hospital population in the 1960s and 1970s), licentiate study in sociology, The University of Helsinki, 1983.
(2) Eason RJ, Grimes JA. In-patient care of the mentaly ill: a statistical study of future provision. Health Trends, 1977;8:13-18.
(3) Weeke A, Kastrup M, Dupont A. Long-stay patients in Danish psychiatric hospitals. Psychol. Medicine, 1979;9:551-556.
(4) Hakkarainen A. Demographic models and the Finnish mental hospital population. In: Proceedings 1982 of the International Conference on Medical Computing. Dublin: Medical Informatics Europe 82, Berlin-Heidelberg, Springer-Verlag, 1982;16:625-631.
(5) Hakkarainen A. Pitkäaikaissairaat psykiatrisissa sairaaloissa. Havaintoja ja ennusteita (Long-stay patients in psychiatric hospitals) Health Services Research by the National Board of Health in Finland No 21. Helsinki 1980.
(6) Räkköläinen V. USP-projekti, Väliraportti. The Schizophrenia Project. Manuscript 1984.
(7) Lehtinen V. Unpublished data April 22, 1983. Subproject of Mini-Finland interview survey of the Social Insurance Institution.

Table 1. The observed No of schizophrenic L-S patients present on Dec.
31, 1980 and two projections: A) according to the Schizophrenia
Project B) according to the old policy

Year of admission	Schizophrenic L-S patients (HA $\geq$ 1 year) present at census		
	Observed Dec. 31, 1980	Projected Dec. 31, 1981	Projected Dec. 31, 1982
I Admitted before 1979	6 188	A) 5 645 [1] B) 5 645	A) 4 799 [1] B) 5 165
II Admitted in 1979	649	A) 474 B) 474	A) 356 B) 356
III Admitted in 1980, plans		A) 400 B) 649	A) 292 B) 474
IV Admitted in 1981, plans			A) 400 B) 649
V Total L-S	6 837	A) 6519 B) 6 768	A) 5 847 B) 6 644
VI Rehabilitation plans	–	A) –400 [1] B) –	A) –400 [1] B) –
VII Total L-S	6 837	A) 6 119 B) 6 768	A) 5 447 B) 6 644

1) All patients to be rehabilitated (400)
belong to the cohorts admitted before 1979

Table 2. The observed No of schizophrenic L-S patients present on
Dec. 31, 1980, the projections A) and B) and the observed
values in 1982

HA group	Observed Dec. 31, 1980	Projected[1] for Dec. 31, 1982	Decrease from 1980	Observed Dec. 31, 1982	Decrease from 1980
PP whose HA $\geq$ 2 years	6 188	A) 5 047 B) 5 995	18 % 3 %	5 690	8 %
New L-S patients whose HA $\geq$ 1 year, but < 2 years	649	A) 400 B) 649	38 % –	623	4 %
Total L-S	6 837	A) 5 447 B) 6 644	20 % 3 %	6 313	8 %

1) e.g. 5 047 = 4 799 + 356 + 292 – 400

TOWARDS A MATHEMATICAL MODEL OF NEUROLOGICAL DISEASES AFFECTING THE EXTRAPYRAMIDAL MOTOR SYSTEM

Gerold Porenta
Department of Medical Cybernetics and
Artificial Intelligence
University of Vienna, Medical School
Freyung 6
A 1010 Wien, Austria

Peter Riederer
Ludwig Boltzmann Institute of
Clinical Neurobiology, Neurochemistry Group
Lainz-Hospital, Wolkersbergenstr. 1
A 1130 Wien, Austria

1. Introduction

Parkinson's disease, a movement disorder affecting the extrapyramidal motor system with akinesia, rigidity, and tremor as main symptoms, was among the first neurological diseases that could be shown to correlate with an abnormal distribution of a chemical substance in the brain. This discovery led to the development of pharmacologically active drugs substantially improving treatment and prognosis of many neurological and psychiatric diseases. Thus, models of the chemical processes in the brain became important for clinical practice.

For Parkinson's disease, post-mortem studies of human brain tissue showed a deficit of dopamine (DA) in certain nerve cells extending from the substantia nigra to the caudate nucleus, two brain nuclei involved in the coordination of the extrapyramidal motor system. During nerve action, dopamine, a transmitter substance, is released into the synaptic cleft and influences the induction of an action potential in the postsynaptic neuron. Therefore, proper nerve action depends on a normal level of dopamine concentration. In therapy, a patient suffering from Parkinson's disease is supplied with an optimal amount of the dopamine precursor L-DOPA that will bring about an increase in nerval dopamine concentration thereby ameliorating some of the motor dysfunctions characterizing Parkinson's disease [1].

For another disease of the extrapyramidal system, Huntington's Chorea, inhibitory nerve cells containing γ-amino butyric acid (GABA) as transmitter substance and extending from the caudate nucleus to the dopaminergic cell bodies in the substantia nigra suffer a partial depletion due to degenerative processes. Contrary to Parkinson's disease where hypokinetic symptoms prevail, hyperkinetic motor dysfunctions are among the characteristic symptoms of this disease. However, substitution therapy as in Parkinson's disease has not yet been achieved. Instead, pharmacological depression of dopaminergic cells is the therapy of choice.

The neural loop between the caudate nucleus and the substantia nigra is completed by excitatory acetylcholinergic (ACh) nerve cells in the caudate nucleus connecting the dopaminergic with the GABA-ergic system. The functional significance of the cholinergic interneurons is considered in the treatment of Parkinson's disease, when anticholinergic drugs are administered to counterbalance a relative cholinergic hyperfunction.

At present, there is to our knowledge not yet a mathematical model suitable to conduct stability and sensitivity analyses of this important neural loop. Thus, we are currently working to develop such a model that should allow to (1) study the dynamic behaviour of the system, especially the interrelation of multiple neurons with feedback effects, (2) simulate pathophysiological states of the extrapyramidal system, and (3) simulate the effects of parameter changes corresponding to certain drug actions.

It is to be emphasized that the model is not aimed at simulating the state of neurons in the basal ganglia of one single patient. Such a model would be difficult to validate as in-vivo measurements of relevant data can hardly be achieved at present. Rather, we develop the model as a research tool that should provide insight into possible cybernetic features of this neural feedback loop and serve as a decision criterium to assess alternative therapeutical approaches directed against dysfunctions of the basal ganglia.

2. Geometrical model

Models of the neural connections of the basal ganglia, often seen as a functional unit, to other areas in the brain as well as models of the neural interactions within the basal ganglia have emerged on the basis of various investigations using different techniques, among them chemical, electrical, or histological methods [2].

From a clinical view the salient feature of diseases affecting the basal ganglia is a severe disturbance of the normally balanced activities of the dopaminergic, acetylcholinergic, and GABA-ergic systems. Accordingly, a sequence of three neurons using dopamine, acetylcholine, and GABA as transmitter substances constitutes the core of this model depicted in Fig. 1.

An action potential in the presynaptic dopaminergic nerve terminal in the caudate nucleus mediates the release of the transmitter substance DA into the synaptic cleft. Subsequently, receptor molecules at the postsynaptic membrane activated by dopamine change the membrane permeability to ions. Whenever the combined effects of activated receptors and external inputs bring the membrane potential to the firing threshold, a postsynaptic action potential is elicited propagating along the cholinergic neuron until it reaches a presynaptic terminal where the synaptic transmission process is repeated. Having passed the cholinergic and GABA-ergic synapses, the action potential reenters the neural loop.

External control mechanisms are modelled as lumped input variables acting at three different locations as indicated by the hatched arrows in Figure 1.

3. Mathematical model

Figure 2 shows a simple model of the transmission process at a neural synapse with five basic compartments: cytoplasmatic transmitter (C), transmitter stored in presynaptic vesicles (V), transmitter within the synaptic cleft (S), free receptor molecules in the synaptic cleft (R), and activated transmitter-receptor complex (RA). For the depicted chemical processes, application of the mass balance theorem to every compartment leads to a corresponding mathematical model, a system of ordinary differential equations either linear or nonlinear depending on the kinetics of the pertinent metabolic pathways.

For a simulation model of the electric activity at both the presynaptic and postsynaptic site, we adopted a system of nonlinear ordinary differential equations describing membrane voltage, and sodium and potassium currents as suggested by Hodgkin and Huxley [3]. To provide for an interdependence between the model parts simulating the electrical and chemical processes, we added equations describing the behaviour of a presynaptic voltage dependent calcium channel [4] controlling the rate of transmitter release. At the postsynaptic site, membrane voltage is controlled through ion channels opened and closed by activated receptors. Each circle in Fig. 2 represents a complete set of equations simulating the electrical state of the membrane. The white arrows show the points of interaction between electrical and chemical processes.

Using kinetic data from the literature [6, 5] as well as data from our own laboratory, we already developed a mathematical model of the acetylcholinergic synapse and implemented a simulation model on the digital mainframe computer of the Technical University of Vienna (CDC Cyber 170-720) using the simulation language ACSL.

Further work will include finishing the descriptions of the dopaminergic and GABA-ergic synapse and simulating the closed loop behaviour of the system taking also into account input from external sources (e.g. telencephalon).

4. References

[1] Birkmayer W., Riederer P.: Die Parkinson-Krankheit. Biochemie, Klinik, Therapie, Springer, Wien New York, 1980.

[2] Dray A.: The Striatum and Substantia Nigra: A Commentary On Their Relationships, Neuroscience 4:1407-1439, 1979.

[3] Hodgkin A.L., Huxley A.F.: A Quantitative Description of Membrane Current and its Application to Conduction and Excitation in Nerve, J. Physiol. 117:500-544, 1952.

[4] Llinas R., Steinberg I.Z., Walton K.: Presynaptic Calcium Currents in Squid Giant Synapse, Biophys. J. 33:289-321, 1981.

[5] Tucek S.: Regulation of Acetylcholine Synthesis in the Brain, J.Neurochem. 44(1):11-24, 1985.

[6] Wathey J.C., Nass M.M., Lester H.A.: Numerical Reconstruction of the Quantal Event at Nicotinic Synapses, Biophys.J. 27:145-164, 1979.

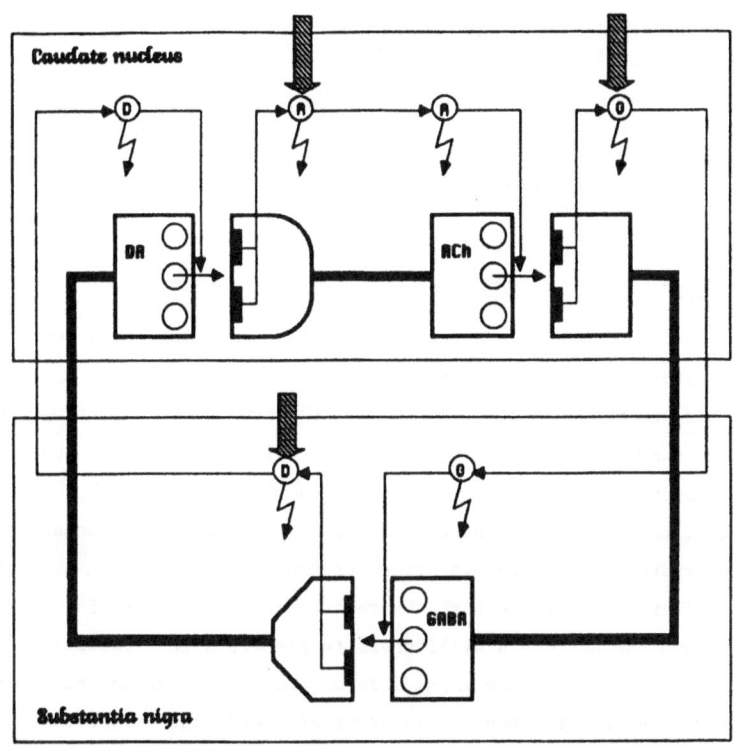

Figure 1. Schematic model of the nigro-striatal feedback loop.
(D, DA, dopamine; A, ACh, acetylcholine; G, GABA;
◯ , presynaptic vesicles; ▮, postsynaptic receptors;
, action potentials; ⬇ , external excitation;)

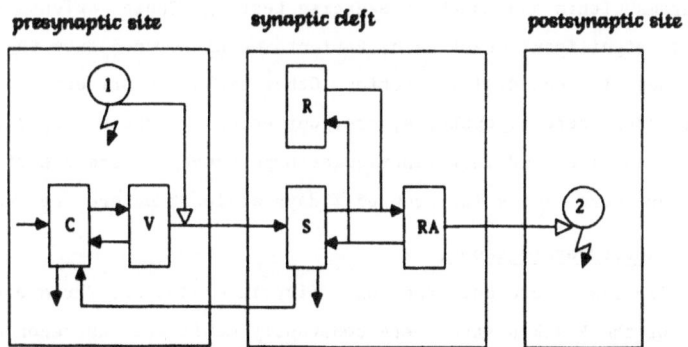

Figure 2. Simple compartment model of a neural synapse.
(C, V, S, cytoplasmatic, vesicular, and synaptic
compartments of the transmitter substance;
R, free receptors; RA, activated receptors;
1,2, pre- and postsynaptic action potentials;)

OPTIMAL SEQUENTIAL STRATEGIES TO EVALUATE PRESENCE AND SEVERITY OF CORONARY ARTERY
DISEASE : AN INFORMATION THEORY APPROACH.

L. Eeckhoudt[x], J.Melin[xx], R. Vanbutsele[xx], J.C.Sailly[xxx], A.Robert[xx], Th.Lebrun[xxx],
C. Brohet[xx], J.M. Detry[xx].
x   : Catholic Faculties of Mons, Chaussée de Binche 151, 7000 Mons (Belgium).
xx : Cliniques Universitaires St.Luc,Avenue Hippocrate 10, 1200 Bruxelles(Belgium).
xxx : G.R.E.S.G.E., Rue F. Baes 1, 59046 Lille Cédex (France).

INTRODUCTION.

The evaluation of coronary artery disease (CAD) is based on 3 sources of information,
i.e. (1) pre-test or prior probability of CAD (P) derived from age, sex, nature of
complaints and presence of risk factors, (2) non-invasive testing such as exercise-
ECG alone (XECG) or combined with thallium scintigraphy (XT1) and, (3) coronary
arteriography (ANGIO) which is the accepted reference method.
Because of the spiraling cost of medical care, cost-effectiveness analyses of
various strategies for the evaluation of CAD are necessary to be performed. In this
study, effectiveness is measured by the reduction in uncertainty following each
strategy and the society's willingness to pay for such a reduction. Cost is
measured in financial terms regardless of the discomfort and risks of each strategy.
Various strategies are compared in terms of their cost-effectiveness; they involve
either an elementary approach or a sequential decision rule.

MATERIAL AND METHODS.

Patient selection .
The study population consisted of 301 consecutive male patients having coronary
arteriograms within one month of exercise testing. These patients were studied
because of significant chest pain. Patients were excluded from the study if they
had evidence of myocardial infarction. Other exclusion criteria were valvular
heart diseases, cardiomyopathies, previous coronary bypass surgery, ECG signs of
bundle branch block and left ventricular hypertrophy or the use of digitalis : the
betablockers were always interrupted 3 days at least before the exercise test.

Exercise electrocardiography.
The exercise tests were performed on a bicycle ergometer. Three orthogonal leads
(X, Y, Z of the Frank system) were constantly monitored and recorded on paper
every minute during the exercise and the first 5 minutes of the recovery. A 20
second-ECG sample was also recorded on a digital magnetic tape at the end of every
minute, at rest, during the exercise and during the 5 minutes of the recovery. The
amount of ST segment depression during maximal exercise was measured 80 msec after
the end of QRS with the PR interval taken as zero reference. ECG was considered

positive if ST segment depression was $\geqslant$ 1 mm.

Myocardial perfusion imaging .

The technique for myocardial imaging has previously been described[1]. During the
same testing session in which the exercise electrocardiogram was performed, thal-
lium-201 (1.5 to 2 mCi) was injected intravenously, 1 minute before maximal exercise. Each patient underwent imaging 5 to 10 minutes after thallium injection under
a Searle Pho-Gamma V camera or an Apex 215 M Elscint camera. Images (250.000
counts) were obtained in the anterior, left anterior oblique 45° and 65° positions.
The stress studies were independently interpreted without computer processing by
two observers who had no knowledge of the clinical, angiographic or electrocardio-
graphic findings.

The results of the thallium perfusion were reported as positive or negative.

Cardiac catheterization .

Selective coronary arteriography was performed using the transcutaneous femoral
Judkins technique. The coronary arteriography was considered abnormal in presence
of a reduction of 50 % or more in diameter of at least one major coronary vessel.
From the arteriographic results, we could determine the true state of the coronary
system for each patient and we considered four levels of severity ("states of the
world") : good health = 0 vessel diseased (VD) or CAD with 1, 2 or 3 VD.

By comparing for each patient the results of the arteriography with those of the
non-invasive procedures, we could derive from our sample an estimate of the probabilities of observing each non-invasive test result (in isolation or in pairs) conditional upon the number of VD.

STATISTICAL METHODS .

For each patient, we obtained from CADENZA[2] the a priori probability of CAD (P) and
we splitted this probability evenly in each level of severity (number of vessels
diseased). Hence, the a priori probability of each patient was characterized by :

$$P(OVD) = 1 - P$$
$$P(1VD) = P(2VD) = P(3VD) = P/3.$$

By using the entropy concept[3], the initial level of uncertainty (IU) was measured
by :

$$IU = - \sum_{i = 0}^{i = 3} P(iVD). \ln P(iVD)$$

When a perfect test is available, i.e. a test measuring exactly the extent of the
disease, the final level of uncertainty (FU) is equal to zero.

As far as non-invasive and less than perfect tests are concerned, we need to know the probability of observing each test result, given the number of vessels diseased. These probabilities have been estimated from our data bank[4] and they are listed in table 1.

TABLE 1

	OVD (n = 67)					2VD (n = 77)			
	T1+	T1-				T1+	T1-		
ECG+	.105	.164	.269		ECG+	.702	.078	.780	
ECG-	.090	.641	.731		ECG-	.169	.051	.220	
	.195	.805				.871	.129		

	1VD (n = 70)					3VD (n = 87)			
ECG+	.571	.086	.657		ECG+	.724	.012	.736	
ECG-	.229	.114	.343		ECG-	.218	.046	.264	
	.800	.200				.942	.058		

By applying Bayes's theorem to these probabilities, combined with the a priori ones, we have completed the probability of observing each number of vessels disea- sed. Conditional upon the test results, we have then obtained the level of uncer- tainty following the test results. Then, the reduction in uncertainty (RU) can be calculated by the difference between IU and FU.

COST-EFFECTIVENESS MEASUREMENTS .

Using Belgian data for illustrative purposes, we obtain the following costs (C) for each test :

$$\begin{array}{lcl} \text{XECG} & : & 3.000 \text{ FB} \\ \text{XT1} & : & 9.000 \text{ FB} \\ \text{ANGIO} & : & 50.000 \text{ FB} \end{array}$$

In order to convert the benefit of a strategy (RU) into monetary units, we have used the willingness-to-pay (WTP) concept. By this concept, we measure the amount of money Society is willing to give up in order to reduce uncertainty by one unit. In this framework, the net outcome (NO) of an elementary strategy is given by :

$$NO = (RU) . (WTP) - C .$$

To evaluate the sequential strategies, we have used the "decision-tree" technique. For illustrative purposes, we have also assumed that WTP = 43.290 BF.

RESULTS .

The NO of different strategies are given in Table 2 for 3 patients with a given prior probability of CAD. The best NO for each patient is underlined.

TABLE 2

Strategy	Exercise ECG	Exercise thallium imaging	Coronary angiography	Net outcome		
				P(CAD) = .3	P = .6	P = .9
I	none	none	none	19.288	2.377	3.160
II	1st	none	none	20.330	4.000	2.068
III	1st	1st	none	20.431	5.305	- 200
IV	1st	none	2nd if*	22.479	9.191	7.000
V	1st	1st	2nd if*	23.498	9.684	1.000
VI	none	none	1st	10.000	10.000	10.000
VII	1st	2nd if*	3rd if*	22.526	10.714	1.000

The "if*" appearing for some strategies means that the corresponding test will be ordered only if it has the highest NO.

COMMENTS .

This cost-effectiveness analysis was applied to three examples of different prevalence of coronary disease. These three examples show that the prevalence of disease strongly influences cost-effectiveness of any strategy. In groups of low and middle prevalence of CAD (P = .3 and P = .6), the best strategies were those using the non-invasive tests on a sequential mode (V and VII). At high prevalence, (P = .9), performing coronary angiography as the only test to evaluate coronary artery disease, is the most cost-effective strategy. A computer program is able to perform this cost-effectiveness analysis for each possible prevalence of coronary artery disease and therefore to guide the physician for selecting the best strategy in an individual patient.

Our data and conclusions have to be interpreted with caution since we have postulated that the severity of the disease was not influenced by the a priori probability; also WTP has been set arbitrarily and different results would be obtained if WTP was modified. Finally we have not discussed the consequences of the CAD evaluation in terms of prognosis and therapeutic decisions.

REFERENCES .

1. MELIN J.A., PIRET L.J., VANBUTSELE R.J.M., ROUSSEAU M.F., COSYNS J., BRASSEUR L.A., BECKERS C., DETRY JM.R. - Diagnostic value of exercise electrocardiography in patients without previous myocardial infarction: a Bayesian approach.

Circulation, <u>63</u>, 1019-1024, 1981.

2. DIAMOND G., FORRESTER J. - Cadenza II : Computer-assisted, diagnosis and evaluations of coronary artery disease. Copyright 1979, Cardiokinetics Inc., Seattle.

3. SHANNON C.E. - A mathematical theory of communication. Bell System Tech. J., <u>27</u>, 397 and 623.

4. MELIN J., EECKHOUT L., VANBUTSELE R., ROBERT A., LEBRUN Th., SAILLY J.C., BROHET C., DETRY J.M. - Selection of diagnostic tests for coronary disease based on a computer-aided determination of their information content. Computers in Cardiology IEEE transaction, in press, 1984.

COMPARISON OF EVALUATION CRITERIA FOR NONPARAMETRIC DISCRIMINANT ANALYSIS

K. P. Pfeiffer, T. Kenner
Physiologisches Institut
Karl-Franzens-Universität Graz
Harrachgasse 21/V
A-8010 Graz, AUSTRIA

INTRODUCTION

Variable selection is a part of the general problem of analysing the structure of
data. For many multivariate problems, like multiple regression, different algorithms
for the selection of a "best" subset of variables according to some model evaluation
criterion are described in the literature (Hocking, 1976). Because of multi-
collinearity of the independent variables the determination of the "best" subset of
variables can become very complex. If stepwise variable selection procedures are
used only "suboptimal" solutions will be found.

Besides the algorithm for selection of the subset an essential question is the
evaluation of the quality of the model. A number of criteria have been stated in
the literature for model evaluation in multiple regression, pattern recognition,
discriminant analysis or computer assisted medical decision making (Hilden, 1978;
Hand, 1981). The criteria are stated in terms of the behavior of certain functions
as a function of the subset of variables.

For many practical applications a large number of independent variables is available
and there may be an uncertainty which of the variables should be included in the
model. Selecting a "best" subset of variables is often a compromise between the
achievement of an optimal fit and the costs of sampling a large number of data.

CRITERIA FOR MODEL EVALUATION

The criterion which should be used for model evaluation should be related to the
intended use. Two types of discriminant analysis (DA) problems can be distiguished.
The aim of _descriptive_ DA is to identify the subtantial different features between
classes. For this type goodness of fit criteria or distance functions seem to be
appropriate evaluation criteria. The aim of _predictive_ DA is to classify future
observations. For this type the results of forced classification or of classification
with doubt of test data or also distance functions seem to be appropriate.

For automatic variable selection algorithms it is necessary that model evaluation
criteria can be compared for different model orders. If stepwise procedures are used
it must be possible to define appropriate stopping rules. Furthermore it should be

possible to weight right and wrong classifications.

It seems also important to notice that model evaluation criteria may be very different from the optimization criterion for model parameter estimation. For example a model may be evaluated by a weighted error or non-error rate whereas the parameters of this model are estimated according to a maximum likelihood criterion. Therefore very often different model evaluation criteria lead to different "best" subsets of variables.

MODEL EVALUATION CRITERIA

In this study kernel functions are used to estimate multivariate probability density functions of the groups. The smoothing factors of the kernel functions for each variable are estimated according to a maximum likelihood criterion parallel to the stepwise selection of the variables (Pfeiffer, 1985).

The quality of the nonparametric discriminant functions is evaluated by criteria which use the information of the estimated probability density functions. To estimate the amount of overlap of the distributions general criteria like Kolmogoroff variational distance or the Kolmogoroff dependence would be very appropriate to evaluate this form of nonparametric discriminant functions. For practical applications the computational work for estimation of these criteria for multivariate distributions and more than two groups becomes very large and therefore simpler criteria are used. Habbema et al. (1978) and Hilden et al. (1978) list some criteria for probabilistic medical diagnosis which can also be applied to nonparametric DA. Some of these criteria like

$$Q_1 = \frac{1}{n} \sum_{i=1}^{m} \sum_{h=1}^{n_i} \hat{f}(\underset{\sim}{x}_{ij}/d_i;H)$$

$\hat{f}(\underset{\sim}{x}_{ij}/d_i;H) \ldots$ is the estimated probability of element $\underset{\sim}{x}_{ij}$ belonging to class d_i

$$Q_2 = \frac{1}{n} \sum_{i} \sum_{j} - \ln(\hat{f}(\underset{\sim}{x}_{ij}/d_i;H))$$

H ... matrix of smoothing factors

$\underset{\sim}{x}_{ij} \ldots$ p-dimensional vector of variables

are very simple to compute and easy to understand, but they do not consider the probability of an element $\underset{\sim}{x}_{ij}$ belonging to an other group then d_i. The scaled quadratic evaluation criterion

$$Q_3 = \frac{1}{n} \sum_{i} \sum_{j} \left[(1-f(\underset{\sim}{x}_{ij}/d_i;H))^2 + \sum_{k \neq i} f^2(\underset{\sim}{x}_{ij}/d_k;H) \right]$$

also takes into account the probability of an element $\underset{\sim}{x}_{ij}$ belonging to class d_k, $k \neq i$.

For many practical applications forced classification is performed and the non-error (NER) or error rate (ER) are used for model evaluation.

Furthermore the classification results may be weighted by a given weight matrix and a loss function is used for model evaluation. The disadvantage of forced classification is the reduction of the information of the probability density function to binary states. To avoid this reduction of the information content classification with doubt can be performed. To take into account the certainity of decisions we propose the following criterion:

$$Q_4 = \frac{1}{n} \sum_i \sum_j v_{ij}$$

with

$$
v_{ij} = \begin{cases}
\dfrac{\hat{f}(\underset{\sim}{x}_{ij}/d_i;H)}{\max\limits_{i \neq k} \hat{f}(\underset{\sim}{x}_{ij}/d_k;H)} - 1 & \text{if} \quad \hat{f}(\underset{\sim}{x}_{ij}/d_i;H) \geq \max\limits_{i \neq k} \hat{f}(\underset{\sim}{x}_{ij}/d_k;H) \\[4mm]
\dfrac{\max\limits_{i \neq k} \hat{f}(\underset{\sim}{x}_{ij}/d_k;H)}{\hat{f}(\underset{\sim}{x}_{ij}/d_i;H)} + 1 & \text{if} \quad \hat{f}(\underset{\sim}{x}_{ij}/d_i;H) \leq \max\limits_{i \neq k} \hat{f}(\underset{\sim}{x}_{ij}/d_k;H)
\end{cases}
$$

$$|v_{ij}| \leq v_{max}$$

For criterion Q_4 an upper limit v_{max} has to be defined. An advantage of this criterion is, that the relation v_{ij} is independent of the model order p and stopping rules, like: if the increase of $Q_4 \leq \varepsilon$ then stop, can be defined.

To evaluate the quality of a model with regard to future data sets, is is necessary to estimate the evaluation criteria from test samples which are independent of the training sample. This separation is achieved by the application of a jackknife or bootstrap procedure and therefore the evaluation criteria in the following example have been computed using jackknife probabilities.

APPLICATION

A group of $n_1 = 32$ male gout patients was compared by stepwise nonparametric DA with a group of $n_2 = 38$ male normouremic control persons. As possible risk factors age, body weight index (BWI), serum lipids, lipoproteins, apo-lipoproteins and ratios of these variables have been examined. Normal kernels are assumed in this study. Instead

of only one smoothing factor for all variables (Hermans, 1982; Hand, 1981) the
smoothing factor of each variable under consideration to be selected for the "best"
model is estimated according to a maximum likelihood criterion (Pfeiffer, 1985).
In tab. 1 the values of different model evaluation criteria of the "best" models,
which have been found by the foreward stepwise variable selection procedure are shown.
Out of all $m = 31$ variables only p= 7 variables have been found to be substantial,
if criterion Q_4 is used for model evaluation and an increase of Q_4 (p+1)/Q_4 (p)$\leq$1.10
has been used as stopping rule. A comparison of Q_4 and tER shows, that the minimum
of tER is achieved for p= 4 and the automatic variable selection procedure would
stop there. Furthermore the difference of the true error rate (tER) and the apparent
error rate (aER) becomes obvious. This example also shows the disadvantages of
criteria Q_1, Q_2 which show a strong dependence on the model order and an adjustment
according to the model order would be necessary if these criteria should be used for
automatic variable selection. Furthermore the dependence of the smoothing factors
of one variable for different models can be seen from table 1 (HDL-phosphol). This
indicates the importance of stepwise estimation of the smoothing factor for each
variable under consideration instead of the assumption of only one constant smoothing
factor for all variables.

Tab. 1: Example of the results of stepwise variable selection according to criterion Q_4

	p= 1		p= 2	p= 3	p= 4	p= 5	p= 6	p= 7
Age								
Body weight index						.774	.774	.774
total TG	.440		.440	.440	.440	.440	.440	.440
HDL-phospholip.		.623	.725	.725	.725	.725	.725	.725
apo AI					.674	.674	.674	.674
apo B							.568	.568
apo AI/HDL-C								.551
apo B/(apo AI+AII)				.572	.572	.572	.572	.572
Q_1	.52	.262	.130	.040	.012	.003	.001	.000
Q_2	.84	1.817	2.400	3.668	4.929	6.341	7.123	8.244
Q_3	.79	.709	.616	.539	.512	.503	.501	.500
Q_4	10.43	6.707	15.589	17.705	20.524	26.958	29.958	33.934
aER	.28	.257	.229	.186	.014	.014	.014	.000
tER	.31	.257	.271	.229	.114	.157	.157	.186

DISCUSSION

To get an impression of the quality of a discriminant function different evaluation
criteria should be considered simultaneously. To use the information content of the
estimated probability density functions for nonparametric DA quality criteria which
use the exact probability values are recommended instead of the frequently used error
and non-error rate. Many clinicians are accustomed to terms like sensitivity, speci-
fitiy, predictive value etc. which are closely related to the yes/no (true/false)
terminology of the error and non-error rate. But these are very rough measures of the

model quality, especially if the number of observations is small. Automatic variable selection algorithms would stop, because the error and non-error rate would not improve, whereas other probabilistic measures would improve if the model order is changed.

Habbema J.D.F., Hilden J., Bjerregaard B.: The Measurement of Performance in Probailistic Diagnosis, I. Meth. Inform. Med., 17/4, 1978, 217-226

Hand D.J.: Discrimination and Classification, Wiley, Chichester, 1981

Hermans J., Habbema J.D.F., Kasanmoentalib T.K.D., Raatgever J.W.: Alloc 80, Dept. of Med. Stat., Univ. of Leiden, 1982

Hilden J., Habbema J.D.F., Bjerregaard B.: The Measurement of Performance in Probabilistic Diagnosis, II. Meth. Inform. Med., 17/4, 1978, 227-237

Hocking R.R.: The Analysis and Selection of Variables in Multiple Regression, Biometrics 32, 1976, 1-49

Pfeiffer K.P.: Stepwise Variable Selection and Maximum Likelihood Estimation of Smoothing Factors of Kernel Functions for Nonparametric Discriminant Functions Evaluated by Different Criteria. Comp. and Biomed. Res., 85, 1985

THREE-DIMENSIONAL SIMULATION OF TUMOR GROWTH AND TREATMENT

W. Düchting and Th. Vogelsaenger
Department of Electrical Engineering
University of Siegen
Hölderlinstr. 3, D-5900 Siegen, West-Germany

ABSTRACT: The main problem discussed in this paper is focused on the question how to simulate three-dimensional tumor growth and treatment in a vascularized tissue segment. The starting points for this procedure are (i) idealized cellkinetic data of normal cells and of tumor cells, (ii) simplified cell-cycle models of normal cells and of tumor cells, and (iii) production and interaction rules of the individual cells. Algorithms and program packages have been constructed describing the spatial and temporal tumor growth. An example of simulating a chemotherapeutic treatment is given. As a result it becomes possible to simulate different kinds of tumor treatment e.g. surgical removal, radiation therapy and chemotherapy prior to clinical therapy and to develop optimized treatment schedules.

1. INTRODUCTION

Control mechanisms play an important role in the growth and development of a multicellular organism. Much investigation done in this area has centered on the role of measuring the kinetics of cell proliferation. In the last few years, there has been a very great increase of introducing mathematical modelling (1,2) and control theory approaches (3) to the field of complex biological processes. The object which is to be modelled in this contribution is an oversimplified homogeneous tissue segment (volume: $1mm^3$) of a fictitious organ containing several capillaries.

2. CELL-CYCLE MODELS

The process of modelling starts with the development of cellkinetic models both of normal cells and of tumor ones describing the regeneration and multiplication of the cell species. For a tumor cell the corresponding cellkinetic model is represented in Figure 1. In contrast to a normal cell a tumor cell is theoretically able to divide infinitely.

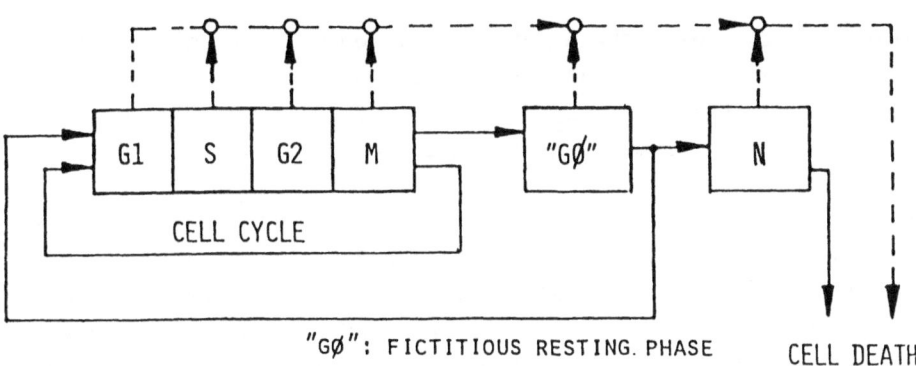

"GØ": FICTITIOUS RESTING PHASE   CELL DEATH
N   : NECROSIS

Fig. 1. Cell-cycle model of a tumor cell

TABLE 1. Relevant cellkinetic data (Cell-cycle time:
$T_C = T_{G1} + T_S + T_{G2} + T_M$; Standard deviation σ)

PHASE DURATION IN HOURS	T_{G1}	σ_{G1}	T_S	σ_S	T_{G2}	σ_{G2}	T_M	σ_M	T_C	$T_{G\emptyset}$	$\sigma_{G\emptyset}$	T_E	σ_E
NORMAL CELL	10	2	8	1	4	1	1	0	23	24	8	16	2
TUMOR CELL	4	1	4	1	1	1	1	0	10	5	2	40	4

In the present simplified model (Fig. 1) it shall pass over to the
fictitious resting phase "GØ" if the distance between the dividing
tumor cell and the microvessels is more than 100μm because of lacking
oxygen supply. From this pool it is normally transferred to the state
of necrosis (N-phase) after the transit time $T_{"G\emptyset"}$. The relevant data
used in this model (TABLE 1) refer back to the cellkinetic literature
(4).

3. INTERACTION RULES

The strategy of modeling used in this paper is listing specifications
and formulating interaction rules both for normal cells and for tumor
ones. For tumor growth the following selected notations may be valid:
- A tumor cell is theoretically able to divide infinitely even if
  there is no empty place available for the positioning of a daughter
  cell. In this case random variables determine the direction of the

dividing tumor cell. The daughter cell generated by mitosis shifts all cells one position farther towards this direction.

- The phase duration (T_{G1}, T_S, T_{G2}, T_M, $T_{"GØ"}$, T_N) of a tumor cell is determined by normally-distributed (Gaussian distributed) random variables.

- The division of a tumor cell is only possible if the distance between a dividing tumor cell and the blood vessels is less than ST= 3 cell layers. All tumor cells living in a larger distance than ST from the capillaries after the next division step pass over to the fictitious resting phase "GØ" and normally to the subsequent phase of necrosis (N-cells).

According to the listed conditions numerous subprogram packages have been developed in the programming language FORTRAN IV, describing the complex cell growth in three-dimensions.

4. SIMULATION OF A CHEMOTHERAPEUTIC TREATMENT

At T=O units of time 11 tumor cells (data s. TABLE 1) are arbitrarily placed in the center of a fictitious tissue segment two layers away from the capillaries. These tumor cells proliferate gradually to form the tumor shown in Figure 2(a). Now the tumor shall be treated by an anticancer drug. It is assumed that all proliferating tumor cells may be killed at T=201 units of time. After an intermediate remission (Fig. 2(b)) a repeated increase of the number of tumor cells can be observed in Figure 2(c). The reason for this behaviour is that all dormant GØ-tumor cells living in a distance less than 3 cell layers from the capillaries have been recruited into the cell cycle again. Therefore a second simulation run delivers the number of GØ-tumor cells as a function of time. The minimum of this curve determines the optimal moment of applying the same anticancer drug for a second time which leads to a more efficient remission of the tumor.

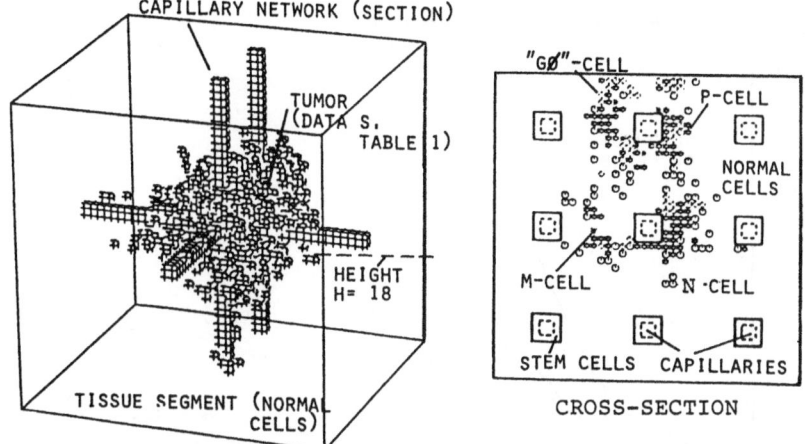

Fig. 2(a). Tumor configuration at T=200 units of time

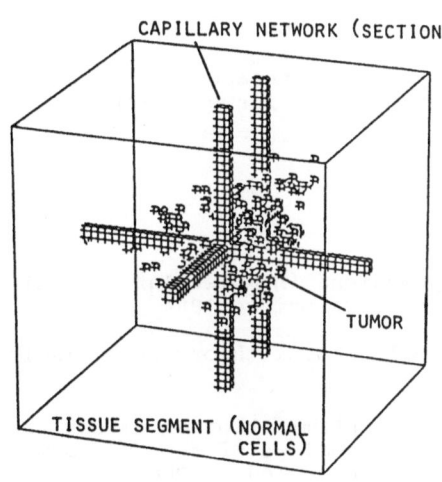

Fig. 2(b). Tumor configuration
at T=250 units of
time after chemo-
therapy at T=201
(Die-out probabi-
lity of the pro-
liferating tumor
cells: 100%)

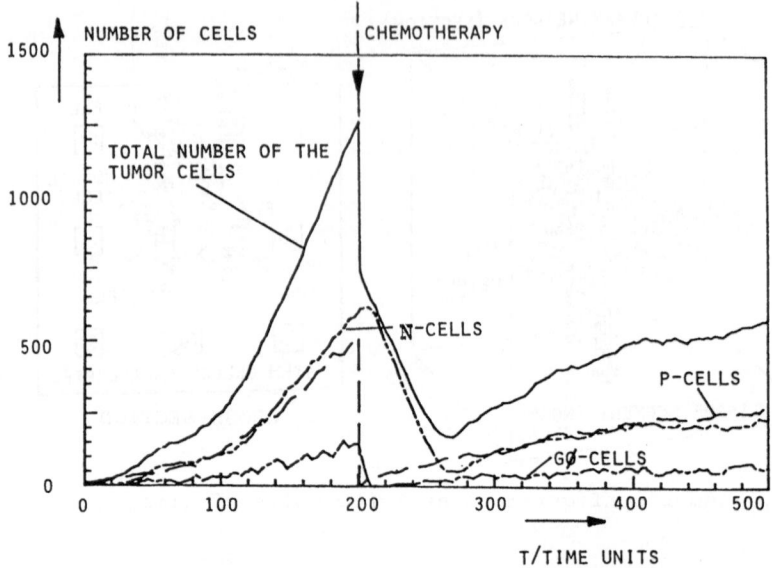

Fig. 2(c). Number of tumor cells as a function of time

Fig. 2(a)-(c). Simulation of a single chemotherapeutic treatment
of a tumor in a vascularized tissue segment

5. REFERENCES

(1) Segel, L.A.: Modelling dynamic phenomena in molecular and cellular biology, Cambridge University Press, Cambridge 1984.

(2) Swan, G.W.: Applications of optimal control theory in biomedicine, Marcel Dekker, New York 1984.

(3) Düchting, W. and Vogelsaenger, Th.: Optimization of cancer treatment by computer simulation. In: Proceedings of the 1984 Summer Computer Simulation Conference, W.D. Wade (ed.), The Society for Computer Simulation, La Jolla/Calif. 1984, pp. 802-807.

(4) Lloyd, D., Poole, R.K. and Edwards, St.W.: The cell division cycle, Academic Press, London 1982.

ACQUISITION AND EVALUATION OF DATA FOR BEHAVIORAL ANALYSIS

Ulrich F. Wellner-Cubasch

6761 Waldgrehweiler, FRG

This paper describes a system for the acquisition and computerized evaluation of observational data. The idea to develop such a system arose when the methods for a project aiming at a quantitative analysis of infant-parent-interaction had to be set up. In regard to the complexity of behavior to be expected and the resulting amount of data systems known from behavioral analysis in primate research could not be employed.

There are three tasks which have to be dealt with:

I.   Finding a reasonable way of describing behavior.

II. Designing and building appropriate hard- and software for acquisition of data as well as for interfacing to a mini-computer.

III. Developing software for management and evaluation of data.

I. A WAY TO DESCRIBE BEHAVIOR

Finding a reasonable definition of "behavior" has to take into account the original meaning of behavior as implied by definitions given by biologists or psychologists, the use of human sense receptors and judgement abilities as measuring instruments as well as all the restrictions that computer processing of such data imposes. SACKETT states that the major problems of measurement in observational research are the limitations of the human observer in regard to reaction time and number of complex discriminations that can be made in real time (1). Any instrumentation will only assist and extend but never replace human judgement abilities; the observer will remain the critical factor. Common strategies for coding behavior (described e.g. in 1,2) often accept an immense loss of information right away especially when complex forms of behavior are to be recorded. In other cases (3,4) the acquisition hardware is not tailored to human capacities thus forcing a definition of behavior directly implying loss of information. We decided on relieving the work of the human observer by restricting the complexity of behavior to be detected. Behavior will thus be regarded as being composed of simple elements; the occurrence of which can be decided upon the observation of a small number of cues. These cues should be well defined by language so that - good training presumed - different observers will be able to decide fast and reliable at any point in time whether a cue can be detected (within- and between-observer reliability > .9). Any more complex behavior may then be expressed as a logical function based on several those elements. Due to this strategy the task of observing behavioral elements may be split among several observers thus increasing performance.

Let some terms be defined in a formal way:

1) A BEHAVIORAL ELEMENT $\widetilde{BE}$ is a time depending binary valued function. To distinguish different $\widetilde{BE}$s an index is appended. $\widetilde{BE}(t) \in \{\emptyset, 1\}$, $t \in (t_0, t_0 + d)$, $d > \emptyset$

2) A <u>CODING SYSTEM</u> for behavior is a vector valued function defined by
   $\widetilde{B}(t) := (\widetilde{BE}_1(t),\ldots\ldots, \widetilde{BE}_N(t))^T \in \{0,1\}^N$. Dimension dim $\widetilde{B}$ = N.

3) The algorithm defining a $\widetilde{BE}_j$ consists basically of a list of observational cues.
   Upon their joint presence $\widetilde{BE}_j(t)$ will take the value one; in all other cases $\widetilde{BE}_j(t)$
   will be zero. The algorithm may thus be regarded as an operational definition of a
   certain behavior. We say that for a point t° in time $\widetilde{BE}_j(t°)$ is <u>OBSERVABLE</u> when
   $\widetilde{BE}_j(t°)$ = 1. We may also look upon $\widetilde{BE}_j(t)$ as a logical variable taking the value
   "true" whenever it is observable. $\widetilde{BE}$s may thus be combined by logical operators.

4) A <u>CATEGORY</u> $\widetilde{C}(t)$ is either a $\widetilde{BE}(t)$ or a (logical) function of a number of $\widetilde{BE}(t)$.
   In the first case it is called an <u>ELEMENTARY CATEGORY</u> $\widetilde{EC}(t)$, in the latter
   case a <u>DERIVED CATEGORY</u> $\widetilde{DC}(t)$.

5) A coding system $\widetilde{B}(t)$ is <u>EXHAUSTIVE</u> when $\widetilde{B}(t) \neq 0$ $\forall$ t. It is <u>EXCLUSIVE</u>
   when $\widetilde{BE}_j(t)$ = 1 implies $\widetilde{BE}_k(t)$ = 0 $\forall$ k $\neq$ j, $\forall$ t .

6) For reasons of digital evaluation the continuous coding system $\widetilde{B}(t)$ is transformed
   to a discontinuous function $\{B_k\}$ defined by $B_k := \widetilde{B}(t_k) = \widetilde{B}(t_0+k \cdot \Delta t)$, k=0,1,...,M.
   That means that $\widetilde{B}(t)$ is sampled at a constant frequency Δt^{-1} . The same applies to
   all $\widetilde{BE}(t)$ involved. For given period of time, sampling frequency, and coding system
   $\widetilde{B}(t)$ we represent the "behavior" observed during that period by a matrix B = (B_{ik})
   with B_{ik} = $\widetilde{BE}_i(t_0+k \cdot \Delta t)$, i = 1,..,n; k = 0,..,M. B is called a <u>BEHAVIOR MATRIX</u>
   BM. The rows are defined by behavioral elements, the columns are defined by the
   state of those elements at uniformously spaced instances in time.

7) Let for a category $\widetilde{C}_i$, a sample index q and w>1: C_{iq} = 0, C_{ik} = 1 for q<k<q+w,
   C_{iq+w} = 0. Such a pattern within a BM is called an <u>EVENT</u> $E_i^{(q+1)}$ beginning at q+1.

Concerning those definitions some remarks have to be made:
How the $\widetilde{BE}$ actually used are constructed cannot be prescribed; this will depend on the
kind of research goal and on practical considerations concerning observability and capabilities of observers. Behavioral elements should not be viewed as being elementary
in a sense that they resemble the smallest undividable units of behavior by which all
more complex forms of behavior can be constructed in a unique way. The set of $\widetilde{BE}$s comprising a coding system should only be elementary in the sense that no $\widetilde{BE}_k$ may be reconstructed as a logical function of the other $\widetilde{BE}_j$, j $\neq$ k; e.g. we demand for independence. The definition of coding system suggested here is a generalisation of definitions
for coding systems used for behavioral research (1,5). In our definition a coding system
is not necessarily exclusive and exhaustive. The lack of those properties has severe
impact on the possible modes of evaluation (1), even though it is possible to transform
any coding system $\widetilde{B}$ to an exclusive and exhaustive system $\widetilde{B}°$. Such a transform will
generally result in increasing the dimensionality of $\widetilde{B}°$ to dim $\widetilde{B}°$ = 2^{n+1} , when
dim $\widetilde{B}$ = n. This will limit the interpretation of data for n above a certain number.
Categories are determined by hypothesises of the research project while the choice of
$\widetilde{BE}$s is explained by practical criteria of observability and simplicity. We therefore
prefer to introduce a distinction between those two entities.

II. ACQUISITION OF DATA

The basic idea underlying the acquisition process is:

1. Each human observer codes a number of $\widetilde{BE}(t)$ by pressing keys of a keyboard. Each key is (temporarily) associated with a certain $\widetilde{BE}_i$. The corresponding key is pressed as long as the $\widetilde{BE}_i$ is observed. The observer is not concerned with sampling.

2. The state of the keys is sampled at a constant rate (10 - 20 Hz, consider reaction time). Thus the columnvectors $(BE_{1j}, \ldots, BE_{Nj})$ of the BM are generated.

3. The columnvectors which resemble bitstrings are recorded sequentially on a mass storage medium or are transmitted directly to a laboratory mini-computer.

The hardware realizing this conception was developed as a portable stand-alone micro-computer. Figure 1 shows its configuration which is essentially a minimum system based on the MC 6809 MPU as described in (6). In addition a keyboard subsystem and a tape subsystem were designed. Special keyboards were built as well.

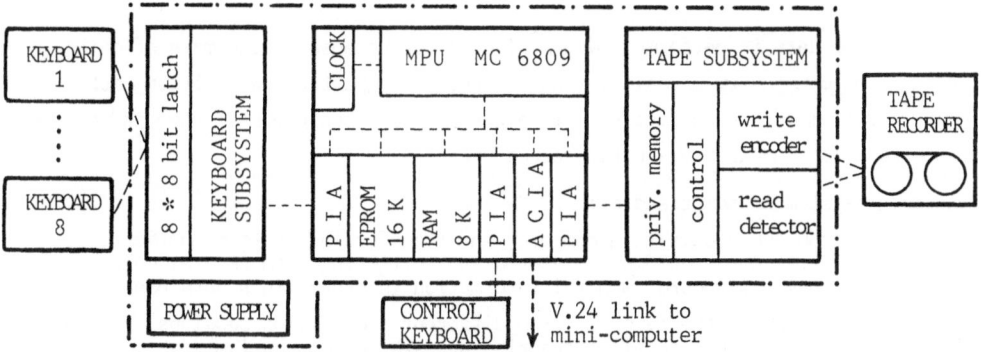

Fig. 1: Block diagram of acquisition mirco-computer

The keyboard subsystem is used to input data from several keyboards, each equipped with 8 keys (which we consider the maximum number of different categories an observer can handle). Because the apparatus is supposed to be used in real life situations in field and not only in laboratory settings, sufficient $\widetilde{BE}$s have to be recorded simultaneously. Therefore 8 keyboards are available (=64 $\widetilde{BE}$s). Whenever more than 64 $\widetilde{BE}$s had to be observed we decided that the situation should be videographed to avoid severe interaction of observers and the observed. The videotape may then be viewed repeatedly generating each time a partition of the BM. When building keyboards it proved to be important to ensure that the keys do not make any noise (click) when being operated because of interference (operant conditioning) with the subjects to be observed.

The tape subsystem was designed to use commercial tape recorders with a speed of 7.5 ips. In write-mode records of 80 bits (64 data bits, 8 bit preamble, 8 bit CRC) are recorded at most every 50 msec (e.g. a sampling rate of 20 Hz); the tape is not stopped between records. The MPU stores the data for one record in the private memory of the subsystem; conversion to bit-serial phase encoded format is then performed by the subsystem itself.

When in read-mode the PLL data recovery circuit of the subsystem will search for a preamble, read the data record to its memory and request service of the MPU via an interrupt. The tape subsystem circuitry is based on the design suggested in (7).

The software is totally contained in EPROM and performs five modes of operation:

1   Read general information and write to tape
2   Read data from keyboards and write to tape
3   Read data from tape and write to V.24 communication link
4,5 Same as 1,2; but write directly to V.24 communication link

The mode of operation is selected by function keys which were placed on a separate control keyboard. There also are keys for the input of digits which allow general information to be recorded. This information consists of experiment and observer numbers and data describing the association of keys and BEs.

III. PROCESSING OF DATA

The processing of data is performed by a mini-computer because of the mass of data involved and the complexity of calculations respectively pattern recognition tasks. Our software system may be subdivided into a general data management system and a number of programs for specific evaluation procedures.

The management system is comprised of:

1. Reading data from the acquisition computer and transferring it to magnetic tape. The behavior matrix BM is columnwise stored as a bitstring with several columns combined in a physical record. General information is stored in a data base.

2. Combining partitions of the same BM (from different acquisition sessions) so that for each sample point in time all categories are stored consecutively.

3. Compressing the behavior matrix by eliminating all-zero rows and replacing alike columns by a special repeat symbol.

4. Creating derived categories by either storing the defining logical expression - which is evaluated whenever such a category is requested - or expanding the BM right away, which will save compute time later on but costs more storage and access time.

5. Extracting portions of the BM (suppression of categories, more coarse time grid) and combining several such portions of different experiments on one real of tape or on disk to diminish compute time for evaluation and comparison later on.

The evaluation system is based on a set of subroutines which allow non-expert users to design programs without knowledge of physical data storage. As an example a user will always reference a category by a unique number or a mnemonic thus determining the row of the BM. The value of the category may either be requested for a certain point in time or relative to the time of the last request. The system will locate the appropriate record and bitposition resp. evaluate the defining expression. This mode of operation will increase compute time in most cases but will enable easier production and service of user evaluation programs.

As an example for a user evaluation program we will give a short description of the CRITERION-DEPENDING-BEHAVIOR-ANALYSIS (CBA) program. This program performs a noninference data description based on the recognition of "events" within the BM. Certain criteria events will be searched for; there may be restrictions imposed on those events (e.g. certain other events must not occur concurrently). The program will then examine which events out of a given set will occur concurrently or in the neighborhood e.g. just before or after the criterion event. For all occurrences of the criterion a symbolic and a quantitative description of those events is given. Furthermore the CBA program will try to construct a "typical" pattern showing relations between the criterion and other events by means of conditional probabilities. These descriptions may give hints to the researcher which behaviors tend to form patterns e.g. depend on one another in some way. We do not give a test of significance of typical patterns. The reason for this shall be made plausible in the concluding remarks:

A number of methods exist for the statistical analysis of the overall, nonsequential aspects of observational data (e.g. 8). These methods are mostly based on the theory of Markow Chains. SACKETT (1) points out that the more difficult problem is the development of <u>practically useful</u> statistical tools for identifying contingent relationships among behavioral categories. The analysis goal is here to identify and test nonrandom conditional probabilities for simultaneously (5) or sequentially (9) occurring patterns. The test of significance commonly used (χ^2) demands for independence between categories resp. samples; but this does not hold true (10). According to KEHL the method of dual stochastic processes (11) leads to construction of reasonable sample space to ensure independence. Unfortunately a practicable method is not yet available (10). The LAG ANALYSIS (12) demands for exclusiveness and exhaustiveness of the coding system thus being of no use to our problem either. So at the moment we restrict all evaluation to a descriptive kind of reduction of data. This is to our opinion the more adequate treatment of behavioral data in those cases where an explorative data analysis is reasonable.

REFERENCES

1 SACKETT G P (1977) Measurement in observational research. In: Sackett G P (Ed.) Observing behavior. Vol 2, Data collection and analysis methods. UPP: Baltimore
2 SACKETT G P, STEPHENSON E, RUPPENTHAL G C (1973) Digital data acquisition systems for observing behavior in laboratory and field settings. Beh. Res. Methods & Instrumentation 5:344-348
3 SAWIN D B, LANGLOIS J H, LEITNER E F (1977) What do you do after you say hello? Observing, coding and analysing parent-infant interactions. Beh. Res. Methods & Instrumentation 9:425-428
4 TORGERSON L (1977) Datamyte 900. Beh. Res. Methods & Instrumentation 9:405-406
5 BAKEMAN R (1977) Untangling streams of behavior. In: Sackett G P (Ed.) Observing behavior. Vol 2, Data collection and analysis methods. UPP: Baltimore
6 MOTOROLA Inc. (1981) M6800/6802/6808 Mikroprozessor Programmierhandbuch
7 MOTOROLA Inc. (1975) M6800 Application Manual
8 GOTTMAN J M (1977) Nonsequential data analysis techniques in observational re search. In: Sackett G P (Ed.) Observing behavior. Vol 2, Data collection and analysis methods. UPP: Baltimore
9 ALTMAN S A (1965) Sociobiology of the rhesus monkey. J. Theo. Biology 8:490-522
10 KEHL D (1976) Die Identifizierung fördernder und hindernder Reize in sequentiellen Beobachtungsdaten. Unveröffentlichte Diplomarbeit. FU Berlin
11 ROMANOVSKY V I (1970) Discrete Markow Chains. Wolters-Noordhoff: Groningen
12 SACKETT G P (1978) The lag sequential analysis of contingency and cyclicity in behavioral interaction research. In: Osofsky J D (Ed.) Handbook of infant development. Wiley & Sons: New York

DIFFERENTIATED EVALUATION OF THE REGULATION AT VARIOUS INTEGRATION LEVELS OF THE HUMAN ORGANISM BY COMPUTERIZED SYSTEM ANALYSIS

J. Michel, H. Cammann, G.-B. Dümde, B. Koch, G. Sch. Vasadze[+],
G. G. Dumbadze[++]
Institute of Medical Physics and Biophysics of the Medical Faculty
(Charité) of the Humboldt University Berlin, Invalidenstrasse 42,
DDR-1040 Berlin, GDR, [+]Central Research Laboratory (CRL) of the IVth
Main Department of the Ministry of Health of the GSSR, Tbilissi and
[++]CRL of the State Medical Institute, Tbilissi, USSR

1. INTRODUCTION

From scientific and health-care aspects, there is an urgent demand
for methods allowing a representative characterization and objective
(diagnostic/prognostic) assessment of the regulatory behaviour (system behaviour) of the human organism under simulated environmental
load. They are necessary for the clearing up of complex regulation
processes as well as of the pathogenesis of regulatory diseases and
for different goals of preventive medicine. Such methods have become
feasible by modern computer technologies. Starting from these requirements, an automated psychophysiological system-analytic investigation procedure was developed, the theoretical and methodical bases
and technical facilities of which have been described in more detail
elsewhere /1/, /2/. Of the comprehensive possibilities opened up by
this computerized method, here especially those of the differentiated analysis of regulation on various integration levels shall be
treated and the insights thus to be gained.

2. METHODS

As the system-analytic procedure has been described in detail elsewhere /1/, /2/, here only its main features shall be presented necessary to understand the results:

a) Program-controlled dynamic investigation with continuous acquisition of relevant biosignals (cp. Fig. 1) and performance parameters under rest conditions and simulated psychic load in terms
   of a jump function (alternative decisions on optic patterns under
   pressure of time). After a period of subject instruction 5 investigation periods follow: rest 1 (R1), reference period (REF)
   for the later load period (stimulus-response regime without alternative decisions), rest 2(R2), load period(LOAD), rest 3(R3). The

R-periods last 3 min each, REF- and LOAD period 5 min each.

b) Automated information exploiting signal analysis to obtain all relevant information of the transmission properties of system elements and the interaction between subsystems. Computation of characteristics as representatives of the behaviour of the different function parameters in the course of investigation. An insight into the type of characteristics is given in Tab. 1 and 2.

c) Formation of effective combinations of characteristics (ECCh) for the classification of subjects according to their psychophysiological system behaviour; presentation and assessment of results in terms of mathematical-statistical models (MSMs) /2/.

Subjects: The results presented here were obtained by investigations in the following groups of subjects:

Group I: 29 men 29 to 40 years of age, clinically healthy;

Group IIA: 28 men 46 to 56 years of age, without symptoms of IHD and other diseases;

Group IIB: 30 men of the same age as group IIA with symptoms of an IHD (Angina pectoris and/or symptoms of an IHD in rest ECG; ruling out myocardial infarction and stroke).

3. RESULTS AND DISCUSSION

Fig. 1 shows MSMs as results of investigations of subjects of groups I and IIA differing only in age, allowing for different integration levels of the organism. Already by means of an ECCh of the parameters of heart function and respiration a quite reliable discrimination of subjects of both age groups is possible (Fig. 1 above). Its reliability is increased by characteristics of the EMG, indicating changes of the muscle tone during investigation and by skin-conductance characteristics as indicators of hypothalamic sympathetic activation (Fig. 1 centre). It much increases if the highest integration level of the CNS is allowed for by EEG-characteristics (Fig. 1 below).

Tab. 1 allows an insight into the physiological background of discrimination. It is of particular interest that, in the three different ECChs, the two highest ranks of selectivity are occupied by the same characteristics, the first rank held by a characteristics reflecting the adaptation of the heart rate under load conditions expressed much less distinctly in older subjects. This result, which is in good agreement with present knowledge, indicates that biological age could be determined reliably by this method.

Fig. 2 shows the respective results of discrimination of the subjects of groups IIA (healthy) and IIB (IHD patients). With the ECCh allow-

ing only for parameters of
heart function and respiration
the discrimination is still unsatisfactory (Fig. 2 above). It
is improved if EMG- and SC-char-
acteristics are included
(Fig. 2 centre) and made much
more reliable by inclusion of
EEG-characteristics (all sub-

Table 1: Description of the six
first characteristics of effective
combinations underlying the MSMs
shown in Fig. 1 in their rank of
selectivity (Rank). Abbreviations:
MV = mean value, WR = wave rate,
CC = correlat. coeff., R1, REF, R2,
LOAD, R3 = investigation periods,
cp. methods, for further abbreviations see legend of Fig. 1)

Rank	Characteristics

MSM Fig. 1 above
1. HR-max. in the 1st third of LOAD minus HR MV of the 2nd and 3rd third of LOAD
2. HR MV of R3
3. HR MV of R2
4. RR recovery quotient in REF = (RR MV of REF − RR MV of R2) / (RR MV of REF − RR MV of R1)
5. HR trend in R3 (SPEARMAN − CC)
6. RR MV of LOAD minus RR MV of R1

MSM Fig. 1 centre
1.-2. as above
3. SC-initial value of R2 minus final value of REF
4. SC-peak-value time in LOAD (time until SC-maximum in the 1st 15 s)
5. RRV MV of REF minus RRV MV of R1
6. HR trend in R3 (SPEARMAN − CC)

MSM Fig. 1 below
1.-3. as centre
4. RR MV of LOAD minus RR MV of R2
5. EEG-THETA WR-rise of trend in R1
6. EEG-BETA2 WR-rise of trend in R1

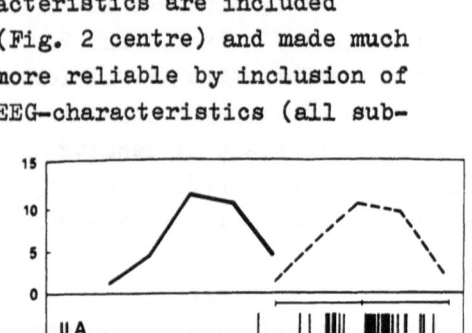

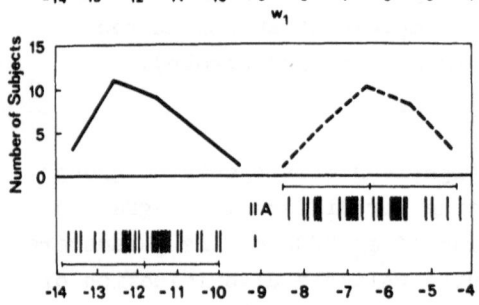

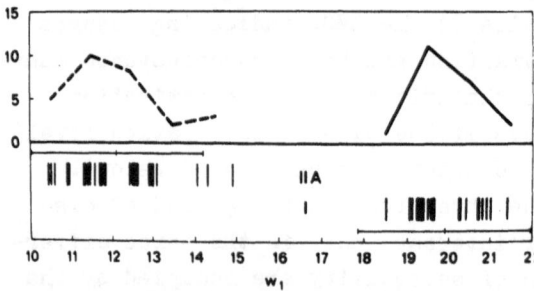

Figure 1: Results of discrimination of subjects of groups
I and IIA by effective combinations of characteristics
(ECCh) of psychophysiological
system behaviour allowing for
different integration levels
of organism. In ECCh the following function parameters
(FP) have been allowed for
and represented by the number
of characteristics in brackets.
Above: 10 characteristics of FP heart rate (HR) (6), heart rate variability (HRV) (0), respiration rate (RR) (2), respiration rate variability (RRV) (2).
Centre: 20 characteristics of FP HR (7), HRV (0), RR (2), RRV (4),
EMG (5), skin conductance (SC) (2).
Below: 14 characteristics of FP HR (3), HRV (0), RR (1), RRV (1),
EMG (1), SC (2), EEG (6).
(For the meaning of characteristics see Tab. 1)

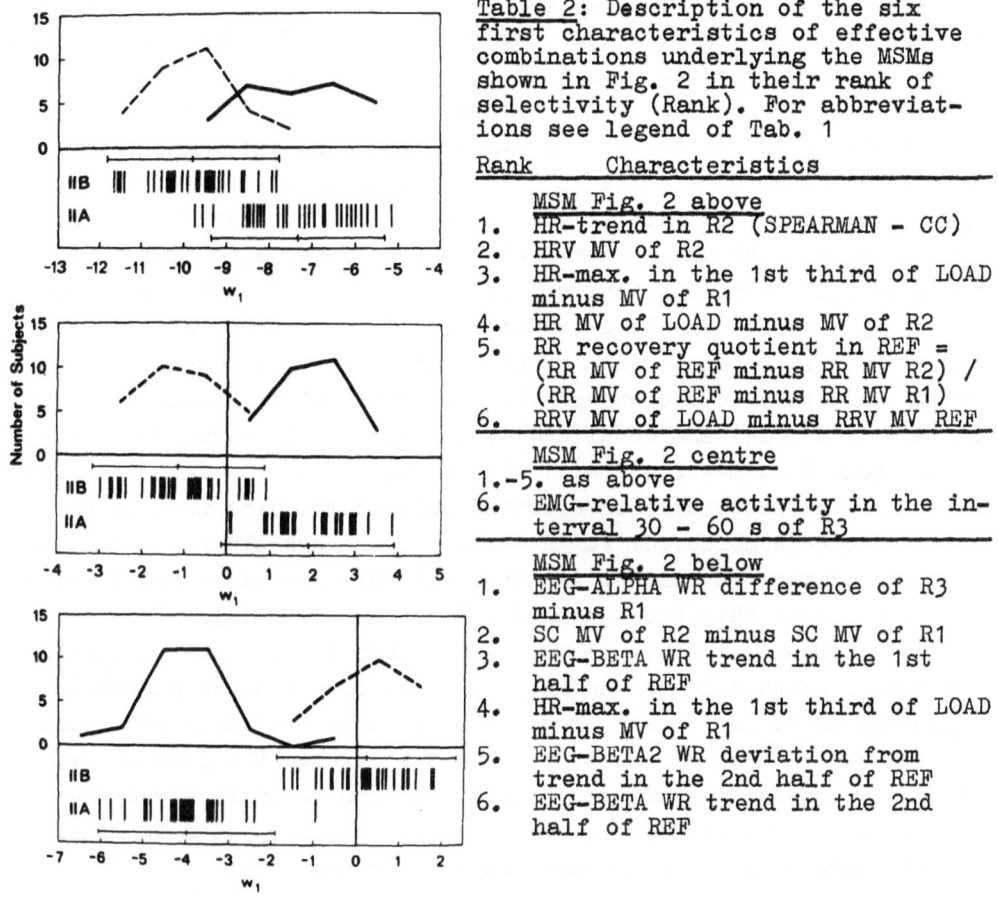

Table 2: Description of the six
first characteristics of effective
combinations underlying the MSMs
shown in Fig. 2 in their rank of
selectivity (Rank). For abbreviations see legend of Tab. 1

Rank	Characteristics
	MSM Fig. 2 above
1.	HR-trend in R2 (SPEARMAN - CC)
2.	HRV MV of R2
3.	HR-max. in the 1st third of LOAD minus MV of R1
4.	HR MV of LOAD minus MV of R2
5.	RR recovery quotient in REF = (RR MV of REF minus RR MV R2) / (RR MV of REF minus RR MV R1)
6.	RRV MV of LOAD minus RRV MV REF
	MSM Fig. 2 centre
1.-5.	as above
6.	EMG-relative activity in the in- terval 30 - 60 s of R3
	MSM Fig. 2 below
1.	EEG-ALPHA WR difference of R3 minus R1
2.	SC MV of R2 minus SC MV of R1
3.	EEG-BETA WR trend in the 1st half of REF
4.	HR-max. in the 1st third of LOAD minus MV of R1
5.	EEG-BETA2 WR deviation from trend in the 2nd half of REF
6.	EEG-BETA WR trend in the 2nd half of REF

Figure 2: Results of discrimination of subjects of groups IIA and
IIB by effective combinations of characteristics (ECCh) of psycho-
physiological system behaviour allowing for different integration
levels of organism. In ECCh the following function parameters (FP)
have been allowed for and represented by the number of character-
istics in brackets (For abbreviations see legend of Fig. 1).
Above: 13 characteristics of FP HR (7), HRV (3), RR (2), RRV (1).
Centre: 18 characteristics of FP HR (3), HRV (1), RR (2), RRV (1),
EMG (10), SC (1).
Below: 19 characteristics of FP HR (1), HRV (0), RR (1), RRV (2),
EMG (2), SC (4), EEG (9).
(For the meaning of characteristics see Tab. 2)

jects of group IIB are correctly and one subject of group IIA wrongly
reclassified - cp. Fig. 2 below). The importance of this result becomes evident by a comparison of the ECChs in Tab. 2. It shows that
allowing for the highest integration level of the organism by including EEG-characteristics, a supplanting of the characteristics of
heart function by those of CNS function from the highest ranks of

selectivity is associated with an increasing reliability of discrimination. Greatest importance is obtained by an EEG-characteristics
reflecting the subject's ability to relax after psychic load, which
is reduced in IHD patients. This result can be considered important
experimental evidence for the hypothesis that, in the development of
IHD, disturbances of the CNS function (disturbances of environmental
adaptation) are of primary (causal) importance. It supports the assumption that, with the system-analytic procedure, also premorbid
states or risky system behaviour with respect to the development of
regulatory diseases can be detected after further optimization. The
results clearly evidence that psychophysiological system-analytic
methods have to take account of the properties of the human organism
as a highly complex and complicated, hierarchically structured dynamic system. This means in particular that, apart from function parameters of the especially interesting subsystems, also such of the
CNS have to be considered. For numerous psychophysiological methods
proposed for various aims of research and for diagnostic and therapeutic procedures this basic demand was not met (see e.g. /3/ and
further references there). In most cases only few peripheral function
parameters, often only HR and HRV, are used to establish generalizing
statements about regulation processes. By the differentiated evaluation of regulation at different integration levels, the limited evidence of one or few regulation parameter(s) can be impressively demonstrated. The results a.o. indicate the possibility of determining
the relevance of function parameters for various aims.

4. REFERENCES

/1/ Michel J: Grundlagen, Methodik und Ergebnisse eines multivariab-
     len dynamischen Untersuchungsverfahrens mit psychischer Bela-
     stung zur quantitativen Erfassung und Differenzierung von Sy-
     stemeigenschaften des menschlichen Organismus - Ein Beitrag zur
     psychophysiologischen Systemanalyse, Dissertation B, Humboldt-
     Universität zu Berlin 1981

/2/ Michel J, Vasadze GSch, Dumbadze GG, Cammann H, Koch B: Mathe-
     matical-statistical Models as a tool for presentation of the
     results of psychophysiological system-analytic investigations,
     in: van Bemmel J, Ball MJ, Wigertz O (eds.): MEDINFO 83 (Amster-
     dam, North-Holland, 1983) 883-886

/3/ Rombouts R: The reproducibility of cardiovascular reactions
     during cognitive tasks, Activ. nerv. sup. (Praha) Suppl. 3
     (1982) 285-294

THE IDENTIFICATION OF A NEW RHEUMATOID DISEASE GROUP
BY MEANS OF MULTIVARIATE STATISTICAL ANALYSIS

H.M.J.Goldschmidt[1],J.den Hartog[2],J.F.Leijten[1],D.Coomans[3] and D.L.Massart[3].

[1]Dept.of Clinical Chemistry and Haematology,Maria Hospital,Tilburg,The Netherlands.

[2]Present address: Pharmacia Nederland b.v., Woerden, The Netherlands.

[3]Farmaceutical Institute, Free University of Brussels, Brussels, Belgium.

A retrospective study was performed on 186 subjects suffering from rheumatic fever, rheumatoid arthritis, lupus erythematosus, gout, arthrosis, osteomyelitis and a group of patients with negative rheuma-serology test results but positive joint complaints. The aim was to examine by means of selected variables the group with negative rheuma-serology test results and positive joint complaints. In order to see if these patients were distinct from the other disease categories or were 'precursor' to one of these disease states. The statistical methods used were: stepwise linear discriminant analysis, k-nearest neighbour method, linear learning machine, hierarchical clustering and principal component analysis.

A definite relationship between the group of patients with negative rheuma-serology test results and those with arthrosis and rheumatoid arthritis was found, while no relationship between this group and the infection processes of osteomyelitis and rheumatic fever could be demonstrated. Approximately 30% of the patients with negative rheuma serology fell into a separate category and may thus represent a new subgroup of rheumatic patients.

INTRODUCTION

Clinical immunology has progressed in the last years with the introduction of more specific and sensitive serological tests for rheumatoid-type diseases e.g. IgM-rheuma factor, IgG-rheuma factor, C-reactive protein. Unfortunately, these as well as the classical tests score a high rate of false positives (up to 40%) and false negatives (up to 20%) compared to the clinical symptoms of rheumatic joint diseases. Therefore, many patients are classified as having rheumatic joint diseases primarily on clinical grounds. Some patients present definite rheumatoid joint complaints but have negative results in a classical rheuma-serology test panel: AST (anti-streptolysine titer), Waaler-Rose test, Latex-fixation test, ANF (antinuclear factor) and PNF (antiperinuclear factor). In these cases, the clinician is tempted to classify the patient as a potential developer of gout. It has also been proposed that a defect in the immunological system is the cause of both complaints and negative test results (1).

In this study we confined ourselves to two related questions. Is the group of patients with definite joint complaints but negative serology test result a separate group with its own character? And, is it a precursor group for one or more disease categories? The application of multivariate statistical methods offers an objective approach of the questions stated.

EXPERIMENTAL

Patients.

From the 186 patients included in this study, 23 were admitted with diagnosis other than rheumatoid diseases but with positive joint complaints and a negative rheuma-serology test panel (NS group). Where the complaint of joint or bone was vague or uncertain, the patient was excluded from the study. Applied medication and subsidiary diagnosis were checked for any coherence and none was found. The NS group was compared with six groups of patients with proven diagnosis and classified according to the ICD.9.CM index (4) (Table 1); a reference group of healthy people with a comparable age distribution was also included.

Variables.

From the medical records of these patients the values of 150 different variables if present were gathered. After the discard of all parameters not available in at least 75% of the patients 39 variables remained, all of a general biochemical, haematological and physical nature. By different feature selection methods we obtained the ten variables most relevant (5): haemoglobin, uric acid, calcium, inorganic phosphate, albumin, alkaline phosphatase, cholesterol, erythrocytes sedimentation rate, bandformed granulocytes and age.

Patient group	Abbr.	Male	Female	Total	ICD.9.CM Index
Rheumatic Fever	RF	8	8	16	711.0 and 711.9
Rheumatoid Arthritis	RA	18	18	36	714.0
Lupus Erythematosus	LE	3	14	17	695.4 and 710.0
Gout	GT	14	7	21	274.
Arthrosis	AR	21	29	50	715.
Osteomyelitis	OS	11	12	23	730.
Negative Rheuma-Serologic test panel	NS	7	16	23	----
Reference	REF	57	29	86	

Table 1. Composition of the selected groups of patients.

Group	A				B			
	SLDA	kNN	LLM	Average	SLDA	kNN	LLM	Average
RF	4.4%	8.7%	1.9%	5.0%	0 %	5%	6%	3.7%
RA	21.7	17.4	13.4	17.5	13.0	8	21	14.0
LE	34.7	8.7	12.1	18.5	8.7	0	12	6.9
GT	8.7	4.4	13.9	9.0	8.7	5	17	10.2
AR	30.4	47.8	56.8	45.0	21.7	39	19	26.6
OS	0.0	13.0	2.0	5.0	0.0	17	8	8.3
NS	----	----	----	----	47.8	26	15	29.6

Table 2. Classification results of the NS group, with (A) and without (B) possible choice for a separate group.

Multivariate statistical methods.

Stepwise linear discriminant analysis (SLDA,2), k-nearest neighbour method (kNN,k=6,3), linear learning machine (LLM,3), hierarchical clustering (3) and principal component analysis (PCA,3).

RESULTS

The rheuma-serologic test results were able to differentiate between several types of rheumatoid and related diseases, e.g. AST correlates with RF, Rose and Latex with RA, and, ANF and PNF with LE. No correlations were found with these rheuma-serology tests and GT, AR and OS. These relations confirmed those known from the literature (6), so the applied multivariate procedures seemed to be sound. In order to avoid reasoning in a circle, the rheuma-serological test results for the NS group are not included since their very classification is based on those results. Comparison with the reference group excluded the possible presence of any malingerers, i.e. the existence of this group as a distinct entity from a group of normals was objectively demonstrated.

Classification criteria were developed (SLDA and LLM) and the NS patients were classified with (A) and without (B) the possible choice for a separate group. In case of the kNN method the training patients consist of six (A) respectively seven (B) categories. The NS patient distribution is expressed as a percentage of their total and averaged (Table 2). Chi-square tests prove that these distributions are significantly different from random frequencies.

Whether the NS patients are considered as a separate category or not, statistical analysis using the three techniques (SLDA, kNN, LLM) demonstrates that they bear virtually no relationship to the OS or RF groupings. On the other hand, they are similar to the patients in the AR and RA groupings. A less certain distinction is permitted in comparison to the LE and GT categories. An average of 30% of the NS patients could be categorized separately. The remaining patients fit a distribution similar to the pattern obtained when no separation of the NS patients was assumed. Similar results were obtained by means of cluster analysis (Figure 1) and PCA (Figure 2). The patients in subgroups A and B are, in general, those who were classified, according to Table 2, in other categories than NS. Subgroup C (30.4%) consists of NS patients that do not belong to one of the other rheumatoid categories. They represent a separate category, a new subgroup of rheumatic patients. The hypothises that the NS patients are gout-precursors could not be substantiated. In fact, looking at uric acid, which is usually considered as the best gout-indicator, again the NS distribution shows no similarity with the gout distribution (Figure 3, Table 2).

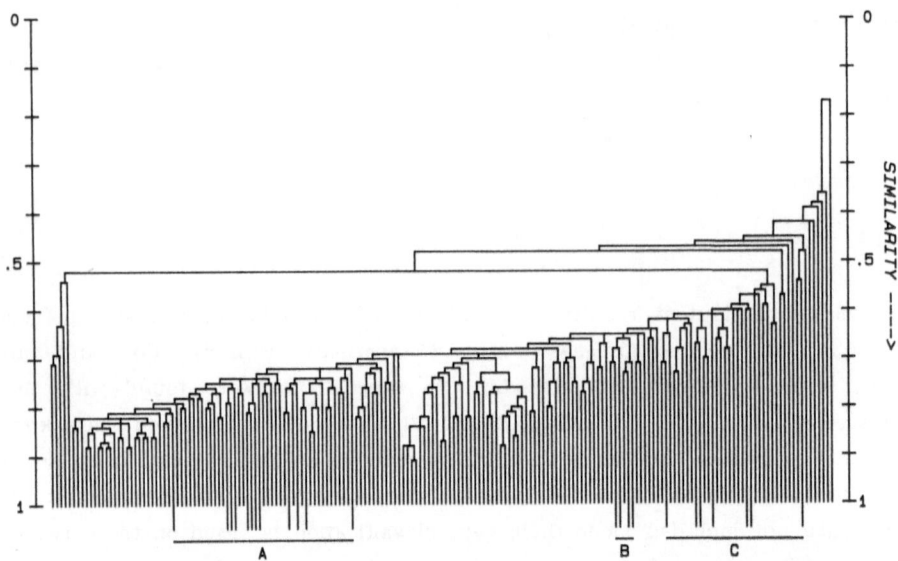

Figure 1. Hierarchical clustering of 186 rheumatoid patients. The 23 NS patients are indicated by the lengthened branches and can be divided into three subgroups A, B and C.

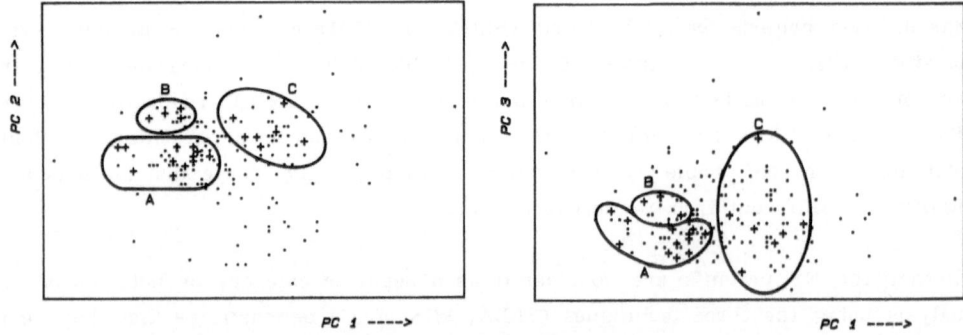

Figure 2. Principal component plots of the plane through PC 1 and PC 2, respectively PC 1 and PC 3 (accounting for 41.5% resp. 34.6% variance). The 23 NS patients are indicated by + and the other patients by . , the three subgroups A, B and C are almost completely identical with those depicted in Figure 1.

DISCUSSION AND CONCLUSIONS

The low percentage of patients in the RF and OS categories tends to eliminate infection as a cause for complaints in the NS group. In addition, the small percentage of patients falling into the gout category argues against their entity as a potential development in the NS patients. The prevalent distribution of the NS patients among the RA and AR categories leads us to believe that these patients might develop either an autoimmune or mechanical type of rheumatoid disease.

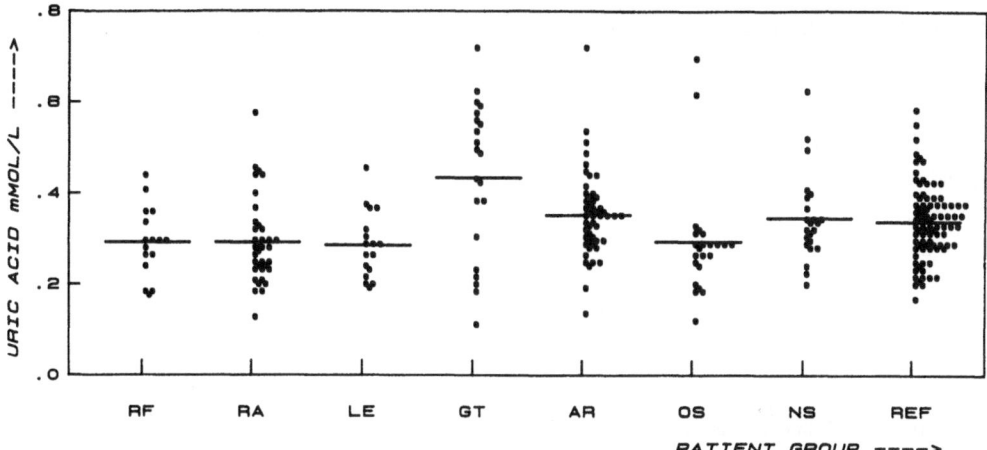

Figure 3. The serum uric acid concentration in mMol/L per patient group. The horizontal bars indicate mean of the distributions. See Table 1 for explanation of abbreviations.

Approximately 30% of the patients with negative rheuma-serology tests and definite joint pain fitted none of the rheumatoid disease categories. This was also illustrated by means of cluster and principal component analysis. These patients are thus classified as NS patients and are distinguishable on the basis of non-serologic tests although their physical complaints are similar to the rheumatoid disease patients. At this moment, we do not have an explanation for these clinical findings. The application of multivariate statistical analysis proved to be of great help in the interpretation of complicated problems such as the quantitative description of a new disease group.

REFERENCES

1. Westendorp Boerma F and Jansz A (1971) Determination of rheumafactors, Labora Clinica, Behringwerke AG., Marburg-Lahn, 3:2
2. Nie NH, Hull CH, Jenkins JG, Steinbrenner K and Bent DH (1975) Statistical Package for the Social Sciences (SPSS), McGraw-Hill, New York, 2nd ed., 434
3. Duewer DL, Koskinen JR and Kowalski BR (1975) ARTHUR available from B.R. Kowalski, Laboratory for Chemometrics, Department of chemistry BG-10, University of Washington Seattle, Washington 98195
4. The international classification of diseases (1978) 9th revision, Clinical modification (ICD.9.CM), Commission on professional and hospital activities, Edwards Brothers, Inc., Ann Arbor
5. Goldschmidt, HMJ, den Hartog J and Leijten JF (1980) The classification of subjects with joint diseases on biochemical and haematological data. Abstracts of the National ABC Meeting, Birmingham, no. 55
6. Eastman RD (1975) Biochemical values in clinical medicine: the results following pathological or physiological change, Whright Ltd., Bristol

A CLINICAL DATABASE FOR THE STUDY OF PROGNOSTIC FACTORS IN BREAST CANCER

J. H. Todd, J. L. Haybittle, R. W. Blamey and D. Pearson
Department of Medical Physics and Surgical Science
City Hospital
Nottingham
United Kingdom

1. Introduction

The treatment of breast cancer has undergone marked changes over the past ten years, based on the statistical analysis of the many factors which may influence the patient's ultimate survival. Most of these factors are present when the patient is first seen at clinic, but other data has to be added as progress following treatment is monitored. The maintenance of an accurate database and the application of the correct statistical analysis is essential for this type of study if maximum information is to be derived and methods of treatment continue to improve (1).

The study of primary breast cancer at the Nottingham City Hospital is one of the largest single centre studies in the world. Over 1200 patients with primary operable invasive carcinoma of the breast have been seen and treated under the care of a single surgeon (RWB). The largest follow-up period is now over eleven years.

This paper describes the implementation of a computerised record system which provides the following facilities:-

a. the recording of clinical data relating to the patient, the tumour and the method of treatment,

b. positive and negative events in follow-up regarding updating local recurrence of the disease, the appearance of distant metastases and treatments,

c. the statistical analysis of the data to study the effect of parameter values on survival or recurrence.

The system we have developed has been in operation for two years and is being used daily by doctors, clerks and scientists.

2. Objective of the System

The objective of the project was to develop a computer system which would provide the clinical research team with rapid statistical analysis of the patient data. The system had to enable:-

a. selection of patients satisfying operator defined criteria,

b. lifetable analysis of the selected patient group by sub-division into sub-groups determined by a parameter value or range,

c. the study of prognostic factors in breast cancer to formulate prognostic indices using multivariate analysis,

d. the software had to be useable by any member of the research team.

3. The Hardware

The hardware is based on the Digital Equipment Corporation's PDP 11/23 processor with 256 kbyte memory and uses two 10 Mbyte Honeywell-Bull exchangeable discs, running under the RT-11 operating system.

4. The Software

a. The Database Structure

Data input, storage and retrieval for individual patients is controlled by a word processing and database manager package, MASS11 (Microsystems Engineering Corporation). MASS11 provides facilities to set up forms for data entry and retrieval. The parameters currently being studied for patients with primary breast cancer is shown in Table 1. Only two forms are used, one to enter the patient into the study and the other to update time dependent parameters, such as survival time or time of death. Individual patient data is updated as soon as it becomes available. If a parameter value is not known then a "not measured" value is entered.

A datafile is generated using MASS11 and is the source of data for statistical analysis. This datafile is regenerated at about six-monthly intervals.

TABLE 1

LIST OF PARAMETERS RECORDED FOR EACH PATIENT

1.	Study number	16.	Oestrogen receptor status
2.	Survival time	17.	Progesterone receptor status
3.	Alive or dead	18.	Adjuvant therapy
4.	Disease free interval	19.	Mode of treatment
5.	Recurrence of disease	20.	Lymph—node classification
6.	Local recurrence time	21.	Tumour type
7.	Presence of local recurrence	22.	Bone metastases present
8.	Axillary recurrence time	23.	Lung metastases present
9.	Presence of axillary recurrence	24.	Viscera metastases present
10.	Age (at presentation)	25.	Prognostic index
11.	Menopause status	26.	Cell reaction
12.	Tumour size	27.	Sinus histiocytosis (1)
13.	Size grading	28.	Sinus histiocytosis (2)
14.	Histological grade	29.	Oestrogen receptor value
15.	Lymph node stage	30.	Progesterone receptor value

b. Statistical Analysis

Statistical analysis of the data requires the operator to define the group of
patients and parameters to be studied. The selection and statistical programmes
have been written and implemented by the authors in FORTRAN.

Selection of Patient Groups

The operator is prompted through the selection routine by carefully designed
screens.

Patient groups are defined by:-

i.   Identifying the number of patients to be selected,

ii. Identifying a parameter and its value that must be satisfied for selection,
     e.g. menopause – post–menopausal. Up to 5 parameters may be ANDed to form
     the patient group,

iii. Identifying a parameter and its range within which the patient's parameter value lies for selection, e.g. age – 40 to 60 years.

Lifetable Analysis

The patient group is sub-divided into sub-groups to compare the survival (or re-currence) time of one parameter value or range with another, e.g. histological grades 1, 2 and 3 can be compared. The time parameter may be survival time, disease-free interval or local recurrence time. The parameter selected for sub-grouping is tested. If it is "not measured" that patient record is rejected. The selected patient records are divided into "withdrawals" and "events" in six-monthly intervals for each sub-group for the lifetable routine (2).

Survival probability for each time interval and sub-group is printed, along with a graphical plot of the survival curves.

Prognostic Factors

After selection of the patient group to be studied, up to 9 parameters may be chosen as covariates in the multivariate analysis. All parameters are tested and if "not measured" that patient record is rejected. A multiple regression method is used to study the relative importance of prognostic factors, i.e. the covariates, to establish a prognostic index which is a more superior predictor of survival time than any single parameter. The application of this method to primary breast cancer has already been described in detail (3).

Manual Data Input

Facility is also provided for the manual entry of data for lifetable and multi-variate analysis as well as other commonly used statistical tests, such as chi-squared, Wilcoxon rank tests, etc.

4. Discussion

The implementation of the clinical database system has enabled the rapid analysis of 30 parameters recorded for each of 1200 patients. Typically, a lifetable analysis of all patients takes less than five minutes, whereas by manual methods this would take two man-days. The speed of identification of patient groups and of analysis has quickened the pace of research and resulted in the rapid testing of hypotheses.

The Prognostic Index is used to determine the appropriate treatment for each patient as it gives a good prediction of clinical outcome. Our own research is aimed at refining the index for survival and studying the factors which determine whether and where recurrence of the disease occurs (4).

From time to time additional parameters are entered into the database. Modifications to the data entry forms or the creation of an additional form to enter the extra parameters is simple. The patient group selection programme only requires the list of parameters (as shown in Table 1) and the number of parameters for each patient to be modified. Thus advances in histology, methods of treatment, etc. may be easily accommodated.

The software is continually being improved and is now in the process of being rewritten in BASIC to run under the CP/M operating system.

References

1. Blamey, R. W., Elston, C. W., Haybittle, J. L., Griffiths, K.: Prognosis in Breast Cancer, The Nottingham Tenovus Trial. Comm. Res. Breast Disease 3: 93-112, 1982.

2. Mould, R. F.: Cancer Statistics. Published by Adam Hilger, Bristol, U.K., 1983.

3. Haybittle, J. L., Blamey, R. W., Elston, C. W., Johnson, J., Doyle, P. J., Campbell, F. C., Nicholson, R. I., Griffiths, K.: A Prognostic Index in Primary Breast Cancer, Br. J. Cancer 45: 361-366, 1982.

4. Ellis, I. O., Hinton, C. P., MacNay, J., Elston, C. W., Robbins, A., Owaihati, A.A., Blamey, R. W., Baldwin, R. W., Ferry, B.: Immunocytochemical staining of breast carcinoma with the monoclonal antibody NCRC-11: A new prognostic indicator. B.M.J. 290: 881-4, 1985.

Simulation of cell kinetics in the intestinal tract

H.P. Meinzer

German Cancer Research Center
Institute of med. and biol. Informatics
Heidelberg, FRG

B. Sandblad

UDAC

Uppsala, Sweden

Abstract

The mucosa of the intestinal tract is well suited for kinetic studies mainly due to
its relatively simple geometric structure, its accessibility and the high proliferation rate. Our computer model controls simulation of spatial, structural and time
aspects. Comparison with published data allows interesting answers to models and speculations in the field. We suggest a theory for the control of proliferation by the
number of generations since leaving the stem cell.

Introduction

A theory of intestine cell dynamics must by necessity be dynamic which means that it
must be formulated as a dynamic model. Furthermore it is important that such a model
allows calculation and prediction of system behaviour under different circumstances.
Only by using a dynamic model it will be possible to interprete the enormous amount
of experimental data available in the correct context, and to suggest further experiments that must be performed for continued theory formulation.

The Biology of the System

The inner wall of the intestine, the mucosa, is a system well suited for studies of
cell kinetics in epithelial tissues. In the intestine the proliferation rates are high
- the tissue is completely renewed within a few days - and the cell structures are
rather simple. The intestine consists of several parts such as duodenum, small intestine (jejunum and ileum), colon and rectum. These parts have partly different cell
characteristics.

The inner surface of the mucosa consists of a set of extending projections. From these
folds the villi are extended. Between the villi there are depressions called crypts.
The crypts are present in all segments of the intestine, while the villi vary in size,
and are not at all present in e.g. the colon. The villi and the crypts are covered by
a cell layer exactly one cell thick. New cells are being born in the lower part of the
crypt and migrate upwards to the top of the villus where they finally fall of the
tissue.

The surface of the crypt-villus system can be devided into four regions or compartments. The cells are born in the two lower compartments, mature in the third compartment and perform their functional activities in the fourth compartment. Cell loss is
assumed to take place in the upper part of the villus, or in the upper part of the
crypt when no villus exists. The cell migration process is similar to that found in
the skin, where cells are born in lower levels, mature while travelling towards the
surface and are finally being worn off.

A widly accepted model for basic cell kinetics is the following. During its life a
cell cycles through four phases, G_1-, S-, G_2 and M-phase. S is the synthesis phase,
G_1 and G_2 are intermediate phases and M is the mitosis phase. During mitosis a cell
is split up into two new cells. Cells in mitosis in the upper part of the proliferation zone have an increasing probability to divide into nonproliferating, maturing,
cells.

In this model of cell kinetics it is necessary to assume the existance of a 'stem
cell', an eternally proliferating and to its position fixed cell. In order to maintain
structure, this 'stem cell' must be located near the bottom of the crypt and the migration of new cells is towards the villus. The crypt bottom is populated with an
other cell type, the paneth cells.

A more complete model of the crypt should also include other types of cells, but this
would not effect the basic kinetic assumptions. This means that we can study the crypt
cell kinetics by a linear model describing one column of crypt cells. Differentiation
and migration are processes with a gradient from the bottom to the top. Several descriptions of crypt cell structures, supporting the assumptions above, can be found
in e.g. [APPL80], and in [CAIR65].

The Crypt Model

Since our model will be used for verification of model hypothesis it must be very
modular, so that new model elements easily can be included. The model therefore exists
in many different versions, and what is described below should be regarded as one
example. The model is based on the assumption of a linear, nonturbulent migration from
crypt bottom towards the villus. In the model a cell is described by:

- its identification (name),
- its position in the crypt column,
- its phase in the kinetic cycle,
- its generation (number of mitosis since 'stem cell'),
- its age (since last mitosis).

The cell cycle dynamics is described by the phase transition time distributions. The
type of distribution can be a normal, lognormal or gamma-distribution.

The phase transition time is a stochastic variable. In the model phase transition times can also be made functions of position.

After leaving the M-phase, a cell splits into two new cells. If the 'split evant' occurs at position i in generation g, the attributes of cells with a position j (with j < i), are not changed, while cells in higher positions are shifted one position up.

The dynamic control of the size of the proliferating zone can be described in two different ways. For the 'slow cut-off' version a model suggested by carnie in [CARN65] has been used. Here the probability for a cell split to result in two new proliferating cells is a function of the location. Our own main contribution in the theoretical field is the 'generation cut-off' model, where we assume that there exists a generation g^{max}, so that when a cell of generation g^{max} is divided into two new cells, these are both nonproliferating. With this assumption we can very nicely simulate experimental results. After last mitosis the nonproliferating cells have a lifetime which is determined by a stochastic parameter of the same distribution as is used for the cell cycle time. When cell death occurs the cell leaves the column, and the length is reduced by one position.

It has been experimentally found that the number of paneth cells in the crypt bottom can vary. This means that the stem cell is not always in a fixed position, but the position is described by a distribution. Such a 'stem cell distribution' has been included in the model so that the simulation results can be compared to experimental results.

Implementation and Execution

The simulation model is implemented as an interactive computer model. It exists in two versions, one written in FORTRAN and one in SIMULA. Together with the model of the crypt cell dynamics, the CRYPT program also contains a set of facilities for design, execution and evaluation of simulation experiments.

A simulation experiment is initiated by the input of model and experiment specification data. Such data consist of e.g.:

Model specification data:
- phase time distribution and parameters,
- lower and upper limits for proliferation cut-off region, or number of proliferating generations,
- life-time of cells after last mitosis,
- paneth- and stem-cell distributions.

Experiment of specification data:
- length of simulation run and intervals between reports,
- start values for random number generators.

During the experiment reports on model behaviour can be shown on a terminal, but normally results are stored for later evaluation.

The design of the model output has been made in order to fulfill the objectives, i.e. to show dynamic properties of the system and to varify/falsify model hypotheses. This means that we calculate such information that is compatible with experimental data normally found in literature. The calculations are sometimes made by 'simulated experiments on the simulated crypt' during execution of the model. Whenever new aspects of the crypt dynamics are studied, it is very easy to extend the possibilities to select appropriate output.

Today we have the following 'output menu' available:

- various single variables such as growth fraction, mean mitotic index, migration and production rates etc.,
- crypt length distribution,
- cell age distribution,
- migration rate over column,
- mitotic index,
- labelling index,
- FLM (fraction of labelled mitosis),
- cell generation distribution over column,
- fraction of proliferating cells over column,
- distribution of number of mitosis per column.

All output information can be shown directly as pictures on a graphic terminal. It is also possible to include stored data from experimental findings in the pictures. In this way it is possible to directly compare experimental results with model results.

Discussion

It has been shown that the basic kinetic behaviour of the intestine crypt cell system can be simulated by the CRYPT model. The purpose of this model is however not only to represent this rather simple structure, but to provide a tool for formulation and validation of hypotheses concerning structural and kinetic dynamics.

The model, as described above, can be used for various studies within its scope of validity. Even so it provides a tool for studies which have no comparison in normal experimental work on dead tissue. With the model, the modelled dynamic behaviour can be studied for 'normal' as well as for 'unnormal' cell growth. Examples of such studies will be published elsewhere.

More important than results is however the methodology as such. It is easy to understand that for formulation of theories of the studied system, it is necessary to use dynamic, structural models. If we want to build models which include dynamic structural descriptions of the crypt and other parts of the intestinal tissues if we want to study transient changes in kinetics or in structures, or if we study control structures which control the dynamic behaviour of the system, then we can not do this in any other way than by using simulation techniques. The system is too complex for any other modelling approach.

This latter problem area, the study of control structures, is probably one most challanging area for future studies. In literature several speculations about control mechanisms for the normal and for different malfunctioning cell systems can be found. To formulate a theory of such mechanisms it is however necessary to study the concurrent effects of a set of interacting control functions. The control functions can be of different biomedical nature and they can be cell internal or external. A model, with a relevant scope of validity, could be developed in the form of a simulation model, and be used for validation of hypotheses concerning such complex and dynamic structures.

References

[AL-D74] Al-Dewachi, H.S., Wright, N.A., Appleton, D.R., Watson, A.J.: The Cell cycle Time in the Rat Jejunal Mucosa. Cell Tissue Kinet 7, 587-594 (1974).

[APPL80] Appleton, D.R.,Sunter, J.P., Watson, A.J.: Cell Proliferation in the Gastrointestinal Tract. Pitman Medical, Bath, U.K., 1980.

[BJER81] Bjerknes, M., Cheng, H.: The Stem-Cell Zone of the Small Intestinal Epithelium. III. Evidence from Columnar, Enteroendocrine, and Mucous Cells in the Adult Mouse. Am.J.Anat. 160, 77-91 (1981).

[CAIR65] Cairnie, A.B., Lamerton, L.F., Steel, G.G.: Cell Proliferation Studies in the Intestinal Epithelium of the Rat. II. Theoretical Aspects. Experimental Cell Research 39, 539-553 (1965).

[CHEN] Cheng, H., Leblond, C.P.: Origin, Differentiation and Renewal of the Four Main Epithelial Cell Types in the Mouse Small Intestine. 1. Columnar Cell. Am. J. Anat. 141, 461-480.

[LEBL76] Leblond, C.P., Cheng, H.: Identification of Stem Cells in the Small Intestine of the Mouse. In Cairnie et al. (eds.): Stem Cells of Renewing Populations. Academic Press, New York, 1976.

[POTT80] Potten, C.S.: Proliferative Cell Populations in Surface Epithelia: Bilogical Models for Cell Replacement. In Jäger, W., Rost, H., Tautu, P. (eds.): Biological Growth and Spread, Mathematical Theories and Applications. Proceedings, Heidelberg 1979. Springer-Verlag, Berlin - Heidelberg - New York, pp. 23-35 (1980).

[TSUB81] Tsubouchi, S.: Kinetic Analysis of Epithelial Cell Migration in the Mouse Descending Colon. Am. J. Anat. 161, 239-246 (1981).

[TUTT73] Tutton, P.J.M.: Variations in Crypt Cell Cycle Time and Mitotic Time in the Small Intestine of the Rat. Virchows Arch. Abt. B. Zellpath. 13, 68-78 (1973).

[WRIG72] Wright, N., Morley, A., Appleton, D.: Variation in the Duration of Mitosis in the Crypts of Lieberkuhn of the Rat; a Cytokinetic Study Using Vincristine. Cell Tissue Kinet 5, 351-364 (1972).

REAL-TIME MATHEMATICAL MODELLING OF PLASMA LEVELS OF I.V. ADMINISTERED DRUGS.

M. RUCQUOI, F. CAMU, E. GEPTS.
Department of Anesthesiology
Academisch Ziekenhuis
Vrije Universiteit Brussel
Laarbeeklaan 101 - 1090 Brussel

Many new compounds devoid of the potentially harmful side-effects of inhalation anesthetics are now widely used. Although most of those new narcotic analgesics, hypnotics and neuro-muscular blocking agents are short-lived, it sometimes remains difficult to determine, measure and maintain a constant level of anesthesia when using discrete reinjections of intravenous agents. Moreover, such reinjections may lead to overdosage.

Aside from the use of various monitoring devices, an understanding of the pharmacokinetics of intravenous anesthetics can provide an additional clue for the optimization of their use. The kinetics of most of those drugs have been successfully fitted to mamillary two or three-compartment models, the kinetic mass balance equations of which are :

$$V_1 \cdot \frac{d}{dt} C_1(t) = -(k_{12} + k_{13} + k_{10}) \cdot V_1 C_1(t) + k_{12} V_2 C_2(t) + k_{13} V_3 C_3(t)$$

$$V_2 \cdot \frac{d}{dt} C_2(t) = -k_{21} \cdot V_2 C_2(t) \qquad\qquad + k_{12} V_1 C_1(t) \qquad\qquad (1)$$

$$V_3 \cdot \frac{d}{dt} C_3(t) = -k_{31} \cdot V_3 C_3(t) \qquad\qquad + k_{13} V_1 C_1(t)$$

The k_{ij}'s can be estimated from experimental data.

The general solution of (1) is

$$C_1(t) = P \exp(-\pi t) + A \exp(-\alpha t) + B \exp(-\beta t)$$

$$C_2(t) = P' \exp(-\pi t) + A' \exp(-\alpha t) + B' \exp(-\beta t) \qquad\qquad (2)$$

$$C_3(t) = P'' \exp(-\pi t) + A'' \exp(-\alpha t) + B'' \exp(-\beta t)$$

π, α, β and the P's, A's and B's being simply arithmetic computed from the known k_{ij}'s.

When injected into the central compartment, a known amount of drug x_o gives a known initial concentration, $C_1(o) = x_o/V_1$, which imposes the initial conditions of the system :

$$P + A + B = C_1(o)$$
$$P' + A' + B' = o \tag{3}$$
$$P'' + A'' + B'' = o$$

A series of BASIC routines have been written, that allow digital and graphical display of the drug levels of the body compartments following one single I.V. injection, according to (2) and (3).

Using the superposition principle, stating that each individual dose of drug is redistributed and excreted independently of every other dose, a simple overlay computing technique is used for simulation of multiple-dose regimens.

The program is organized in 4 modules :

(1) management (updating and data retrieval of a little data bank of kinetic constants)

(2) storing of drug single bolus amounts, entered at the keyboard

(3) updating of the blood level predictions

(4) graphical display (x/t plot or model representation).

The program is currently run under DOS on an IBM personal computer with 256K core memory. Used in the operating theatre in real-time, it allows an estimation of the current plasma levels of the various drugs administered. Moreover, with time acceleration simulation, extrapolation in the future of their decline and the simulation in time of an additional bolus are made possible.

Used with time acceleration or reversal simulation, it allows teaching of pharmacokinetic principles.

It can be used for any drug, provided its kinetic constants are known.

SYSTEMATIC DEVELOPMENT OF A HOSPITAL INFORMATION SYSTEM WITH DISTRIBUTED DATA- AND METHODBASE SYSTEMS: THE AACHMED PROJECT

A. Winter, R. Haux and K.-P. Schleisiek

Abteilung Medizinische Statistik und Dokumentation der RWTH

Pauwelsstraße, D-5100 Aachen

Federal Republic of Germany

Summary: For the Aachen Hospital a concept for a distributed computer-supported information system will be presented. The concept is based logically on distributed data- and methodbase systems (DMBSs) and physically on a set of computers being connected by a local net. As a particulary important DMBS a central information component with a relational database management system is used. This DMBS is, in part, implemented on a database machine. The properties of the concept will be discussed.

Keywords: Hospital information systems; data- and methodbase systems; local area networks.

1. Introduction

Computer-supported hospital information systems are often characterized by having (semi-) autonomous, independently developed application systems (see e.g. Sawinski et al., 1985), and, as Reichertz (1982) pointed out, it is expected that there will be even a growing proliferation of such dedicated and task-oriented systems. However, because of several reasons (Langefors, 1974), there is a need for structuring such systems in order to efficiently provide information and therefore to help to improve the patients' treatment.

In this paper we will briefly point out our system design for the hospital at the Aachen University of Technology. We try to consider the local requirements ((semi-) autonomous systems, especially an application system for medical documentation (Drießen, Raab and Stoll, 1985), availability of a local area network). Our basic (and quite simple) idea is, to model the computer-supported part of the hospital information system logically as a set of (semi-) autonomous data- and methodbase systems which can be interfaced. In order to efficiently provide information a standardized data-communication between these systems will be offered and supported. The AACHMED (computer-supported part of the AAchen MEDical Information System) is an open system, which enables adding, changing or omitting of data- and methodbase systems. Within AACHMED

1. medical and administrative tasks can be integrated,

2. the systems can remain as autonomous as possible, therefore

3. the responsibility of data storage and acquisition can remain at the 'owner' of the data.

Due to this properties, especially due to an increased user's responsibility for his data it can be hoped that data quality can be improved.

Related approaches can be found in Peterson and Isaksson (1982).   Schneider (1982) outlines the complexity of this task, which, in our opinion, can particulary be solved, if the single parts of the whole system can be kept small and - as Wirth (1974) stated for program development - 'intellectually managable'.

2. Hospital Information System

2.1 Logical View

On the logical level AACHMED consists of a set of data- and methodbase systems which are interconnected with a logical net (figure 1). A data- and methodbase system (DMBS) consists of a database and a methodbase. The database and the methodbase are managed by a data- and methodbase management system (DMBMS, figure 2). The DMBMS can activate methods (implemented as programs) of the methodbase and access to data structures of the database. For a more precise definition of a DMBS see Haux (1983). With the logical net, the DMBSs can be interfaced. AACHMED, as the computerized part of the Aachen hospital information system, serves for providing information. The databases can contain medical records, administrative data, laboratory data etc. . The methods can acquire, update or retrieve data.

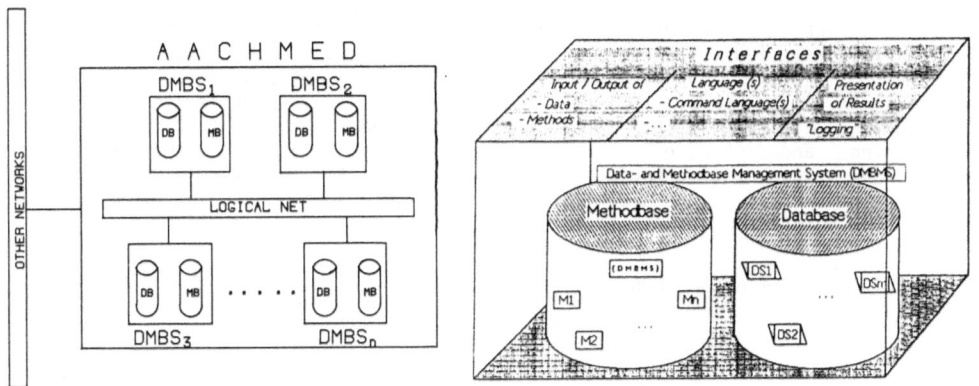

Figure 1: AACHMED, logical view.

Figure 2: Structure of a data-
and methodbase system, (DS:
data structures, M: methods).

Let us briefly mention that such a set of DMBSs with a logical net can itself be
seen as a DMBS and that Wirth's well-known technique of stepwise refinement can be
used in this environment, too. The above mentioned approach can also be formalized,
in order to define and obtain criteria for well-structuredness, especially if the
databases are based on the relational model (Codd, 1979), and if we use concepts
like variables, types and values (as is demonstrated for relational databases in
Schlageter and Stucky, 1983 and for DMBSs in Haux, 1983).

2.2 Physical View

On the physical level AACHMED can be regarded as a set of computers, terminals and a
local area network, where the DMBSs and the logical net have to be suitably mapped
on (figure 3). Note that several DMBSs can be implemented on one computer and that
a DMBS can also use several computers. The logical net is not only implemented by
the local area network but also, e.g., through file exchange, if two DMBS run on the
same computer.

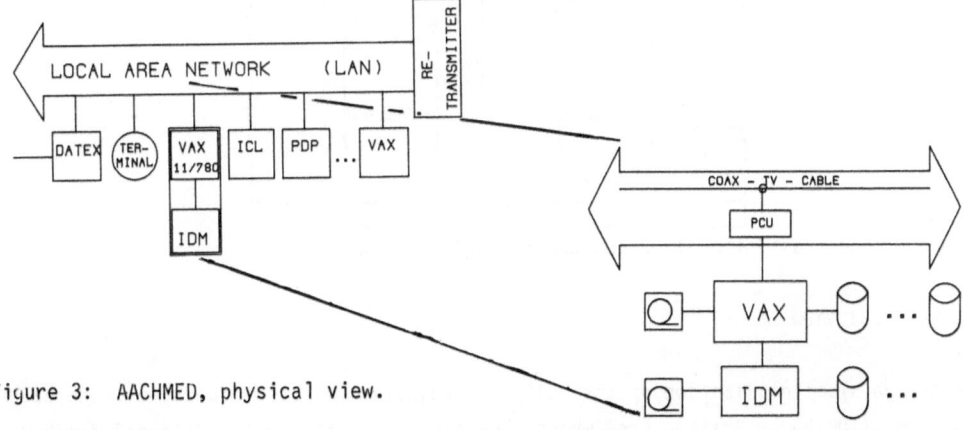

Figure 3: AACHMED, physical view.

For a local area network (LAN), as it is used, excellent physical conditions are provided inside the Aachen Hospital, as with the construction of the building a CATV-net was installed. This cable is used for broadband communication by means of a CSMA/CD protocol, where packets are switched between so called packet communication units (PCUs). These PCUs (Local Net 20) provide communication standards up to level 5 of the ISO-OSI model (see e.g. Fink, 1982), which means establishing and keeping so called "sessions" between any pair of terminal and/or computer connected to a PCU. Hence, for interfacing DBMSs through the local-area-network nothing but the communication-programs have to be provided. For external interfacing a DATEX-connection is planned.

3. Central Information Component

3.1 Logical View

For structuring the exchange of data between DMBSs a special DMBS - a central information component (CIC) - is offered to the users. The CIC provides standardized data communication between the DMBSs and stores data which are needed globally, i.e. by several users. Stimulated by Eckert (1984) we designed a special data structure, the so-called pick-up box (PUB). Every time a user- (or a DMBS-) specified event occures in the CIC, the CIC deposits a corresponding notice into a specified PUB. The user, or DMBS, respectively, authorized to read the PUB can pick-up the data (figure 4). E.g., if some biochemical tests (SGOT, SGPT,...) for a patient are ordered, the order is put in the corresponding PUB of a laboratory DMBS. With this CIC, especially with its possibility of providing asyncronous, transaction-oriented processing, we try to keep the DMBSs as autonomously as possible.

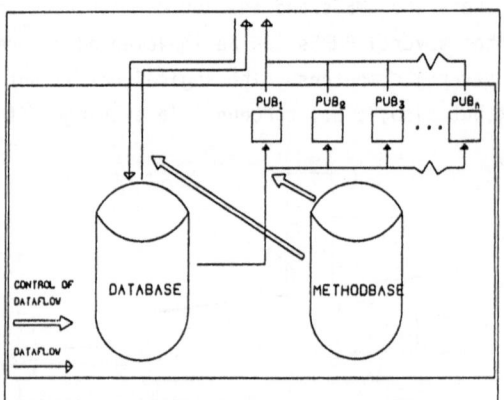

Figure 4: Central information component, logical view.

3.2 Physical View

For the physical realization of the CIC a dedicated database machine has been selected (IDM 500, Britton Lee),which achieves an efficient relational database management by dedicated hardware and implemented software for data definition and manipulation (figure 3). The database machine serves a host, which is a VAX 11/780.

4. Discussion

A logical view via elements like logical net and distributed DMBSs seems a well feasible method for describing the computer-supported parts of a hospital information system. By that logical view a central information component can be modelled and implemented quite easily, which provides standardized data-communication and asynchronous data processing. Data protection (security and privacy) and quality are intended to be improved by keeping data and the responsibility for the data at the data owner, as far as possbile. The system's availability is improved by keeping the connected DMBSs as autonomously as possible.

Acknowledgements: Thanks are due to U. Eckert, Heidelberg, whose experience and critique strongly influenced our ideas. This work has been supported by the Deutsche Forschungsgemeinschaft.

References

Codd, E.F. (1979). Extending the database relational model to capture more meaning. ACM Trans. Database Syst. 4, 397-434.

Drießen, H., Raab, F., Stoll, U. (1985). AACHMED: Benutzer- und Systemhandbuch - Version II. Technical report, Abt. Med. Statistik und Dokumentation, RWTH Aachen.

Eckert, U. (1985). Das Heidelberger Klinikinformationssystem - Kopplungskonzept und Erfahrungen. Manuscript of a talk, given at the Aachen University of Technology.

Fink, R.L. (1982). A status report on local net technology. Peterson, H.E., Isaksson, A.I. (eds.).Communication networks in health care, 51-60. Amsterdam: North-Holland.

Haux, R. (1983). Statistical analysis systems - construction and aspects of method design. Stat. Software Newsl. 9, 106-115.

Langefors, B. (1874). Information systems. Rosenfeld, J.L. (ed). Information Processing 74, 937-945. Amsterdam: North-Holland.

Peterson, H.E., Isaksson, A.I. (eds., 1982). Communication networks in health care. Amsterdam: North-Holland.

Reichertz, P.L. (1982). Future developments of data processing in health care. Meth. Inform. Med. 21, 55-58.

Sawinski, R., Möhr, J.R., Wiederspohn, J., Koch, A. (1985). Design and prototyping of components of a hospital information system. Submitted for publication.

Schlageter, G., Stucky, W. (1983). Datenbanksysteme: Konzepte und Modelle, 2nd edition. Stuttgart: Teubner.

Schneider, W. (1982). Why and how to use communication networks in health care - the systems analytical background. Peterson, H.E., Isaksson, A.I. (eds.).Communication networks in health care, 91-100. Amsterdam: North-Holland.

Wirth, N. (1974). On the composition of well-structured programs. ACM Comp. Surveys 6, 248259.

Record Linkage in Cancer Registration

T. Broz, Dr. E. A. Clarke
The Ontario Cancer Treatment and Research Foundation
7 Overlea Boulevard
Toronto, Ontario M4H 1A8
Canada

INTRODUCTION

Ontario is the most populous province of Canada with a population of approximately 8.5 million and covers an area of more than one million square kilometres. The Ontario Cancer Registry is operated by the Ontario Cancer Treatment and Research Foundation which is a statutory organization funded by the Ontario Ministry of Health. The Foundation operates Regional cancer treatment and research Centres in seven major cities within Ontario. Approximately 50% of all cancer patients in Ontario are referred to these Centres.

There is no legal requirement to register a case of cancer in Ontario although the Foundation, under an act of the provincial legislature, has the mandate to collect and compile information on all cancer cases in the province. It has, therefore, been necessary for the Foundation to use sources of information other than the records of patients treated at its Centres to create a population-based Registry.

Sophisticated computer techniques have been developed by the Foundation to create cancer registrations from the 175,000 records received annually from various sources. Two principle systems used in the registry will be described in "Record Linkage" and Case Resollution".

RECORD LINKAGE

Hospital information on all patients is provided to the Ministry of Health in machine readable form by an independent organization called the Hospital Medical Records Institute. Legally, every hospital in the province must provide this information on every patient discharged. Hospital information on cancer patients is extracted from this file by the Ministry and is then forwarded on magnetic tape to the Foundation.

RECORD LINKAGE - Cont'd

The Registrar General in Ontario is responsible for recording all births, marriages and deaths in the province. Annually, the Foundation receives a computer file of all deaths from that source.

Paper copies of pathology reports on specimens diagnosed as malignant are voluntarily forwarded to the Foundation by ninety-five percent of pathology laboratories in the province. Information from these reports is abstracted and coded by Registry staff and entered directly into the computer using an on-line system developed by the Foundation.

The same patient may be recorded in more than one of these files and often more than once in the same file. Thus a patient who is admitted to hospital twice in one year, has a biopsy taken and is treated at one of the Foundation's Centres, will appear in the hospital file, the pathology file, and in the Foundation patient file. To register every patient only once, requires linking all records pertaining to the same patient. In many areas of the world this is done manually. However, because of the volume of reports received by the Ontario Cancer Registry, together with the fact that there is no unique identifying number in Ontario, the Registry uses a computerized record linkage system. A Generalized Iterative Record Linkage System (GIRLS) was developed by Statistics Canada in conjunction with the National Cancer Institute of Canada. A schematic representation of the system is shown in Figure 1.

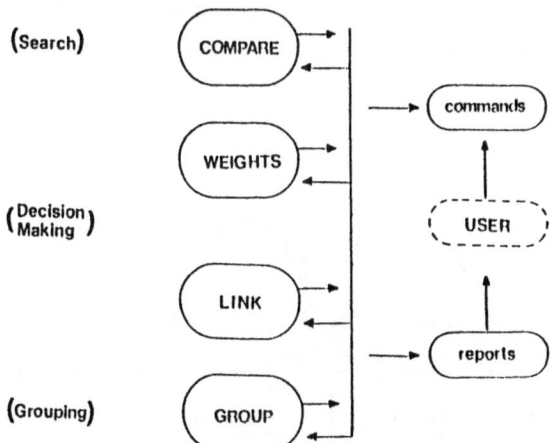

FIGURE 1 - GENERALIZED ITERATIVE RECORD LINKAGE SYSTEM (GIRLS)

RECORD LINKAGE - Cont'd

In the first phase, records are compared to each other and pairs of records which appear to belong to the same patient are identified as potential links. Further computer processing examines only these potential links.

The weight phase evaluates the quality and significance of agreement and disagreement between individual data items on the pair of records involved in a potential link. A numeric score known as a "weight" is assigned to the result of the comparison of each item and these individual weights are then added together to obtain a total weight for the potential link. The greater the total weight the greater the probability that the two records linked by the pro- gramme belong to the same individual. Using the total weight, the link phase classifies all links into three categories: definite, possible and rejected. In the group phase, records belonging to the same individual are formed into groups. Thus, if record A links to record B and record B links to record C, then records A, B, and C are all identified as being the same group and are considered to belong to the same individual.

The word iterative in the name GIRLS refers to the fact that it is possible and actually advisable to repeat this process more than once. This permits the system, with the help of the user, to re- view previous observations and improve the results of the linkage by assigning more precise weights. The distribution of the number of links compared to the total weights is shown in Figure 2.

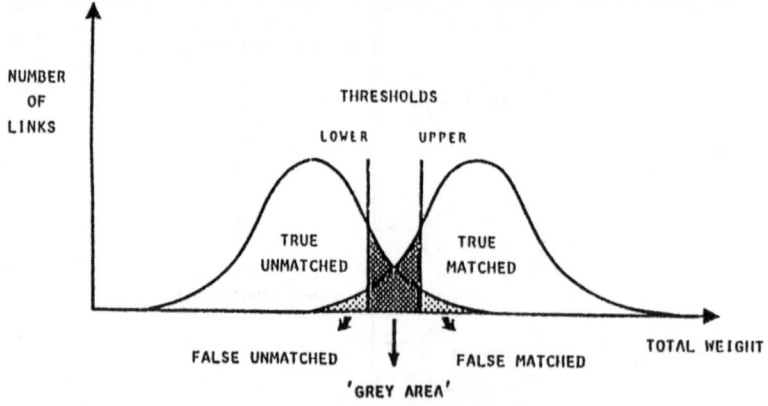

FIGURE 2 - DISTRIBUTION OF THE NUMBER OF LINKS BY TOTAL WEIGHT

RECORD LINKAGE - Cont'd

   The majority of links tend to cluster around the highest and
lowest weights. The area between these two clusters is called
"the grey area" and generally contains the fewest number of links.
These links are reviewed manually and the human decision overrides
the decision of the computer. Manual resolution minimizes the
number of false links and missed true links.

   Many data items may be used in comparing two records during the
linkage process but no single data item is essential. Name, sex,
date of birth, and health insurance number (which refers to a family
not an individual) are frequently used. In general, the more information used for comparison in the records, the better the results of
the linkage.

   Linkages of files are performed in sequence. Hospital reports
are first internally linked, then linked to pathology reports. The
resulting file is linked to previous incidence data and provides
provisional incidence data. More specific information about site,
histology, treatment, and stage of disease, is provided by linking
this file to records of patients seen at the Foundation's Centres.
Finally, the linkage with the death file provides information on the
number of cases reported by death certificate only, and provides a
method of inactive follow-up for patients in the Registry.

   The patient identifying information on all patients in the
Registry is used in linkages with other cohorts of individuals for
studies in cancer etiology and for monitoring cancer risk in occupational groups. The existence of the data in machine readable form
and the experience of the Registry in using computerized record
linkage techniques facilitates the task of undertaking cohort studies
of this nature.

CASE RESOLUTION

   The linkage process identifies patients; however, in order to be
able to report cancer cases rather than patients, the Registry uses
a computer programme known as "Case Resolution" which was developed
at the Foundation. Case Resolution examines all the records for one
patient, determines the site of disease, the histology, the date of
first diagnosis and method of diagnosis.

CASE RESOLUTION - Cont'd

The Case Resolution programme will also identify multiple primary
tumours occuring in the same individual. The philosophy of the
Ontario Cancer Registry is that a second tumour occurring in the same
patient is considered metastatic unless shown otherwise. The site of
a second tumour must be in a different 3 digit rubric according to
the International Classification of Diseases. The morphology of the
second tumour must also be different from the first. The time
interval between the occurrence of the second tumour and the first
is not taken into account.

The case resolution programme consists of several phases. First,
it identifies the most likely site of cancer, then all records
supporting or confirming the selected site are associated together.
A composite case record is created by selecting the best information
available from the associated records. Using a complex set of rules
which take into account the source of each record, results are
verified by checking for consistency between the selected site,
histology, sex and age. In the final phase, cancer case records are
counted and summarized to create the cancer incidence data for the
province.

DISCUSSION

A major issue concerning the reliance of the Registry on computer
techniques is the quality of the incidence data generated. The
Ontario Registry results have been compared to data published by the
long standing population-based of Saskatchewan and Connecticut and
were found to be compatible. Two internationally accepted indices
of reliability have been used in this comparison. These are "deaths
in the period," which is the ratio of mortality to incidence, and the
proportion of cases identified by death certificates only.

Finally, cancer incidence rates have been compared between
Jurisdictions and it was found that Ontario rates are similar to
those of Connecticut and New York and higher than those of
Saskatchewan, Iowa and Utah. This is explained by the fact that
Ontario like Connecticut and New York has a predominantly urban
population where as Saskatchewan, Iowa and Utah are more rural.

CONCLUSION

In conclusion, in a population of eight million, covering an area of more than one million square kilometres, computer techniques, including record linkage, provide the only practical and economic method of cancer registration. Computer applications lead to greater consistency and therefore greater accuracy. As the data are computerized, analyses are facilitated. The methods and systems used by the Ontario Cancer Registry are also applicable to the establishment and maintenance of other disease registries.

REFERENCES

Hill, T. "Generalized Iterative Record Linkage System." Special Resources Sub-division, Systems Development Division, Statistics Canada, 12-K R.H. Coats Building, Tunney's Pasture, Ottawa, Ontario K1A 0T6, 1981.

Howe, G., J. Lindsay. "A Generalized Iterative Record Linkage System For Use In Medical Follow-up Studies." *Comput Biomed Res* 14 (1981): 327-340.

Newcombe, H. "Record Linking: The Design of Efficient Systems For Linking Records Into Individual and Family Histories." *Am J Hum Genet* 19 (1967): 335-359.

Newcombe, H., J. Kennedy, S. Axford, A James. "Automatic Linkage of Vital Records." *Science* 130 (1959): 954-959.

Newcombe, H.B., M.E. Smith, G.R. Howe, J. Mingay, A. Strugnell, J.D. Abbatt. "Reliability of Computerized Versus Manual Death Searches In a Study of Eldorado Uranium Workers." *Computers Biol Med* 13 (1983): 157-169.

Smith, M., H. Newcombe, R. Dewar. "Automated Nationwide Death Clearance of Provincial Cancer Register Files - The Alberta Cancer Registry Study." In Alvey, W. (ed). *Statistics of Income and Related Administrative Record Research*, 1983. Washington, DC: US Treasury, IRS (Statistics of Income Division), 1983; 43-52.

FROM HOSPITAL-BASED TO POPULATION-BASED TUMOR REGISTRATION: PRIORITIES FOR AN EVOLUTIONARY DEVELOPMENT

Ch. Thieme, D. Hölzel, G. Schubert-Fritschle

Department of Medical Statistics and Data Processing, University of Munich, FRG (Head: K.K. Überla)

Registries play an important role in the cancer statistics information system of every country. Objectives which are usually or frequently aimed at include: measurement of the cancer load in terms of morbidity and/or mortality; support and evaluation of primary or secondary prevention; and measurement of the efficacy of cancer care, i.e. diagnosis, treatment, follow-up (1).

Interdependence of population- and hospital-based registries

The primary task of population based registration is the measurement of cancer incidence. The minimum set of items required for this purpose includes age at diagnosis, sex, place of residence, and ICD diagnosis, as compiled in (2) for almost 110 registries. Some population-based registries collect considerably more information about each case.

For many countries, hospitals are the most important data sources for population-based registries (PBRs) (1,3). If there are both PBRs and hospital-based registries (HBRs) in an area, they may act independently of each other, or cooperate through data exchange. Points of contact and possibilities of such cooperation are shown in fig. 1.

Typically, the HBR is located at a surgical department or hospital. It collects details on diagnosis and primary treatment, and, sometimes, carries out follow-up procedures. Thus, the items relevant to incidence statistics may be transferred from the HBR to the PBR.

Institutions which are never or not always involved in primary diagnosis and treatment may also establish HBRs, although the lack of primary information may be discouraging. In fig 1, the items that are likely to be missing in either type of HBR, are marked with dashed lines. In the latter case of a radiology- or oncology-based registry, data transfer

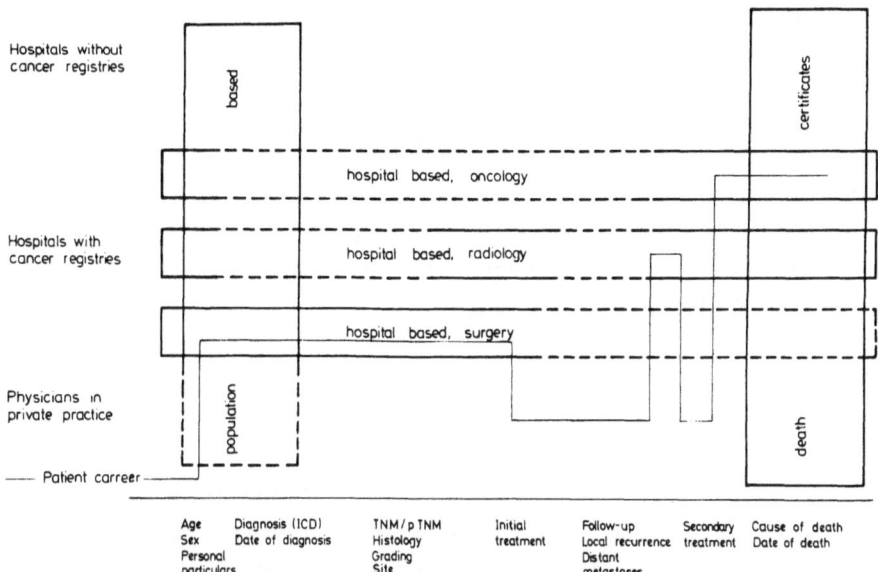

Fig. 1: Interdependence of the data from population-based registries, hospital-based registries and death certificates. Dashed lines indicate cases (population-based) or items (hospital-based) missing for structural reasons. The completeness of cancer statistics may be improved through cooperation or synthesis of population- and hospital-based registries.

from the PBR to the HBR might be helpful to overcome structural data gaps. Moreover, data exchange between HBRs of the former and latter type could be achieved using the PBR as a "data bus".

The screening of death certificates is another requirement which PBRs and HBRs have in common. The routine screening of these records by a PBR might be useful to complete the end-results statistics in the HBRs.

Worldwide cancer statistics show that incidence data of high quality can be gathered even without such intensive interregistry cooperation. On the other hand, record linkage for data from various sources is inevitable for the description of the natural history of disease and the reporting of end results. This is why in several countries efforts are being made towards closer cooperation between the different types of registries. In the American SEER (Surveillance, Epidemiology, and End Results) program (4), for example, the cooperation between both types of registries has largely been achieved, the background of this success being the high density of registries in the U.S.. In particular, it is estimated that 60 to 70% of all cancer patients in the U.S. are registered in one of the over 1,000 HBRs. (3).

Current position and objectives of the Munich Cancer Registry (MCR)

In contrast to the situation in the U.S., the density of PBRs and/or HBRs in the FRG is low. Fig. 2 shows the location of the two PBRs and of the cancer centers where some effort is made towards hospital-based cancer registration. For the region of southern Bavaria, the MCR focuses its attention on both incidence and end-results reporting. It is intended to implement a coherent system of end-results and incidence statistics within one registry which makes use of and gives support to the necessary multi-disciplinary treatment strategies.

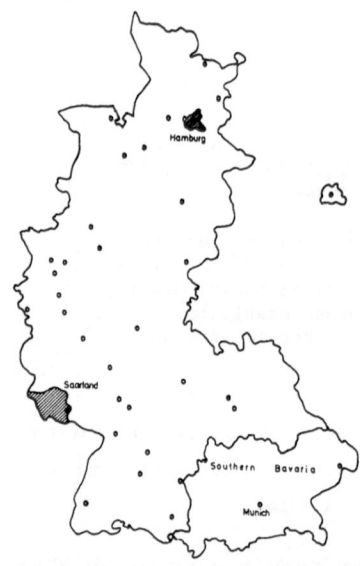

Established in 1978, the MCR has so far collected data on 31,000 patients. At present, the growth rate is 6,000 new patients and 10,000 items of follow-up information per year. Data are mainly gathered from 40 hospitals and cancer departments. Data processing is carried out on a large-scale computer (SIEMENS 7762). The data base system used was developed at our own department (5).

The structure and objectives of the MCR are shown in Fig. 3. Yet the MCR is not population-based; it may be seen as a multicenter-hospital-based registry. For each participating hospital, the MCR takes over the tasks of a HBR. Differences between the hospitals (e.g. university vs. others) lead to different demands. Therefore, flexibility of software and organization is necessary

Fig. 2: Population-based registries for about 5% of the population of FRG. At the cancer centers, efforts are made towards hospital-based registration.

for the MCR. This flexibility is achieved by means of highly modular data evaluation procedures which can easily be combined according to the needs of the hospitals concerned.

On the other hand, information on one particular patient collected from different sources, can be linked without the support of any third institution. Moreover, a synopsis of the patient is possible without explicit record-linkage procedures, as the data structure of the MCR is patient-oriented, and record linkage is done during the update procedure.

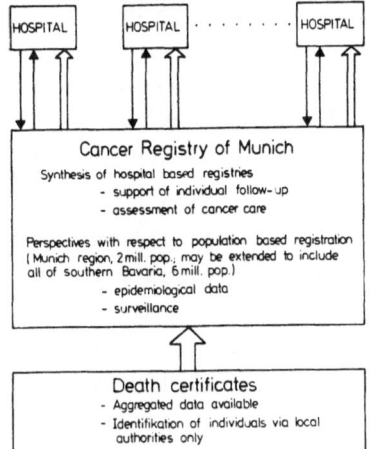

Fig. 3: Structure and aims of the multicenter-hospital-based Munich Cancer Registry.

—→ Data exchange on particular patients between the hospitals via registry.

⟹ Transfer of aggregated data such as life-tables or mortality rates.

Thus, in the normal situation - multidisciplinary treatment and follwo-up -, the synthesis of several HBRs into one yields more complete data records and more recent information for the participants. This capability of the MCR can be used as an aid to individual patient care and also as a support for the statistical analysis.

At the request of the institutions involved, the hospital-limited data evaluation will be abandoned in favor of a more comprehensive analysis taking in the data from all of these hospitals. This may be done to raise numbers (e.g. data from 2 surgeries) or to enhance the completeness of data (e.g. data from surgery and radiology).

Further steps towards a complete system of cancer statistics

This status quo is seen as a starting point towards a more complete system of cancer statistics in southern Bavaria. As a second step, it is intended to make better use of the aggregated mortality data. For the MCR, mortality data are useful to estimate the percentages of population in the various parts of southern Bavaria that are already covered by the MCR. The maintenance and analysis routines required in connection with the handling of mortality data can be used at a later time also for the incidence data which are essentially of the same structure.

From the viewpoint of mortality statistics, the estimation of cancer incidence can be improved by linking the mortality rates with the corresponding probabilities of cure derived from the MCR.

Access to individual death certificates constitutes a further step of the intended development. As discussed above, the screening of these records is important for complete end-results statistics and essential to population-based cancer registration. As this information is not computerized, manual record linkage will be necessary for the evaluation of death certificates. It is hoped in addition that existing legal barriers in the FRG can be abolished in the future.

After this phase of development the population reference for the Munich region may be easily achieved. The resulting incidence statistics permit regional and temporal comparisons. At the same time, the case-number basis for epidemiological studies is broadened. It should be mentioned here that case control studies are already being conducted, two of them having reached the evaluation stage.

An extension to the whole of southern Bavaria with the aim of achieving a comprehensive surveillance for this region will call for a simplification of our present tumor-specific documentation concept as an alternative for minor hospitals. The screening of death certificates for all of southern Bavaria might pose problems in so far as the acces to them will be via numerous local authorities.

Conclusions

We looked upon the lack of any registry in this area as an opportunity to examine the advantages of an integration of hospital- and population-based tumor registration. A simultaneous approximation to the equal-ranking goals of epidemiology and end-results reporting seems to be possible. In view of the moderate infrastructure available, each of the already complemented or envisaged expansion stages will probably afford attractive utilization options for the MCR.

This is seen as an evolutionary process which will probably lead to a complete data base of high quality. It is felt that on this path some of the criticism of registries referring to the clinical uselessness of their data collection can be refuted. Our first steps seem encouraging.

References:

1   Waterhouse, J.A.H.: Strategies for the development of a coherent cancer statistics system. World Health Stat. Quarterly 33 (1980) 185-196

2   Waterhouse, J.; Muir, C.; Shanmugaratnam, K.; Powell, J. (Eds.): Cancer Incidence in five Continents - Volume IV, IARC-Scientific Publications (42), Lyon 1982

3   Smart, C.R.: The role of tumor registries in cancer etiology and management; from: Cancer prevention in clinical medicine (Ed.: G.R. Newell), Raven Press, New York, 1983

4   Ries, L.G.; Pollack, E.S.; Young, J.L.,Jr.: Cancer patient survival: Surveillance, epidemiology, and end results program 1973-1979. J.N.C.I., 70 (1983) 693-707

5   Hölzel, D.; Eckel, R.: MINDIUS Programmbeschreibung. Technical Report of the Department of Medical Statistics and Data Processing, University of Munich, FRG, 1977

Address of the authors:
ISB / Klinikum Grosshadern, Marchioninistr. 15, D-8000 München 70

RTO - A MANAGEMENT SYSTEM FOR A COMPUTERIZED CANCER REGISTRY

M. Montella, F. Antignani, G. Di Lucca, V. Toglia
Istituto Nazionale Tumori "Fondazione Pascale" Napoli - ITALIA

ABSTRACT

The computerized system RTO (Registro Tumori Ospedaliero), which has been created in
the National Institute for Cancer Research and Treatment of Naples (3.500 in-patients,
6.000 hospital admission per year), is aimed at a Hospital Cancer Registry.
It is implemented on SPERRY-1100/60, EXEC-8 O.S., in COBOL language, using the
DPS/1100 package (Display Processing system designed for the management of
display-oriented transactions in an online environment).
The system is also planned to select and transfer automatically statistical relevant data
in standard files handled by GENSTAT (General Statistics) package for biostatistical and
epidemiological data analysis.

INTRODUCTION

The hospital cancer registry is based on directions of W.H.O. and its aims are:
a) **supply current statistical data about the activity of National Cancer
Institute (e.g. relative rates of case, places of origin and socioeconomical
distribution of patients);**
b) **management of a better assistance for in-patients with lower costs;**
c) **connection of in- and out-hospital assistance;**
d) **simplification of patient follow-up and clinical trials;**
e) **supply case-control studies data base;**
Setting up the computerized hospital cancer registry we tried not to modify hospital
routinary activity by using a fit daily activity schedule.
Fondamentals of this schedule were:
- **daily registration of admitted patients for each ward;**
- **interview with each patient by an ad hoc questionnaire;**
- **tracing each patient clinical data from medical record at discharge;**
- **data quality control and coding;**
- **data storage.   (Fig. 1)**
The data recording card of the register was divided in three parts: the first part
comprises personal and social data; the second part data related to clinical treatment;
and the third part laboratory investigations. For coding purpose we used the
International Classification of Diseases for Oncology ICD-O (W.H.O. 1976 GENEVE) as used
by Lombardy (Varese Province) Cancer Registry; for non cancer in-patients we also use
the 9TH revision of I.C.D.; while job coding was based on Bureau International du
Travail Classification Internationale des Professions (GENEVE 1968) adapted by
"Istituto Centrale di Statistica" Roma.
The RTO system scheme was planned by a logical analysis method applicable to
relational data base, but also effective in non data base environment, to fulfil needs of
independence, integrity and non-rendondancy of data.

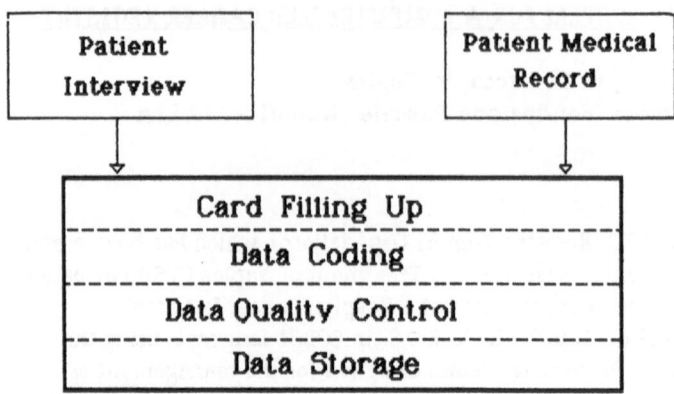

Fig. 1

SYSTEM DESIGN

On the basis of requirements and data analysis we identified three logical entities each
of them with its homogeneous own attributes and its internal Keys:
- "PAZIENTE" (patient's sociopersonal data);
- "RICOVERO" (clinical data);
- "ESAMI DI LABORATORIO" (laboratory investigation data).   (FIG. 2,3,4)

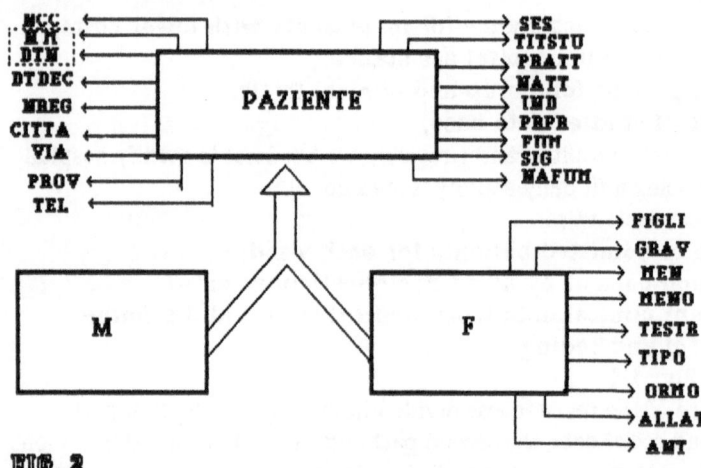

FIG. 2

NREG	RTO number	TITSTU study degree	FIGLI sons
NCC	medical record number	PRATT current job	ALLAT breast feeding (months)
NN	name and surname	NATT current job years	MEN menarch age
DTN	date of birth	IND industry	MENO menopause age
SES	sex	PRPR previous job	TESTR estrogenic therapy
CITTA town	FUM smoke	PRPOST before after menopause
VIA address	SIG cigarettes-day	GRAV first pregnancy age
PROV provence	NAFUM smoke years	TIPO contraceptive use
TEL telephon number		ORMO contraceptive therapy

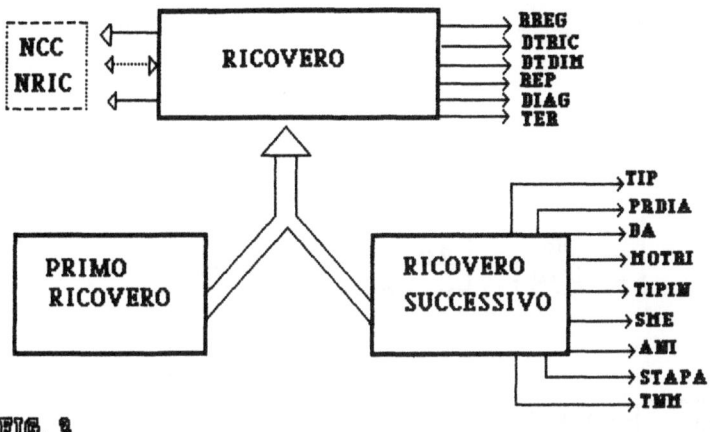

FIG. 3

BREG	RTO number	PRDIA	clinical history
NCC	medical record number	DIA	former diagnoses date
RIC	hospital addmission number	MOTRI	addmission diagnoses
DTRIC	hospital addmission date	TIPIN	operation
DTDIM	disgharge date	SHE	metastases
REP	vard	AMI	follow-up years
DIAG	diagnosis	TIP	patient clinical state
TER	therapy	TMM	T.M.M.

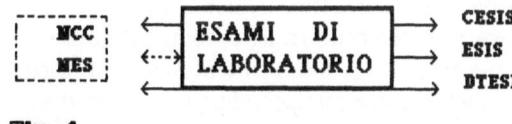

Fig. 4

THE ENTITY IS COMPOSED BY RADIOLOGICAL, HISTOLOGICAL AND BIOCHEMICAL INVESTIGATION DATA .

The entity "PAZIENTE" has an ISA hierarchy too : male or female, this one has further attributes. The entity "RICOVERO" has an ISA hierarchy: first hospital admission or following ones .
By joining the three logical entities and working out ISA emerging hierarchies we were able to get logic data system view.   (Fig.5)

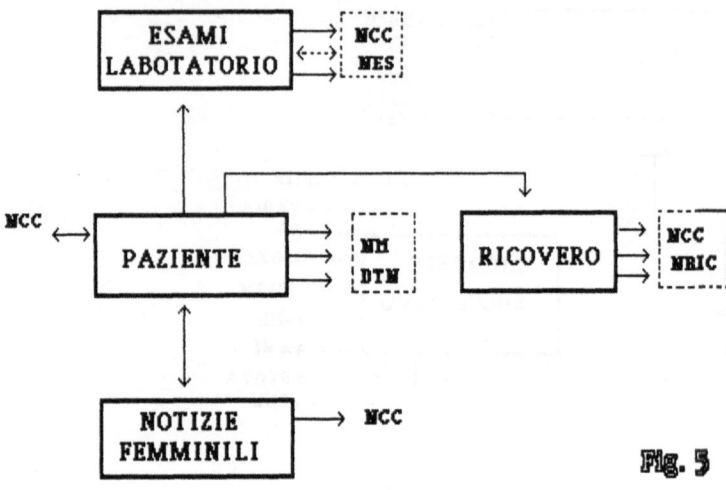

Fig. 5

Elaboration of ISA hierarchies required a new logical entity "NOTIZIE FEMMINILI"
(female data), which is linked up with the entity "PAZIENTE".On the contrary the second
hierarchy was worked out as a sigle entity "RICOVERO" which comprises the attributes
of first hospital admission and follow-up.

The picture scheme shows the logical view of the system with all its entities, their
attributes and their associations.

The Fig.6 shows the files architecture. The whole system is hinged on patient's personal
data file which is an indexed file. We can get access to it by patient medical record
number or by patient's name and date of birth. All other files (which are index filetoo)
make reference to this one. Particularly every record concerning a woman produces a
corresponding record in female data file, the access to it is the patient medical record
number. For each record in personal data file there are corrisponding records in the
hospital admission and laboratory investigation files. We can get access to them by a
key maked up by patient medical record number and admission or laboratory
investigation number. These keys are automatically and progressivaly associated to
each record when we insert a new hospital admission or a new laboratory
investigation.

SAme coding and decoding tables, necessary for a system optimization and its best use,
settles up the whole data system. (The figure shows some tables for job, diagnosis and
pathology examination code)

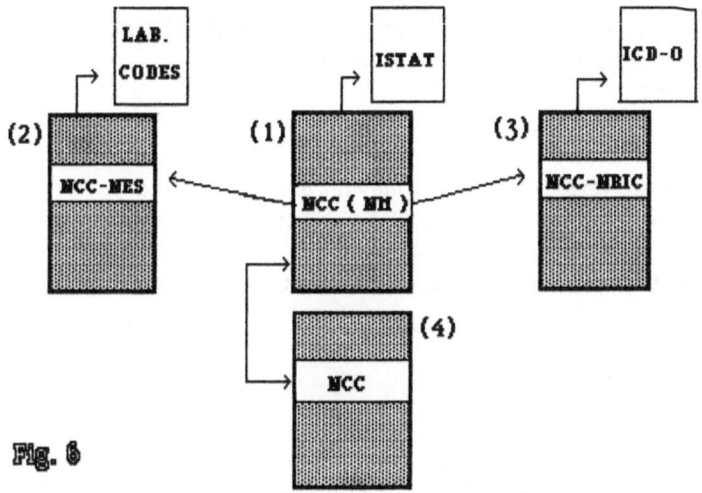

Fig. 6

1) patient personal data file 2) laboratory investigation file 3) clinical data file 4) women data file

SYSTEM FUNCTIONS

The system handling procedures carry out the following functions presenting them as a menu':

1) Data input

Data insertion of each admitted patient's personal, social and clinic data is interactive by video-terminal screen. By using the software utility DPS-1100 some displays are produced for data insertion . These displaies are runned by COBOL procedures. The operative procedure is made simple enough to be operated by a non specialized operator;   We forecast a set of dynamic controls and messages in the different fields to minimize error opportunity.

Data inserion is divided in two different operations according to whether it is a first hospital admission or a following one. In the first instance patient's sociopersonal data are required and,by the following displays the clinical data of first hospital admission. In following hospital admission are required only clinical data of this admission. When necessary, it is possible to modify the socio-personal data, using a specific function. All data are inserted after coding.

2) Patient data inquary

By using patient's name and date of birth or his medical record number we can get all data we need in real time. Data are showed on terminal as a series of displays with all data decoded.. It is possible to distinguish an inquiry function of patient socio-personal data with a stepwise exhibition of several hospital admissions and a display function of laboratory investigation data. It is also possible to print every display with its data by a hard-copy function using an interactive printer.

3) Update

It is possible to update wrong data by a specific procedure. By selecting this procedure we can get access to wrong data by a key: patient medical record number or patient's personal data. We can get also access to a single hospital admission or laboratory investigation directly by a key given by hospital admission number.

4) Decodified file report

This function prints a list of all decodified patient data.

5) Statistical analysis

This procedure selects, in the various files, data relevant to statistical and epidemiological analysis storing them in specific files to be processed by statistical packages. (Fig. 7)

In the National Cancer Institute of Naples we use the Genstat package of ROTHAMSTED EXPERIMENTAL STATION.

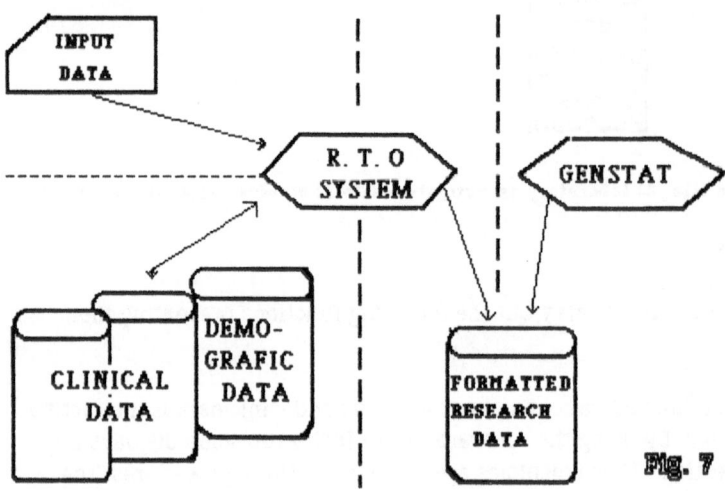

Fig. 7

CONCLUSION

After a three year of computerizzed hospital cancer registry soucessful instalation, the RTO system as stored 10.500 patients and 18.000 hospital admission data.
In the very next future is uor purpose to set up a network with other hospital registrie.

REFERENCES

Bracchi G., Martella G., Pelagatta G. : Tecniche di organizzazione degli archivi. ISEDI 1980
Bracchi G., Martella G., Pelagatta G. :Sistemi per la gestione di basi di dati. ISEDI 1980
Ceri s.: Progettazione di base dati. CLUP 1980
ISTAT Classificazione delle professioni, 1981
Mclemman R., Muir C., Stenitz R., Winkler A. : Cancer registration and its techinique
IARC scientific publication N. 21, 1978
WHO Manual of international classification of descase - 9th revision, 1975
WHO International classification of desease for oncology (ICD-O), 1976

A HEALTH DATABASE AS A TOOL FOR RELATING MEDICAL AND ENVIRONMENTAL-HEALTH DATA

Gj. Deželić, J. Kern, S. Vuletić, and N. Deželić
Andrija Štampar School of Public Health, Medical
School, University of Zagreb, 41000 Zagreb,
Yugoslavia

INTRODUCTION

In comprehensive health care programs, such as programs for fighting chronic non-infectious diseases in population groups (1), a huge amount of data is generated, being by nature multidimensional and showing complex relationships. In such programs the principles of data acquisition and generating information should be as follows (adapted from Ref. 2):

1. person specific, *i.e.* able to describe health problems, attributes, events, activities and outcomes in terms of numbers of individuals possessing them;
2. population-based, *i.e.* having capacity to make comparisons within and among different living space localities;
3. problem-oriented, *i.e.* having capacity to identify, label, classify and count inhabitant-, household-, settlement--problems;
4. provider and user specific, *i.e.* serving at present but able to be changed later;
5. process specific, *i.e.* having capacity to identify inter-ventions, enables monitoring and quality control;
6. time specific, *i.e.* having capacity to follow events;
7. practical, *i.e.* allowing easy access and use of a computer.

It is obvious that several types of data should be collected in order to satisfy the above principles: medical, health-environmental, demographic, sociological, *etc*.

The problems of this kind can be solved by organizing data into databases, as these collections of interrelated data, having low and controlled redundancy, allow fast and efficient information production and retrieval in various health applications (3,4).

There are many reports in the use of database technology in the health care domain, but they are tackling predominantly problems of information production from medical documentation (5). Few reports are dealing so far with databases on environmental-health data, and these are predominantly oriented to the monitoring of atmosphere, water and soil pollution. There was an attempt to link health data with data on environmental exposure (6), but this has been done by using existing sequential files created from health statistics data.

Such an approach can hardly meet all requirements postulated by the above principles. On the one hand, the list of environmetal indicators has to be expanded from those oriented to environmental pollution to indicators on housing, economic, social and cultural factors, and on the other hand, it should be possible to link such environmental data to personal data in order to make possible interventions in each specific case of medical prevention and treatment.

It is the aim of this work to design a database suitable for studying the influence of environmental factors on population health, but also for fulfilling tasks in health care of population groups and individuals by providing health professionals with necessary information in their daily preventive and curative work.

METHODS

The database POPUL has been designed as a CODASYL-type network model and implemented under DMS 1100 in the UNIVAC 1100/42 computing system of the University Computing Center, Zagreb. The software for database loading was written in COBOL, and information retrieval is performed by using both MACRO procedures and conversational queries of the DMS QLP (Query Language Processor).

Data loaded into POPUL has been collected in a local rural community in the northwestern part of Croatia (Belec in the commune of Zlatar Bistrica). The community encloses 11 villages, 681 households and 2633 inhabitants. Data for 77% households and more than 90% of inhabitants has been included so far.

RESULTS

The conceptual design of POPUL is shown in Fig. 1. The database consists of 12 entities linked with simple and complex relationships. For the sake of user's convenience some redundant relationships have been preserved in order to increase the database operability (*e.g.* settlement - household and settlement - address, inhabitant - household and inhabitant - address).

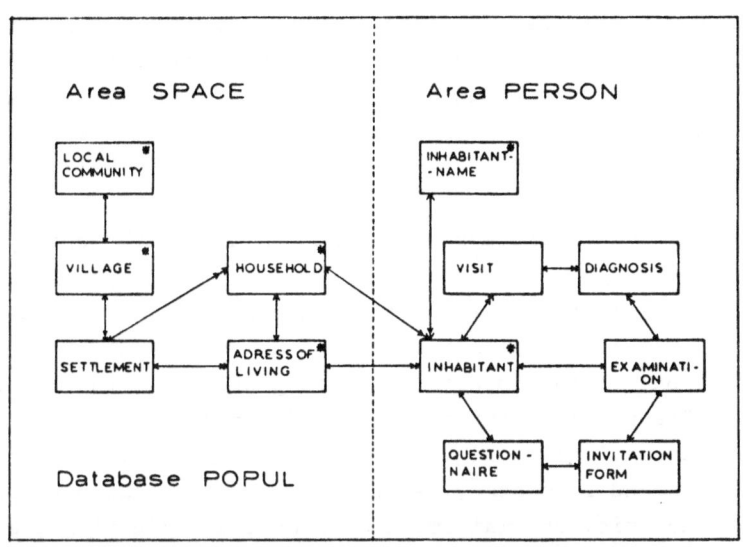

Fig. 1. The conceptual design of the database POPUL;
"*" directly accessible entities, "↔" 1:1
relationship, "↤↦" 1:n relationship

Andrija Stampar School of Public Health   Basic Health Unit
Z a g r e b   B e l e c

                    I N V I T A T I O N   F O R M

ID NO.: 0000000000057   DATE OF INTERVIEW: 030684
NAME: K.   I.   YEAR OF BIRTH: 931
ADDRESS: Belec 62   SETTLEMENT: Spoljari

QUESTIONNAIRE DATA

CHRONIC COUGH: yes
TREATED OF HYPERTENSION: no
MOBILITY: mobile
CAUSAL BLOOD PRESSURE: I   20.0/12.0 (kP) [150/090 (mm Hg)]
                           II   21.3/12.0 (kP) [160/090 (mm Hg)]
                          III   21.3/12.0 (kP) [160/090 (mm Hg)]
ARRHYTHMIA: no

REMARKS:

==
SCHEDULED FOR EXAMINATION: 100984
==

Fig. 2. A typical example of the invitation form produced
        automatically from the database POPUL by fulfilling
        the criteria P_{sist}.GE.18.7 AND/OR P_{diast}.GE.12.0

The entities in the area SPACE contain data describing general characteristics of localities and housing, such as water supply and quality, solid waste disposal, indoor and outdoor space as well as amenities and sanitation of housing. The entities in the area PERSON contain general data on inhabitants, and data on some chronic disease problems in the population (the entity QUESTIONNAIRE) and on visits to the general practitioner office serving the community (the entity VISIT).

So far the questionnaire attributes are oriented to the recognition of the hypertension problem in the population because this has been reported as one of the important health problems in the Belec population (1). For persons with indicated hypertension an invitation form is issued automatically (Fig. 2) and a thorough health examination by the specialists and laboratory is performed. Other health problems, like chronic bronchitis, rheumatism, and intestinal infections, are to be included into the database. The visit data is now being prepared for loading. Both the attributes from this entity and from specialist's examination will serve for the evaluation of population's morbidity data collected in the entity DIAGNOSIS.

DISCUSSION

The database POPUL proved to satisfy the principles listed in the Introduction. Its person specificity reflects in the ability of the basic health unit team (doctor, nurse) to get information on each inhabitant as well as on a population group. It is population-based as it allows comparisons among population groups living at different localities. The depiction of various health problems is possible by asking simple queries and the planning of necessary interventions is well supported.

Although logically encompassed in respect to medical and health-environmental data, many details have to be solved in future development. The list of environmental indicators has to be elaborated in order to define attributes related to the characteristics of the locality (like weather conditions, land and landscape quality, existence of surface water, *etc.*), to the space relationships (like accessibility and quality of health and other services, existence and quality of roads, *etc.*) and to the socio-behavioral factors (7). It is also possible to introduce data capable of giving genealogical information. In that case a more sophisticated database security system has to be implemented guaranteeing privacy of each individual's data.

The most important feature of the database POPUL is the integration of data on individuals and space. It is, therefore, possible to correlate environmental data with aggregated data of population groups, and *vice versa* to inspect the environmental factors (ecological and sociological) under which an individual lives. Knowing the health risks connected with these factors, the health unit team might obtain necessary suggestions for possible prevention and intervention measures on a microlevel.

In conclusion we can emphasize that the key problem in preparing and analyzing medical and health-environmental data is how to transform "data" into "information" and such "information" into "intelligence" to help and guide the doctor as a decision-maker. We have to concentrate our efforts to the creation of data ensembles that will help the above mentioned process (data - information - intelligence) on the local, basic health care level. This certainly demands linkage of the database with some expert systems capable to help solve problems which may arise in local communities. Future research has to explore the possibilities of such development.

REFERENCES

1. Vuletić S. (with 18 coauthors), A Comprehensive Programme for Fighting Chronic Non-Infectious Diseases in Basic Population Groups - The Belec Study. I. Evaluation of the Extent of the Problem (orig. in Croatian), Lij. vjes. 106:443-447,1984.

2. White K.L. A New Look at Health Information, World Health Forum 4:368-373,1983.

3. Sauter K. Medical Databases - Conceptual and Technical Aspects, Proc. Medical Informatics Europe '81, Toulouse, Lecture Notes in Medical Informatics, Vol. 11, Springer-Verlag, Berlin-Heidelberg-New York 1981, pp. 58-65.

4. Deželić Gj. The Organization of Databases for Health Records Processing, Proc, 8th Intern. Congress on Health Records, Pre-Papers, Vol. 2, The Hague 1980, pp. 236-243.

5. Wiederhold G. Databases for Health Care, Lecture Notes in Medical Informatics, Vol. 12, Springer-Verlag, Berlin-Heidelberg-New York 1981.

6. Sjöström A., Westerholm P. Liaison of Environmental Exposure Data with Morbidity Data, in: Information Systems for Health Services, Public Health in Europe No. 13, WHO Regional Office for Europe, Copenhagen 1980, p. 115.

7. Urban Environmental Indicators, Organization for Economic Co-Operation and Development, Paris 1978.

PERFORMANCE IMPROVEMENTS OF RELATIONAL DATABASE SOFTWARE RECONSIDERED
FOR MEDICAL APPLICATIONS

Piotr J. Jasiński
Computer Centre
Technical University of Poznań
60-965 Poznań, Poland

SUMMARY

In the past few years relational databases became a popular tool in medical applications. The paper is an attempt to evaluate time performance problems from the point
of view of medicine-specific types of queries and microprocessor technology applied.
Some corresponding ideas of join operations scheduling and support of selection processes are discussed in details. The considerations deal with the implementation of
relational database software oriented to medical, particularly clinical research
applications.

1. INTRODUCTION

In the 80's one can observe an increasing popularity of relational methodology applied to the design and use of medical databases. This trend is reflected in the
architecture recommendation for systems supporting statistical studies [1], clinical
research oriented databases (e.g. [2]), common general patient databases (e.g. [3])
and more sophisticated applications (e.g. processing of free-text medical narrative
[4]).   Nowadays, it seems that database users positive feed-back motivation or -
alternatively - frustration, depends heavily not only on the feasibility of query
formulation but also on the time efficiency of query processing. Time - oriented
meaning of efficiency is even more important due to extremaly deep evolution of the
technology applied. In the 70's a number of fundamental investigations on relational
databases performance were reported but their typical hardware kernel were big mainframes (e.g. IBM System 370). At present, in microprocessors environment we have to
face problems resulting from slow CPUs and time-consuming I/O operations (conventionally used floppy disks may decrease average access time up to an order of magnitude).

Apart from hardware consideration we should note that the nature of medical applications differs significantly from the most commonly investigated commercial, office
-oriented examples [5]. Essentially, queries concerning individual entities are
relatively rare. Instead, queries of global nature are the most frequent, requiring
correspondent processing of a large portion of a database. Then, intorerably slow
processing of queries has been reported [3,4].

The aim of this paper is to describe the philosophy of some corresponding ideas of
performance improvements, developed for query processing of ReDS (Relational Data
System) software project implemented on LSI-11 16bit based microcomputers (for
details of basic design see [6]).

2. ORGANIZING PLAN OF ALGEBRAIC OPERATIONS

In a current version of ReDS query language [7], union, difference, intersection,
theta-join and some forms of domain algebra have been introduced but the structure
of a single query is still best suited to the class of "select-join-project" expre-
sions. From this point of view the greatest attention is paid to natural join which
constitutes the most characteristic and useful operation of relational database algebraic interface. Although very efficient merging scan algorithm (a part of sort -
merge) was applied as implementation technique, the time of join processing is
linear to the cardinalities of operand and result relations and represents dominant
component of the total query processing time [8,9]. Well-known and intuitively obvious approaches, adopted in ReDS software consist in performing all selections as
early as possible [10]. (Nota bene: reducing operand relations cardinalities is more
efficient than reducing their width via project operations).

The following example illustrates the tuning of time performance by means of an analysis of operand and intermediate relations cardinalities and proper sequencing of join operations. Having at his disposal a very simple yet practical database with the schema:

PATIENT (pat-no, admission-date, sex, age, state, discharge-date)
PROBLEMS (problem-no, pat-no, problem-code, discharge-state)
DRUGS (therapy-no, pat-no, start-date, problem, drug-name, days, dose)
CHARACTERISTIC: PROBLEMS of PATIENT, DRUGS of PATIENT,
DESIGNATION: PROBLEMS from DRUGS via problem,
the user is interested in receiving the following data: age and sex of patients treated with propranolol longer than 9 days, together with dosages, problems for which this drug has been administered and patient's state at discharge.

To obtain the answer desidered data from all three relations are needed and because the schema is cyclic there are three possible sequences of join operations. From our own AMI database system [2] we can use the following real parameters: for each 1.000 tuples in relation PATIENT expected cardinalities of relation PROBLEMS and DRUGS are 3.340 and 9.180 tuples, respectively. The value "propranolol" of an attribute drug-name has selectivity 3.27% itself; together with conjunctive selection condition (days > 9) selectivity can be approximated at the level of 1% (i.e. ca. 1% of tuples satisfies selection condition defined). Having such numbers, and assuming simultanous selection during merging scan the join of PATIENT and DRUGS should be performed first because it gives the smallest intermediate (temporal) relation (of 918 tuples approximately) and - consequently - minimal time of whole user request processing. A corresponding plan of algebraic operations (see Figure 1) is practically ruled by the user who is assumed to have some degree of understanding of the nature and complexity of the processing ordered.

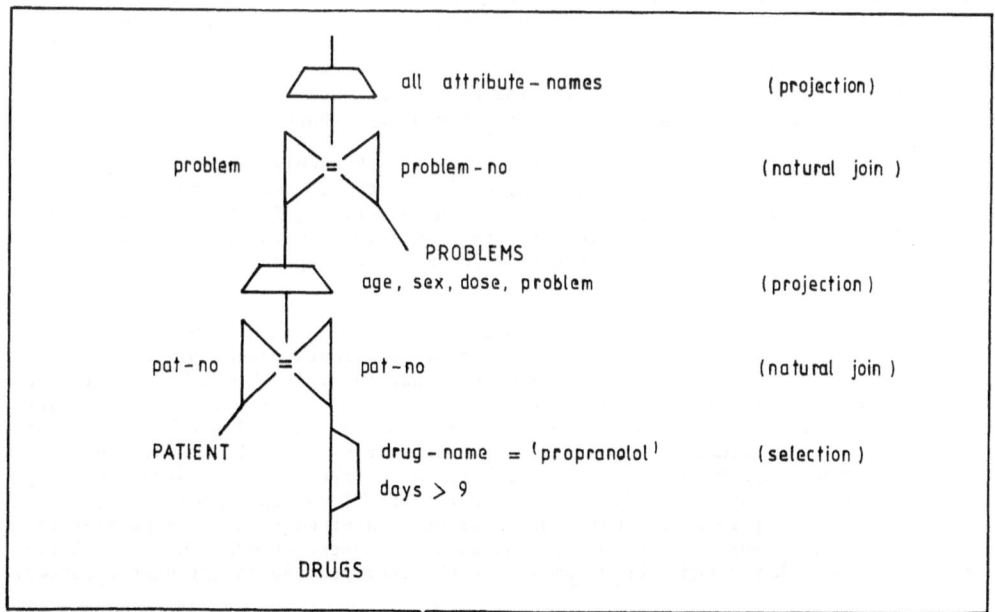

Figure 1. Plan of algebraic operations for exemplary request of data

In ReDS query language we can formulate the whole task as follows:
CREATE PROPRANOLOL-PATIENTS (age, sex, problem, dose) FROM PATIENT & DRUGS
      WHERE drug-name = "propranolol" AND days > 9.
SELECT age, sex, problem-code, dose, discharge-state FROM PROPRANOLOL-PATIENTS &
                                                        PROBLEMS.

For typical end-users (physicians, secretary) an alternative JL (join-less) query
language is proposed; then, at the cost of smaller retrieval power and temporal relations unavailability the user may deal with database system in terms of attributes
only. For example presented, the query takes the form of:
RETRIEVE age, sex, problem-code, dose, discharge-state IF drug-name = "propranolol"
                                                        AND days > 9.
and the sequence of joins is optimised automatically, from the point of view of
system' response time.

3. DESIGNING EFFECTIVE INVERTED STRUCTURES

Further noticable performance improvements are possible through the use of supplementary inverted structures (indexes). In office-oriented applications indexes are
usually implemented for all key attributes and this approach reduces dramatically
the number of I/Os for queries concerning individuals (parts, orders, e.g [5]).
The question in medical, particularly in research-oriented applications, concerns
rather non-key attributes and is of highly non-deterministic nature.
In clinical and research-oriented applications delection of patients groups, performed accordingly to the criteria defined by physician constitutes a kernel task
of the whole processing.

Precise calculations show that in the query CREATE (see Section 2 of this paper)
the use of appropriate inverted structures (for drug-name and days) may reduce the
time of processing to approximately 40% of the time when join is computed via merging scan with concurrent serial scan selection. This particular result is a good
one but the example is optimistically tendentious. When inverted structures are
used to support selection the reduced time of join on selected tuples only must be
increased by the following extras:
- time of inverted structure (secondary index) inspection,
- time of tuples retrieval, which per tuple is usually longer than in sequential
  scan mode,
- time of creating intermediate relation(s) with all the tuples selected.
The use of inverted structures is advantagous if the total time of processing is
markedly shorter than in the case of simple scan selections. Roughly speaking, in
typical implementations, when the selectivity of attribute value is relatively low
(to say, over 30%), inversion is not useful and may even degrade the system' time
performance.

In an efficient design of inverted structures there are two main problems. Firstly,
we should note that some attributes or/and certain attribute values may be of less
interest or may not appear at all as selection conditions. It should be underlined,
that in medical applications of databases the assumption of uniformity of attribute
values in queries is not realistic. Secondly, medical databases describe human populations where the values of the majority of the attributes included have nonuniform distributions. Moreover, some attribute values are strongly correlated (e.g.
see data on age, sex and mortality taken from former AMI database project [2]).
Instead of making a priori, estimated assumptions we decided to use non-parametric
techniques, i.e. extensive sampling of real database installations. The basic motivation for approach was that non-parametric techniques provide the highest accuracy.

For continous observation of attributes' values incidence in queries a distinct
software component of ReDS system, the so called Usage Monitor, is being introduced.
Usage Monitor serves to analyze characteristics and complexity of each consequtive
query processed and aggregates these data in the form of performance-oriented parameters, since the begining of database installation.
No special software tool is needed for database contents monitoring. All necessary

and adequately precise data can be made available through the periodical sampling, i.e. the use of a set of specifically formulated queries in which previously developed non-relational functions like HISTOGRAM and SCATTER-PLOT remain intensively used.

Table 1

Attribute values in queries	Stored values of attributes		
	uniform distribution small set, low selectivity	uniform distribution big set, high selectivity	non-uniform distr. high selectivity of some values
uniformity of all attribute values	U	R(c)	R(p)
prevalence of certain atribute	P(p)	R(p)$^{*)}$	R(p)$^{**)}$

U – inversion useless
R – inversion highly recommended
P – inversion probably useful
c – complete; inversion for all elements of attribute value set (domain)
p – partial; inversion for a subset of attribute value set
*) partial inversion for a subset of values of an attribute whose prevalence is observed in user's queries
**) partial inversion for these values of an attribute, which appear most frequently in queries and are sufficiently selective

Table 1 compromises the simplest, non-formalized presentation of "decision table" for efficient choices and design of inverted structures, based on queries and database monitoring.

4. FINAL REMARKS

It has been observed that the nature, characteristics and performance significance of selection processes in medical databases has not been paid adequate attention to [11]. The presented software facilities of queries and database contents monitoring allow the total cost of creation and maintenance of inverted structures (secondary indexes) to be kept as low as possible. At the same time the user of the database receives maximal time performance improvements of selection processes. This is useful not only for join-type queries but for queries concerning a single relation, also. In addition, database contents sampling provides current values of parameters used in joins optimisation (cardinalities, selectivities, see Section 2 of this paper).

The facilities provided within ReDS software are believed to fill to some degree the gap between the current investigations on databases performance [12], micros and their use in medical applications of databases [13].

ACKNOWLEDGEMENTS

This work has been partly subsidized by the Polish Academy of Science (under contract No. 10.8.8.04.02) and this support is gratefully acknowledged.

REFERENCES

[1] Klonk J, Rassmann B.: The architecture of a data processing system to support statistical studies. Med.Inform., 1984, Vol. 9, No. 2, 125-134.

[2] Jasiński P.J., Krug H., Szymańska M.: Database system for research in clinical cardiology: development retrospection and application.In: Computers in Cardiology 1983 (Aachen), IEEE Computer Society Press, 123-126.

[3] Göhring R.: Operating experience with the relational patient database (to appear in Medical Informatics).

[4] Chi E.C., Sager N., Tick L.J., Lyman M.S.: Relational data base modelling of free-text medical narrative. Med.Inform., 1983, Vol. 8, No. 3, 209-223.

[5] Chamberlin D.D. et al: Support for Repetitive Transactions and Ad Hoc Queries in System R. ACM TODS, Vol. 6, No. 1, 1981, 70-94.

[6] Jasiński P.J.: Project of self-contained relational database software: design and clinical applications outline. In: MIE 84, Lecture Notes in Medical Informatics, 24 Springer-Verlag (Berlin), 1984, 194-199.

[7] Jasiński P.J.: ReDS - design of algebraic query language processor with definition, retrieval and powerful domain algebra capabilities. Paper submitted to the 8th International Seminar on Database Management Systems (1985).

[8] Merrett T.H.: Why Sort-Merge Gives the Best Implementation of the Natural Join. Technical Report SOCS-81-37, McGill University, Montreal, October 1981.

[9] Bitton D., DeWitt D.J., Turbyfill C.: Benchmarking database systems: a systematic approach. Computer Science Technical Report No. 526, University of Wisconsin-Madison, December 1983.

[10] Smith J.M., Chang P.Y.-T.: Optimizing the Performance of a Relational Algebra Database Interface. Comm. ACM, 1975, Vol. 18, No. 10, 568-579.

[11] Jasiński P.J.: Data systems in cardiological departments: an overview of literature (to appear in Medical Informatics, 1985, Vol. 10, No. 3).

[12] Christodoulakis S.: Implications of certain assumptions in data base performance evaluation. ACM TODS, 1984, Vol. 9, No. 2, 163-186.

[13] Leven F.J., Stoll Ch.: Features of micro data base systems and their impact on applications in health care systems. In: MIE 82, Lecture Notes in Medical Informatics, 16, Springer-Verlag (Berlin) 1982, 784-790.

DISTRIBUTION TECHNIQUE AND PERFORMANCE OF RELATIONAL DATABASES IN DECENTRALIZED HEALTH CARE ENVIRONMENTS

Z. Królikowski   and   M. Szymańska
Computer Centre   Institute of Cardiology
Technical University   Academy of Medicine

Poznań, Poland

ABSTRACT

Decentralized information systems developed in the last years and supporting the operation of hospitals, have certain specific features. In this paper we propose a selection of the most suitable, in our opinion, techniques of data distribution and optimization of queries, considering the specifics of decentralized systems in health care environments. Throughout the whole paper the methodology of distributed relational databases has been applied uniformly.

1. INTRODUCTION

Distributed database systems (DDS) offer several attractive advantages against centralized databases. These advantages include increased data reliability and faster, localized access to data and have particular importance in health care environment. In the last years, many computerized distributed systems for management, storage and retrieval of medical information have been developed [2,7,9].

In this paper we will try to look at the most common approach used in data processing in decentralized health care environment, from the point of view of performance. Our consideration will be focused on distribution techniques and query processing evaluation. The paper is organized as follows: Section 2 presents functionally decomposed network structure of health service institution; in Section 3 database distribution techniques best suitable for supporting medical services operation, are presented as well as the evaluation of query optimisation methods. Finally, Section 4 summarizes the major points of this paper.

2. NETWORK STRUCTURE OF HEALTH SERVICE INSTITUTION

The practice of the last years has proved the idea of distributed relational database to be the most suitable for supporting medical services. Many information systems oriented to clinical data storage and retrieval at hospital level, contains three main groups of information [2, 7, 9], stored at the sites of distributed system (fig. 1).

This structure, in most general terminology of Spector approach [9], consists of the following components:
- central information - a set of all the information of administrative, statistical and epidemiological interest, obtained from each patient during his consequtive contacts with the institution in question,
- ward information - all necessary information (separately for each ward) concerning individual patient i.e. age, sex, diagnosis, observation, treatment, etc.
- technical departments information - a complete set of all relevant information for each autonomic department (laboratory, biochemistry, pathology, radiology,pharmacy).
It is obvious that each ward site has to cooperate, less or more frequently, with technical departments. On the other hand, the data resources of the central site are updated and managed on the basis of

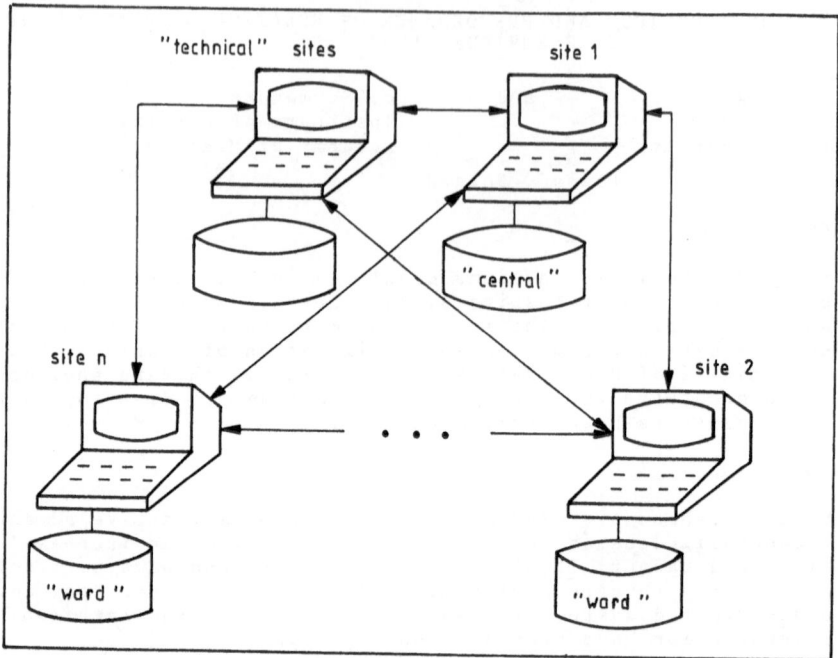

Fig. 1. Recommended structure of health service institution system

data adequately selected from all other sites. Moreover, it is to be noted, that during the hospitalisation of a patient, he can be transferred from one hospital ward to another. For this reason corresponding operations of data transfer between ward sites must be available.

3. PERFORMANCE OF DISTRIBUTED RELATIONAL DATABASES IN HEALTH CARE ENVIRONMENTS

The data distribution techniques adopted in distributed database system have high significance for system efficiency. It has been shown, that in medical applications the partitioning of complete relations between suitable sites as well as horizontal and vertical partitioning are useful from the point of view of data availability [4]. However, investigations on experimental DDS have proven the vertical partitioning of relations into particular computer sites to have degraded the efficiency of the whole distributed system [5, 8]. The horizontal partitioning of relation reduces the efficiency of the system to a lesser degree. This method, however, requires transmitting relations tuples among the system's sites which can result in a time delay. Most papers dealing with distribution strategies propose the relation as the main distribution unit. In view of this recommendation isolation of patient administrative data and their storage at one determined site (site 1 - central administration - see fig.1) should be the first main principle. The same should concern relation design at other sites. It should be noted, however, that such performance-oriented relation distribution needs some level of data replication (e.g. between ward sites and laboratory sites).

The other important problem influencing the efficiency of a DDS is the problem of query optimization. The selection of appropriate plans of executing queries depending on their own parameters and data base characteristic allows to obtain essential reduction of the time of query execution. So far, some methods of a query execution plans generation in DDS have been developed. These methods have been elaborated assuming the relational operations execution to be negligibly short in comparison to the time of data transmission. However, the latest measurements made in experimantal DDS [8], have proven that the relational operation execution times are not negligibly short. They often are the overriding component of the total time of query execution. The main reason is that modern distributed systems in health care environments and in other applications are designed using microcomputers of relatively small computing capabilities. On the other hand, transmission subsystems efficiency are substantially increasing. Therefore, it seems necessary to introduce a model strategy of query optimization taking into account specific conditions of health care institutions. Developing a new analytical model of query execution cost in a DDS should be a first step in this direction. In the model suggested all real cost of query execution have been considered. The model has layer structure corresponding to the structure of distributed database management systems and phases of query processing. In [1,5] it has been proven, that query optimization methods developed previously, can result in an increase of query execution cost in DDS due to the changes of the system's cost interrelations in health care environment. The results of the investigations, reported in detail in [1, 5], give a firm foundation for developing a new strategy for query optimization in DDS. The application of the model developed could contribute to an increase of distributed database efficiency in systems supporting health care service.

4. SUMMARY

In this paper we attempt to draw attention of DDS designers to the two, in our opinion, most essential problems ruling the efficiency of information systems in health care environment i.e. selection of data distribution techniques and query optimization. Some solutions have been proposed, which seem to be most suitable from the point of view of practical experiences and latest theoretical consideration. The application of the methods proposed in the design and implementation of distributed data systems for health care service should result in improving time performance, better efficiency of the whole systems and user's satisfaction.

REFERENCES

[1]   Cellary W., Królikowski Z., Morzy T., Analytical model for performance evaluation of transactions in distributed database systems, Eighteenth Annual HICSS Conf., Honolulu, Hawaii, 1985 (paper available from authors).

[2]   Bianchi E., Blardi P.S., A model of information system oriented to clinical data storage and retrieval at hospital level, In: MEDINFO 83, North-Holland (Amsterdam) 1983, pp. 1143-1145.

[3]   Gardarin G., A unified architecture for data and message management, Report SCH-I060, Inst. de Programmation, Paris, 1979.

[4]   Jasiński P.J., Relational approach to clinical databases: experience and perspectives, In: MEDINFO 83, North-Holland (Amsterdam) 1983, pp. 1094-1097.

[5]   Kaiser P., Distributed databases - some problems and questions,
      Intern. Seminar on Architecture of Database Management Systems,
      Dec. 3-7, 1980, Zaborów, Poland.

[6]   Królikowski Z., Towards improved strategies of query processing
      in distributed database systems, Ninth Symposium in Informatics,
      Jahorina, Yugoslavia, 1985 (paper available from authors).

[7]   Rickmann H., Kuehn H., Pietrzyk P., Laboratory data processing
      with three coupled computer systems, In: MEDINFO 83, North-Holland
      (Amsterdam) 1983, pp. 1151-1155.

[8]   Rolin P., Rapport Sur la compage de mesure de performance du pro-
      totype Sirius-Delta, Rapports de Recherche No. 175, INRIA,France,
      1982.

[9]   Spector M., Elgard M.C, Gremy F., Project analysis of a hospital
      information network: total or partial integration of existing ap-
      plications, In: MEDINFO 83, North-Holland (Amsterdam) 1983,
      pp. 1147-1151.

MEDICAL RECORD OF ONCOLOGY PATIENTS

L. Fernández, M. Azcue, A. Martín, A. Molina and M. Borges
National Oncology Institute, Havana, Cuba

In this paper we will show the design of the computer system for the
medical record of oncology patients. The system is modular and it
has particular information for each clinical department and for each
localization of cancer. It also contains general information of all
the patients.

INTRODUCTION

The increase of the life expectancy and the mean age of the population
together with the industrial development have brought malignant diseases occupied the second place as causes of death in Cuba and one of
the highest rates in our continent (1,2).

Local Hospital Registry has as its essential element a file for all
cancer patients seen, and its main functions are to ensure that case
records contain sufficiently detailed information for statistics and
management purposes (3).

The medical record of oncology patients in the National Oncology Institute is our automatization objective.

This document has the most important characteristics of cancer patients who was admitted in the hospital. The functions of this system
are to collect, store, process and communicate relevant information
in order to satisfy scientific and administrative requirements for
different levels of the Centre.

The computerized medical record was designed to be relationed with the
other applications in the hospital as control of beds, appointment
procedures, drug system and other technical departments.

GENERAL CHARACTERISTICS OF THE SYSTEM

This system was designed for a Cuban minicomputer CID 300-10 in Pascal
programming language. Facilities of Pascal have been profited in the
definition of files. Gentab (4) was created as a parametric program
in the edition of general outputs. Standardized rates, cumulative
rates (5) and special statistical methods are used in the performance
of the system.

The system was designed with the following modular conception:

- Patient identification: This is a general task for all patients admitted in the hospital.

- Clinical Departments: We take in this module information about anamnesis, diagnosis, treatment and follow up.

- Tumor localization: Particular information about the characteristics of the tumors are taken in this step as clinical examination, diagnosis results, pathological status etc.

- Follow up module: The functions of this task are the control of the attendance of patients and the evaluation of the efficacy of treatment.

OUTPUTS

We wanted to explain the outputs in relation to their principal goals.

- General Information: It is the systematic information about general characteristics of patients: age, sex, clinical stage, primary site and TNM.

- Particular Information: It will offer to the clinical departments specific information of patients: metastasis, histological type, risk factors etc.

- Follow up studies: Survival figures of all cancer localizations by clinical stage, treatment, histological type etc. will be analyzed. We will use Kaplan Meier, log rank and Cox tests (6,7,8).

CLOSING REMARKS

All data are taken directly in face of patients. A close relation with the National Cancer Registry (9) has been planned. A performance data base for oncologic research is a very important goal to be obtained. This system can be applied in retrospective studies and in trend analysis of selected groups of data in order to provide support for the research and clinical needs in a Cancer Centre.

REFERENCES

1. Ministerio de Salud Publica. Informe Anual. Cuba 1977.

2. OPS/OMS. Las Condiciones de Salud en las Americas. 1973-1976. Public Cientf No 364, 1978.

3. Pedersen E. Some Uses of the Cancer Registry in Cancer Control. Brit. J. Prev. Soc. Med (1962), 16, 105.

4. Gentab. Programa Generados de Tablas. Dpto. Análisis y Automatización. Instituto de Oncología. Cuba. 1984.

5. Doll, Rand, Smith P. Comparison between registries: Age-Standardized Rates in: Waterhouse J., Muir C. et al. (eds) Cancer Incidence in Five Continents, Volume IV, Lyon (IARC Scientific Publications Nr 42), 1982.

6. Kaplan E.L. and Meier P. Nonparametric Estimation from Incomplete Observations. J. Am. Stat. Assoc. 53 (1958), 457-481.

7. Crowley J. and Breslow N. Remarks on the Conservation of Parameters in Survival Data. Biometrics 31 (1975), 957-961.

8. Cox D. Regression Models and Life Tables. J.R. Stat. Soc. B, 34 (1972), 187-220.

9. Registro Nacional de Cáncer. Instituto de Oncología y Radiobiología. Ministerio de Salud Publica. Cuba.

THE BRITISH CHILD HEALTH COMPUTER SYSTEM

Dr. Colin H.M. Walker* (Chairman), Mr. Michael J. Rigby** (Vice-Chairman)

Child Health Computing Committee (Great Britain)

* Consultant Paediatrician,   ** Regional Service Planning Officer,
   Department of Child Health,   Mersey Regional Health Authority,
   Ninewells Hospital and Medical   Hamilton House,
      School,   24 Pall Mall,
   Dundee, DD1 9SY.   Liverpool,   L3 6AL.
   Scotland.   England.

Introduction

The British Child Health Computer System has been developed under the control of the Child Health Computing Committee (CHCC), with the program being produced by the Welsh Health Technical Services Organisation (WHTSO). As a result an extremely flexible yet comprehensive system is available for any Health Authority in Great Britain to use.[1,2] Pilot testing of the last major component of the system was completed in late 1984. Already the majority of Health Authorities use the Child Register and Immunisation Modules; approaching 10% use the Pre-School Module (released for general use in 1984); and considerable interest is being shown in the School Health Module (available for general use from late 1985). This is the latest stage in 20 years of British experience of computer applications in preventive Child Health Services.

Objectives and Background

The British approach to health care gives considerable emphasis to preventive services, yet the social philosophy of the country gives emphasis to freedom of choice. Management of preventive services for children must respect these principles, yet ensure that individual children are not disadvantaged, particularly as those children in family environments giving highest risk are least likely to be brought forward. These services therefore require techniques which encourage uptake, and identify those children not attending or who have a medical need for special care. Such scheduling and record keeping is - in principle - an ideal computer application,[3] though decisions about record contents and definitions are more difficult.

The first British application in this field was in 1962, in West Sussex, with a system to schedule immunisation appointments for children under 5 years of age, to record the results, and to highlight defaulters.[4] Thereafter, a number of other Authorities developed their own local systems, with considerable variety of approach as well as of computer hardware. As such systems proliferated, problems were caused when individual children moved, or as staff moved between Authorities. Also of concern was that, in general, those Authorities dealing with the greatest volume of difficult social problems could least afford to develop such systems.

Foundations for a National System

The preparation for a major reorganisation of the British National Health Service in 1974 gave opportunity to prepare for a national system.[5] In that reorganisation all-purpose Area Health Authorities were created, to be responsible for hospital, preventive, and other community services. All had access to ICL mainframe computers at Regional Computer Centres.

The Government's Department of Health & Social Security commissioned the National Computer Centre (NCC) to produce an overall blue print for a national system and to prepare the programs for the initial functions.

The Basic Concept

NCC proposed four independent yet interlinked modules – the "sun – satellite" principle. The Child Register Module forms the "sun" which is needed to operate any of the other modules. The "satellites" are three service delivery modules – for Immunisation, Pre-School Health, and School Health. Each participating Health Authority decides which of these three modules it wishes to use, though any child within the Authority will have one comprehensive medical record on the computer system.

NCC obtained experience of a number of different immunisation systems then operational, and produced the first programs for the Child Register and Immunisation Modules. WHTSO was then asked to maintain these programs, and to complete the further developments.

The Child Register

The Child Register contains key identification information including forenames, surname, address and general practitioner. Individual records are generated from the statutory Notification of Birth. For children moving at later ages, a broadly similar form is used to create a new local record.

When the record is initially loaded onto the Child Register, the system generates the unique link number used to identify the child within the system. This link number comprises a code for the Health Authority, date of birth, a Soundex code based upon the surname, sex, a suffix used if two records would otherwise have an identical key, and two check digits. This identifier is used on the comprehensive master index, on labels produced for Health Visitor records, and all turn-round documents relating to the child.

The Child Register is updated whenever identification information about the child changes. A code indicates whether the record is an active one for a current resident, that the child has left, or any other appropriate record state.

Immunisation Module

In principle, the operation of the Immunisation Module is straightforward. Each Authority decides on one or two immunisation schedules which it will use for children aged up to five years; it also decides the treatment centres. Each treatment centre then determines the frequency and times of its immunisation sessions, which of the two schedules will be used, and which of a range of appointment methods it will use.

Authorities choose between a policy of obtaining legal consent soon after birth, or alternatively at attendance for each new course of prophylaxis. The Health Visitor obtains from parents details about the immunisation they wish their child to receive and the location they wish to attend.

On a weekly or fortnightly basis the computer program determines which children are due for an appointment, whether their treatment centre has a session, and whether they can be accommodated within it. From this selection and matching, appointments are allocated, appointment cards are produced, and lists of children called for are sent to each treatment centre. After the session immunisations given, and any known reasons for non attendance are recorded. Unfortunately, because of continued failure to obtain a standard format between pharmaceutical manufacturers, it is currently not possible to computer-record the batch number. The system informs Health Visitors of children who have failed twice to attend without reason, and it calculates payments due to general practitioners.

Pre-School Module

CHCC supervised the design and production of this module from first principles. There being less experience in applying computers to health surveillance, the first stage was to examine the limited number of systems then available, and also to assess the objectives of Pre-School Health Surveillance systems. From this was determined both the information base necessary, and the scheduling arrangements required to meet the needs of different Health Authorities. The computer programs were completed on schedule in mid-1981, but the CHCC felt field testing was essential before general release. Despite some delay in obtaining ethical approval to the pilot running, trials started in mid-1982 and lasted for six months. The trials were successful, but suggested certain further developments which were built into the system, which was available for general use from January 1984.

The Module applies the same principles as the Immunisation Module, but has greater facilities and a larger data base. It commences with comprehensive information from the Neo-Natal Discharge Form where this is used. This form was designed in parallel with the system, but can be used by Authorities not using the computer; conversely, the computer can operate without the neo-natal information. The form contains key data about the ante-natal period, the labour, and the post natal period until the child is discharged from hospital; these were agreed with the Royal College of Obstetricians & Gynaecologists and the British Paediatric Association.

Scheduling is very similar to the Immunisation Module, except that each Authority can operate three different schedules. Moreover, within those schedules the Authority decides the contents of each examination and the category of professional staff who will undertake it. Additionally, for any child, at any examination the examiner can request a special recall after any interval.

There are three main components to the data base for the individual child:-

1. The results of each surveillance examination within nine standard and three locally-determined categories.

2. Significant diagnoses are recorded for each child, using the British Paediatric Association Supplement to the International Classification of Diseases. These diagnoses are individually flagged if they become historic rather than current, and also if they are significant for the dental treatment of the child.

3. Other indicators helpful to the health care of the child are recorded, including future recall dates.

The trials of the Module confirmed that scheduling produces a higher attendance rate.[6-8] Much more significant though, is the creation of an epidemiological data base for all children. This enables children with special needs to be identified, changes in health can be monitored, and particular patterns of health care or screening evaluated.

School Health Module

This Module was similarly designed from first principles, and was piloted from September 1983 to May 1984. The evaluation was successful, and the Module will be available for general use in September 1985.

This Module consists of a series of linked sub-routines, of which an Authority can use any combination. Medical examinations are recorded in a similar way to the Pre-School Module, though the examinations are normally undertaken at school. Immunisations due are scheduled on an individual course basis, with the consent form showing previous history and also recording the antigen subsequently given. A range of surveillance routines is provided, including testing of vision and hearing, and dental inspections. These each provide recall and referral facilities, as well as feeding information to the main medical record.

Apart from extending by 10 years the age range of children covered and adjusting to the school environment, the main further aspect of this module is linkage with educational activity in schools in two main ways. First, Education

Authorities are asked to share in the creation and maintenance of the Child Register. Secondly, and specifically under the control of the school doctor individually for each child, the system can produce a card to the Head Teacher indicating any special management requirements which the child will have in school as a result of health needs. This information will not include clinical information, but will give helpful advice. Detailed issues resulting from this inter-professional and inter-authority collaboration remain to be resolved at national level, but it is essential for the well being of children.

Confidentiality and Security

At an early stage CHCC developed its own confidentiality and security protocol, which has the approval of the British Medical Association. The three ethical principles upon which it is based where endorsed in the House of Commons by the Secretary of State for Social Services.[9] The protocol indicates procedures to be adopted within Computer Centres, at Administrative Centres, and at operational level within the Health Service. More recently, the Data Protection Act 1984 has added statutory safeguards.

Computer Hardware

The system was initially designed for batch operation on Regional ICL mainframe computers, as this was the only technology available to all Health Authorities. This is becoming dated, and technological aspects are now being updated.[10] Also, Regional networks are being developed which will permit local data capture and on-line interrogation.

The next stage proposed by the British Computer Policy Committee is the development of the approach to cover other community health functions. This may include transferability to other hardware.

Conclusion

The British Child Health Systems is a case-study of objective design, collaboration[11,12] and evaluation, and as a result it is becoming widely used. CHCC is committed to ensuring the system is updated and developed when necessary, and recognises that training support is vital for successful utilisation. A powerful facility is now available for preventive health care scheduling and recording, and for epidemiological analysis.

REFERENCES

1. Walker, C. H. M., British Medical Journal, 285: 1671, 1982.

2. Walker, C. H. M., British Medical Journal, 287: 1400, 1983.

3. Rigby, M. J., Health and Social Services Journal, 92: 1044, 1982.

4. Galloway, T. McL., Medical Off icer, 109: 232, 1963.

5. Department of Health and Social Security. Management Arrangements for the Reorganised National Health Service. HMSO. London, 1972.

6. Chesham, I., Rigby, M. J., & Shelmerdine, H. R., Health and Social Services Journal, 85: 293, 1975.

7. Bussey, A. L., & Holmes, B. S., Lancet, 1: 450, 1978.

8. Bussey, A. L., & Harris, A. S., Community Medicine, 1: 29, 1979.

9. Hansard, House of Commons, 26th May, 1978. Col 809-9.

10. Walker, C. H. M., British Medical Journal, 281: 90, 1980.

11. Rigby, M. J., Health Trends, 13: 97, 1981.

12. Department of Health and Social Security. Steering Group on Health Services Information (Chairman, Mrs E. Körner) - 5th Report to the Secretary of State. HMSO. London, 1984.

MICROCOMPUTER IN THE HOME CONTROL OF DIABETES IN A CHILD

M. Kataja
National Public Health Institute
Helsinki, Finland

Introduction

Microcomputers are often advertised to be useful in helping with book-
keeping or similar home activities. When a microcomputer is at hand,
truly useful home applications seem to be quite rare. In our family
the computer is used mainly for writing, for maintaining some lists
where a sorting procedure is essential, and in controlling the treatment response of a diabetic child.

Juvenile diabetes is caused by an autoimmunization process which de-
stroys the beta cells of the spleen. Short after the onset of diabetes
the spleen functions partially so that exogenous insulin is needed
much less than later when the spleen does not function at all.   The
progression of this autoimmunization process during the first two to
three years after onset requires continuous monitoring of the insulin
response while adjusting the dosage. The purpose of the control system
described later is to help the doctor and especially the child's
mother to maintain the correct insulin dosage.

Theory

In the human organism, blood sugar level is controlled by a complex
system of hormones. Insulin is the most important hormone in transmitting glucose from extracellular space into the cell. The normal metabolism maintains blood glucose levels within rather narrow limits
(some 3.5 to 5.5 millimoles per litre) to avoid hypoglychaemia (low
blood sugar) and hyperglychaemia (high blood sugar). Normally insulin
is used to lower the blood sugar and glucose is produced in the liver
to raise it. If the blood sugar level is much too low, glucagon is
used to raise the glucose concentration and, in the opposite situation
kidneys pass excess glucose to urine.

In diabetes the normal control mechanism do not function; therefore the blood sugar level is controlled principally by diet and physical exercise. These factors are matched to the insulin level rather than matchin the insulin to these factors. The individual's insulin response is quite unique; This causes a need of personalized insulin dosage. The response is also disturbed by other factors. Among these infection is the most serious producing a temporary greater need of insulin.

Blood sugar may be monitored directly by taking blood samples from finger-tips or indirectly by measuring urine sugar. The direct method is more accurate but being invasive it is not used regularly in children.

Sugar is normally not secreted to urine but at levels above the "kidney threshold" (9..10 mmol/l) sugar is released with a speed roughly proportional to the concentration. Although these parameters may vary among individuals, they remain nearly constant within an individual. This fact provides the basis for indirect control of the child's diabetes.

When the amount of excess sugar passed to urine is measured, an indication of the blood sugar level during the collection period is obtained. More precisely, this amount is a time integral of the function K$\ast$(blood sugar $\triangle$ kidney threshold), where the operator $\triangle$ denotes the MODUS-function (A$\triangle$B = A-B if A>B and A$\triangle$B=0 otherwise). The constant K, needed to match the units, is obtained by a careful series of simultaneous observations of blood and urine sugar. This is normally accomplished in the hospital immediately after diagnosis of diabetes as part of the procedure to find the proper diet and dosage of insulin.

Excellent treatment balance may be obtained by injecting rapid insulin before each meal. In this case there may be no secretion of sugar to urine for a long time. For children, this approach is undesirable because the probability of deep hypoglychaemia is dangerously high.

Home control by means of urine samples

The normal Finnish procedure for child diabetics is to take four urine measurements daily and to observe the percent sugar concentration as well as the ketones. Usually, a quite convenient stix method is used.

In our case this procedure was altered so that all urine is monitored by recording the **time**, the **amount**, and the **concentration** on a special for developed for this purpose. Actually, we have a continuous collection of these records from the beginning of our daughter's diabetes. Initially I used the data in hand calculations to determine the secretion speed, but quite rapidly I took advantage of a computer. The program was originally written in FORTRAN but I transtaled it to BASIC to operate on my CP/M machine at home.

The purpose of the control procedure is to calculate the mean secretion of sugar to urine as a daily average in 20 minute steps. The collection time is normally a calendar month but the procedure may be used for an uninterrupted period of time from two days to several months. Two week periods are useful after changes in insulin dosage.

Techniques

The program is written so that the input is prepared by a WordStar word processor, one line for each day beginning about 8 a.m. There is no strict input format, numbers may be separated by spaces or commas. Each line contains:

- day identification (number in month)
- one or more observation pairs: Time and amount of sugar
- checksum of sugar secreted during the day.

The first two lines of data used in the example were:

```
1  11.1 8  14.5 2.6 16.3 0.1  18.1 0  21.3 0.5  7.4 0.7  11.9
2  11 2.4  17  0.9  20.4 0.1   7.0 2    5.4
```

The program calculates the secretion profile by assuming a constant secretion speed over the whole collection period (after the preceding observation). The number of observation pairs in our case is normally 5 or 6. On the form, there is space for 7 daily observations, but during infections as many as 10 measurements may be required.

The program produces a table of hourly secretion means and a histogram, as shown in the figure on the next page. The data entry, test run, corrections and the final calculation take normally 20 minutes.

Summary

The program fulfils well its original purpose in the home control of diabetes in one family member. It is also clearly the most useful task carried out by the home computer.

Home Follow Up of a Diabetic

Time	g/h	Time	g/h	Time	g/h	Time	g/h
1	0.12	7	0.25	13	0.40	19	0.47
2	0.12	8	0.15	14	0.58	20	0.37
3	0.12	9	0.88	15	0.66	21	0.45
4	0.25	10	0.68	16	0.63	22	0.36
5	0.25	11	0.68	17	0.58	23	0.17
6	0.25	12	0.40	18	0.50	24	0.13

Mean secretion g/h December, 1984

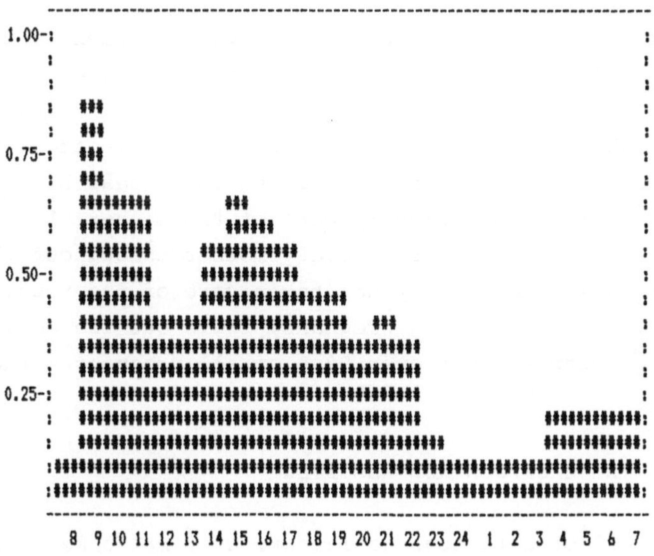

```
     ---------------------------------------------------------
1.00-:                                                        :
     :                                                        :
     :                                                        :
     :   ###                                                  :
     :   ###                                                  :
0.75-:   ###                                                  :
     :   ###                                                  :
     :   #########      ###                                   :
     :   #########      ######                                :
     :   #########   ############                             :
0.50-:   #########   ############                             :
     :   #########   ################                         :
     :   ################################    ###             :
     :   #####################################                :
     :   #####################################                :
     :   #####################################                :
0.25-:   #####################################                :
     :   #####################################   ############:
     :   ######################################   ###########:
     :#################################################################:
     :#################################################################:
     ---------------------------------------------------------
        8  9 10 11 12 13 14 15 16 17 18 19 20 21 22 23 24  1  2  3  4  5  6  7
```

Figure 1. Actual example from December, 1984.

CONGENITAL MALFORMATIONS - INFORMATION SYSTEM AND ITS USE

Anneli Ruusinen
The National Board of Health
Siltasaarenkatu 18 A, 00530 Helsinki, Finland

1. INTRODUCTION

Notification of congenital malformations detected during the first
year of life has been compulsory in Finland since 1963. The reports
on defects detected in liveborn infants are completed by information from death certificates for all deceased children and stillborn
from the 28th week of gestation. Towards the end of 1984 22 105
malformed cases have been reported from 1.5 million births. This
gives the incidence of 1.5 per 10 000 births.

It has been estimated that about 70 % of the malformations detected
during the perinatal period are notified, mainly the minor defects
remaining unreported. In addition, about one third of the malformations remain undetected at birth and immediately thereafter. The
Maternity Welfare Centres (an activity of the local health centres)
are responsible for the post-delivery care of the mother. At the
centres detailed records are kept on every mother throughout the
pregnancy. The midwife who usually has taken care of the routine
examination and interviews during pregnancy fills out the notification report. The centres cover over 99 % of all pregnant mothers.

2. THE STRUCTURE OF THE CASE/CONTROL REGISTER

The information collected through notification of malformations
also serves special studies. For this purpose, since 1964, certain
marks or indicator defect have been chosen for more detailed epidemiological investigations and for continuous case/control studies.
The indicator defects should be clearly defined, easily detectable
at birth and severe enough to focus the clinician's attention.
Following defects have been selected for special analysis: defects

cleft and the structural malformations of the skeleton excluding
congenital dislocation of hip, clubfoot and other questionable
anomalies. All these structural malformations are believed to
be traceable to impaired organogenesis during the first trimester
of pregnancy. For each study mother a pair control case is chosen,
i.e. a mother whose delivery has taken place immediately before
the study mother's delivery in the same health centre district.
Information as well as blood samples are obtained from the control
mother exactly as from the study mother. The interview of the case
mother and the control mother is carried out by the midwife at
the local health centre. The parametres gathered from the primary
notification report, eventual death certificate, the interview
questionnaire and the antenatal record are transmitted on magnetic
tape.

Since 1981 a special study on congenital heart defects has been
in process. The project on heart defects started as an evaluation
project. The items in the interview have been supplemented and
several control cases have been selected for each defect case. The
control cases have been selected at random from live born healthy
infants. The control cases are chosen by computer from the infants
born at certain dates. The system enables a more efficient use of
the multivariation methods in analyses than the system of merely
one study/one control case.

There are plans for the new system to be taken into use for all
study cases in the register within two or three years.

The reasons for focusing the special study on congenital heart
defects have been that only few investigations have been carried
out on the causes of heart defects and it seems evident that
external factors play a major role in the developing of the heart.

3. THE USE OF THE REGISTER

The register on congenital malformations has two main purposes:

1. To serve as a monitoring system and
2. To serve as a data resource on the incidence and as a basic
   material for further studies.

The number of cases and different types of notified malformations
are followed by monthly statistics. The statistics by geographical
regions and by type of malformations are the regular statistical
data. The Finnish Register is a member of an international organization: International Clearinghouse for Birth Defects Monitoring
Systems. Through the Clearinghouse, the national projects (program
directors) can quickly evaluate changes observed in their data
by making rapid comparison between their baseline and current
rates and those of other monitoring systems. The Clearinghouse
is an independent organization and negotiations are taking place
to obtain an official relation with WHO as a non-governmental
organization. The primary source of communication and the core
of the Clearinghouse activities are quarterly reports which are
produced less than five months after the end of a calendar quarter.
Data on eleven selected conditions are regularly reported to the
Clearinghouse. These selected conditions are anencephaly, spina
bifida, hydrocephaly, cleft palate, cleft lip, esophagcal defects,
hypospadias, limb reduction deformities, omphalocele and Down
syndrome. They were selected for routine international comparisons
because most of them are regarded to have a multifactorial etiology
in which the environment may play some role, most of them are
clearly defined, they are usually diagnosed shortly after birth
and they occur in sufficient numbers for reliable baseline rates
to be calculated from 100 000 births, which is the minimum baseline
requirement for full membership in the Clearinghouse. The rates
are given for the observed number of each malformation per 10 000
births. The expected number of cases in each program is calculated
by applying the baseline rates to the total number of births
(O/E-ratio). In addition there are some joint studies going on
between individual programs e.g. multimalformed infants and specific subgroups of limb reductions.

Especially the pair register serves as a source for further
studies and comparative surveys. Many valuable studies particularly concerning the medicament during pregnancy have been performed.

As an example of the co-operation between the register in the Nordic countries is a study on the hospital treatment of certain malformed babies. The material consists of the notified cases on four determined diagnosis (spina bifida, cleft palate and cleft lip, atresia and stenosis, Down syndrome) under the period of 5-6 years (1977-). The cases will be identified from the material of hospital patient registers. The purpose is to find out how these children have overcome.

4. EVALUATION

The register on congenital malformations has proved to be one of the most feasible registers for the studies to find means to prevent defects both nationally and internationally. Usefulness will increase when the new method of several control cases will cover all study cases and when the birth register as a part of register on patients discharged from hospitals will start in the beginning of 1986. The register on all infants (discharged from hospitals) will give both supplementing and comparation material to the malformation register and it gives information of circumstances during pregnancy and delivery and treatment during hospital care period.

REFERENCES

1. Aro, T. Incidence secular trends and risk indicators of reduction limb defects. Health Services Research by the National Board of Health in Finland, 31. Helsinki 1984

2. Banister, P. Evaluation of vital record usage for congenital anomaly surveillance. In: Hook EB, Janerich DT, Porter IH, eds. Monitoring, birth defects and environment. The problem of surveillance. New York: Academic Press, 1971:119-136.

3. Bjerkedal T, Bakketeig LS. Surveillance of congenital malformations and other conditions in the newborn. Int.J Epidemiol 1975; 4:31-36.

4. Chen R. A surveillance system for congenital malformations. JASA 1978; 73:323-327.

5. Czeizel A. The Hungarian congenital malformation monitoring system. Acta Paediatr Acad Sci Hung 1978;19:225-238.

6. Dessemond M, Boschetti R, Mamelle N. Systematic registration of malformations (Fre). J Genet Hum 1975; 23 (suppl):50-57.

7. Ericson A, Källen B, Winberg J. Surveillance of malformations at birth: a comparison of two record systems run in parallel. Int J Epidemiol 1977;6:35-41.

8. Flynt JW Jr, Ebbin AJ, Oakley GP Jr, Falek A, Heath CW Jr. Metropolitan Atlanta congenital defects program. In: Hook EB, Janerich DT, Porter IH, eds. Monitoring birth defects and environment: the problem of surveillance. New York: Academic Press, 1971:155-158.

9. Flynt JW Jr. Trends in surveillance of congenital malformations. In: Janerich DT, Skalko RG, Porter IH, eds. Congenital defects: new directions in research. New York: Academic Press, 1974:119-128.

10. Hill GB, Spicer CC, Weatherall JA: The computer surveillance of congenital malformations. Br Med Bull 1968; 24:215-218.

11. Hultin H. Registration of congenital malformations (Fin). Kätilölehti 1971;76: 398-399.

12. International Clearinghouse for Birth Defects Monitoring Systems, Annual report 1982

13. Klemetti A. Registry for congenital malformations (Fin). Duodecim 1971;87:1409-1411.

14. Klemetti A, Saxen L. The Finnish register of congenital malformations. Health Services Research of the National Board of Health in Finland, Helsinki, 1970.

15. Klingberg MA. Epidemiologic methods in research of congenital malformations (Ita). Riv Ist Sieroter Ital 1968;43:269-286.

16. Kucera J. Preparation of international system for follow-up of congenital defects; WHO (Cze). Cesk Pediatr 1973;28:270-271.

17. Källen B, Winberg J. Multiple malformations studied with a national register of malformations. Pediatrics 1969;44:410-417.

18. Källen B, Winberg J. A Swedish register of congenital malformations. Experience with continuous registration during 2 years with special reference to multiple malformations. Pediatrics 1968;41:765-776.

19. Ruusinen A. The Finnish Register of Congenital Malformations. A Review of the Matched-pair Register in 1970-1977. A working paper for the fifth working conference of birth defects in Hungary 1978.

20. Saxen L, Klemetti A, Härö AS. A matched-pair register for studies of selected congenital defects. Am J Epidemiol 1974;100:297-306.

21. Saxen L. Newborn Monitoring. In: Shepard TH, et al, eds. Methods for detection of environmental agents that produce congenital

defects. Amsterdam: Elsevier, 1975:205-219.

22. Tikkanen J, Heinonen O.P., Leppo K, Epämuodostumarekisteriä uudistetaan. The renewing of the register on congenital malformations. Suomen Lääkärilehti 1984; 7:512-515.

23. Tikkanen J, Heinonen O.P. Etiology of congenital heart disease. Manuscript 1984.

24. Weatherall JA, Haskey JC. Surveillance of malformations. Br Med Bull 1976;32:39-44.

HANDLING OF THE NOTIFICATIONS ON CONGENITAL MALFORMATIONS IN FINLAND

USE OF REGISTER OF LOW-BIRTH-WEIGHT INFANTS FOR THE EVALUATION OF ADIPO-
SITY INDICES.

*J. B. GOUYON, **F. A. ALLAERT, **N. DEBBAS, **L. DUSSERRE,
*J. L. NIVELON, *M. ALISON.
* Hôpital d'Enfants de DIJON (Pr M. ALISON - Pr J. L. NIVELON)
** Service d'Informatique Médicale (Pr L. DUSSERRE)
Boulevard Maréchal de Lattre de Tassigny 21034 DIJON CEDEX - FRANCE -

INTRODUCTION

Recently Roland-Cachera and al. established reference curves for the
adiposity index W/H^2 between 1 month and 16 years of life. This adiposity index is reliable method to assess indirectly the development of
fat mass in infants. Moreover, Miller and Hassanein (1) established reference curves for another adiposity index W/H^3 at birth according to
gestational age. Villar and al. (2) suggested that W/H^3 at birth correlates with subsequent growth in weight and height among hypotrophic
full term infants. References graphs for W/H^2 index are only available
after the first month of life and index W/H^3 for neonatal period. We
have studied the development of the adiposity index W/H^2 between 3 and
18 months of life among low-birth-weight (L.B.W) infants (less than
2500 g) according to their weight and W/H^3 index at birth.
The concept of hypotrophia (birth weight below the 10th percentile according to the gestational age) is more widely used by obstetricians
and paediatricians than the Rohrer's index (weight/height^3) which is an
adiposity index. However Walther and Ramaekers (3) had recently suggested that an index W/H^3 below the 10th percentile had a higher predictive value of neonatal morbidity than hypotrophia.
We used data prospectively gathered within a larger study regarding assessment of development of L.B.W infants.

MATERIALS AND METHODS

Weight and height at birth and corrected chronological age of 3, 6, 9,
15-18 months were available for 300 infants included in the general
framework of a prospective study on the assessment of perinatal care
and postnatal development of L.B.W newborns (4) of various gestational
ages. On the whole, 400 items were available on the perinatal period
and 55 new items on the first 18 months of life for each newborn. So, in
order to obtain an homogeneous sample the infants with perinatal or
postnatal diseases affecting growth were excluded from the study. The
criteria for exclusion were : twins, children of diabetic mothers,
newborns affected by embryofetopathy, chromosomic abnormalities, severe

congenital malformations, RH incompatibility. Twins were the main criteria for exclusion (n= 70). On the whole the study included 2 samples :
190 infants (100 girls) for the evaluation of adiposity indices and 222
infants for the estimation of the predictive value of neonatal morbidity of the W/H^3 index.

We have previously described the methodology used for storing and compiling the data about the perinatal and postnatal period (4). In summary, up to 400 items about maternal past-history, pregnancy, birth and
neonatal diseases can be prospectively collected for each newborn hospitalized in our neonatal unit. Data are compiled on a micro-computer
HP 45B. The data allow us to obtain regular evaluation about the quality of care in our unit (5). From the 3rd to the 48th months of corrected chronological age, general practitioners and paediatricians collect
data on growth and neurological development of these infants and send
this information to us for compilation. Informed consents are obtained
from the parents.

- The gestational age was estimated according to the obstetrical data
and the Dubowitz score.

- The corrected chronological age modifies the postnatal age in case
of prematurity and allows us to compare growths of infants with various
gestational age at birth (corrected age in weeks = postnatal age in
weeks - 41 gestational age in weeks).

- Weight and height were determined at birth and later by the regular
doctors at the corrected chronological ages of 3, 6, 9, 15-18 months.
At birth the weight and height were compared to the reference graphs of
Leroy-Lefort (compiled for the French population) and those of Usher-
Mc Lean (6, 7) more widely used. Hypotrophy is defined by a weight be-
low the 10th percentile.

- The weight indices (W/H^3) were compared to the Miller Hassanein
reference graphs (1).

- At the chronological age of 3, 6, 9, 15-18 months the adiposity indices W/H^2 were interpreted in relation to sex by using Rolland-Cachera
references graphs recently compiled for the French population.

RESULTS

1- Rohrer index W/H^3 and hypotrophy at birth (table 1)

The percentage of hypotrophy at birth amongst the 190 infants studied
is different according to the references used : 40 % with Usher and
Mc Lean graphs and 69 % with those of Leroy-Lefort (p < 0.001). However
the average W/H^3 index is not influenced by the choice of weight references when the newborns are divided in four groups : eutrophic babies
with W/H^3 index ⩾ 10th percentile, hypotrophic babies with W/H^3 index

$\geqslant$ 10th percentile, eutrophic babies with W/H^3 index < 10th percentile and hypotrophic babies with W/H^3 index < 10th percentile.

2- Evolution of the adiposity index W/H^2 of eutrophic and S.G.A infants (table 2).

Amongst both sexes, the average adiposity indices of the S.G.A and eutrophic infants are not different beginning with the corrected age of three months. Meanwhile, amongst the S.G.A boys, the frequency of adiposity indices W/H^2 < 10th percentile increases between 3 and 6 months and between 3 and 9 months. This evolution is significantly observed amongst the S.G.A girls either between 3 and 9 months or 3 and 15-18 months.

3- Predictive value of the Rohrer's weight index (W/H^3)

Among 222 newborns studied for the evaluation of predictive value of W/H^3 index : 61 % were premature ; 40.5 % were hypotrophic according to Usher and Mc Lean's graphs ; 36.5 % had W/H^3 index lower than 10th percentile. Table 3 shows that the low W/H^3 index had a better value for hypothermia than hypotrophia ; but no differences were obtained for hypoglycemia, hypocalcemia, non conjugated hyperbilirubinemia, neonatal respiratory distress, apnea and low Apgar indices.

COMMENTARY

All the adiposity indices evaluate the proportion of the fat mass, accepting the fact that the lean mass remains constant for a given height. The adiposity index W/H^2 fulfills at best the conditions of good index of fat mass in both sexes (8). Physiologically the W/H^2 index curves indicate a reduction of corpulence between 1 and 6 years and an increased before one year and after 6 years (8).

In our study the average W/H^3 index among S.G.A and A.G.A groups is not influenced by the type of references used to define these groups. An index W/H^3 below the 10th percentile at birth reduces significantly the frequency of an W/H^2 index up to the 10th percentile between 3 to 18 months of corrected chronological age. The S.G.A infants had an increased frequency of low W/H^2 indices until 9 months for boys and 15-18 months for girls in comparison to a reference group of adapted for gestational age infants.

So these changes of adiposity indices W/H^2 among the S.G.A infants during a period (first year of life) of physiological increase of height of adipocytes, urges further study regarding the period of multiplication of adipocytes with a rapid development of fat mass observed after 6 years of life (9, 10).

Table 1. Average weight index for each group according to the reference weight classifications of Usher-Mc Lean (U-McL) and Leroy-Lefort (L-L).

SD : Standard deviation
NS : Non Significant

Breakdown \ Gestational age		30 à 33 weeks				34 à 37 weeks				38 à 41 weeks			
		n	A	SD	value of p	n	A	SD	value of p	n	A	SD	value of p
Eutrophics at weight index ≥ 10th perc.	U-McL	19	2,35	0,235	NS	58	2,44	0,17	NS	9	2,49	0,17	-
	L-L	15	2,39	0,242		33	2,47	0,19		1	-	-	
S.G.A at weight index < 10th perc.	U-McL	2	1,9	0,08	NS	12	2,03	0,09	NS	33	2,12	0,15	NS
	L-L	5	1,96	0,08		26	2,03	0,09		36	2,13	0,14	
Eutrophics at weight index < 10th perc.	U-McL	6	2,02	0,06	NS	20	2,06	0,10	NS	3	2,21	0,05	-
	L-L	3	2,03	0,07		6	2,11	0,09		0	-	-	
S.G.A. at weight index ≥ 10th perc.	U-McL	0	-	-	-	6	2,38	0,13	NS	22	2,5	0,18	NS
	L-L	4	2,18	0,09		31	2,38	0,11		30	2,5	0,18	
TOTAL		27				96				67			

Table 2. Average weight index for the boys and the girls from 3 months to 15-18 months. (according to Leroy-Lefort).

SD : Standard deviation
NS : Non Significant

♂

Age	n	A	SD	Breakdown	x^2 test or Fischer	n	A	SD	Breakdown	x^2 test (p)	TOTAL
		EUTROPHICS					S.G.A.				
3 MONTHS	25	161,33	14,54	≥ 10e perc. 22 / < 10e perc. 4 (NS)	(NS)	47	158,86	14,81	≥ 10e perc. 40 / < 10e perc. 7	p<0,05	72
6 MONTHS	21	167,22	16,50	≥ 10e perc. 17 / < 10e perc. 4 (NS)	(NS)	41	163,64	16,36	≥ 10e perc. 26 / < 10e perc. 15 NS	p<0,05	62
9 MONTHS	20	168,47	13,31	≥ 10e perc. 18 / < 10e perc. 2 (NS)		29	166,50	17,08	≥ 10e perc. 19 / ≤ 10e perc. 10	NS	49
15-18 MONTHS	12	166,82	12,82	≥ 10e perc 11 / < 10e perc. 1		18	167,16	11,77	≥ 10e perc. 15 / ≤ 10e perc. 3		30

♀

Age	n	A	SD	Breakdown	x^2 test or Fischer	n	A	SD	Breakdown	x^2 test (p)	TOTAL
3 MONTHS	19	154,08	14,46	≥ 10e perc. 17 / < 10e perc. 2 (NS)	(NS)	65	154,73	13,82	≥ 10e perc. 56 / < 10e perc. 9	NS	84
6 MONTHS	16	156,85	14,15	≥ 10e perc. 13 / < 10e perc. 2 (NS)	(NS)	44	159,97	13,65	≥ 10e perc. 34 / < 10e perc. 10 NS	p<0,01 p<0,05	60
9 MONTHS	11	168,56	12,18	≥ 10e perc. 9 / < 10e perc. 2 (NS)		39	161,40	17,04	≥ 10e perc. 23 / < 10e perc. 16	NS	50
15-18 MONTHS	7	171,18	16,5	≥ 10e perc. 6 / < 10e perc. 1		23	157,23	11,26	≥ 10e perc. 15 / < 10e perc. 8		30

Table 3 : Breakdown of hypothermia and hyperbilirubinemia according to
weight index and birth weight.

	Weight index		Birth weight	
	< 10th perc.	≥ 10th perc.	< 10th perc.	≥ 10th perc.
Hypothermia (< 36°)	(34.24 %) vs (19.2 %) p < 0.05		(24.7 %) vs (26 %) NS	
Hyperbilirubinemia (≥ 100 mg/l	(28.3 %) vs (45.4 %) p < 0.05		(25.4 %) vs (46.7 %) p < 0.01	

REFERENCES

1- Miller HC, Hassanein K (1971) Diagnosis of impaired fetal growth in
   newborn infants. Pediatrics 48 : 511-522.
2- Villar J, Belizan JM, Spalding J, Klein RE (1982) Post-natal growth
   of intrauterine growth retarded infants. Early Hum Dev 6 : 265-271.
3- Walther FJ, Ramaekers LHJ (1982) The ponderal index as a mesure of
   the nutritional status at birth and its relation to some aspects of
   neonatal morbidity. Acta Paediatr Scand 71 : 436-440.
4- Allaert FA, Gouyon JB, Dusserre L, Cinquin P, Couillault G,
   Nivelon JL, Alison M. The setting up of a system of self evaluation
   in a newborn unit. Preliminary results. Medinfo 1983, Van Bemmel/
   Ball/Wigertz. Ed IFIP, IMIA. North Holland. 1983, 2 : 659-662.
5- Gouyon JB, Allaert FA, Brichon P, Debbas N, Traore E, Dusserre L,
   Nivelon JL, Alison M. Psychomotric development of Low-Birth-Weight
   infants. Methods and preliminary results. In Third International
   Conference on System Science in Health Care, Munich. Ed Van Eimeren W,
   Engelbrech R and Flagle ChD. Springer-Verlag Berlin Heidelberg New-
   York Tokyo. July 16-20 1984, 581-583.
6- Leroy B, Lefort F (1971) A propos du poids et de la taille des
   nouveau-nés à la naissance. Rev Franç Gynec 66 : 391.
7- Usher R, Mc Lean F (1969) Intrauterine growth of life-born caucasian
   infants. J Pediatr 74 : 901.
8- Rolland-Cachera MF, Sempe M, Guilloud-Bataille M, Patois E,
   Pequignot-Guggenbuhl FP, Fautrad V (1982) Adiposity indices in children. Am J Clin Nutr 36 : 178-184.
9- Hirsch J, Batchelor B (1976) Adipose tissue cellularity in human obe-
   sity. Clin Endocrinol Metab 5 : 299-311.
10- Häger A, Sjöström L, Arvidsson B, Björntord P, Smith U (1977) Body
    fat and adipose tissue cellularity in infants: a longitudinal study.
    Metabolism 26 : 607-614.

QUALITY CONTROL OF THE OBSTETRIC CARE WITH THE AID OF SPECIAL PURPOSE
COMPUTERS FOR FETAL HEART RATE MONITORING AND PERINATAL DATA BASE

V. Kariniemi and J. Rosti
Department of Obstetrics and Gynecology, Salo District
Hospital, 24130 Salo, Finland

Introduction: Attempts to benefit the recent development in computing technique
are being made in several obstetric units. Especially the vast amount of data
obtained from the fetus by electronic monitoring of fetal heart rate (FHR) and
uterine activity in cardiotocography (CTG) has focused the interest of modern
obstetricians in computers. CTG-recordings are mostly evaluated visually, but
some authors have claimed that a proper computer program might be superior to
human eye in recognition of the FHR patterns. It is generally accepted, however,
that visual evaluation of FHR variability is extremely difficult (1,2). Yet FHR
variability is one of the most important parameters describing the function of
the fetal nervous system. November 1st, 1983 the Perinatal Data Base of Salo
District Hospital was founded. Simultaneously, quantification of FHR variability
by microprocessorbased small computers was started as a screening method during
labor. This report is to describe some recent experience obtained by the system.

The purpose of the study:
- to find out the physiological background and environmental factors
  which have effect on FHR patterns during labor
- to improve the quality control of the obstetric care
- to study which data during pregnancy and labor are worth storing in
  the data base

Methods:

Quantification of FHR variability is performed with the aid of two special-
purpose computers, which are connected to the conventional Hewlett-Packard
CTG-monitors. The computers are made of microprocessors and they can process
any kind of electromagnetic heart signals (3,4). In practice the first screening
analysis of FHR variability is done 2 to 3 weeks before the expected date of
delivery. It is done from a five-minute sample of abdominal fetal electrocardiogram. If this antepartal recording of fetal electrocardiogram (FECG)

fails, as it does in about thirty per cent, a conventional nonstress CTG
by ultrasound is recorded. During labor the intrapartal analysis of FHR variabi
lity is started by abdominal FECG, and continued by direct FECG, if the
abdominal signal is too noisy. Ultrasound is needed only in 1% of labors.

The analysis of FHR variability is a modification of the method proposed by
Yeh et al (5). In this method a statistical analysis of fetal heart intervals
and interval differences is made on-line. The computers print two indices of
FHR variability, the interval index (II) describing the long term component
and the differential index (DI) describing the short term component of FHR
(5). According to our previous studies, II measures mainly the fetal arousal
level (4), and DI the integrity of the autonomous nervous system, which are
affected by fetal oxygenation, maternal smoking and medication (6-9). The main
principle in our method is, that only those interval differences, which are
smaller than five beats per minute, are included in the analysis.

The Perinatal Data Base of Salo District Hospital is weighted on cardiotoco-
graphic findings. The indices of FHR variability from the antepartum period
and from the last six hours of labor before delivery are stored in the memory
of a computer at the Computing Center of Helsinki University Central Hospital.
The mothers are allowed to move freely about in the delivery room from time
to time if they wish. During such periods they are disconnected from the
monitors. The visual evaluation of CTG patterns is done by the first author
by counting the number of late and variable decelerations. These figures and
47 other clinical data are stored. Between 7 a.m. and 9 p.m. a sample of
blood from the umbilical vein is collected to determine the environmental
factors which might affect the acid-base balance of the blood flowing towards
the fetus.

The statistical analysis of the collected material is done by the BMDP system
of the University of California.

Subjects:

From the 1st of November 1983 to the end of March 1985, the data from 902
newborn are included. The material is unselected, except for 15 complicated
pregnancies, which were admitted to the University Hospital.

Results:

Annual statistics of the obstetric unit can be obtained directly by BMDP-program
2D. Two methods of fetal heart rate monitoring, analysis of fetal heart rate variability through abdominal fetal electrocardiogram (AFECG) or trough abdominal and
direct FECG, can be compared by BMDP program 3D (Fig 1). The effect of one environmental factor, smoking on fetal heart rate variability can be studied by
"cleaning" alcohol consumption from the material (Fig 2). The possible synergistic
effect of smoking and alcohol on the fetus and placenta can be determined by the
two-way analysis of variance (BMDP program 7D, Table I). The effect of maternal
medication during labor can be studied also by analysis of variance (BMDP-program
4V, Fig 3).

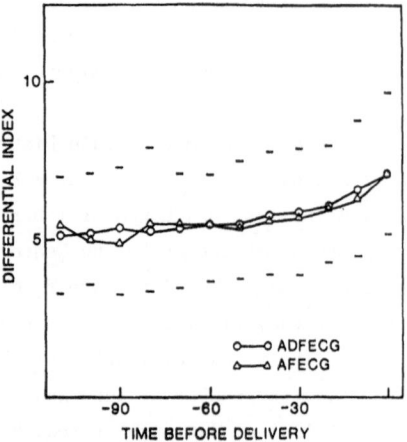

Fig 1. The mean ($\pm$SD) beat-to-beat variability of fetal heart rate during last two
hours of labor of 99 fetuses measured by
abdominal and of 527 fetuses measured by
abdominal and direct (ADFECG) fetal electrocardiogram. The means were compared
by BMDP program 3D. The differences were
not significant. The result indicates
that the same reference values can be
used, whether the indices have been
measured by abdominal or direct method.
(differential index (5) = beat-to-beat
variability of fetal heart rate)

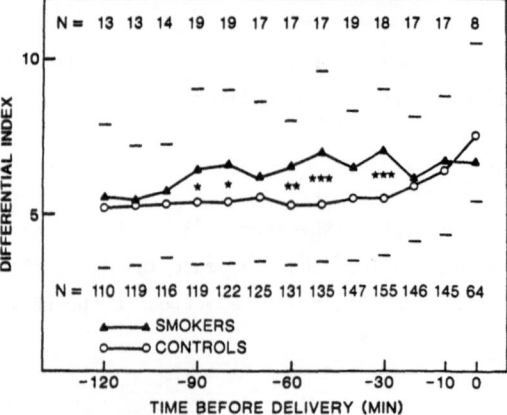

Fig 2. The mean ($\pm$SD) beat-to-beat
variability of fetal heart rate
of 41 smoking and of 281 nonsmoking
mothers who denied alcohol consumption during pregnancy. The means
were compared by BMDP program 3D.
*=$p<0.05$, **=$p<0.01$, ***=$p<0.001$.
(differential index (5) = beat-to-
beat variability of fetal heart
rate)

Table I

Means ($^{\pm}$SD) of birthweights, placental weights and placental/birthweight ratios
according to the smoking and alcohol consumption habits of mothers.

	A	B	C	D		
Smoking	−	−	+	+	p	Bonferroni
Alcohol consumption	−	+	−	+		
N	535	76	77	27		
Birthweight (g)	3708$^{\pm}$520	3716$^{\pm}$557	3601$^{\pm}$439	3386$^{\pm}$557	A-D	**
Placental weight (g)	558$^{\pm}$115	565$^{\pm}$111	572$^{\pm}$101	538$^{\pm}$148		NS
Placental/ (%) birthweight ratio	15.1$^{\pm}$2.4	15.3$^{\pm}$2.3	15.9$^{\pm}$2.4	15.7$^{\pm}$2.4	A-C	*

Fig 3. Mean ($^{\pm}$SD) interval
and differential indices
of fetal heart rate (5)
before and after paracer-
vical blockade among 42
fetuses in labor. The
increment of the interval
index is significant.

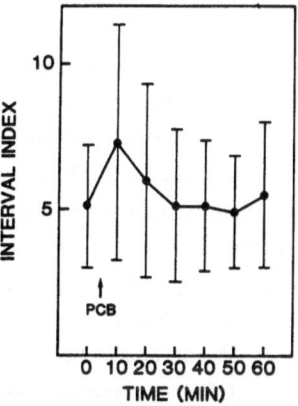
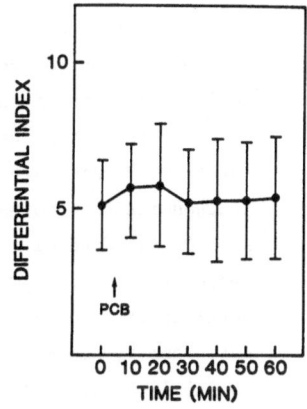

Discussion:

Continuous analysis of fetal heart rate variability during labor and screening
of antepartal fetal heart rate variability, with the support of Perinatal Data
Base have proved their value during 15-month period. New information from the
fetus has been obtained. The data in Table I indicate that the main effect of
smoking alone on the fetoplacental unit is the increment of placental/birthweight
ratio, instead of formerly reported low birthweight. Alcohol consumption with
smoking, on the other hand, is the real factor which has a decreasing effect on
birthweight. It is interesting to note that although the acute effect of smoking
on fetal heart rate variability is decreasing, the chronic effect is opposite,
increasing (Fig 2). We consider this to be a chronic effect of smoke to the fetal
nervous system. A formerly often used medication to relieve pain during labor,
intramuscular pethidine, has been avoided since it was observed to associate with
hypoxia and metabolic acidosis in the umbilical vein (10). Paracervical blockade
on the other hand did not associate with acidosis and its effect on fetal nervous
system is not a depressive one, rather an arousal effect (Fig.3).

References:

1. Kariniemi V. Evaluation of fetal heart rate variability by a visual semiquantitative method and by a quantitative statistical method with the use of a minicomputer. Am J Obstet Gynecol 130:588, 1978

2. Escarcena L, McKinney RD, Depp R. Fetal baseline heart rate estimation. I. Comparison of clinical and stochastic quantification techniques. Am J Obstet Gynecol 135:615, 1979

3. Kariniemi V, Katila T, Laine H, Ämmälä P. On-line quantification of fetal heart rate variability. J Perinat Med 8:213, 1980

4. Kariniemi V, Siimes A, Ämmälä P. Antepartal analysis of fetal heart rate variability by abdominal electrocardiography. J Perinat Med 10:114, 1982

5. Yeh S-Y, Forsythe A, Hon EH. Quantification of fetal heart rate beat-to-beat interval differences. Obstet Gynecol 41:355, 1973

6. Stange L, Rosen KG, Hökegard KH, Karlsson K, Rochlitzer F, Kjellmer I, Joelsson I. Quantification of fetal heart rate variability in relation to oxygenation in the sheep fetus. Acta Obstet Gynecol Scand 56:205, 1977

7. Kariniemi V, Ämmälä P. Short-term variability of fetal heart rate during pregnancies with normal and insufficient placental function. Am J Obstet Gynecol 139:33, 1981

8. Lehtovirta P, Forss M, Kariniemi V, Rauramo I. Acute effects of smoking on fetal heart rate variability. Br J Obstet Gynaecol 90:3, 1983

9. Kariniemi V, Ämmälä P. Effect of intramuscular pethidine on fetal heart rate variability during labour. Br J Obstet Gynaecol 88:718, 1981

10. Kariniemi V, Rosti J. Intramuscular pethidine assciated with metabolic acido sis in the newborn. (submitted)

THE COMPARATIVE INVESTIGATION OF THE CAUSALITY RELATED TO THE PREMATURITY IN THE NEW-BORN POPULATION

Benedek Srajber[1] and András Paksy[2]

[1] Computer Service for State Administration, Budapest, Hungary

[2] Ministry of Health, Budapest, Hungary

Introduction

The rate of the perinatal mortality is relatively high /19 ‰/ in Hungary. This is closely related to the proportion of the new-borns weighing less than 2500 g. /LBW-infants/ or having less than 37 weeks of pregnancy /preterm babies/. These babies were considered as "premature" infants. We have tried to discover the causality of the prematurity in such a way that we compaired two fundamental categories of the normal new-borns and the premature infants surviving 6th day.

Material and Method

From 1972 to 1980 we experimented a methodology for the complex analysis of the causality related to the prematurity. The programsystem is called PERINAT. It consists of seven main modules /FIGURE 1/.

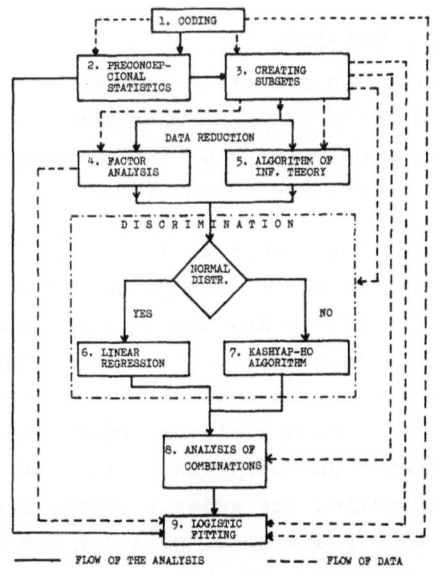

FIGURE 1: MODULES OF PROGRAMSYSTEM "PERINAT"

The first time we applied our program system to the representative
sample of the Hungarian new-born population /30.000 cases, 127 fac-
tors/ in 1971. The procedure was repeated for the total new-born population /144.000 cases, 94 factors/ in 1981. Antropological /e.g. sex
of the offspring, maternal stature, maternal age/ and social /e.g. per
capita income, maternal education, marital status, employment/ and obstetrical /e.g. birth order, abortions/ and gestational /e.g. EPH Gesto-
sis, hyperemesis, smoking habits/ factors were taken into consideration.

At both of investigations the steps of the processing were as follows.

Step 1   We utilize the module hypothesis and as a first approximation
        we determine about 50 factors having significant influence on
        the prematurity.

Step 2   We perform the data reduction /modules 4,5/ and obtain about
        20 important factors /or group of factors/.

Step 3   The normal and premature categories are separated by the mo-
        dules 6 or 7. Each of the factors taken into account gets a
        weight corresponding to its own importance.

Step 4   We compute the fidocial intervals pertaining to the combina-
        tions of the 6-9 factors of greatest importance.

Step 5   The module 9 produces the different curves of the intrauterine
        growth.

Results and Short Interpretation

The most substantial results are given in the form of tables and figures. The Table 1/a and Table 1/b summarize the computed data in the
Step 1,2,3 and contain some aspects of the evaluation and give a starting point to the interpretation of the results.

It is clear from both of our investigations, that the complications
during pregnancy and delivery, the too young and too old parents, the
decreased professional activity and the marital status of the mother,
the high number of the previous life-borns or pregnancies, the low
educational level and the manual employment of the parents, the disadvantageous social environment as well as the disease during pregnancy
have significant influence on the prematurity. The complication group
containing placenta anomalies has great significance, because of the
placenta praevia and the abruption of placenta and the preterm amni-
orrhexis.

TAB. 1/a: THE MOST IMPORTANT FACTORS AND THEIR WEIGHTS GAINED BY THE STEPS 2,3. REPRESENTATIVE SAMPLE, 1971. RELIABILITY OF DECISION: 76 %.

ORDER	IDENT.	INFLUENCING FACTOR	WEIGHT
1.	20	IV. Complications during the pregnancy and delivery WHO codes	0,470
2.	24	Number of the liveborns	0,340
3.	26	Number of the artifical interruption	0,333
4.	27	Number of spontaneous abortions	0,307
5.	62	Marital status of the mother	0,235
6.	101,102	Mother's smoking habit in the first and second half of the pregnancy	0,207
7.	22	VI. Complications during the pregnancy and delivery WHO codes	0,204
8.	96	Symptoms of pregnancy /Edema, Proteinuria, Hyperemesis/	0,122
9.	88	Non specific disease before pregnancy	0,105

TAB. 1/b: THE MOST IMPORTANT FACTORS AND THEIR WEIGHTS GAINED BY THE STEPS 2,3. TOTAL POPULATION SAMPLE, 1981. RELIABILITY OF DECISION: 75 %.

ORDER	IDENT.	INFLUENCING FACTOR	WEIGHT
1.	94/1,2,3,5	The father is dependant	0,183
2.	77/1, 86/1	Too young parents	0,135
3.	82/8,9 84/10,85/1	Decreased professional activity of the mother /dependant, house-wife/	0,038
4.	78/1,3,4	Marital status of the mother /not married, widowed, divorsed/	0,021
5.	77/5,6 86/4,5,6	Too old parents /mother > 35, father > 40/	0,021
6.	23/1,2,3	0-2 presences at the pregnants' care	0,018
7.	8/4,15/4	High number of the liveborns and the pregnancies /≥ 3/	0,016
8.	11/1	All of the previous liveborns were less then 2500 g.	0,010
9.	80,81,83, 85,88,89, 91,93	Low educational level and manual employment of the parents	0,008
10.	21/2,3; 24	Complications and treatment in hospital during the pregnancy	0,003
11.	19/2,3; 19/9	Previous liveborn within one year or over eight years	0,001

A substantial conclusion can be drawn from the "Symptoms of pregnancy /Edema, Proteinuria, Hyperemesis/" obtained great weight. Our results

indicate that vomiting during pregnancy has to be taken into consideration more seriously than it used to be.

The arteficial and spontaneous abortions got great weights /Step 3/ in
1971, but it was not so in 1981. The importance of the abortions has
decreased. The corresponding intrauterine curves proved the same statement in both of cases. The reason is to be given by our obstetricians.

The 1th, 6th, 8th and 11th factors in the Table 1/b proved to be great
important and got relatively high weights. Earlier the attention wasn't
sufficiently turned to these influencing factors.

As regards the Step 5 we produced the curves of intrauterine growth
for every important factor. We pointed out the changes of the intrauterine standards during the ten years period. For example in 1981 there
is a small decreasing in the intrauterine growth both in weight and
length. In 1971 the weight of 2.500 was reached at the half of the 36th
gestational week, but in 1981 it happend exactly at the second third
of the 36th week. The percentiles of the male new-borns are above the
curves of the females /FIGURE 2/.

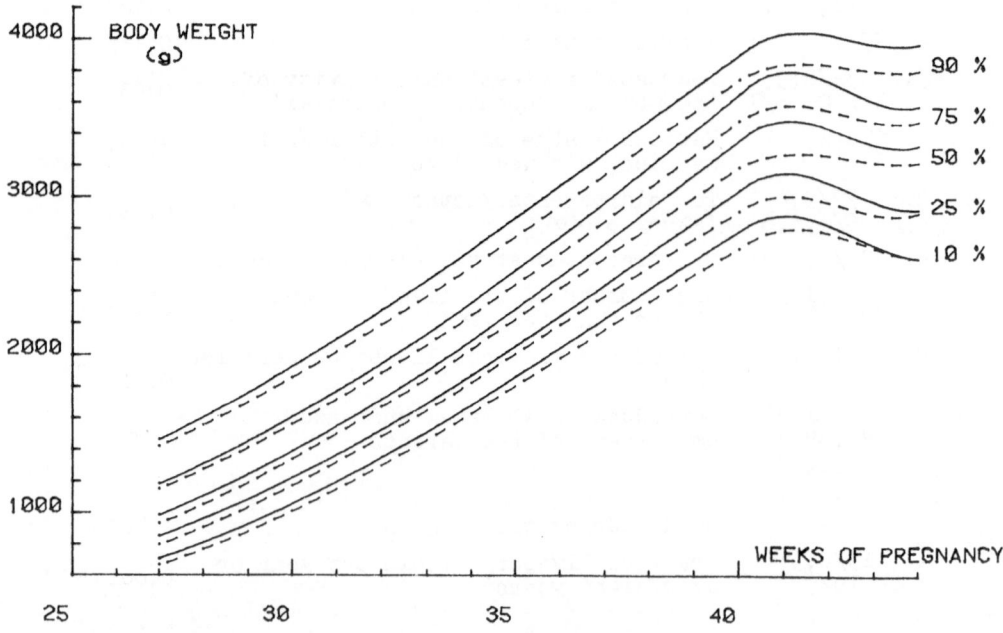

FIGURE 2: INTRAUTERINE GROWTH OF THE FEMALE AND MALE NEWBORNS
/PERCENTILES, 1981./

The interpretation of the combinations caused some difficulties, but it was very useful for us. /The number of the combinations in the case of 5 factors: 232./

Conclusion

We processed two nation-wide materials and found out a lot of factors influencing prematurity. The most important factors /with highest weights/ and their combinations may be responsible for the premature infants and implicitly for the high percentage of the mortality.

Acknowledgement

We are highly grateful to Miss Á. Tasnády, Mrs G. Farkas, Mrs M. Németh, Mr J. Sebők and Mr L. Sánta for their effectual co-operation.

References

1. Altman, D.G. and Colles E.C. Assesing birthweight for dates on a continuous scale. Ann. Hum. Biol. 7/1980/35-

2. Carr-Hill, R.A. and Pritchard C.W.: Reviewing birthweight standards, Brit.J.Obstet.Gynecot. 90/1983/718-

3. Duncan, E.H. et al.: The causes and prevention of stillbirth and first week death I. The evidence of vital statistics, J.Obstet. Gynecol. Brit.Emp. 59/1952/183-

4. Hogue, C.: Low birth weight subsequent to induced abortion, Amer J. Obstet. Gynecol. 123/1975/675-

5. Sebők,J., Paksy,A., Srajber,B., Kiszel,J., Dabóczy,Á.: Causes of Prematurity /1980/, Wissentschaftliche Zeitschrift der Humbold-Universitat zu Berlin, Math.-Nat.R.XXIX 5/6.

6. Sebők,J., Paksy,A., Srajber,B., Kiszel,J., Molnár,A.: Medical, Social and anthropological Factors Influencing Intrauterine Growth, /1980/, Wissentschaftliche Zeitschrift der Humboldt-Universitat zu Berlin, Math.-Nat.R.XXIX 5/6.

7. Shah, F.K. and H.Abley: Effects of some factors on neonatal and postneonatal mortality, Milbank Memorial Fund. Quart. 49/1971/33-

8. Simonovits,I. et al.: Secular trend in birth length and birth weight of newborns in Hungary 1920-1972, Acta.Paed.Acad.Sci.Hung. 16/1975/97-

9. Srajber,B.: Programsystem for the multifactorial investigation of the national surveys, Információ Elektronika 5/1982/268-275

10. Thomson, A.M. et al.: Assesment of fetal growth. J. Obstet.Gynecol. Br. Commonwolth. 75/1968/903-

<u>EVALUATION OF A CHILD DEVELOPMENT PAEDIATRIC EXAMINATION SYSTEM</u>

Dr. J. S. Dodge,
Rugby Health Authority,
24 Warwick Street,
Rugby, CV21 3DN
England.

<u>INTRODUCTION</u>. Developmental screening has traditionally been provided in the English health service by general practitioners and by community health doctors working in health authority clinics.   A system of developmental screening which relies on the casual attendance of the parents and child without any standardised monitoring system has been found to be ineffective and inefficient in the early discovery of remedial defects and it is also ineffective in the identification of children with special educational needs. (1)   The criteria for a good developmental screening system are firstly that each and every child should be examined at approximately the appropriate time: secondly, that there should be a mechanism for identifying children who fail to attend and an endeavour to trace them and to persuade them to attend for examination.   Thirdly, that there should be a clear process of referral for specialist advice, and fourthly there should be a recall system so that those children where there is a doubt as to the result of any tests can be reassessed. Fifthly, the results should be recorded in a systematic manner so that they can be understood by other health professionals and at subsequent examinations, and sixthly that the tests themselves should be of proven value, sufficient to indicate whether further action is necessary but not so numerous as to preclude their application to all children and with a repeatability giving consistent results.   A final criteria is that those health professionals conducting the tests should be competent and experienced: this competence requires appropriate specialist training.

In 1977 the Warwickshire Area Health Authority introduced a computerised child health programme.   This initially comprised an immunisation module but was quickly expanded to include a developmental pre-school examination module.   In the schedule of examinations for this latter module children are examined at 6 weeks and 9 months by a doctor; at 18 months by a health visitor; at 2 years and 3 months by the health visitor and doctor combined; at 3 years and 3 months by the health visitor. There is also a 4-year check, the primary objective of which is to assess the child's special educational needs, if any.   The Warwickshire Child Health Computer Programme has always been fully available to general practitioners: currently about 50 per cent of children are immunised through the computer scheme by their general practitioners, but 95 per cent of children receive their developmental examinations in the health authority clinics.

DOCUMENTATION.   In the developmental screening programme there is a common format to
the computer-produced medical record which is produced in advance of the examination.
Appointment cards are supplied to the appropriate health professionals who arrange
their own appointment programme.   The computer-produced record forms for the examinations are colour coded, a different colour being used for each examination.
A facility for a 'recall' examination is provided which enables a child to be recalled
either by the doctor or the nurse for re-examination of a particular aspect of the
series of tests.   The computer forms are in two sections and each section has two
parts.   The first part of the form contains the standard identification of the child,
giving name, address, general practitioner and health visitor and specifying when the
examination is to be done and who is to do it.   The second part of the first section
is devoted to communication of appropriate information either found at previous
examinations or, in the case of the first (6 weeks) examination, a review of the
perinatal data concerning that child.   The first part of the second section is
concerned with information from the examination.   The tests used are the 'Mary
Sheridan tests' (2), the results of which are interpreted as the outcome of a block
of tests and are recorded as satisfactory, unsatisfactory or doubtful.   The implication of a satisfactory examination is that the child can proceed to the next stage:
an unsatisfactory examination is generally a clear indication for referral, whereas
a doubtful result indicates the advisability of a recall examination to confirm
normality or otherwise at a later date.   The examiner records the results of the
present examination as satisfactory, unsatisfactory or doubtful using the letters S,
U or D as appropriate (Fig. 1).

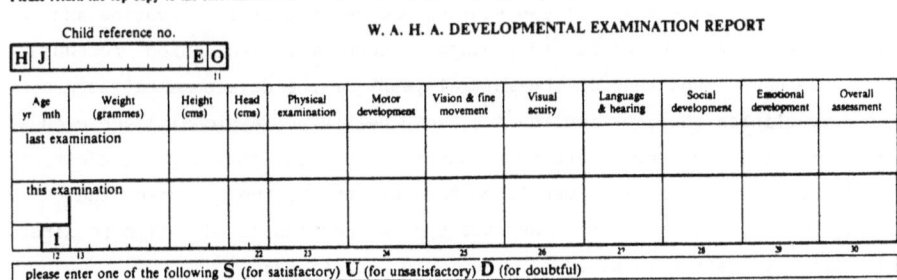

Figure 1.

Notes are not recorded in the computer record but diagnoses are recorded.   The final
part of the second section requires the examiner to indicate one of three possibilities,
the child is either declared satisfactory and passed on to the next examination; as
unsatisfactory and is referred to a defined specialist, or is recorded as "doubtful"
and a recall examination is arranged.   We have found that this type of final section
serves to concentrate the mind of the examining health professional so that a

definite decision is made regarding the future care, or otherwise, of the child.

EVALUATION.   Evaluation of the developmental screening programme is carried out as
a continuing process and concentrates on two aspects: efficiency of the process and
effectiveness of the screening system itself.   The use of this computerised
programme to provide service and operational management information has already
been described (3).   This is an important aspect of the total information system
as it makes efficient provision of the service easier and more readily evaluated.
Failure to attend for the examination can be followed up and a high overall rate of
attendance achieved.   Evaluation of the effectiveness of the examination occurs in
two stages - the medium and the long term.   A routine print-out is prepared for
each clinic and shows the number of attenders and the number who should have attended.
The results in each block of tests are summarised and the number of defined diagnoses,
with their ICD coding, the number of referrals for a consultant's opinion, and the
number of recalls for doubtful findings are given.   There is a separate print-out
for each stage of the series of six examinations and the set is produced each
quarter.   This provides the basis for a first stage evaluation, not only by the
managers of the service, but by the clinic staff themselves.   Self-evaluation by
the latter, with appropriate assistance, is likely to be more effective in modifying
the system towards greater effectiveness than an evaluation imposed from above which
is often perceived as threatening and is thus counterproductive.

The standard reporting system was developed because of a steadily increasing number
of requests for 'one-off' analysis programmes.   The system is the best amalgamation
of the generally desirable that one can achieve and because it is a routine and not
a special programme is much cheaper to produce.   Economy in evaluation procedures is
important.   We have found that in the initial years of the developmental screening
programme some clinics (and, by implication, some health professionals) achieved a
much greater recall or referral rate than others.   This can provide an indication
to the health professionals with overall responsibility for the programme the
desirability of in-service education and the type of continuing education required.
The longer term evaluation is based on a series of questions:

     (a)   What remedial defects have been found and have they been
          dealt with satisfactorily?

     (b)   Is there any indication of defects being missed (and found at
          a later date)?

     (c)   Are children with special educational needs identified at an
          appropriate early date?

The format of the record with a common and agreed system of tests and the standard-
ised recording of the results of these in groups enables us to analyse the
sequential progress of all children through the screening examination system without
too much difficulty.   In addition, those with special needs can be followed up.
This latter aspect of evaluation obviously extends over a greater period than is the
case with the investigation of the other questions and a record in readily
retrievable format is an absolute necessity.   Evaluation procedures need to be
built into the system and a satisfactory aspect of the present programme is that the
intention to evaluate, which was expressed in the design stage, is now being realised.

It is entirely proper for all screening procedures to be questioned and it is
absolutely necessary to evaluate and audit any system which is supposed to achieve
a better health status.   However, another factor has recently become apparent:
in times of decreased resource, the urgent tends to take priority over the important,
and although prevention is said to be better than cure, it does not necessarily
attract adequate resources.   It is necessary to justify the results of a screening
programme in order to retain resources, let alone attract new ones.   The computerised
programme has enabled us to evaluate the effect of the system, particularly with
regard to the new Education Act which requires a much greater precision with regard
to the definition of children with special educational needs.   The greater efficiency
of the computerised developmental examination programme has enabled us to undertake
a great deal of the preliminary assessment of the child with a minimum of difficulty.

REFERENCES

(1)   Drillien C. and Drummond M.   Developmental Screening and the Child with
       Special Needs.   William Heinemann, London.   1983.

(2)   Sheridan M.D.   The Developmental Progress of Infants and Young Children.
       No. 102 in the Reports on Public Health and Medical Subjects.   H.M.S.O.   1968.

(3)   Dodge   J.S.   Use of a Computerised Child Immunisation Programme to provide
       Service Management Information.   Proc. Fourth World Conference on Medical
       Informatics.   ed. Van Bemmel J.,   Ball M.J. and Wigertz O.   p. 1276.
       Elsevier Science Publishers B.V. Amsterdam.   1983.

A COMPUTER BASED SYSTEM FOR OPTIMAL BLOOD INVENTORY CONTROL.

P.Å. Andersson, J.O. Hildén, G. Liedén, J. Styf, O. Wigertz.
Linköping University Hospital, S-581 85 Linköping, Sweden

Introduction

In the ideal blood bank there should be no outdating and no shortage of blood. Without taking special actions, however, it is impossible to achieve that state in any blood bank. Recycling of blood units from hospitals with high percentages of outdating to hospitals with many transfusions is an accepted and effective method of reducing outdating. Several descriptions of computer based systems for redistribution between blood banks have been published (ref 1, ref 2). In the last few years rapid progress in blood banking has been made, e. g. new ways of storing red cells (SAGMAN - saline suspended red cells without plasma, extended storage time, (ref 3)), and new techniques in pre-transfusion testing (type and screen - no direct test donor/recipient, (ref 4)). Computers for supporting laboratory management and for storing laboratory information have been introduced in an increasing number of blood banks. These new techniques have cre-ated new possibilities for inventory management. By means of computer simulations we have studied the effects of adopting these new techniques in blood banking, including local blood inventory optimization and planning the drawing of blood. Based on experience from computer simulations, a computer based system for optimal blood inventory control has been developed.

Materials and Methods

A simulation model, including all routines from drawing blood to storage and distribution, has been developed. This model is built on manually collected data from our region (about 1 million inhabitants). These data cover all inventory changes in 11 blood banks during a period of 5 weeks. The collected data have been statistically analyzed and appropriate statistical distributions have been fitted to them. At the time when this data-collection was carried out, no recycling of blood occurred in the region and only whole blood, with a maximum storage time of 35 days, and ordinary crossmatching were used. Three parameters - outdating, mean age of blood at transfusion and shortage of ABO-identical blood at reservation - have been studied. Analysis of the collected data showed that the total outdating in the region involved 16.7 % of the blood drawn, the mean age at transfusion was 18.2 days, and the shortage of ABO-identical blood at reservation was 22 units per week.

An optimization model including special-purpose optimization algorithms has been developed. The optimization routines consider the actual inventory situation and available
information concerning the blood donors, together with the estimated, parameter-con-
trolled demand distributions, in a computerized blood bank inventory system. The optimization routines form the basis for planning of the inventory inflow. The simulation
programs have been constructed in such a way that they can be used for evaluation of
both the optimization model and as a guideline for undertaking a number of changes in
different blood bank routines. The simulations are based on an equal risk of shortage
of blood at reservation in each simulated case. The complete results are not presented
here.

In the present work we have studied the effects on the three previously mentioned parameters in different situations and in hospitals of different sizes for a period of 30
weeks.

Based on the results of the simulation, a computer based blood inventory control system has been designed. Along with the simulation module and a statistical supervision
module, an optimal inventory control 'package' of routines has been developed and is
currently installed at the blood bank at Linköping University Hospital.

Results

Simulations with our optimization algorithms for local blood inventory control has
shown an average reduction of outdating to 7.8 % (of total inflow) for whole blood and
7.2 % for SAGMAN blood. The mean age at transfusion was 15.8 days for whole blood and
15.1 days for SAGMAN blood. ABO-shortages at reservation were 26 per week for whole
blood and 147 per week for SAGMAN-blood. A comparison with the figures from the data
collection period (5 weeks) will not be quite adequate (16.7% outdating, 18.2 days mean
age at transfusion and 22 ABO-shortages per week) as the time-series of demand values
are different (although they are samples of common statistical distributions). With
hypothetical, ideal regional co-operation - centralizing all inventories in only one
inventory - the outdating would only be reduced to about 5 % (same figure for whole
blood and SAGMAN blood).

With the introduction of new blood banking techniques (e. g. type and screen procedures and extended storage time), the outdating can be further reduced in each blood
bank, independent of its size, by 40 - 60 % for the type and screen procedure and by
30 - 50 % for an extra sixth week of storage (based on results from simulations). This
will reduce outdating to very close to zero.

Our local inventory control system is designed with the following system
specifications:

A necessary, fundamental condition is an existing computer based blood bank information system with:

- data on donors and their donations.

- blood inventory database showing actual inventory situation.

- reservation routines with recording of bags reserved and transfused/released for
  every request for blood.

Based on this ordinary blood bank information which is stored in the computer, a dynamic process will update the parameters to obtain a proper adaptation to appropriate
statistical distributions. The statistical supervision updating procedure is automatically executed each time the user asks for periodic preplanning of the drawing. The
statistical supervision can be described in the following way:

A new method similar to exponential smoothing for computing moving averages has been
developed. This updating scheme is combined with an estimation of the parameters characterizing the statistical distributions involved, in regard to the special distribution properties. These distributions are evaluated by the application of the good-
ness-of-fit tests to the collected data. The updating involves automatic supervision
of the prediction errors which arise when the averages are used as prognoses, and an
alarm function if the assumed distribution shapes are questionable.

The requisition frequency depends on the day of the week. The number of units per requisition is influenced by the kind of reservation: for acute or planned transfusion.
The reservation times depend on the weekdays included in the period from reservation to
planned transfsuion and possible return. The transfusion probability is dependent on
the reserved number of units and on the kind of reservation - acute or planned.

Input for the inventory control system will be:

- maximum drawing capacity for each day in the period to be planned.

- minimum drawing to ensure drawing of blood from donors with blood groups which are
  seldom required (automatically retrieved from donor information and determined by a
  parameter for number of weeks since last call-up for donation of blood).

- inventory levels (each ABO and Rh group) for free units.

- inventory levels (each ABO and Rh group) for reserved units not used on the planned
  transfusion day.

- prognosis for reservation demands (based on weighted dynamic updating of the appropriate demand distributions).

- risks of shortage, first an average risk of shortage in free inventory, and secondly
  an average risk of shortage of ABO identical blood at reservation (if the blood bank
  needs to limit transfusion of non identical ABO group). These risks can be tested in
  the simulation model and situations when shortage occur can be analyzed in order to
  choose acceptable risks.

- percentage of reserved blood which is transfused. The statistical supervision considers different transfusion rates for different prereservation times. These figures
  are automatically calculated by the system.

The control system must also know which procedures are used at reservations, e g. reservation time before release to another patient, reservation procedure before planned
day of transfusion, week profile for drawing blood, etc. Other parameters which must be
known are the time lag from call-up to donation and time of blood drawing to the point
when all tests are validated so the units will be free for transfusion.

Output from the inventory control system will be:

- recommended inventory levels for each day and for each blood group during the
  preplanned period.

- recommended drawing for each day and for each blood group during the preplanned
  period.

If the blood bank is able to follow the recommended drawing (which can be controlled
by special call-up routines on the local computer, which either produce lists with
telephone numbers or call-up cards to be sent to selected donors), co-operation concerning blood inventories is of little interest. If the number of drawings diverges
considerably from that which is recommended, the desirable inventory levels can be
reached by redistribution. This type of co-operation between blood banks in a region
is not based on regular transports, but is a question of economy and good relations
between blood banks.

Our optimal blood inventory control system at Linköping University Hospital is beeing
installed on a VAX 11/750 and will be tested in routine use at the blood bank. System

programs are written in Standard Digital MUMPS and the optimization routines, the statistical supervision module and the simulation module are written in Fortran for high portability demands. Results from the use of this prototype system will be published later.

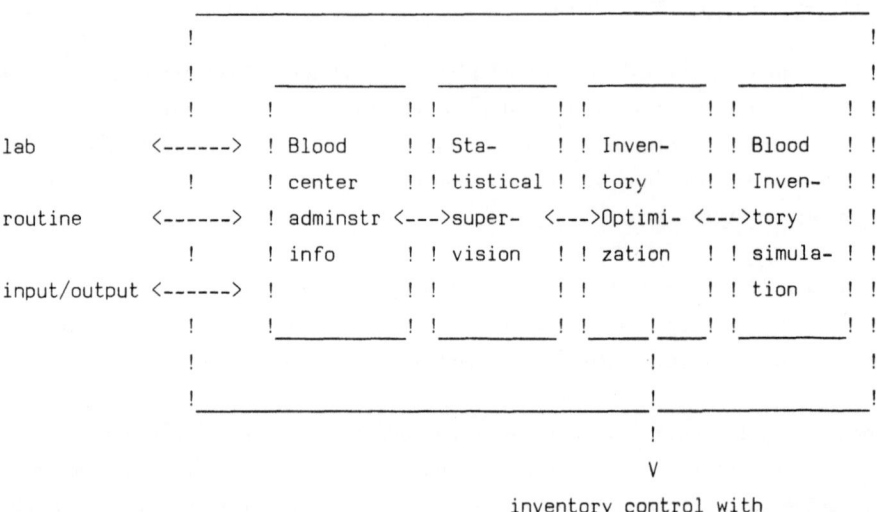

inventory control with
output of desirable drawing

Conclusion

Outdating can be reduced considerably through introduction of new blood banking techniques rather than through regional co-operation. If new techniques - including the described 'package' for automatic inventory supervision, statistical analysis and optimization algorithms - are used, the outdating can be reduced to very close to zero, even for smaller hospitals, without any risk of shortage of blood at transfusion.

References

1 - E. BRODHEIM, G. PRASTACOS. PBDS: A decision support system for regional blood management. Management Sci. 1980, 26, p. 451 - 463.

2 - G. PRASTACOS. Blood inventory management: An overwiev of theorei and practice. Management Sci. 1984, 30 p. 777 - 800.

3 - C. HÖGMAN, O. ÅKERBLOM, K. HEDLUND, I. ROSEN, L. WIKLUND. Red cell suspension in SAGM medium. Vox Sang. 1983, 45, p. 217 - 223.

4 - H. HEISTÖ. Pretransfusion blood group serology. Transfusion 1979, 19, p. 761 - 763.

MULTILAB - A FOURTH GENERATION LABORATORY INFORMATION SYSTEM

Esa Soini
Department of Data Processing
Helsinki University Central Hospital
Helsinki, Finland

"What can be made simple,
 must not be made complicated"

Occam's razor

SUMMARY

Helsinki University Central Hospital changed in the beginning of 80's radically its data processing policy and introduced new methods of software development. A new laboratory information system has been developed with these fourth generation tools, which consist of MUMPS programming language, a data dictionary driven application generator, several utility programs and prototyping. This laboratory system has been tested in six different laboratories.

INTRODUCTION

Information technology has been applied in the clinical laboratories since early 60's. During three decades hundreds of laboratory information systems have been developed. Unfortunately many of them are in use only in the laboratory, where they were developed. Commercial supply of flexible and cost-effective laboratory information systems has been insufficient in many countries.

Computers have evolved rapidly during the last decades. Even small laboratories can afford the use of micro computers. The progress of programming methods has been modest in the shadow of astonishing hardware development. Now, at last we are getting better software methods. These so called fourth generation programming tools consist of very high-level programming languages, report generators, graphics languages, parameterized application packages and, above all, application generators (2).

What will be the impact of these new methods in laboratory information systems? Is it really possible now to develop systems without programming?

This presentation will discuss these issues in the development of new laboratory information system in Helsinki University Central Hospital (HUCH). HUCH is a very large hospital with 200 wards and 2600 beds, but actually it consists of several rather independent clinical units. There are 11 clinical laboratories in our hospital and they differ very much from each other. The largest laboratory in Meilahti hospital produces over 2 million patient tests annually and the smallest unit in the Psychiatric Clinic only 20.000. Thus HUCH is a very suitable place to test the flexibility of a laboratory information system.

FOUR GENERATIONS OF LABORATORY INFORMATION SYSTEMS

The first laboratory information system in Finland was introduced in Tampere Central Hospital in 1967. This first generation system was totally batch based. Punched cards were used in data input and all lists were produced with a line printer in computer room. The system was programmed in Fortran and run on an IBM 1130 computer.

The second generation laboratory information system was developed in Helsinki University Central Hospital in the beginning of 70's. It was largely based on the previous system. On-line interfaces for laboratory equipment and use of terminals were the major enhacements. The system was run on an IBM 1800 computer.

In 1975 HUCH acquired a Honeywell-Bull 66/20 mainframe and a NOVA 830 mini computer. The on-line system was converted to the NOVA computer and the rest of the laboratory system to the Honeywell central computer. We programmed this third generation system mainly in Cobol and introduced a sophisticated IDS/I data base management system for all patient related information. Although terminals were used in all time-critical parts of the system, it was still essentially a batch based system.

This third generation system was efficient, but technically complicated. It soon became also too expensive to develop further and implement to other laboratories. The main architecture of the system and the software tools were obviously inadequate. Thus in 1980 we carried out a thorough investigation to choose a new strategy and methods for information system development. We then made the decision to develop a fourth generation laboratory information system based on distributed mini computers and to use ANSI Standard MUMPS as the main programming language.

The development of the new laboratory system was started in 1982. Our goal was to develop a system that could be implemented without extensive work to different clinical laboratories. The planning of the system lasted about one year. Then we developed a prototype of the system, which we started to test in different laboratories in summer 1984. The final system has been developed based on the experiences of this testing and we have started to implement it now. The new system will be totally in use in several laboratories by the end of 1985.

This new system was named MULTILAB.

MAIN FEATURES OF MULTILAB

In the development of MULTILAB system we could utilize the fifteen years of experiences in the field of laboratory information systems in Finland. On the other hand the evolution in laboratory functions and equipment as well as the new data processing technology have strongly influenced the development of our new MULTILAB system. Some of it's main features are

*   MULTILAB is totally terminal oriented and all it's functions can be used at distributed work stations; it emphasizes data communication between hospital units and has a sophisticated electronic mail system

*   MULTILAB is very easy to use, user interface is consistent and it is always possible to ask on-line help from the system

* MULTILAB includes a complete and up-to-date manual of laboratory tests and functions

* MULTILAB is a complete laboratory information system; it helps in every phase of laboratory work from test requests to statistics; it can manage all kinds of laboratory tests and results in simple numerical form, free text or graphics

* MULTILAB is open and modular, it can be used only partially, as a centralized or a distributed system or even without a patient administration system

* MULTILAB does not require any special EDP personnel

TECHNICAL SOLUTIONS IN MULTILAB

MULTILAB is to a great extent independent of the computer system. According to the type of the laboratory it can be run on a single user micro computer or a multi computer system with hundreds of work stations.

COMPUTER   The MULTILAB computer must be provided with a ANSI Standard MUMPS programming system. There are practically no other requirements for the computer system.

WORK STATIONS   The MULTILAB system does not use any special features of terminals. A work station can be a simple terminal or a micro computer.

ON-LINE SYSTEM   Laboratory equipment can be interfaced directly to the laboratory computer, via a CRT-terminal or via a pre-processing micro computer. The choice depends naturally on the type of the laboratory equipment.

In order to keep the MULTILAB system simple to maintain we have used standardized programming methods in development. This principle guarantees also a consistent user interface to the system.

MULTILAB is based on a set of hierarchical software tools:

MUMPS   ANSI Standard MUMPS is one of the four standardized programming languages, which guarantees a high degree of independence of computer equipment. MUMPS has also proved to be a simple and efficient tool in interactive system development.

FILE MANAGER   File Manager is a MUMPS-based application generator and information management system. It was developed by George F. Timson in Veterans Administration, USA (3). We built the prototype of MULTILAB using File Manager as a main tool minimizing thus programming efforts. All data structures and files in MULTILAB system obey File Manager conventions. Thus they are very flexible and can be managed by File Manager modules if necessary.

DISPLAY MANAGER   Display Manager is a tool for interactive forms
                   management. It was developed in Kuopio University
                   Computing Centre. Many health care organisations in
                   Finland have standardized the user interface in
                   their interactive systems. The use of Display
                   Manager makes the creating of input display forms
                   easy and guarantees a consistent user interface in
                   all systems.

SYSTEM MANAGER   System Manager creates a logical structure for a
                   group of MUMPS modules. It manages system structure,
                   user/terminal oriented data security, system
                   follow-up and error handling. It provides those
                   system management functions that are common to all
                   on-line systems. System Manager was developed in
                   Helsinki University Central Hospital (1).

EVALUATION

The development of the MULTILAB system has proceeded via several
phases: survey of the laboratory functions in our hospital -> planning
of a new system -> development of a prototype system -> testing and
evaluation of the prototype system -> creation of the final system ->
user training -> implementation of the final system in different
laboratories. The whole project has lasted over three years. There
have been some ten people in the project group, four systems analysts,
two instructors and four laboratory experts.

Compared to the previous laboratory information system projects the
users' share of the work has now increased. On the other hand coding
has considerably decreased. With these new software tools we were able
to develop a complete prototype of the system without extensive
programming. The prototype was rather inefficient in use of the
computer resources, but it has been very flexible to change according
to the testing experiences.

Although the MULTILAB system is easy to use, it changes the lives of
hundreds of people in our hospital. Thus there is a demand for a
extensive training programme. It takes more than a year to complete
the training of all nurses, laboratory technicians, clerks etc., who
will use the MULTILAB system in a large hospital. The teaching of the
technical use of the system has not been so important, but the new way
of thinking and the management of changes in the whole work
environment.

According to our experiences the total time to plan, develop and
implement a laboratory information system, has not shortened.

The prototype of the MULTILAB was tested in three different
laboratories in Helsinki University Central Hospital and in three
laboratories in Helsinki City hospitals. Each laboratory evaluated the
function of the system and suggested necessary changes for it. The
test laboratories found out errors and deficiencies in the system. It
has taken some three man months to correct the errors and to make the
improvements in the system. The evaluation of the MULTILAB system has
led us to the conclusion, that this system can be implemented to
different laboratories without re-programming.

DISCUSSION

The evolution of the information technology was very fast in the 70's. We acquired new computers, efficient multiprogramming operating systems, structured programming languages, smart communication protocols and almighty data base management systems. The computer systems became very powerful, but at the same time highly complicated and vulnerable. Every branch of the computer science demanded a special expert and nobody was able to manage the whole system.

The user of a laboratory information system longed for the simple systems of the previous generation and cursed the technical "progress" that had led to this expensive dead end.

In Helsinki University Central Hospital we have tried to solve this problem by turning back to simple and cheap computer technology. We are using distributed, task-oriented mini computers, simple terminals and conservative data communication technics. The key factor in our data processing policy has been the use of uniform and efficient software tools. We have totally abandoned our previous programming methods. All our systems analysts use the same high level system tools and thus no-one is irreplaceable.

With these new software tools it is possible to develop a comprehensive laboratory information system with a small systems staff. The problem is the implementation of the system. It still takes plenty of time and training. The implementation of a laboratory information system in a new laboratory can be difficult, but much more difficult it is in a laboratory that already has a computer system.

Despite the progress during the four generations of laboratory information systems in Finland, the pioneer times in this field are not yet over. Still the laboratories depend on EDP personnel when implementing computer systems. Perhaps the next generation of laboratory information systems reaches the goal, that Wexelblat states (4): "The third generation makes us work for the computer, the fourth generation will help us work for ourselves, the fifth generation ought to do the work for us".

REFERENCES

(1)   Koskimies, J.E.K., SYSTEM MANAGER - a Tool for MUMPS Application Programmer, MUG Quarterly, 1982, 3:30-33.

(2)   Martin, J.E., Application Development without Programming, Addison-Wesley, 1984.

(3)   Timson, G.F., The File Manager System. Proceedings of the Fourth Annual Symposium on Computer Applications in Medical Care, 1980, 1645.

(4)   Wexelblat, R.E., Nth Generation Languages, Datamation, 1984, 9:111-117.

"MATHEMATICAL CHROMATOGRAPHY" - RESOLUTION OF OVERLAPPING SPECTRA IN GC-MS

Erkki J. Karjalainen and Ulla P. Karjalainen
Department of Clinical Chemistry, University of Helsinki,
and United Laboratories Ltd., Helsinki, Finland

Abstract

Pure spectra are rarely found, when complex biological samples are subjected to analysis by gas chromatography/mass spectrometry. Most of the spectra are weighted sums of several pure spectra. We have developed a new method - "mathematical chromatography" - to isolate the pure spectra. The raw data are obtained by repetitive scanning of mass spectra during a gas chromatographic run. Basically the method uses regression analysis to solve alternately for the concentrations and mass spectra of different compounds. Because the absolute magnitude of the spectra remains unknown, all solution spectra are scaled to have a vector length of unity. The method yields reproducible results typically in less than 20 iterations. No previous knowledge about any spectrum is required. The method can be applied to any two-dimensional spectroscopy.

Introduction

Gas chromatography (GC) is the method most often used when complex volatile biological samples are analyzed (1-3). The number of components found in one run is very large although the requirement for volatile derivatives limits the total number of different molecules. Molecular overlap is the normal situation in all profiling studies. Capillary columns have markedly improved the separation but still the GC peaks do not always represent single molecules.

The information capacity of the GC instrument is increased by adding a mass spectrometer (MS) as a specific detector. This gives an additional dimension to solve the overlap problem. It is possible to register a mass spectrum from every GC peak. However, when the peak is not pure, the collected spectrum is some combination of the component spectra.

To aid our studies for the doping analysis of human urine samples, we developed a method, that can find the component peaks and their mass spectra in partial chromatographic separations having considerable overlap. This problem has earlier been studied by several groups using a variety of methods; factor analysis (4-6), generalized inverse method (7), libraries of previous analyses (8, 9) etc. These methods have required manual intervention by the analyst. However, for true automation the method should be as self-contained as possible. Our procedure does not require operator intervention.

Experimental section

Sample preparation. The conjugated steroid fraction from human urine was extracted and processed according to Kuoppasalmi and Karjalainen (10). The XAD-2 was, however, replaced by Sep-pak® (Waters Associates, Milford, MA), and bacterial ß-glucuronidase (Boehringer, Mannheim, FRG) was used instead of the Helix Pomatia extract.

Gas chromatography / mass spectrometry. A HP 5995B GC-MS (Hewlett-Packard, Palo Alto, CA) with a 12.5 m long capillary column (cross-linked dimethyl silicone fused silica, i.d. 0.2 mm) was used. The initial temperature in the oven was 200 °C. The temperature was increased 2 °C/min to 280 °C. Mass spectra were collected every 1.8 seconds in the continuous scan mode where all measured spectra are stored on a floppy disk.

Data processing. The spectral data were transferred to an Eclipse S/250 computer (Data General, Westboro, MA). The spectra were mathematically analyzed using the new algorithm. The method solves alternately the problem for the mass spectra and concentrations. The solutions are constrained to be positive. The procedure is started with random concentrations or spectra. After the solution was found, the results were printed out in a graphical report using a Versatec 1200A printer/plotter (Versatec Inc., Santa Clara, CA). The programs were written in Fortran 5 and Business Basic, and they run under RDOS operating system. The graphical output utilizes a special vector-to-raster converter (VRC 400, Versatec Inc.) to speed up the conversion of the plotted vectors to the final raster form.

Results

The total abundance data from GC-MS is shown in Figure 1. It shows the sum of the intensities of masses in each scanned spectrum. Below the total abundance plot tick marks show the positions of the resolved spectra. The number of components (64) clearly exceeds the number of chromatographic peaks in the plot.

Figure 2 shows the concentration profiles of two highly overlapping components. The maximum of the smaller compound (a) is situated one scan earlier than that of the larger compound (b). Figure 3 shows the original mass spectra corresponding to the maximum of each compound (scans number 199 and 200). The mathematically resolved spectra are shown in Figure 4. From run to run the reconstructed spectra are very reproducible.

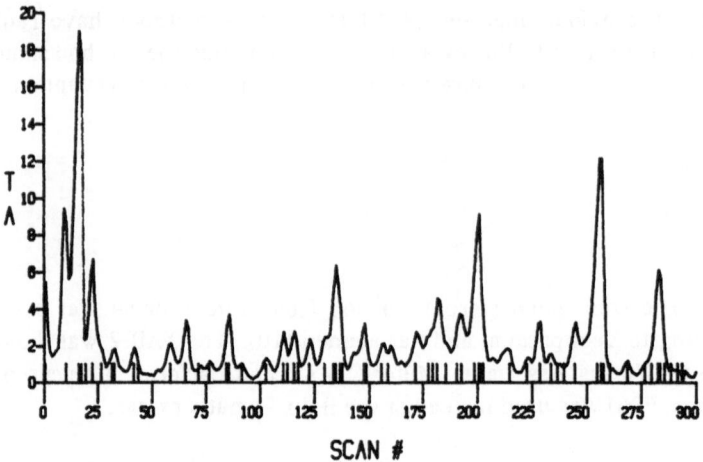

Figure 1. Total abundance of mass spectral scans during a GC-MS run.
The tick marks on the horizontal axis show the maxima of resolved compounds.

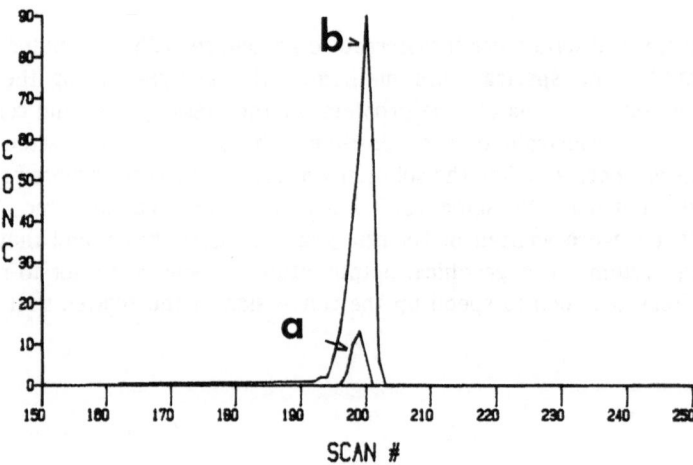

Figure 2. Two resolved compounds with a high degree of overlap.

One component always present is "background". It consists of electronic noise as well as of any real components which continuously reach the detector ("chemical background"). Its concentration is relatively constant on the time scale. The mass spectrum of the "background" varies according to the sample run on the gas chromatograph. If the sample contains just a small amount of material the spectrum consists mainly of electronic noise. When there is relatively much material in the injected sample the "background" spectrum shows also m/e peaks which correspond to some chemical entities derived e.g. from silylating reagent.

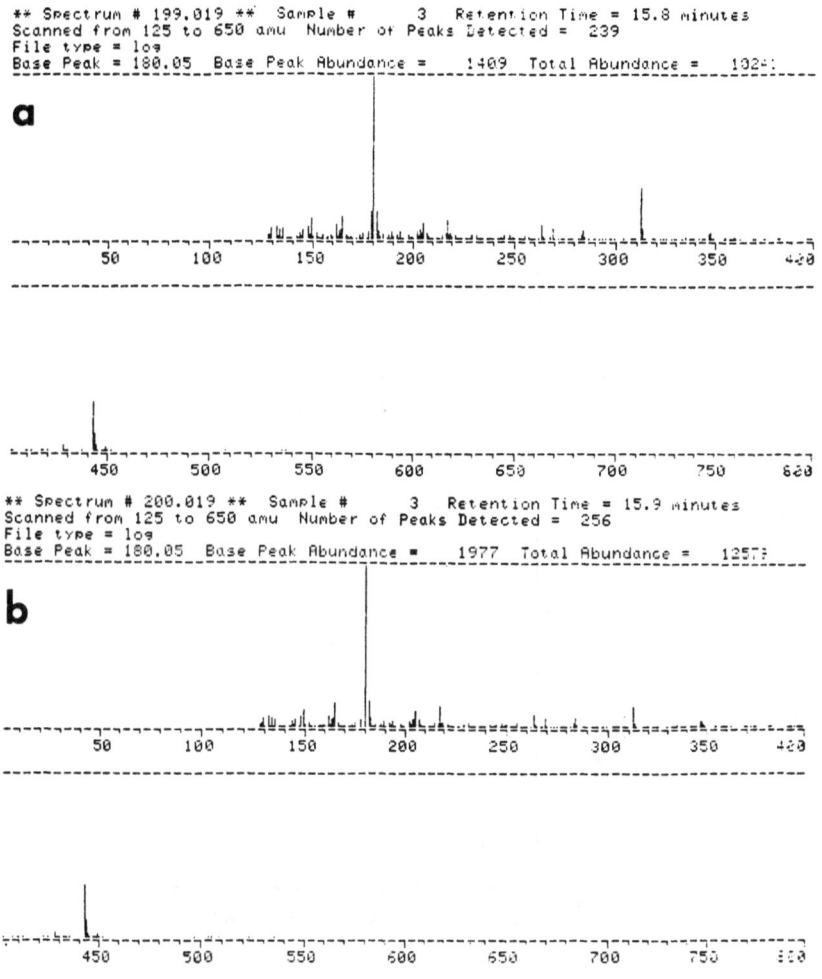

Figure 3. Original mass spectra at the time points corresponding to the maximum of each of the two overlapping components.

Discussion

The new method offers a very useful complement to classical isolation procedures. For the first time, the complete GC-MS run can be totally dissected into its components. The spectra of the pure molecules sum up to form a type of ionisation balance. Because the totality of the observations has been accounted for, there is much less chance of missing some component.

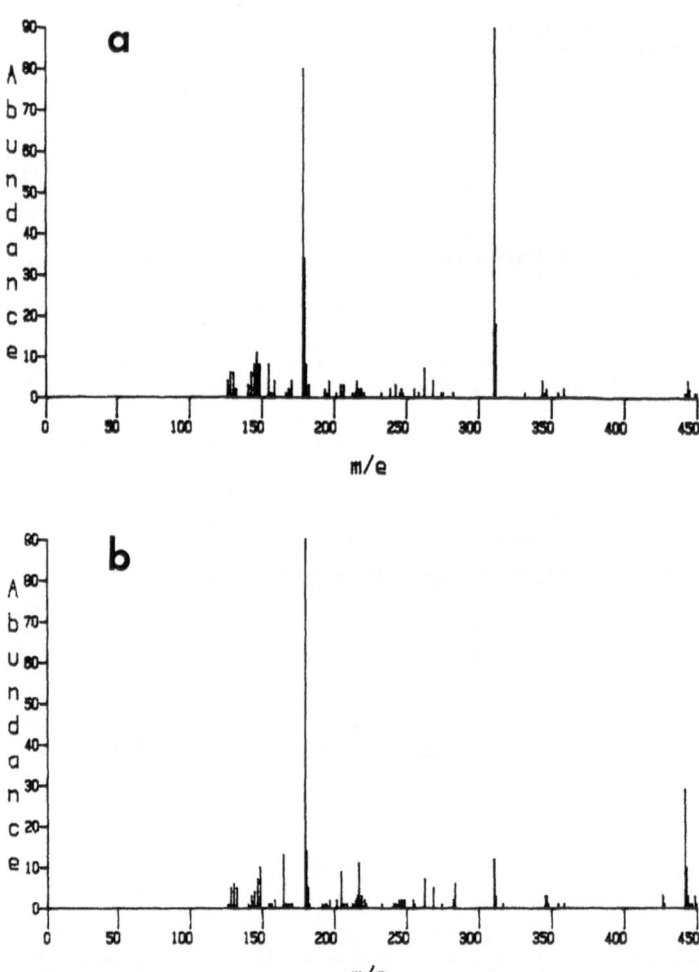

Figure 4. The mathematically resolved pure spectra.
The upper spectrum (a) corresponds to the smaller compound and the lower spectrum (b) to the larger one.

The normal method for getting pure spectra has a number of cumbersome steps that are necessary to physically isolate the molecule of interest. If the physical separation is inadequate, there is carry-over from the neighboring components. The spectra come to contain fragments that are not originating from the molecule in question. "Mathematical chromatography" isolates the spectra in the computer, not on the chromatographic column. The improved result shows up as a reduced number of ions that are present in the final spectrum. The better quality of the spectra can also be seen as more precise isotope ratios.

The new method is applicable to all problems in GC-MS. The same mathematical ideas apply equally well to mass fragmentography or SIM. It is obvious that the idea can be applied to any form of two-dimensional spectroscopy, where one or both of the axes can be physical separations. The constraints have to be somewhat modified for each spectroscopy but the key idea of successively applying two ortogonal regression analyses remains the same.

The gain in information can be utilized in a number of ways. We can measure more molecules than before. Compounds that have been hidden under other peaks can now be found. When known mixtures are analyzed for their concentrations, the chromatograms can be made shorter in time with less physical separation than before. The resolution lost by the shorter runtime is recovered in the computer with a gain in speed of analysis. Another way to utilize the improved information is to use smaller sample loadings. This results in less contamination and less frequent cleaning of the mass spectrometer. As the quality of the spectra is improved, library search methods can be made more effective. Rapid forward searches can be safely used as the background has been fully eliminated.

The new algorithm works in a stable fashion and rapidly converges to the final results. The main variable parameter used in the program is the number of molecules that is present in a given chromatographic run. The problem is automatically solved a number of times with different values for this parameter until the correct number is found.

The algorithm sets no limit to the number of components that can be analyzed in a single set of measurements produced in a chromatographic run or spectroscopic analysis. For a component to be identified, at least two original spectra should contain it. Most of the literature seems to consider cases with a very low number of components, typically two or three overlapping components (11). In the present method, hundreds of components can be analyzed in a single sample. A further advantage of the new method is the fact that no spectrum libraries are needed for the analysis to work.

Summary of the new method

1) The method provides for a mass balance of pure components. All new components are easier to find.
2) The method is universally applicable to all types of molecules that can be analyzed in GC-MS.
3) The method is applicable to all types of two-dimensional spectroscopies.
4) Less preliminary purification of the sample is needed.
5) The number of molecules measured in a single GC run increases.
6) The number of observed masses (m/e) in each spectrum is smaller in processed spectra than in original spectra.
7) Isotope ratios can be determined more precisely.
8) There is less contamination of the mass spectrometer due to the lower sample loading.
9) Chromatographic runs can be speeded up as more overlap can be tolerated.
10) As the cost of computing goes down, it is relatively more economical to do "mathematical chromatography" than separations by physical chromatography.

Acknowledgements

We would like to thank Mr. Antti Leinonen, B. Sc. for his help in GC-MS data collection. Also thanks are due to Dr. Christoph Bannwart for bringing up the word "mathematical chromatography" as a description of the new algorithm.

References

1) Issachar D, Holland JF, Sweeley CC. Metabolic Profiles of Organic Acids from Human Plasma. Anal Chem 1982; 54:29-32.
2) Liebich HM, Pickert A, Stierle U, Wöll J. Gas Chromatography-Mass Spectrometry of Saturated and Unsaturated Dicarboxylic Acids in Urine. J Chromatogr 1980;199:181-9.
3) Muskiet AJ, Fremouw-Ottevangers DC, Wolthers BG, de Vries JA. Gas-Chromatographic Profiling of Urinary Acidic and Alcoholic Catecholamine Metabolites. Clin Chem 1977; 23:863-7.
4) Halket JM. Factor Analysis of Repetitively Scanned Spectra in Gas Chromatography-Mass Spectrometry. The number of components in partially resolved peaks. J Chromatogr 1979; 175:229-41.
5) Tway PC, Love LJC, Woodruff HB. A Totally Automated Data Acquisition/Reduction System for Routine Treatment of Mass Spectroscopic Data by Factor Analysis. Anal Chim Acta 1980; 117:45-52.
6) Malinowski ER. Obtaining the Key Set of Typical Vectors by Factor Analysis and Subsequent Isolation of Component Spectra. Anal Chim Acta 1982; 134:129-37.
7) Sharaf MA, Kowalski BR. Quantitative Resolution of Fused Chromatographic Peaks in Gas Chromatography/Mass Spectrometry. Anal Chem 1982; 54:1291-6.
8) Baty JD, Wade AP. Analysis of Steroids in Biological Fluids by Computer-Aided Gas-Liquid Chromatography-Mass Spectrometry. Anal Biochem 1974; 57:27-37.
9) Costello CE, Hertz HS, Sakai T, Biemann K. Routine Use of a Flexible Gas Chromatograph-Mass Spectrometer-Computer System to Identify Drugs and Their Metabolites in Body Fluids to Overdose Victims. Clin Chem 1974; 20:255-65.
10) Kuoppasalmi K, Karjalainen U. Doping Analysis in Helsinki 1983. The first IAAF World Championships. Clinical Chemistry Research Foundation Library 1984; 1:1-40.
11) Osten DW, Kowalski BR. Multivariate Curve Resolution in Liquid Chromatography. Anal Chem 1984; 56:991-5.

COMPUTERIZED INTERPRETATION OF H P L C CHROMATOGRAMMS BY MEANS OF

ABSORBANCE RATIO METHOD AND DERIVATIVE SPECTROSCOPY.

U.Wellner and H.K.Biesalski
Institute of Physiological
Chemistry II
University of Mainz , FRG
Saarstr.21   D6500 MAINZ

As in other chromatographic processes it is the aim of high pressure
liquid chromatography (HPLC) to identify the components of a mixture,
whereby there may be some information on the class of substances in
question.The analytical procedure can shortly be desribed as follows.
The mixture is injected in a mobile phase (solvent) and passes a column
where the separation takes place.The separated components leave the
column at different retention times.A following detection device
generates a signal as a function of concentration (chromatographic peak).
Usually the components are identified by relating retention times of
external standards to the times of occurence of chromatographic peaks.
A system for the computer aided evaluation of such chromatograms was
developed by the authors (1). That system was designed in such a way
that all components of the mixture to be analyzed are supposed to separate completely, e.g. only chromatograms with distinct peaks were allowed,while overlapping peaks are rejected by a checking algorithm.
An inevitable shortcome of this algorithm is,that total overlapping of
peaks - which result in a single peak (with undetectable shoulders) -
cannot be recognized ,so that it was the responsibility of the HPLC-
operator to ensure the absence of such envents.
The case of overlapping peaks - partially or even totally - occurs for
example in adsorption chromatography on pure silica columns when retinyl-
esters are to be separated (2,3).A separation of these substances which
will yield a chromatogramm acceptable by the evaluation system is not
impossible but will require an immense analytical effort.It was shown
by the authors that with a mobile phase hexane:diisopropylether (98.5:
1.5)separation will be achieved in a closed recycling system not before
48 hours of equilibration of the mobile phase and column over Al_2O_3 .
The recycling system is necessary to ensure constant solvent strength
of the mobile phase and constant adsorption capacity of the column which

will be significantly altered in case of contamination by water (4).
Beforehand it is not known to the HPLC-operator whether such an effort
will have to be undertaken at all ,e.g.whether there are several retinyl
esters contained within the mixture to be analyzed. If only one ester
is present in biological samples (mainly retinyl palmitate) a more
simple and less time consuming HPLC precedure can be employed. In this
paper some methods are described which will allow the operator to decide about the purity of peaks,e.g. decide wether several substances
co-chromatograph or not.These methods form the theoretical background
for an enhencement of our computerized identification system.No redesign
of the system is necessary but two more modes of operation are added.
These modes will be activated and included within the common analytical
procedure whenever there are any doubts about the purity of peaks.
All three methods to be introduced are based on absorption spectra
S (λ) recorded at various points of the chromatographic peak. The methods
are:

1. Analysis of spectra
2. Derivative spectroscopy
3. Absorbance ratio method

1. For purity testing of a peak by spectral analysis a UV or fluores-
cence spectrum is recorded preferably at the maximum of the peak.This
spectrum is compared directly by pattern recognition methods (e.g. visual inspection , distance calculation) to spectra of the pure substances in question. Decisions are possible when typical differences be -
tween the spectra of the pure substances exists at all , e.g. when the
extinction coefficients $\varepsilon_i(\lambda)$ differ sufficiently. In such a case the
compound spectrum of a compound peak will in general differ from the
spectrum of any of the pure substances. Dissimilarity will thus give
hints to the presence of impurities.In case of retinyl esters there
are no remarkable differences between the spectra of the different esters.

2. To amplify slight differences in spectra S(λ) derivatives of the
original signals can be formed (5). Performing comparison of the se cond
derivative d^{2}S(λ) is called derivative spectroscopy. For this procedure
it has to be ensured that the signal S(λ) is smooth in refernce to
noise induced by the detection device. In case of small absorption differences ,when a high amplification has to be used to generate a meaning
output signal , such noise cannot be avoided. Therefore an appropriate
smoothing algorithm (e.g. digital filtering) has to be implemented .
The derivatives are digitally calculated from the filtered signal.

This procedure will work because the frequency of noise lies well a-
bove the meaningful frequency components of the signal $S(\lambda)$. The second
derivatives of the spectrum of the peak to be tested are compared to
the second derivatives of the spectra of the external standards similar
to spectral analysis. For purpose of detecting differences between
derivatives the second derivative of a pure substance is examined for
characteristic minima indicating local maximum or shoulder in the original spectrum. Two values of the wavelength λ are thus determined. A
characteristic measure is obtained by forming the ratio $q = d^2 S(\lambda_1)/$
$d^2 S(\lambda_2)$. According to the law of Lambert-Beer the concentration of the
substance is just a scaling factor in $S(\lambda)$; therefore concentration is
canceled in q. For any peak in question the same ratio q is formed
in order to test whether the peak is pure or not. For comparison to
different external standards different values of λ_1 and λ_2 are choosen.
choosen. As an example we take the spectrum of a pure substance (retinyl-
palmitate) and of the same substance but contaminated (retinylstearate).
The second derivatives show two distinct minima, so that λ_1 is chosen
as 300 nm and λ_2 as 350 nm. The ratio q for the pure substance is
0.360 while for the impure it is less (6). In the programm system the spectra and their second derivatives as well as information about chracter-
istic values of λ are stored in a data base, so that the operator is
only concerned about the class of substances in question.

3. The third method - the absorbance ratio - for purity testing works
on the original spectrum $S(\lambda)$ again, but the information is increased
by taking spectra at different points of the chromatographic peak, preferable in the middle of the leading edge, the maximum and the middle
of the trailing edge (7). To obtain these spectra the HPLC process is
modified by using the stop-flow mode. For each spectrum the pump is
stopped, the spectrum taken, digitized (wavelength resolution of about
0.05nm , amplitude resolution 10 Bit) and recorded by the computer .
Each spectrum will thus be represented by 4000 data points. The pure
substances are treated in the same way to obtain reference spectra .
Then a number of characteristic figures are calculated for each pure
substance in the following way : For a set of wavelength $\left\{ \lambda_1 \cdots \lambda_n \right\}$
the corresponding values of $S(\lambda)$ are determined and ratioed; this will
yield a set of ratios $\left\{ q_1 = S(\lambda_1)/S(\lambda_2) , q_2 = S(\lambda_1)/S(\lambda_2) \cdots \cdots \right\}$
For a pure substance these ratios are independent of when the spectrum
was taken, e.g. at which point of the peak. This depends on the cancel-
lation of concentration by forming ratios. The variability of those
quotients in an experimental situation is indeed very small (8).

Quotients q_i^* obtained for a peak to be analyzed are compared to the reference q_i. Any deviation above the normal variability (which is determined when calculating the reference quotients) between q_i^* and q_i give strong indication for impurity. It has to be pointed out that some q_i and q_i^* may be equal even when impurities are present. This will happen if the extinction coefficient functions involved are by chance equal at the corresponding λ_j , λ_k . Furthermore it is important that the variation of absorbance within the spectra recorded is sufficient , e.g. the concentration of the substance has to be high enough; for trace analysis the method will not yield a reliable result. We suggest that the variation of absorbance should be at least twenty times the calibration error.

Some concluding remarks on instrumentation :
The methods described may be applied whenever a variable wavelength detector with scanning mode (Beckman 165 , Perkin Elmer LC55 ,Perkin Elmer 650 10S) is implemented in the HPLC apparatus.
Obtaining spectra by the stop-flow method does not impose severe re-quirements on the computing equipment used. Most scanning detectors can be adjusted down , e.g. 1-2nm/sec scan speed which will result in a sampling rate of 20-40 Hz. This will even allow saving of the data records on disk at real time.
Apart from the calculations required for testing the programm modules should provide for showing spectra and derivatives on a display .
This is very useful for the learning phase of the system when pure substances are chromatographed in order to obtain reference data.

Apart from the methods described here classical signal analysis of the spectrum using Fast Fourier Transform suggests a further tool for de-termination of the number of components under a strongly overlapped peak (9). Concerning the method introduced by METZGER (10) for gas chromatography its applicability to HPLC has still to be examined .

Literature
1 BIESALSKI HK,WELLNER U Computer aided evaluation of HPLC (High Pressure Liquid Chromatography) with fluorometric detection. Lecture Notes in Medical Informatics 16:64-69 (1982)
2 ROSS AC Separation of long chain fatty acid esters of retinol by high performance liquid chromatography. Anal.Biochem.115:324-330 (1981)

3 PAANAKER JE , GROENENDIJK GWT Separation of geometric isomers of retinyl ester , retinal and retinol , pertaining to the visual cycle, by high performance liquid chromatography. J Chrom 168:125-132 (1979)

4 BIESALSKI HK , HAFNER G , BÄSSLER KH Separation of long chain fatty acid esters of retinol in biological samples using isocratic adsorption chromatography (HPLC) . To be published

5 O'HAVER TC Potential clinical applications of derivative and wavelength modulation spectrometry. Clin Chem 25:1548-53 (1079)

6 BIESALSKI HK , WELLNER U Qualitative analysis of chromatographic peaks by derivative spectroscopy. To be published

7 JOST R , MACLEAN W , STOVEKEN J Confirmatory identification of HPLC peaks using absorbance ratios at several wavelength. Chrom Newsletter 4:1-4 (1976)

8 HEIN H , JÖSTER R Die Leistungsfähigkeit des photometrischen Detektors LC55 mit variabler Wellenlänge beim Einsatz in der Hochdruck-Flüssigchromatographie. Appl.Chrom.28 (1977)

9 MALCZEWSKI ML , GRUSHKA E Multiple peak recognition in high per - formance liquid chromatography by fast fourier transfromation. J Chrom Sci 19:187-194 (1981)

10 METZGER HD True peak area separation of overlapping peaks in gas chromatograms by means of a process computer. Chromatographia 3:64-70 (1970)

PATIENT ADMINISTRATION AND ON LINE RADIOIMMUNOASSAY DATA REDUCTION

USING A MICROCOMPUTER.

GREGOIRE L., PEETERS T.L., and VANTRAPPEN G.R.

Gut Hormone Lab, Dept. of Medical Research,

University of Leuven, Gasthuisberg, Leuven B-3000 Belgium.

1. Introduction.

The most important equipment in a radio-immunoassay laboratory consists of nuclear counters. Manufacturers have responded to the increased use of their instruments for radio-immunoassay, first by incorporating computing facilities into them, next by linking them to a microcomputer. A counter-computer combination is indeed a flexible combination, but if the computer is fully dedicated to the counter, the computer hardware is mostly idle. We have developed a software package for a microcomputer-counter combination, in a multi-user multi-tasking environment. The package involves all aspects of administration and data reduction.

2. Configuration.

We use an IBM PC XT (512 K) running under the OASIS-86 operating system (from OASIS-Technologies Inc., Lafayette, Ca., USA) which is a fully multi-user multi-tasking system including such features as a 4 printer spooler, task priority system, file and record locking. Up to four nuclear counters can be connected via a code activated switch (Black Box, Pittsburgh, Pa., USA) connected to one serial port. The program controlling this switch runs in background and is also responsible for starting specific programs overnight (such as printing reports, status survey). In our laboratory another serial port is used for an additional workstation (VISA-50, Geveke Elektronics, Relegem, Belgium), and two parallel ports serve two printers. If required this configuration can be extended to maximum 4 workstations.

3. Software.

3.1 Overview.

The programs of our package are divided into four "environments", each one representing a particular aspect of the tasks performed in the lab (see figure 1).

```
"Labbank"     "Patient"     "Assay"        "Counter"

ANALYSIS      ENTER         INFO
PROTOCOL      MODIFY        MANUAL
DOCTOR        SEARCH        AUTO
              REPORT        WORKSHEET
              BILL          UNLOAD
              SAMPLE        QUALITY CONTROL
```

Figure 1. Programs and their "environments".

All information related to the workload of a particular lab, for example assay protocols, is stored in the Lab data bank by using a set of programs called "Labbank", while all tasks related to patient administration, are performed by the "Patient" programs which form and use the Patient data bank. Data transfer from the counters to the computer and other activities connected with the operation of the counters are under separate control ("Counter" programs) and require no user intervention. The "Assay" programs assemble assay protocol, sample identification and counter data, perform, eventually automatically, all calculations, print the results and store them in the patient data bank.

3.2. Labbank.

The number and type of compounds which a laboratory determines does not change every day. Similarly the protocol used for the determination of a certain compound is fairly constant, and many protocols have even parts in common. Finally, even the "clients", i.e. the doctors sending samples to the lab, form a relatively constant set. To avoid the repeated introduction of the same information every time an assay is performed, all such information ("labbank") is stored on disk. The labbank must be constructed before assays can be calculated, but any kind of information can always, and easily, be changed.

With program ANALYSIS information about the analyses performed in the lab is stored in the computer. This information includes a code number, name, abbreviation, molecular weight, concentration units, normal range, health insurance code, cost and a few other items. Normally an analysis refers to the determination of one compound in one sample, but one code can also refer to a group of determinations (example thyroid function tests), or to a dynamic test, in which case labels for the different samples can be defined. With program DOCTOR names, addresses and registration numbers of doctors can be stored, while program PROTOCOL stores all data required to transform counter results into concentrations (number and concentrations of standards, single or duplicate determinations, etc..).

3.3.Patient.

Samples received in the lab for analysis are numbered consecutively and using program ENTER all information required for further processing is entered in the computer and stored on disk. This information includes sample number, patient identification, name, address and registration number of the doctor to which results will be reported, analyses asked for. Optionally information relevant to the analysis to be performed can also be stored (sex, age, weeks of pregnancy, date last period, sampling time). After analyses are completed, results are automatically transferred to the patient data bank. Using program MODIFY all information present in the patient data bank can be corrected.

Several other programs use the information present in the patient data bank, for patient administration. Program REPORT generates reports either for patients with all analyses completed, or for a defined group of analyses. For urgent analyses, reports can be generated automatically after assay calculation. Program BILL prepares a list of all analyses to be billed, with all information required by law. Program SEARCH rapidly retrieves information about one patient (for example to answer a request by phone about results). This program can also generate alphabetical or sequential lists of the contents of the patient data bank. For a single patient a full "patient history" can be prepared. Program SAMPLE generates a list of all patients for which a request has been made for a particular analysis or a combination of analyses.

Both data banks (patient and laboratory information) reside on disk, together with programs, counter data etc... The files are organized so that there is room for 99 analyses, 99 protocols, 200 doctors and 30000 patients. The use of programs MODIFY,SEARCH and SAMPLE (access to patient information) is protected by passwords.

3.4. Counter Operation.

After the radio-immunoassay (or other) procedure has been performed samples are counted in the radioactivity counter. Normally operation is on-line, i.e.

results obtained by the radioactivity counter are directly transferred to the computer. Transfer of data is guided by signals from the counter, and is supervised by the program responsible for the code activated switch , which comes down to the fact that the operator doesn't have to worry about it.

3.5. Assay.

Program INFO displays on the screen an overview of assay processing. Figure 2 is an example of an output generated by INFO. The first column is the identification given to the assay, by the operator. If the radioactivity counter signals the presence of a new programnumber, but the operator has not yet defined a worksheet, the assay is listed as UNKNOWN. The second column shows the status of the assay. An assay can be either PRINTED, COUNTED, COUNTING, LOADED, UNLOADED, CANCELLED, or REPEAT. The assay status is the result of operations in the computer or in the counter, or of an operator intervention.

A PRINTED assay has been fully processed. However, assay calculations can always be restarted (for example after correcting a point of the standard curve). An assay scheduled for reprocessing is labeled REPEAT. If error conditions arise during assay processing this is shown by the label CANCELLED. Assays for which the programs have all information, except counter data, are LOADED. The meaning of COUNTED or COUNTING is clear. UNLOADED refers to meaningless counter data (no processing required), LOCKED that an equipment failure occurred during processing (power failure of the counter for example).

```
*************************************************************************
*********          LABMAN  ASSAY  INFO  RELEASE 1.0        ***********
*************************************************************************
Date: 19-03-85                                          Time: 14:02:27
=======================================================================
         ASSAY      COUNTER  FILE          ASSAY      COUNTER  FILE
  NAME   STATUS     Nr Prg    Nr    NAME   STATUS     Nr Prg    Nr
-----------------------------------------------------------------------
MOT-78   INVALID    2  7      1    T3U-134  PRINTED   2  3      14
UNKNOWN  UNLOADED   1  2      19   GAS-158  REPEAT    2  8      4
CEA-66   UNLOADED   2  7      2    MOT-80   COUNTED   1  3      11
MOT-79   CANCELLED  2  1      15   T4-128   LOCKED    1  8      10
T3U-34   PRINTED    1  8      20   UNKNOWN  COUNTING  1  3      6
GAS-152  PRINTED    1  5      17   MOT-81   COUNTED   1  7   1  3
GAS-137  PRINTED    1  9      8    TSH-23   COUNTING  2  6      13
T3-159   PRINTED    2  4      7    PGE-58   LOADED    1  5      12
TSH-21   PRINTED    1  4      5    GLU-62   LOADED    1  8      18
INS-56   PRINTED    1  5      9    MOT-91   LOADED    2  3      16
=======================================================================

W)ORKSHEET  ;  A)UTO  ;   M)ANUAL  ;   U)NLOAD  ;   I)NVALID  ;
```

Figure 2. Screen from INFO.

The third column codes the counter in which the assay resides. The fourth column gives the counter program number. The last column designates the file used for storing the counter results. There are 20 files used for this purpose. When all 20 have been used the first one is automatically cleared allowing the storage of counter results of the next assay and so on. However, unprocessed data will never be cleared. When an assay must be calculated all information required by the program can be quickly assembled by linking protocol, counterdata and patient information together. This process is performed in the "Assay" environment by program WORKSHEET. The construction of a worksheet is extremely simple. The operator gives the codename of the protocol, the counternumber and the programnumber of the counter. Automatically the worksheet is constructed. It will contain a copy of the protocol present in the "Labbank" files and a list of all patients to be assayed for this compound obtained from the "Patient" files. The operator can edit any item present in the worksheet. He can change the protocol, add or delete patients etc..

Calculations are performed by the programs AUTO or MANUAL. If AUTO is used, all identified assays will be automatically executed in the order in which they were counted, then assays will be calculated as soon as they are counted. AUTO can be set overnight, so that the next morning results will be already available for all assays counted overnight. With program MANUAL execution of the assay is under operator control. This not only means that the order in which assays are calculated can be selected, but also provides the possibility of intervention in the calculation process itself. During processing by MANUAL the standard curve is computed first and the results are displayed in tabular form. The operator has then the option to cancel any further computations, to continue or to continue after making some changes.

The mathematical and statistical background of the calculations is beyond the scope of this paper. Suffice to say that radio-immunoassays can be calculated using smoothed cubic spline, polygonal interpolation or four parameter logistic. Quality Control parameters (including results for target samples) are stored for the last fifteen executions of every protocol. They can be listed, displayed or used for QC evaluation.

FOURTH GENERATION LABORATORY SYSTEM

P-A. Andersson, S. Hansson, A. Kapiris, S. Lindstedt, G. Lundqvist, and R. Nordberg
Department of Clinical Chemistry, Gothenburg University, Sahlgren's Hospital, S-413 45
Gothenburg, Sweden

System development

During the period of 1970-1975 we developed two laboratory computer systems at
Sahlgren's Hospital, one for chemistry and one for haematology. They were based on two HP
2100 CPU's (32K and 16K) with 24 and 5 Mbytes discs, tapes, printers and card readers. All
development was done in the laboratory and a small group of programmers was established.

This has been regarded as the first generation laboratory system, based on real time
operating systems.

About 1975 it had become obvious that furhter development required (a) a time-sharing
system, and (b) an online data acquisition system. An HP 3000 CX was therefore bought,
which in 1976 was exchanged for an HP 3000 series II.

A completely new software was written for this system. One of the main features of the
new system was the use of an advanced database system. Together with great number of
other facilities this became regarded as the second generation laboratory system.

The opening of the new laboratory at the East Hosptial introduced a unique possibility to
design a laboratory computer system, based on the experience from Sahlgren's Hospital. A
new philosophy for data acquisition was introduced which will be described below. This
development led to a dialogue based system which, via asynchromous terminal connectors was
connected with a data collection system. The data collection system consisted, and still
consists, of micro computer instrument interfaces and a front end computer. A data base
constituted the central part of the whole system. With these improvements the third
generation laboratory system was a fact.

The fourth generation

An analysis of the different tasks running on the laboratory computer shows that most of
them are of administrative types. The idea that one needs a computer with a more
technically oriented operative system for laboratory applications is nowadays recognized as a
misjudgment. There are, after the data collection and evaluation which is of technical nature,
numerous steps of administrative type in which the results are treated both before and after
they are reported to the requesting wards. The existence of a computer in the laboratory is
today also used by the laboratory management to get support in plain administrative routines
like inventory, supply, budget and personnel planning etc.

The intention with the application software system has been to make it easy for the
users to maintain and modify it. It is therefore based on standard HP 3000 system software.

The software is also transferable between different types of HP 3000 models, making it possible to select a computer model that fits the size of the laboratory.

CRT-routines

The interactive routines at the CRT-terminals are reached through a menu with entries which are branched. The operator is guided in each entry by a display form. The forms in which the operator is supposed to key information are inversley displayed and the cursor is automatically located in the right position. The field between the registration fields is protected; any attempt to try to write anything outside these fields will fail.

In order to avoid unnecessary registrations the computer itself adds as much information as possible. Thus when the patient identification number has been registered by the operator, the computer checks if the patient is registered before; if this is the case, the computer adds the name of the patient, the ward where the patient is treated and the name of the doctor who is treating the patient. The computer then asks the operator if this information is still valid (which has been found to be the case in more than 90% of the cases).

Retrospective searches for old results per patients, editing of patient information, verification of collected measurement data etc. are examples of other interactive CRT-routines.

Front end computer

The main task for the front end computer is to maintain communication with the instrument interfaces, II:s, and with the main computer and to buffer and switch data in both directions. The various tasks of the front end computer are described below.

Communication between II and the front end computer. It maintains communication with the II:s and stores analysis results and execute commands, such as retrieval of request information.

Buffering of data from II:s. Incoming data from the II:s are mainly analysis results. These are buffered in the front end computer to make it possible to transfer them to the main computer via a low priority port. This means that these transfers do not disturb other main computer activities. A consequence of this is that a very fast response is obtained for the interactive routines at the CRT-terminals.

Front end computer is equipped with a mass storage device in order to maintain data acquisition even when the main computer is down.

Request handling. Request information is transmitted to front end computer from main computer and enables, at demand, the front end computer to send this information to the specific instruments or work stations.

Instument Interfaces

The instrument interfaces are constructed to achieve the best possible flexibility in order to adapt them to the various instruments and working sites. Thus, both software and hardware are constructed in a modular way to simplify the adaption and future changes due to system developments.

591

The various tasks for the II:s are instrument communication, protocol conversion, buffering of results, operator communication, and communication between the II:s and the front end computer/main computer.

Laboratory databases

In this generation of the laboratory system we have splitted the laboratory database into five more or less independent databases.

The major advantage of this split is to make the system more modular, easier to maintain and easier to integrate with other systems, or subsystems. The laboratory system has now the following databases

patient database   long time storage database   production statistics database
laboratory work database   control samples database

The patient database contains patient identification number, name, ward and category.

The laboratory-work database is the heart of the system. The database has the following main data sets

analysis definitions   analysis combination definitions
reference areas   working lists definitions
orders and results.   actual working lists
different types of comments like error text   control sample definitions

The long-time storage database contains laboratory records that have been reported. The structure of this base is a subset of the orders and results in the laboratory work database.

The control-sample database contains results of control samples and truncated patient means. The purpose of this base is the long term statistical rewiev for determination of quality production statitics.

The production-statistics database contains number of analysis per customer distributed on routine or emergency samples and month.

From this database the system produces-production reports sorted on customers or analysis. It is also possible to include routines for charging of certain orders.

Reporting routines

The reports are obtained either via batch routines initiated by the software system or interactively via CRT or printing terminals.

Batch Reporting

Daily reports. When an analysis, consisting of one or several result parameters, is completed (including eventual transformation calculations), it is filed in sequential order in a report generating system. The file for results to be reported is subdivided depending on:
1. Type of analysis
2. Category of customer
3. Category of patient
4. Special information registered at the reception of the test specimen or any combination of the points above.

Results pertaining to an emergency sample or other test results which may lead to immediate treatment of the patient are reported directly as they are ready either on the customers local printer as soon as they are ready on a special printer at the laboratory.

The result reports are sorted and printed on command or at certain fixed hours during the day. Most reports are printed on a lineprinter, while some are printed on printers located in different places within the laboratory or in the wards. The selection is governed by type of analysis/customer.

Cumulative reports. When an analysis has been reported in one of the above mentioned ways its results are transferred to a cumulative register in the database. (The results are stored on discs during various time intervals depending on which analysis or patient category it belongs to.) A cumulative report consists of all results from all analysed samples for one patient arranged in chronological order. The cumulative reports are then generated from this register.

The cumulative reports are normally generated only once or twice a day. A cumulative report for a patient is generated depending on (a) whether any new sample has been analyzed since the last cumulative report was generated, or (b) whether a cumulative report has been specially ordered for one patient.

Graphical reports. Certain analyses, with time dependent reference values, are best reported in graphical form. This type of cumulative list in analog form gives the best overview of trends in the results but the relatively slow speed with which they can be produced limits the use of this type of reports. The introduction of laser printers might be the future solution to this limitation of graphical reports.

One graph may also cover a combination of analyses.

Interactive Reporting

The software initiated result reporting complements the interactive result reporting routines at the CRT-/printing terminals (sometimes supported by a plotter). The purpose is that these routines should be used for data retrieval from the register of test under process as well as from the long-term register for any specified patient.

All of the software initiated as well as the interactive report routines allow addition of the following: 1. Reference intervals (as a function of sex, age, drug intake, pregnancy stage etc). 2. Asterisk (or any other equivalent mark) for indication of pathological results. 3. Comments in free text format. 4. Exchange of results with text (For example coagulated, <10, colour: red).

Quality control

Special routines for calculation, statistics and hypothesis tests of the results obtained from the analyses of quality control specimens are continuously running as background jobs. Special programs are coupled to these routines for display and printouts of the various quality control/samples per analysis.

The results obtained from the analysis of these quality control samples are stored in one of the registers of the database. From this register it is then possible to make special studies of certain prarameters over longer time intervals in respect of quality control samples identification, analysis, index, date (-interval), time (-interval) and analysis result.

The identification of a quality control sample is built and treated like a patient identification number. The combination of the quality control identification number and an analysis code makes it possible to retrieve data from the quality control result register with a very short response time.

The time interval for storage of a single result of a quality control measurement varies with respect to what is relevant for that specific analysis. For a low fequency analysis there is normally no summary. For more frequent analyses the single results are stored for one week, then converted and stored as a statistical summary containing number of results, sum of results, square sum of results etc.

Time dependent trends can be presented graphically as, for example, in "cusum"-plots.

The patient results are stored in the same way as the control samples and are daily reduced to mean value for the group.

Production statistics

The function covers accumulation of the number of analyses carried out per customer, updating of register of customers regarding their account etc, and processing of quantitative production statistics from which the debiting is produced. Production statistics also include routines for report generation.

The quantitative production control accumulates the number and cost for produced analyses per customer, type of analysis and stores it in the "production register" of the database. Updating of the production files is normally done during those hours when the computer is least busy.

The different routines in this laboratory's administrative part of the computer system can be summarized in the following routines: 1. Updating of customers. 2. Generation of lists of customers. 3. Generation of production statistics.

These routines are interactive routines which are initiated periodically. Generation of production statistics and invoicing is normally only done once a month. The output consists mainly of two parts. In the first part costs are arranged according to account numbers. It shows number of analyses delivered during the last month as well as accumulated for the year, and the cost for this. The other part is arranged according to analyses and gives costs both for the last month and accumulated for the year.

Sampling (i.e. drawing of a blood sample) is treated in the same way as an ordered analysis in the administrative routines.

Routines for automatic invoicing have been made and are being used in one of the installations.

Within hospital mainframe communication

The HP 3000 family has a number of facilities to communicate to other computers which give the laboratory system the opportunity to communicate with other systems, such as a patient administrative system and an economic system or other laboratory systems.

OUPA - PATHOLOGY DATA MANAGEMENT SYSTEM
OF OULU UNIVERSITY CENTRAL HOSPITAL

Seppo Sutinen, Pekka Lassila, Ulla-Maija Karjalainen
Departments of Pathology and Data Management
Oulu University Central Hospital
SF-90220 OULU, FINLAND

Although data management systems are widely accepted in the clinical laboratory, their application to anatomic pathology has lagged far behind. Two technical problems seem to lie at the root of this difference; (1) the large quantities of text to be stored for long periods in anatomic pathology laboratories, and (2) the construction of diagnostic expressions to be transformed into code form to allow an efficient retrieval of cases by diagnostic label (Ulirsch 1984). However, recent advances in automated coding and decreases in costs of the equipment have now made the computer both practical and feasible for the management of anatomic pathology data.

The pathology data management system of Oulu University Central Hospital was developed on the basis of a previous data management system which had been effective in the Department of Pathology, University of Oulu from 1964 to 1979, and which, after a major revision, had continued since that as the pathology data management system of the Oulu University Cental Hospital. Another major revision began in January 1984 and progressed so that an on-line activity could be started on November 5, 1984. This system, which was named OUPA, is a conversational time sharing system, in which the user and computer discuss through the terminal. It is an integral part of the total data management system of the hospital. OUPA performs functions connected with daily laboratory routine, diagnostics and patient care, administration, teaching and research.

Installation and software

The central processing unit is a Digital VAX 11/750 computer with 5 megabytes of memory, located in the department of data management with two Digital RA 81 disk storage units, each with 456 megabytes of memory. A Digital TU 80 tape recorder is used for safety copies. The central computer is also used by the clinical laboratory and connected with three other similar units through a local network. In the pathology department there are five display terminals and an additional two will be installed next year. This year the system includes two dot matrix printers and a combined typewriter-printer. An additional daisy wheel printer is planned to be purchased next year. The programming language was FAS (Finnish Assembly Language) and the program used in developing was PETO (a general terminal operation program) both developed by the Finnish State Computer Centre, Helsinki, Finland.

Goals

The principal goals of the system are listed in Table 1.

Table 1. Goals of OUPA.
----
1. Daily laboratory routine:
   - Assign accession numbers for all specimens received and autopsies
     requested, and generate complete and accurate daily logs of them.
   - Keep an accurate record of the results of investigations performed
     and later, generate pathology reports using word processing.
   - Transfer data between pathology and other departments.
2. Diagnostics and patient care:
   a. Biopsy and cytology:
   - Consolidate different parts of the same operative specimen if
     various parts (e.g. frozen section, metastatic lymph nodes, and
     primary tumor) are received at different times.
   - Provide the pathologist with diagnoses of all specimens from this
     patient examined previously.
   - Allow immediate access to the status or the diagnosis of a specimen
     for telephone inquiries by physicians or nursing personnel.
   - Ensure that all specimens are signed out in due time.
   b. Autopsy and morgue:
   - Allow immediate access to the status of a death occurred in the
     hospital (e.g. time of death, scheduled time of medical/forensic
     autopsy, time when the corpse may be/has been given out, the
     status and prosector of medical/forensic autopsy, etc.) for
     telephone inquiries by physicians, family members, undertakers or
     public authority.
3. Administration:
   - Monitor the amount of work performed by individual pathologists in
     order to correctly divide the work load between full time and
     different part time workers.
   - Monitor the total work load of the laboratory in order to correctly
     aim the resources available.
   - Automate the billing process
   - Prepare statistical reports for hospital administration or public
     authority.
4. Teaching and research:
   - List all specimens and diagnoses for patients to be presented at
     interdepartmental conferences.
   - Retrieve cases for illustrative purposes.
   - Retrieve all specimens and diagnoses for patients on whom malignant
     or suspicious cells (Papanicolaou classes III to V) have been seen
     in cytologic specimens.
   - Facilitate retrieval of cases in which photographs have been taken,
     tissue deep-frozen, or electron microscopy performed.
   - Provide a retrieval system with reliable data for retrospecive
     studies (e.g. by diagnosis, sex, age, year etc.).
   - Allow statistical studies to be performed on the material.

Operational principles

General. Self-advisory programs are used by regular laboratory
personnel as normal daily routine. Specialized data input personnel is
not required. Keeping record of specimen accessions and input of
administrative data are carried out as a single work step. OUPA assigns
the accession numbers for all specimens received and autopsies requested
replacing the time-honored manual log books by printed daily lists of
specimens to be filed. Only the accession number is written manually on
the request sheet and specimen containers, as well as the date of
arrival and name of the pathologist to whom the specimen is assigned on
the request sheet. Using the social security code of a patient OUPA has

access to his or her demographic data included in the data pool of the patient administration. Provided the social security code on the request sheet is correct, this practically abolishes the possibility of typing errors during input because no more data for patient identification need to be typed. However, if no correct social security code is available, the system accepts any temporary code, written twice in identical way. But in order to retrieve the patients previous specimens a correct social security code is imperative. In addition, all codes entered into the computer are translated into Finnish frases and displayed for the user to verify.

At present, the pathologist's report is typed on paper by a secretary and only the free text diagnoses with SNOMED codes or the cytologic classes are entered into the computer. Our plan is, however, to start the generation of the reports by word processing next year, after which a separate work step for input is no more needed. And as soon as possible OUPA will be extended to transfer the reports to the patient floors and requests for examinations to the pathology department.

Diagnostic expressions. Diagnostic expressions are entered into and retrieved from OUPA in free text form. A diagnostic expression has two parts: 1) anatomic site with topography code, and 2) structural change with morphology code. Autopsy diagnoses also include a code expressing their weights as causes of death, i.e. immediate, antecedent or underlying cause of death, an illness contributing to death or an additional finding (Sutinen et al. 1974). Otherwise the language and wording used are free. For cytology the class will usually suffice, but it is also possible to enter free text diagnoses as for biopsies. A SNOMED code is entered together with the free text diagnosis. They are used to generate a dictionary of synonymes. After that has been compiled OUPA will take care of encoding, too.

Dictionary of synonymes. Although retrievals of diagnostic expressions for the care of an individual patient are possible without any dictionary of synonymes, such is needed for hierarchic retrievals, e.g. by anatomic site, organ system or pathologic process (Aller et al. 1977). In order to generate the dictionary SNOMED codes are used as keys. Expressions used with the same SNOMED code are retrieved, clearly erroneous words are corrected and the correct diagnoses are taken into the dictionary as synonymic expressions. Later, when an expression appears that is not included in the dictionary, OUPA asks what code would be appropriate. Possible typing errors and misspelling are first checked by a secretary. After that a SNOMED code is given to the expression by a pathologist or, if an appropriate code does not exist, a new code is generated.

Files

The principal files are shown in Table 2.

Table 2. Principal files of OUPA.

Name of file   Content

Specimen files: All specimens by accession numbers
- Biopsy (B)   with demographic, administrative and
- Electron microscopy (E)   diagnostic data as date of arrival,
- Consultation (C)   social security code, hospital, floor
- Cytology (S)   quality of specimen/organ, pathologist
- Gynecologic cytology   cytology/morgue assistant, consulting
  (N,J,G)   pathologists, number of blocks or slides
- Immunology (F,V)   additional stains, stored, photographed,
- Cytogenetics (K,M,P,X)   illustrative case, diagnoses/results of
- Autopsy (O,L)   examination/cytologic class
  (Total 15 files)

Examination file   Kinds of examinations performed with codes
                                  in groups
                                  Allowed delays, billing and work load
                                  data

Quality file for cytologic   SNOMED topographic codes for
specimens   specimens

Additional stain file   List of regular and laborious
                                  stainings

Pathologist file   Pathologists, cytology and morgue
                                  assistants with codes

In addition the files of patient administration are used.

Functions materialized

Input. Accessioning of the specimens/autopsies and input of
administrative data are performed as a single work step. OUPA assigns
the accession numbers. Input of diagnoses/results is performed
separately after the reports are typed.

Output. Daily lists of specimens received printed by OUPA have replaced
previous manual log books. For autopsies and immune histochemistry
lists of examinations are also being printed monthly. Each pathologist
receives daily a list of specimens assigned to him/her with the results
of all previous examinations of the same patients. The results from
1978 to 1982 are given as SNOP codes, those from 1983 to November 4,
1984 as SNOMED codes and those thereafter both as free text diagnoses
and SNOMED codes. The results of cytologic examinations are given as
Papanicolaou classes. For interdepartmental conferences, the results of
all examinations of any given patient may be retrieved using the
patients social security code. Lists are prepared weekly of those
examinations that are not signed out in due time, first to the
pathologist concerned, and second to the chief of sevice.

For administrative purposes, the amount of work performed by each
pathologist is computed monthly, as well as the total amounts of all
examinations performed at desired intervals. Reports to the Finnish
Cancer Registry are prepared automatically and all specimens and
diagnoses for those patients on whom malignant or suspicious cells have
been found cytologically are retrieved at desired intervals. In
addition, illustrative cases of given diseases and materials for

retrospective studies are retrieved by diagnosis on request.

Billing of other hospitals and private patients as well as payments for part time pathologists are performed on the basis of computed output of OUPA.

Updating of all files is performed by the regular clerical pesonnel of the pathology department.

Functions to materialize later

Monitoring the deaths occurring in the hospital and taking care of the file of photographic slides will materialize in spring 1985. Generating the pathologist's reports by word processing is planned to be started in the beginning of next year, and transferring data between patient floors and pathology department slightly thereafter. The synonyme dictionary for diagnostic expressions is intended to be in operation latest 1987.

References

Aller, RD, Robboy, SJ, Poitras JW, Altshuler, BS, Cameron, M, Prior, MC, Miao, S, Barnett, GO: Computer-assisted pathology encoding and reporting system (CAPER): An on-line computer system developed at the Massachusetts General Hospital. Am J Clin Pathol 1977;68:715-720.
Sutinen, S, Koskinen, P, Vastamäki, R: A method for automatic storage and retrieval of alphabetic autopsy diagnoses coded by computer. Lab Invest 1974;30:762-766.
Ulirsch, RC: Status of anatomic pathology data management systems. Arch Pathol Lab Med 1984;108:884-887.

SOME MEDICAL INFORMATICS FOR MEDICAL STUDENTS?

J.R. Möhr and R. Sawinski
Institute for Medical Documentation, Statistics & Data Processing
University of Heidelberg, Heidelberg, D6900, F.R.G.

Abstract: The experience with a minimal resource introductory course to medical informatics (MI) for medical students in the second year of clinical education is summarized. The course consists of four times ninety minutes of lectures including a modest amount of demonstrations. Emphasis is put on motivating the students for the subject by giving an overview of theoretical concepts and applications. This primary goal was reached while at the same time the knowledge could be only moderately increased, hopefully to a level which will permit the students to progress on their own.

1 Introduction

In some countries good success has been reported with offering comprehensive and well designed courses in medical informatics (MI) to medical students at various levels (5, 6, 7, 8). In many others, the subject seems still to be neglected in medical curricula. In the Federal Republic of Germany, a small amount of biometrics and medical informatics is a mandatory part of the medical curriculum since 1973. However the courses and textbooks are with few exceptions (9) still heavily dominated by aspects of documentation and biometrics, and the allotment of time to both subjects in the curriculum is very restricted (2 hrs of lectures and practical exercises per week during the first clinical year (1st semester), 4 times two hours during the second clinical year within a practical course in medical ecology (4th semester)). In Heidelberg it was therefore decided to offer the students a choice of close to a dozen different subjects during the ecology course, thereby enabling us to treat several subjects in small groups somewhat more comprehensively (e.g. clinical trials, epidemiology, logical foundations of diagnosis etc.).

Since the summer semester of 1983, the authors have offered an introductory overview in medical informatics (MI) in this context, the reason being that contrary to biomathematics, there had not been a prior introduction to MI. The experience with this course, which since has been conducted seven times, will be summarized in the following.

2 Structure of the course

The course consists of four sections:

A Definition, characterization of MI based on (1, 2, 6)

B Technical foundations; functional computer architecture, from bits to languages, user interface, selection criteria for computers.

C Demonstrations

C1 LAB DEMO Interpretation of Calcium Metabolism Data using a

BASIC Program on a micro computer (4)

C2 HIS DEMO Demonstration of a fourth generation hospital

Information system with emphasis on application surface (3)

C3 OFFICE DEMO: Demonstration of Apple LISA™ Office

Computer System with emphaiss on functional spectrum and iconic manipulation

C4 STATISTICS Demo: Demonstration of application of statistical packages (SAS™) with

emphasis on the gain obtainable from correct application of such systems.

D Medical Office Computing: Survey of state of the art, future prospects, social implications.

(This part takes only 60 minutes, the final 30 minutes being devoted toan examination.)

The structure outlined evolved continuously, the basic concept having been decided, after an initial survey in the first hour of such a course showed that the students had essentially no idea of computer applications in medicine and their fundamentals. Contents of the individual sections, especially the demonstrations were varied considerably. Also the location of the demonstrations was varied several times placing them first, second or third while maintaining the sequence A, B, D for the remaining sections.

3 Student sample and examination

The examination was intended to survey the knowledge of the students as well as their attitude towards the course through a few (4-6) questions to be answered by free text for each section. The knowledge assessment part contained three questions, asking the students to characterize 1) Different types of computer applications in medicine, 2) Selection criteria for computer systems, 3) Computer applications considered to be problematic.

A fourth section asked the students to characterize eight computer related buzzwords. All were considered to represent a level of technical knowledge helpful in reading popular articles and advertisements on computers. Three had not been treated during the course (artificial intelligence (only course A), structured programming (only course B), modem, systems analysis) and were included in order to assess the level of knowledge of the group prior to course attencance (control questions). Five had been treated during the course (operating system, computer language, byte, direct access storage, peripheral devices) and were used to test the level of knowledge acquired during the course (test questions). Both sets of questions were assumed to be of equal difficulty and discriminating power.

Answers were rated as 0 if wrong, 1 if the association was correct or an acceptable example was given and 2 if a satisfactory comprehensive characterization was given.

In the attitude section, a first question asked students whether they considered it necessary to busy themselves further with MI and to give a reason for their reply. Other questions to be answered by free text, concerned strong and weak points of the course, the sequence of sections A through D etc.

Finally this section contained a question where students were asked to rate 1) the relevance of the material of the course 2) the amount of material covered 3) the usefullness1 of the handouts 4) each part of the demonstration on a five point seale, usually from -2 (bad) over 0 (indifferent) to 2 (good). Due to the variation of course contents and the assessment instruments only the results of the final two courses conducted in Nov./Dec. 1984 will be reported below with some reference to the experience with earlier courses.

Students during the wintersemester were free to choose among 12 different offers. The main selection criterion seems to have been compatibility with other curricular duties, - in part due to very scant information on goals and contents of the course prior to making the choice. Therefore the students taking one of the two courses (referred to as A and B) may be fairly representative of the current student population.

Course A was delivered predominantly by J.R.M., course B. by R.S.. Contents are considered to have been identical due to extensive information exchange during previous courses. Students had ben told that their performance in this examination would have no effect on their curricular career, since the goal was to improve the course. All examination results were evaluated by J.R.M.

4 Results

Courses were regularly attended by over 90% of enrolled students (22 course A, 27 course B), partly due to checking attendance. Student involvement was fair, in particular section D usually provoked lively discussions.

4.1 Assessment of knowledge

All students in course A and 70 to 75% in course B were supposed to have answered these questions correctly by identifying several aspects in a structured manner. At the beginning of the course only some students associated applications in medicine like statistical evaluation or support of special investigations (e.g. CT, ECG). (Knowledge concerning problem prone applications had not been checked).

Figure 1 shows that in course B 9% of the answers to control questions were considered satisfactory while a fraction of 26% was obtained for in course A for such answers. Similarly only 40% of answers to test questions were considered correct in course B while in couse A a fraction of 67% was achieved. Only some 20% of answers were considered wrong in both courses.

4.2 Assessment of attitude towards course

Hundred percent of students in course A and all but 2 students in course B expressed that they felt it was necessary to busy themselves further with MI, mostly because of a general trend, or because they expected some utility of this technology for themselves. Comments concerning the improvements for the course were mostly encouraging, many asking for more in more time, for optional add on courses, for more possibility for hands on experience. One quarter objected to the examination. Similar attitudes were evident from the ratings attributed to the various course qualities. Interestingly, the demonstration of the intrepretation of laboratory data, which was delivered by a clinician and emphasized medical aspects, received consistently the highest ratings among the demonstrations. The sequence of the course components was rarely commented.

In summary then, the primary goal of motivating the students and providing them with an overview seems to have been achieved while the conveyance of knowledge was limited especially if the very modest demands are taken into consideration.

Figure 1 Effect of Course on knowledge of participants.
Responses to 3 Control questions and 5 test questions given by 22 participants of course a and 26 participants of course B are compared to assess gain in knowledge.

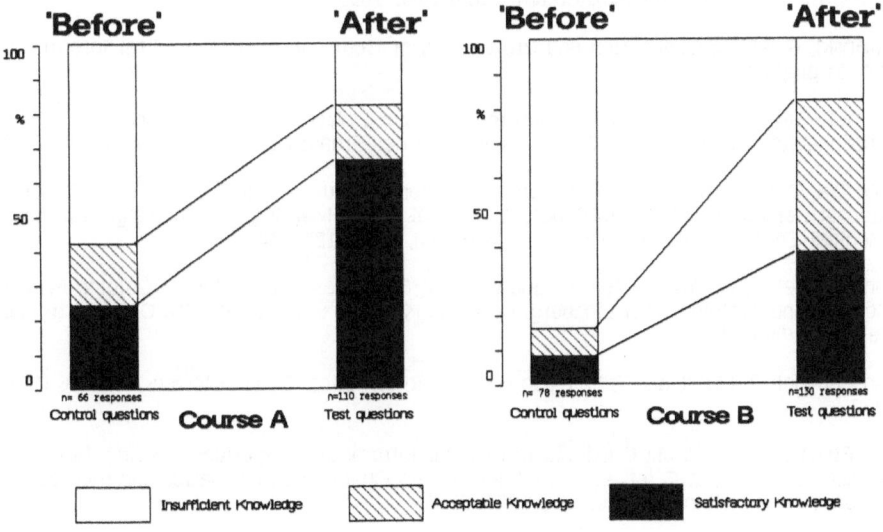

5 Discussion

The results reported are based on a number of rather weak assumptions: representativety of the student sample for our students, of the questions for the knowledge before and after the course, comparability of the two sets of questions, willingness of the students to disclose their knowledge, comparability of contents and presentation mode in both courses. Most of them may be violated in some way or other. Still the results seem to show clearly that the level of "computer literacy" of the students is extremely low initially and can only be raised moderately with the amount of effort put in by the students and ourselves. The increase achieved may be related to prior knowledge, to general intellectual capacity, motivation, influence of the teachers – factors which one would assume anyway, while the results in this respect are not conclusive.

However it seems evident for us that our future colleagues can be interested in the subject of MI. This fact is relevant in face of the common experience in more biomathematics oriented teaching endeavours where commonly attendance rates drop from 50% initially to less than 10% finally unless severe enforcements are applied. We propose therefore that –where ressources with respect to time, personnell, technical suport etc. do not permit more elaborated approaches– a course of the described type may serve to provide a basis, from which the students are able to carry on by themselves, and that this is better than scaring them away from our field for the rest of their lives by too high demands.

References:

(1) Möhr, J. R.: Trends, Effizienz und Effekte medizinischer Informatik im Krankenhaus. Bayr. Int., 5 (1983) 25 – 28

(2) Möhr, J. R.:Training and Education in Medical Informatics. In van Bemmel et al. (eds.): MEDINFO 83 (North Holland: Amsterdam, 1983) 1030-1035

(3) Sawinski, R. et al.: Conception and Prototyping of Components of a Hospital Information System. In preparation.

(4) Schmidt-Gayk, H. et al.: Tischrechnerprogramm zur Erfassung von Störungen des Calcium- und Phosphatstoffwechsels, der Nierenfunktion und der Ernährung. Med. Techn., 97 (1977) 98-106

(5) Tuinstra, C. L., Verweeen, A. A.: Information Science in the Medical Curriculum: Principles and Practice at Leiden University. In Pagès, J. C. et al. (eds.): Meeting the Challenge: Informatics and Medical Education. (North Holland: Amsterdam, 1983) 127-134

(6) Van Bemmel, J. H.: The System behind Medical Computer Applications - Guiding Principles for Courses and Training -. In Lindberg, D. A. B., Kaihara, S. (eds.): MEDINFO80 (North Holland: Amsterdam, 1980) 546-547

(7) Van Bemmel, J. H., et al.: Training in Medical Informatics. Comp. Biomed. Res.: 16 (1983) 414-432

(8) Van Bemmel, J. H. et al.: Curricula in Medical Informatics: Experience During Ten Years in Amsterdam. In Pagès, J. C. et al. (eds.): Meeting the Challenge: Informatics and Medical Education. (North Holland: Amsterdam, 1983) 55-65

(9) Wingert, F.: Medical Informatics (Springer: Berlin, Heidelberg, New York, 1981)

COMPUTING IN DIALYSIS UNITS: HOW TO ENGAGE AND TRAIN ALL MEDICAL STAFF WHEN INTRODUCING COMPUTING IN PATIENT CARE?

B. Lindholm, L. Johansson and Y. Gustavsson.
Department of Renal Medicine and Karolinska Institute, Huddinge University Hospital, S-141 86 Huddinge, Sweden.

Enormous amounts of clinical data accumulate over months and years in patients with chronic renal failure. The medical supervision often includes over 50 different time-varying clinical and laboratory parameters. It is virtually impossible to keep track of all these data with conventional records even if these are well-organized and used with discipline (Gordon et al 1983). As a result nephrologists have been among the first physicians to use computers in patient care (Stead 1984). There are by now several reports on successful applications of computer technology for the handling of clinical data in dialysis and transplantation units (Pollak et al 1977, Gordon et al 1983, Knapp 1983, Morgan and Will 1983, Pollak et al 1983, Stead et al 1983, Stead 1983, Taylor and Sells 1983, Trimbel et al 1983, Wing et al 1983, Stead 1984). However, it is also known but less well-documented that many medical computing projects have failed when transferred from a research base to clinical practice (Stead 1983). One reason for such failures may have been a frustrating and unsuccessful dependence on computer experts with whom clinical staff have had difficulty communicating; such problems have been particularly severe in large, "mainframe" projects, which use a central computer (Gordon et al 1983). In recent years many of the difficulties inherent in early computer technology have been eliminated. Software has become more and more user friendly. Furthermore, improved computerized medical records systems (Pollak et al 1983, Stead et al 1983) and clinical database systems for handling of numerical data in dialysis and transplantation units (Gordon et al 1983) have been developed. Although this has solved many of the problems concerning computing per se the introduction of computer technology in the clinic may lead to other problems including difficulties to integrate the new technology within the existing organizational framework. Furthermore, problems may arise if nurses and other users are not well-informed about the purposes and functions of the computer system.

In this report we describe our experiences in the introduction of a multi-terminal computer system which links several dialysis units in a renal clinic. We emphasize the need to involve and train all categories of the staff already at an early stage during the computerization process.

Background and definitions of problems

Our centre is responsible for the treatment of patients with end-stage renal diseases in a population of about 1.6 million. Due to improved patient survival there is a continuous accumulation of patients on renal replacement therapy; this is a world-wide experience (Wing et al 1983). The difficulties to predict and plan for the treatment of all patients was an important reason to initiate a regional database system; this need was also appreciated by the health authorities in the Stockholm region. Furthermore, we need to produce regular reports both to the European Dialysis and Transplantation Association Registry (EDTA) and to a national registry; when performed manually this work takes several months to complete. Another reason for introducing computing was a need to evaluate the results of different therapies for research purposes as well as for the routine "production control" at our clinic. Thirdly, each dialysis session results in large amounts of data. Since more than 30 000 dialysis sessions are carried out each year enormous amounts of data accumulate. Thus, we needed a computer system for the storage and retrospective retrieval of data for individual patients and for groups of patients. Fourthly, our centre consists of several geographically separated dialysis units. Since the internal postage service may be slow and since patients records often must be transported rapidly between the different units, e.g., when patients develop acute complications, we needed to improve the transfer of vital patient data between the units. Last but not least we felt that computing could improve the quality of medical decisions and relieve the medical staff from some of the time-consuming manual handling of data which would give more time for the care of the patients.

Planning for the introduction of the system

Already at an early stage during the planning process we began a continuous cooperation with representatives from the different categories of our staff (physicians, nurses, auxilliary nurses and secretaries). All of the staff, in total about 170 persons, would be affected by the computer system. We wanted all users to participate in the planning process, not only a few interested physicians. This was felt as desirable first of all because the goals of the project had to be decided, and also because the planning of all specific items would be more relevant if the users could define what they expected the system to do for them. The initial planning process of our computer project was characterized by a continuing dialogue between the users and computer experts, representatives from the regional healths authorities etc. During this phase we could integrate ideas about: (1) what computer systems could do (according to the computer experts), (2) what we could afford (according to the health authorities), and (3) what we (the clinical users) wanted the system to do. The most obvious problem during this work was communication difficulties because the different parties tended to use their own specialized professional language. However, this problem was partly solved when we established a small working team which included two nurses, one nephrologist and one computer expert (Fig 1). This group could "translate" messages between the different interested parties, negotiate with administrators, representatives from trade unions and companies etc.

After about one year the specific aims of the project were defined in detail and we could then proceed to buy and install the necessary hardware and software. However, due to financial problems and other administrative difficulties it took us another one or two years until all of the equipment was there. The working team (Fig 1) played an active role in coordinating this work.

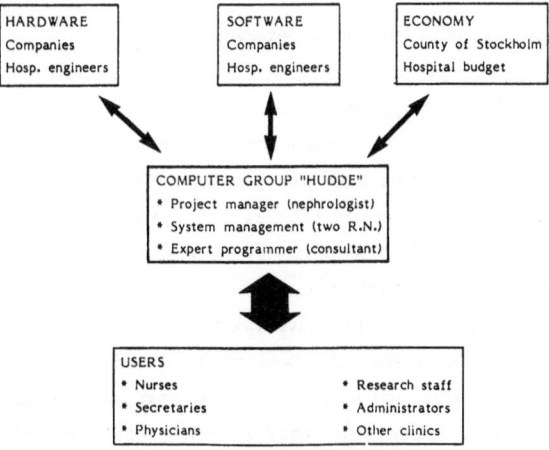

Fig 1. The organization of the computer project.

Description of the system

The current system operates on a PDP 11/24 (Digital Equipment Corporation)
using the RSX 11M operating system. It has a secondary storage capacity of 280
MB. Five peripheral working stations are used, two of these are connected via
the telephone network. The software includes a commercially available package
(Clinical Data System, (CDS), Clinical Computing Ltd, London) which originates
from the renal unit at the Department of Medicine, Charing Cross Hospital
Medical School, London University. The CDS system is a computerized clinical
database system that maintains records of numerical data. It also stores demographic data and a time-oriented event list. Sophisticated graphic and administrative routines display multiple values simultaneously either in the native
form or in transformed state (products, reciprocals, quotients etc). There are
enquiry and report programs; specific questions can be stored and used whenever required. A key feature of the CDS system is that it eliminates the need
for traditional programming procedures. Its data and graphics processing
facilities can be configured by the existing staff at the renal unit. Therefore the system could be modified according to the local needs and standards
at our unit. This work, and the maintenance of the system including most
organizational and technical tasks, are performed by two specialized nurses in
our clinic (Fig 1). The database system has been linked to a statistical
package (Hässle STAT-PACK) which enables us to evaluate the clinical data
statistically without having to re-feed data manually. The CDS system has been
described in detail earlier (Gordon et al 1983).

Training of users and building up a database

The introduction of the computer system followed three steps: (1) training of
nurses, auxillary nurses and secretaries, (2) these were responsible for the
daily input of clinical data for all patients, and (3) the introduction of
physicians as users of the system (Fig 2.). The two nurses in the working team
(Fig 1) have instructed all users on an individual basis. Since most of the
staff had become familiar with the aims of the system already at an early
stage of the project most of them have been motivated to learn how to use it.
At present, more than 80 users have been trained and use the system routinely.
In case of problems the users contact the two specialized nurses in the
working team. Each user among the staff is responsible for the entries of data

for "their" patients. Thus, the rather unrewarding and time-consuming work to build up the database has been shared by many; the average daily time for this work is about 10 min per user.

The value of the clinical database is depending on the quantity, and the quality, of the information which is stored in accessible computer memory. By now, our system contains information of about 1 500 patients. The rate of data input corresponds to about 20 -30 Megabytes per year. Since most of the data is fed into the computer by the medical staff the quality of the data can be checked continuously. Furthermore, one or more pre-set minimum and maximum levels for each parameter are included so that when a parameter deviates from the pre-set levels the system warns the user automatically.

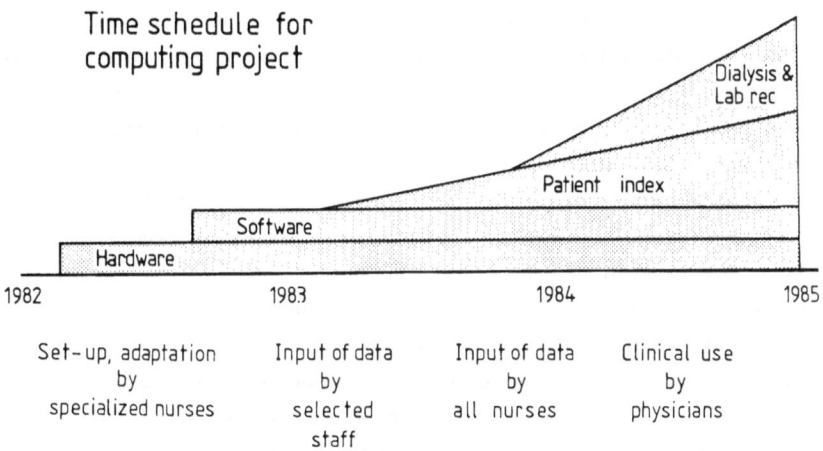

Fig 2. The time-consuming process to organize a clinical computing project. Note that the physicians were the last users to be trained.

The last step in the process to introduce computing in the clinic was the training of physicians. The benefits of computing is perhaps most obvious for this group of the users. This reflects the fact that the system offers the physicians large amounts of clinical data, which can be used in their clinical work or for research purposes. The benefits to the nurses, on the other hand, have to be weighed against their efforts to feed the data into the computer, and many nurses have felt that computing represents an additional burden in their daily work.

Concluding remarks

Perhaps our most important experience so far is that the process to introduce computing in clinical practice is very time-consuming (Fig 2). However, the computer system has now been established and has been shown to be a valuable tool in the clinical work, in research, for various administrative tasks and as a method for communication between different units. The costs involved appear to be acceptable; the average computing cost per each dialysis session is about one US dollar, and the total costs constitute 1 -2 % of the total budget.

The organization of our computer system is characterized by a large degree of decentralization and active participation of both the medical and the administrative staff. An organizational adaptation has been necessary in the clinic to meet the demands of the new technology. However, we have been able to carry out this project without employment of computer experts or specialized administrative clerks. Instead, two nurses have gradually been trained in various aspects of computing. They are now the system managers of the project and the nurses and other users contact them if problems arise during the routine usage of the system. These regular contacts with all the users may often be very productive; every day new ideas and suggestions about various improvements of the system are proposed by the medical staff. Thus, the improvements of the software and its applications appear to be a never-ending process. Innovations in the field of computing in our clinic have important bearings on the clinical work, and vice versa. On the whole, the clinical work has to be organized in more uniform and "logical" way than earlier. This adaptation is of value not only because it makes computing easier but also because the organization of the clinical work may improve.

References

Gordon M, Venn JC, Gower PE, de Wardener HE: Experience in the computer handling of clinical data for dialysis and transplantation units. Kidney Int 24: 455-463, 1983

Knapp MS: Computing, mathematics and the nephrologist. Kidney Int 24: 433-534, 1983

Morgan LB, Will EJ: Selection, presentation and interpretation of biochemical data in renal failure. Kidney Int 24: 438-444, 1983

Pollak VE, Buncher CR, Donovan ER: On-line computerized data handling system for treating patients with renal disease. Arch Intern Med 137: 446-456, 1977

Pollak VE: Computerization of the medical record; use in care of patients with end-stage renal disease. Kidney Int 24: 464-473, 1983

Stead WW: Evolution of technology bring computers to the bedside. Kidney Int 24: 436-437, 1983

Stead WW, Garret Jr LE, Hammond WE: Practicing nephrology with a computerized medical record. Kidney Int 24: 446-454, 1983

Stead WW: Using computers to care for patients with renal disorders. M.D. Computing 1 (5): 42-50, 1984

Taylor GT, Sells RA: Microcomputers for renal units. Lancet 1: 1366-1367, 1982

Trimble IM, West M, Knapp MS, Pownall R, Smith AFM: Detection of renal allograft rejection by computer. Br Med J 286: 1695-1969, 1983

Wing AJ, D'Amoro J, Lamm LU, Selwood NH: Evolving methodologies in computerized European Registries. Kidney Int 24: 507-515, 1983

INTEGRATING STATISTICS IN MEDICAL INFORMATICS: A LECTURE ON
STATISTICAL ANALYSIS SYSTEMS

R. Haux
Abteilung Medizinische Statistik und Dokumentation der RWTH
Pauwelsstraße, D-5100 Aachen
Federal Republic of Germany

Summary: In this paper I will try to point out the necessity of
giving lectures in statistical analysis systems, and that this can
only be done when basic knowledge in the field of informatics and
statistics is available. The structure of such a course is given and
experiences in lecturing the course to different audiences are
reported. Integrating statistics and informatics, as it is needed
here, seems to be especially successful in curricula focussing on
medical applications such as the Medical Informatics curriculum at
the University of Heidelberg/Heilbronn Polytechnical School.

Keywords: Statistical analysis systems; education; computational
statistics; medical informatics.

1. Statistical Analysis Systems

Statistical analysis systems, like BMDP, SAS or SPSS (for references
see Francis, 1981), are widely used in medicine. They serve as a
valuable tool for statistical data analysis, especially if there are
studies were the sample sizes are large, the data management is
considerable and/or the amount of descriptive, exploratory data
analysis is high. This can be the case for epidemiologic studies,
controlled clinical trials, long term observational studies, studies
with multi-center designs etc. . Users of statistical analysis
systems are physicians or other scientists, who should have basic
knowledge in applied statistics, as well as statisticians.

2. The Need for Lectures on Statistical Analysis Systems

Through the wide use of statistical analysis systems we also have to
observe that these systems sometimes give wrong or ambiguous results
to the user especially to the untrained one, who is not very firm in
statistics and in using the system correctly.

As Nelder (1977) states: "Most current programs will not give the
user any explicit warning that anything is wrong ... . The
uncritical use of ... procedures ... is tending to bring the
subject of statistics into disrepute."

Besides the criticism of the existing statistical analysis systems
there is also an intensive discussion concerning future developments,
especially when artificial intelligence methodology is applied in
order to extend these systems to statistical expert systems.

Zelen (1983) outlines possible shortcomings in this development.   He
describes such "automatic data analysis systems" in the following
way: "The user will input a set of 'stylized' questions dealing with
various hypotheses or models.   The system will choose one or more
appropriate data analysis techniques and give the answer ..." and he
states "I do not welcome this future, as I believe it will stifle
individual innovations on particular problems.".

What we have to keep in mind are two facts: (1) that there is a
strong need for such systems and (2) that the development of such
systems as well as, partially, their appliction is not a trivial
task.

If we do not want to teach only the use of a special, existing
statistical analysis system, but if we also want to analyze the
structures of such systems and investigate their   construction
principles, we need knowledge from the field of informatics and from
the field of statistics.

Teaching only the application of a statistical analysis system, i.e.
learning the command language, getting familiar with the operating
system etc. concentrates on the user of such a system as e.g.   on
the physician mentioned above.   This is of course necessary for
applying a system and is done by the system distributors, by
departments for medical informatics and statistics and by computing
centers.   Within such a course, however, we do not have the
possibility to discuss the problems and shortcomings as mentioned in
the preceding section - in the same way as we cannot sufficiently
discuss possibilities to overcome the shortcomings of FORTRAN in a
FORTRAN course; therefore courses on programming methodology and/or
on compiler construction are appropriate.

Within informatics, or computer science, respectively, we especially
need knowledge in program development and database systems theory and
technics. Within statistics we need basic knowledge in experimental

design as well as some experience in applying statistical methods.

These requirements - knowledge in informatics and statistics - can be fulfilled within statistics curricula (including lectures in informatics) and in informatics curricula forcussing on medical applications (Haux, 1984) - because medical statistics/biometry is a substantial part of the application field. Examples are the curriculum medical informatics at the University of Heidelberg/Heilbronn Polytechnical School (Möhr, Leven and Rothemund, 1982) and curricula in computer science with medicine as subsidiary subject (for an overview on such curricula in the Federal Republic of Germany see Reichertz and Koeppe, 1982).

In the Heidelberg/Heilbronn curriculum probability theory, mathematical foundations of statistics and biostatistics are taught. So basic knowledge in estimation and test theory as well as experience in the application of simple statistical tests exists in any case, besides, of course, the fundamentals of computer science.

3. A Lecture on Statistical Analysis Systems

According to the above mentioned requirements, such a lecture should be placed at the graduate level. A proposal for such a course is now given. If differs heavily from the above mentioned courses for users; it differs also from statistical computing courses as described in Chambers (1977) and in Kennedy and Gentle (1980), were nearly only (but extensively) algorithmic aspects are discussed.

The aims of the course are: to impart basic knowledge in
1. the design and in
2. the evaluation of statistical analysis systems and also (but not only) in
3. the application of existing systems (user's level as well as programmers's level).

The course is divided into the following parts:

(1) Basic knowledge

The first part of (1) deals with terminology and concepts for data- and methodbase systems (as is outlined in Haux, 1983). Using this terminology, we can define statistical analysis systems and point out the differences to database systems, statistical database systems, application systems etc. .

We are now able to describe some existing systems and can give examples for their application. This is done for the widely used systems BMDP, SAS, SPSS(X) and, depending on the time available, for S (Becker and Chambers, 1984) and for the database management system SIR which is frequently used for statistical applications in medicine.

(2) System design - part I

This part is dealing with design aspects for statistical analysis systems. The importance of a sufficient data type and data structure type concept is shown. Using a controlled clinical trial as an example, it is demonstrated that, as an appropriate and high quality tool, a statistical analysis system has to support the user's data analysis by (1) executing the analysis conscientiously with as little effort to the user as possible and (2), in order to ensure a high quality analysis, by supervising the analysis in a constructive manner.

As a 'by-product' or appendix of part (2) we can also discuss the data (-base) design for studies to the extent as described in Holle and Leibbrand (1985).

(3) Program development for statistical data analysis

Here, in a first part, it is pointed out what has to be especially considered for the design of methods (programs) for the methodbase of a statistical analysis system. Besides some general aspects, the detection of faulty data, the time complexity of some statistical algorithms, numerical problems and other subjects are discussed. Here it can be seen that easy and efficient program development is strongly dependent on the system design.

In the second part of (3) it is shown how program development within an existing statistical analysis system can be done. As an example SAS is used and a so-called (SAS-) procedure is developed and implemented.

(4) System design - part II

Being now acquainted with the knowledge of (2) and (3) we can discuss two additional aspects of system design. The importance of a well-structured methodbase (in analogy to a well-structured database) can be shown. Secondly the possibilities of artificial intelligence techniques for statistical analysis systems - i.e. the extension of statistical analysis systems to statistical expert systems - is raised. Here it is neccessary to show the misuse of these techniques, which can easily happen when the statistical methodology is not sufficiently understood by the system designer.

(5) Requirements for statistical analysis systems

On the basis of the work of Francis (1981) and Hultsch et al. (1978) criteria for the evaluation of statistical analysis systems are summarized.

4. Some Experiences

Several times the course, as described in section 3, has been lectured during 1983 and 1985. It has been given by the author to graduate students in medical informatics (University of Heidelberg/Heilbronn Polytechnical School) to computer science students with subsidiary subject medicine (University of Technology Aachen) and to statistic students (University of Dortmund).

The course, as I believe, is successful if there are two basic foundations: sufficient knowledge in informatics and familiarity with the problems occuring in (medical) statistics. Because of the frequent demand of being familiar with such systems in their future work as professionals, the students were interested in learning the application of such systems and could be stimulated to discuss the problems of system design in order to construct a valuable tool for the user.

Medical informatics curricula seem to be one appropriate location to give such a lecture. Here a fruitful basis could be established for research and development of statistical analysis systems, and in computational statistics in general - a field where the integration of statistics and informatics is needed.

References

Becker, R.A. and Chambers, J.M. (1984). Design of the S System for Data Analysis. Comm. ACM 27, 486-495.

Chambers, J.M. (1977). Computational Methods for Data Analysis. New York: Wiley Publ. Company.

Francis, I. (1981). Statistical Software: A Comparative Review. Amsterdam: North Holland.

Haux, R. (1983). Statistical Analysis Systems - Construction and Aspects of Method Design (Part 1). Stat. Software Newsl. 9, 106-115.

Haux, R. (1984). Integrating Statistics in Computer Science Education. To appear in: Proc. Europ. Symposium on Biostatistics/Medical Statistics, October 22-26, 1984, Berlin, GDR.

Holle, R. and Leibbrand, D. (1985). Data Design for Clinical Trials. To appear in Stat. Software Newsletter 11, No. 1.

Hultsch, E., Jannasch, J., Krier, N., Sund., M. and Victor, N. (1978). Requirements for program systems used for statistical data analysis. Stat. Software Newsl. 4, 3-30.

Kennedy, W.J. and Gentele, J.E. (1980). Statistical Computing. New York: Dekker.

Möhr, J.R., Leven, F.J. and Rothemund, M. (1982). Formal Education in Medical Informatics - Review of Ten Years Experience with a Specialized University Curriculum - . Meth. Inform. Med. 21, 169-180.

Nelder, J.A. (1977). Intelligent Programs, the Next Stage in Statistical Computing. Barra, J.R. et al. (eds.). Recent Developments in Statistics, 79-86. Amsterdam: North Holland.

Reichertz, P.L. and Koeppe, P. (eds., 1982). Ausbildung in der Medizinischen Informatik. Berlin: Springer.

Zelen, M. (1983). Biostatistical Science: A Look into the Future. Biometrics 39, 827-830.

A POSTGRADUATE MEDICAL EDUCATION DATABASE

John S Bryden and Linda B Boyle
Postgraduate Medicine
University of Glasgow
GLASGOW
G12 8QQ
United Kingdom

The adequate supply of suitably trained doctors for senior posts is of concern to every country in the world.

Although doctors are numerically small as a percentage of all caring professionals, because of the doctor role in key health decision-making, every nation must ensure both an adequate supply of doctors and that their training is adequate.

Much of their postgraduate education has, in the past, been caught up with medical mystique and only in recent years have planned training programs become well delineated. In the UK, a Royal Commission proposed and Westminster ratified a structure where National councils would supervise and Regional Postgraduate Deans would implement planned programs of training. (Ref 1)

Any post diploma training of doctors has to marry the service needs of hospitals and clinics with the academic needs of the trainees - often this marriage produces contented bedfellows - but a hospital may wish to exploit young doctors as essential "pairs of hands" or academic training may move those in training towards esoteric sidelines for removed from day to day clinical practice.

National or regional committees may express strong views on how the training should be structured, but little or no information is available to assure the quality of the training in terms of the centralised guidelines.

Scotland, although quite a small European country with 5.2 million population, has however had several centuries tradition of producing high quality medical graduates, of giving them quality immediate postgraduate experience and of exporting around three quarters of its medical graduates, many to England, Wales and Ireland, but also to almost every country in the world. (Ref 2)

In the West of Scotland, both undergraduate and postgraduate medical education are based on the five-centuries old Glasgow University. It serves both the industrial conurbation around the city along with the agricultural counties in the West and South West of Scotland as well as the adjacent inner and outer islands: in all, a catchment population of about 3 million with between 5 and 6,000 doctors of whom around 1,650 are normally in training.

The West of Scotland postgraduate medical and dental education has a strong participative specialty orientated committee structure to support it, led by a Postgraduate Dean.

Despite this, Timbury, a former Glasgow Postgraduate Dean, in working reports (Ref 3) highlighted the lack of meaningful information about the collective progress of young doctors and propounded the need for the use of information technology to improve the quality of the information.

Viner, Lees and Dick (1982), described their MEDICS scheme based on one of the London regions (Ref 4). Visits to this scheme found it to be of a highly dedicated quality but that it had been very slow to develop. We did however, build much upon their existing work.

Careful appraisal suggested that we needed data on the doctors, on the posts they held and on the history of these doctors and these posts.

Would we only gather "head count" data or should it be personalized around identifiable doctors? Just as Heasman and Acheson in the sixties (Ref 5 & 6) showed that meaningful data about hospital care could only be produced around identifiable patients, it is our view that similarly meaningful data about doctor's training needs to be tied around named participants. This does mean that the data held becomes much more sensitive and procedures have had to be developed for its "holding" that are described later in the paper. By the time that the authors were responsible for the development, albeit superficial, decisions had been taken about the funding. There was only sufficient funding for 8-bit microcomputer technology. The theoretical file structure was sized and decisions made to purchase from the UK manufacturer, Comart, an 8-bit multiboard system which runs under Digital Research's networking system known as CP/NOS. It provides 2 hard disk drives, a magnetic tape streamer for back up and 2 lines for communication to the Glasgow University mainframe computer (an ICL 2976) for statistical and similar major number crunching work.

Because of previous experience of one of the authors, (JSB), Ashton Tate's DBase II has been used as the software throughout. Our experience has confirmed that this is an appropriate "language". It allows, on the one hand, easy use by the non-sophisticated computer user to create databases and access the information and, on the other hand, has proved adequate for our computer professional support to produce reliable software.

In the UK, an administrative census is completed on all doctors at the end of each September. Although this only holds limited information, it seemed to offer us a good starting point. We obtained from this census magnetic tapes for each of the 6 Health Boards that comprised our catchment area. It seems so simple to transfer data. We had to access to a "black box" approach which took data from magnetic tape and dumped it on a compatible floppy. So simple - but it caused endless problems. For example, although DBase II will accept data from a wide range of formats, the tape to floppy converter we were using dumped data in huge blocks which were too big for DBase. Software had to be written to break up the data acceptably: for one large health authority the file was so long that it was more than one floppy in length - the standard conversion system had not foreseen this problem - back to source for this data - redivided onto 2 tapes: once the data was on the machine, some random checks revealed that my senior colleague's name and some others, including my wife's, were missing from the file - mistakes in the parameters in selecting the appropriate records.

From one health authority we found no juniors at all - it had not been noticed that a complete group was missing. Despite all these "glitches", the main files were begun with over 4,000 doctors involved.

Our training programs, especially for the more junior doctors, are built up around jobs of only 6 months tenure. Almost every young doctor changes post each 31st January and 31st July. This means at least 1,500 doctor changes and the same number of post changes each year, split into 2 huge peaks.

Our approach has been essentially low cost. Perhaps in an ideal world each of the 153 employing institutions might have had a work station directly linked to us, but this was neither financially nor logistically desirable. In each hospital there is however, a "girl-friday" (Ref 7)

who processes these doctor movements. One of us, (LBB), has developed
close contact with them and this ensures that a relevant photocopy of
each doctor's documentation arrives at the database office. Only by
such human relationships is it possible to improve the data quality.
One approach might have been to have introduced standard documentation
on which each institution was forced to submit the data. Although the
database was related to our monopoly state Health Service, we nevertheless had to negotiate with this large number of potentially independent
data sources - any bar to the free flow of information was to be avoided.
As a result of the free approach, we receive all the data within a few
weeks of each changeover date.

Software must also allow for human frailty. Our updating procedure has
to allow for random arrival of the notifications of the filling and
emptying of posts. Often we are told that Doctor X has now filled post
Y before we know that Doctor Z has vacated the same post Y to allow for
the arrival of X. Equally, Doctor A may have filled post C before we
know that he or she has left the previous post B. Our updating allows
for this and places such temporarily displaced doctors in a file known
as "Limbo"!

Doctors will ultimately be identified by their UK General Medical Council
(GMC) registration number. We are attempting some record linkage between
a GMC tape and our own data. Until this is complete and until the GMC
number is more widely used, we use a computer generated number along
with the surname and date of birth. If need be, however, we do hold a
second surname to allow for both maiden and married but also because
some doctors (especially those from overseas) may use shortened versions
of their legal name. Posts are also given an identifier. This has
become a 10 digit component number joining together a series of codes
already in use nationally.

These 2 long files of the database are interlinked with;
a) an archival file which holds details of moves of doctors and through
posts,
b) a file of each of the patterns rotational placements,
c) files of each of the last 2 years of Glasgow medical school undergraduates,
d) files of agreed planned appointments to junior interm posts for the
coming 2 academic years,
e) working "look-up table" files to interlink standard codes and their
translations.

This database has now been developing at the time of writing for over 18 months with 3 of the 6-monthly changeovers having been recorded. Plenty of data has been pouring in; what has been coming out? A synopsis file, to capture a point prevalence, is now not far short of a megabyte in size. Statistical analysis on 8-bit microcomputers although feasible for small files, is well nigh impossible for such a database. The system when designed however, was aware of such limitations and the synopsis files are passed by land lines to the University mainframe.

Like other UK universities, this offers access to a whole range of sophisticated software packages. Many of these allow solely for remote on-line job entry along with batch processing.

We have found however, that the conversational version of SPSS - the so-called SCSS allows for very sophisticated statistical analysis but with real time access. (Ref 8) This allows an interactive approach to data analysis, especially through the ability to look at a window-full or snapshot of the data.

Until this database has existed for the possible 10 years that it may take the average doctor to complete his training, we will not have the full picture but already tabulations are highlighting new facts about the training.

Such a database is seen both by doctors and employers as holding sensitive information. An already successful technique is Scotland has been to have a publicly identified and personally responsible data-holder for clinical data. This we have used for the PIMMS scheme. The data holder has, as a sounding board, a Steering Committee. In addition both to reassure the doctors and improve the quality of the information, each doctor is about to receive a turnround document showing his or her data.

Much hard personalized work has been involved in implementing this database on the education of doctors. It continues to show that only with this effort does one produce high quality information.

References

1   Royal Commission on Medical Education 1968;   UK HMSO.

2   Duncan A. Memorials of the Faculty of Physicians and Surgeons of
    Glasgow 1599-1850 1896;   124

3   Internal Communication. Scottish Council for Postgraduate Medical
    Education 1983.

4   Viner RS, Lees W, Dick GWA. A Regional Medical Manpower and Training
    Information System. Community Medicine 1982; 4:108-112.

5   Acheson ED. Medical Record Linkage. Meth Inform Med 1969; 8:1-6.

6   Heasman MA, Carstairs V. In Patient Management in Scotland. Brit
    Med Jnl 1971; 1:495.

7   Defoe D. The Life and Strange Surprising Adventures of Robinson
    Crusoe. London: W Taylor 1719.

8   S.C.S.S. Manual. Published by McGraw-Hill

AN EXAMINATION AND EDUCATION SYSTEM FOR
CLINICAL DISCIPLINES OF MEDICINE

J.Janecki,B.Blaszczak

Polish Academy of Sciences,
Institute of Biocybernetics and Biomedical Eng.,
Laboratory of Medical Informatics,
00-020 Warszawa, ul.Rutkowskiego 12,
POLAND.

1. SUMMARY

An examination and education system for clinical disciplines
of medicine provides an efficient method for testing the state of
students'or doctors' knowledge. An examination consists of the
following tests :

> basing on the patient's data and symptoms some essential
> investigations should be chosen, then a diagnosis should
> be selected and finally a proper treatment method should
> be chosen.

Each choice could change the score / negative points are allowed /
and is always followed by comments. The kind of this system response
might depend on several former choices / so called dependent responses /. Items in the presented lists are displayed in a random order
which is generated for each test execution.

Up to 16 students might be simultaneously examined by system
running on the SM4 computer / PDP 11/40 /.

2. TEST STRUCTURE

The aim of a test is to make the student solve problems similar to the real life ones. Each test consists of an introduction and three decision stages.

The introduction contains the student's situation / "you are in the street", "you are at the hospital", etc./ and short summary of the patient's case.
The three decision stages are :

- the investigation stage : choose an investigation method
      which results will affort possibilities for diagnosis,
- the diagnosis stage : choose the proper diagnosis basing on
      the results of the former stage,
- the treatment stage : choose the adequate treatment method.

Each choice is made by typing in the selected number when presented with numbered lists.

The described test structure was given in /1/. However, basing on /2/ and our own experiments, the following new elements were incorporated :

- the student's situation as a part of the introduction,
- the score,
- the dependent responses,
- the random order of items in the lists.

Details are given below.

The system responds to any choice by the comments and by the number of points / positive or negative /. The lists of choices with the corresponding comments were worked out by the experienced physicians and were adapted by the computer staff. Both proper and wrong choices were included, so only few choices lead to the next stage :

- the diagnosis stage must be preceded by the proper investi-
      gation program,
- the treatment stage must be preceded by the correct diagnosis.

The test structure is shown in fig.1.

An additional question " Are the collected data sufficient for further procedure ? " is asked on the path between the investigation and diagnosis stages. This question enables further investigations

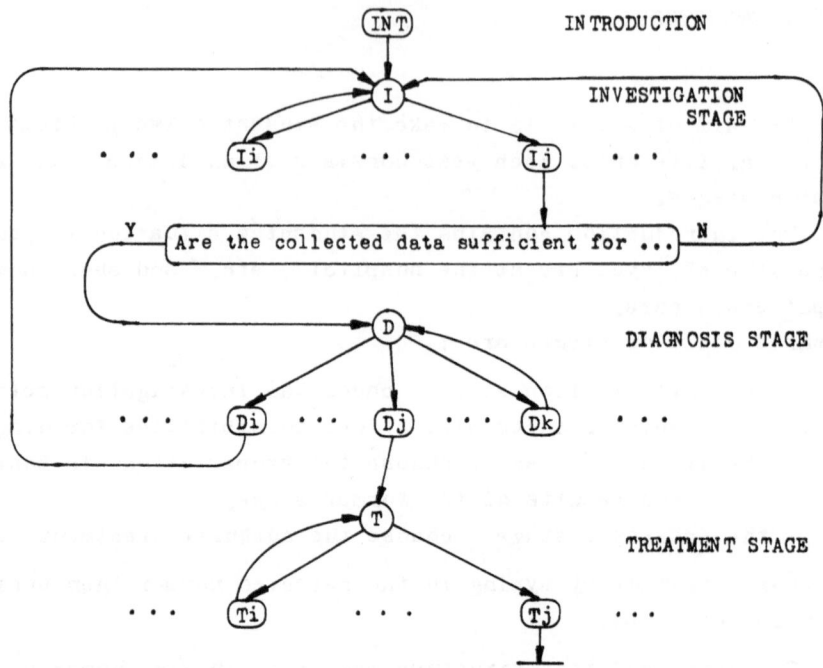

Fig.1. Test structure.

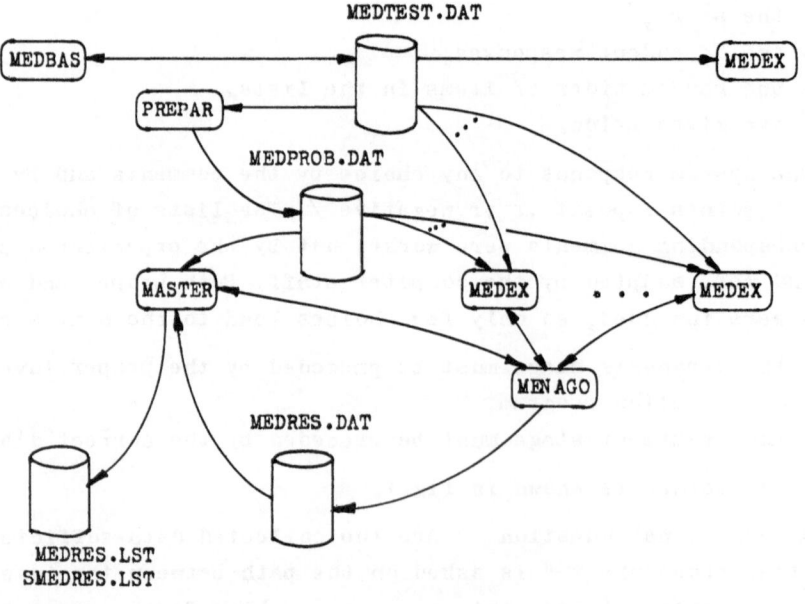

Fig.2. System structure.

if desired. Similar question could be found in /1/, too.

There are many paths through the test as it is shown in fig.1.
To enable different system responses in each case, the dependent response facilities have been incorporated. A response conditioned by
a path in the test graph is called a dependent response. The types of
conditions are as follows :
- an exactly defined part of a path in the graph,
- a set of vertices which should be previously visited,
- " is this decision made as a first one / on this stage / ? ",
- " is this decision made as a following one / on this stage /?".

Several dependent responses might be connected to a choice. This produces different responses depending on the previous choices.
For example,when fetal death is suspected, the X-ray examination selected as a first one is a mistake and selected as a final investigation
would be perfect.

The traditional multiple choice tests suffer from an important
disadvantage : numbers of the correct answers could be learnt by
heart without any understanding. In our tests, items in the lists
are displayed in the random order. Evidentlly, in spite of this,the
proper path could be quickly found and learnt by means of multiple
test execution. But now the whole procedure is remembered rather than
the numbers of proper choices - the educational object is secured.

3.SYSTEM STRUCTURE

The system has been developed to enable the storing,maintaining
and executing the set of medical tests.The system structure is shown
in fig.2.

Tests are stored in a specialised data base called test base
/ MEDTEST.DAT file /.Each test is assigned to a division and to a
difficulty level.

An examinating program MEDEX provides the execution of the
tests in one of the following modes :
- "study" mode : any test could be chosen and solved,
- "examination" mode : the tests of the examination set have
                            to be solved.
An sufficient number of the examination sets could be created with
the aid of PREPAR program.Only the description of the examination
set structure must be passed to PREPAR / numbers of tests of each

division and level /. The tests are chosen in a random way.
MEDPROB.DAT file contains examination sets .

The examination course is controlled by the teacher with the aid
of the MASTER process. The intertask cooperation and examination sets
distribution is handled by the MENAGO process. Students are examined
by the MEDEX processes. They introduce themselves to the system and
then solve the given tests.

The gained scores are displayed in two following ways :
- short list : contains personal data and gained scores
/ per cents of the max. score/,
- full list : additionally contains the scores gained on
the particular stages of the succeeding
tests.
The system runs on the SM4 computer / PDP 11/40 / under the RSX-11M
operating system. The programs were written in FORTRAN IV to achive
machine independence and easy implementation on various machines.
The SEND/RECEIVE mechanism is employed.

4. CONCLUSIONS

The system has been presented to many physicians who show a
great interest in our results. Extensive comments to all paths seem
to be one of the most important features of our system. The most
precious is the ability of giving comments to the whole sequences
of choices - the computer system feature only. Thanks to it, the
system teaches the complicated, multistep procedures rather,than
the simple implications.

Our experiments indicate the necessity of more flexible test
structure with variable number of stages. The one-stage test corresponds with classical multiple choice tests. The demand for the
additional "introductory diagnosis" stage could be satisfied in a
four-stage test.

References.

/1/ Spannbauer P.M.: "Computer-assisted medical diagnosis",Internat.
Clinical Products Review, Nov 1983,pp.60-64.
/2/ Dr.Verbeek : personal communications,MIE'84,Brussels.

EDUCATION AND TRAINING OF MEDICAL STUDENTS IN STATISTICS AND MEDICAL COMPUTING

J.Zvárová
Department of Social Medicine, Medical Faculty, Charles University
Karlovo náměstí 32, 121 11 Prague 2, Czechoslovakia

INTRODUCTION

The new concept of teaching social medicine at the Medical Faculty, Charles University in Prague is focused on concrete and contemporary tasks of the Czechoslovak health services and care of people's health. Medical students learn both the conception of health protection in Czechoslovakia and the role of medicine in medical preventive activity (1). In view of scientific and technical progress there arise new requirements on knowledge and skills of physicians what is needed in order to understand properly health care problems and services.This task is becoming increasingly important with the information explosion and increasing use of more and more powerful computers. Considering the variability of all biological, clinical and laboratory measurements it is clear that in every field of medicine arise problems which cannot be successfully solved only by deterministic way of thinking. Therefore thinking based on a sound understanding of statistical principles and methods is essential in medicine and health care.

THE AIM OF TEACHING STATISTICS AND MEDICAL COMPUTING

The aim of teaching statistics to medical students might be defined as "to equip medical students with the knowledge, attitudes and data handling skills necessary for their future jobs as community oriented physicians" (2). In Czechoslovakia the teaching statistics and medical computing is a part of social-medicine studies. In the third pre-clinical year, medical students are taught about statistical principles and methods of statistics and their application to medical practice. The examples used to illustrate the statistical principles and methods are taken out of medical practice with respect to the stage of students medical knowledge. The ground that is covered in a basic programme of statistical principles and methods is as it follows (3).

1. Introduction to the role of statistics in medicine and health care. Basic statistical concepts, scales of measurement, sampling methods, sampling errors.

2. Types and stages of investigations, e.g. planning, collecting data, data processing, data presentation in tables, graphs and charts, data interpreting.

3. The concept of probability, probability calculations, random variable and probability distribution (normal, binomial, Poisson).

4. Measures of central tendency and location (mean,median,mode),measures of variation (range, percentils, variance, standard deviation).

5. Statistical inference. Point estimation and confidence interval. Tests of significance, their use and interpretation (t-tests, χ^2 - tests, non-parametric tests).

6. The concepts of association and causality, measures of regression and correlation. Introduction to the time series.

7. Rates and proportions. Standardization of rates (direct standardization, indirect standardization). Introduction to use computers in medicine and health care (digital, analog, hybrid).

All these statistical concepts and methods are taught with use only elementary mathematical knowledge and the emphasis is put on the problem formulation and the interpretation of the results obtained. As a part of teaching social medicine in the fifth clinical year of medical studies, health statistics including demography and vital statistics is involved. Social medicine studies in the sixth clinical year of study are devoted to solving problems from medical and health care practice in which students use all their knowledge and skills attained during their social medicine studies including statistical and computing abilities.

THE EVALUATING OF STUDENT LEARNING

Traditional teaching combined with modern methods of programmed teaching can considerably increase the effectiveness of nowaday university teaching. To reveal imperfectness in student's knowledge and skills, react on them in due time of the teaching, turns out to be one of the university lecturer's tasks (4). For this reason it is necessary to perform evaluation of the educational process.

Further we will discuss in more details one method for evaluating of student's basic statistical knowledge in the third pre-clinical year of social-medicine studies (5).Student's knowledge is verified by means of the examination programme used during the seminar at the end of term. Each of the students receive a card with three examples concerning statistical methods application in medicine. The triple of the given examples is different for any of the students and 50 alternatives have been elaborated. Together with the card each student obtains all necessary statistical tables and the preprint form for putting down the results. Using the overhead projector students are informed which partial problems to solve and how to put their results down in the form. Every student puts 24 items down that belong to his variant of the examination programme. The examination programme contains no multiple choice questions and thus the probability of a random choice of the correct answer is considerably reduced. The evaluation of the programmed examination is performed by comparing with correctly filled in forms for respective variants. The total obtained result is expressed as a value of the gross score for each of the students. The results obtained by the examination programme are demonstrated on the sample of 370 students (academic year 1981/82) and on the sample of 267 students (academic year 1982/83). Some basic characteristics of the examination programme are displayed in the following figures and tables.

Table 1: Difficulties of separate items in both samples of students

Item number	Difficulty Q(%) 1981/82	1982/83	Item number	Difficulty Q(%) 1981/82	1982/83
1	30.0	29.6	13	27.6	17.2
2	20.3	17.2	14	10.3	9.0
3	39.5	37.5	15	22.2	6.7
4	30.8	38.9	16	24.1	27.7
5	0.8	1.9	17	23.8	27.3
6	4.6	5.6	18	10.8	10.5
7	38.9	20.6	19	11.4	9.7
8	37.0	21.7	20	19.5	13.5
9	11.4	12.0	21	7.3	8.6
10	68.4	47.6	22	16.5	4.1
11	36.5	49.8	23	33.0	27.0
12	11.6	5.2	24	34.9	23.2

Table 1 presents total difficulties of separate items in both samples
of students. Using difficulties of separate items the difficulty of
the total examination programme was evaluated to be $\bar{Q}$ = 23.76 % (academic year 1981/82) and $\bar{Q}$ = 19.67 % (academic year 1982/83).In Figure 1
the distribution of gross score values for both samples of students,
with the main peaks shifted to the right, are depicted. This shift
here is desirable as the results of the examination programme are used
not only as one of the bases for confering credit but also as the criterion to sit for the social medicine exam ahead of the schedule. So
the programme should differentiate more in the class of better respondents.

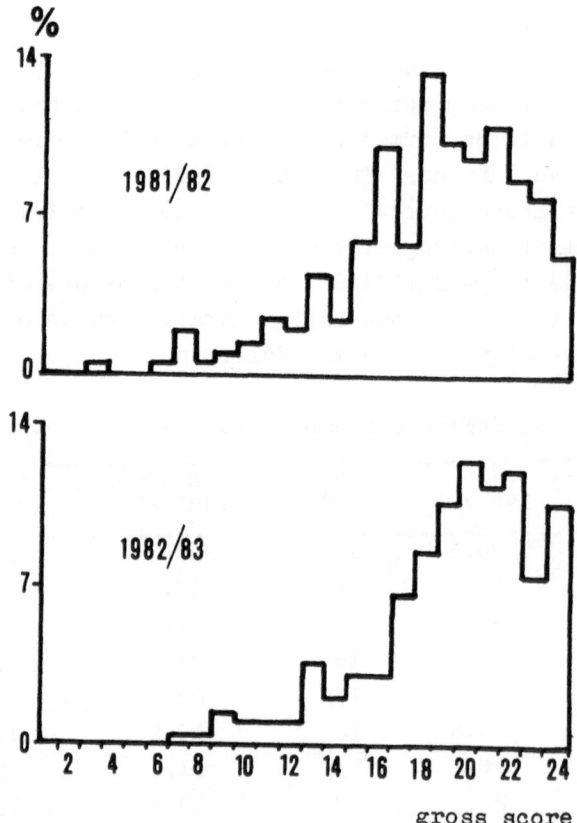

Fig.1: Distribution of gross score values

In Figure 2 separate items are plotted according to the decreasing
values of the difficulty index P = 100 - Q.

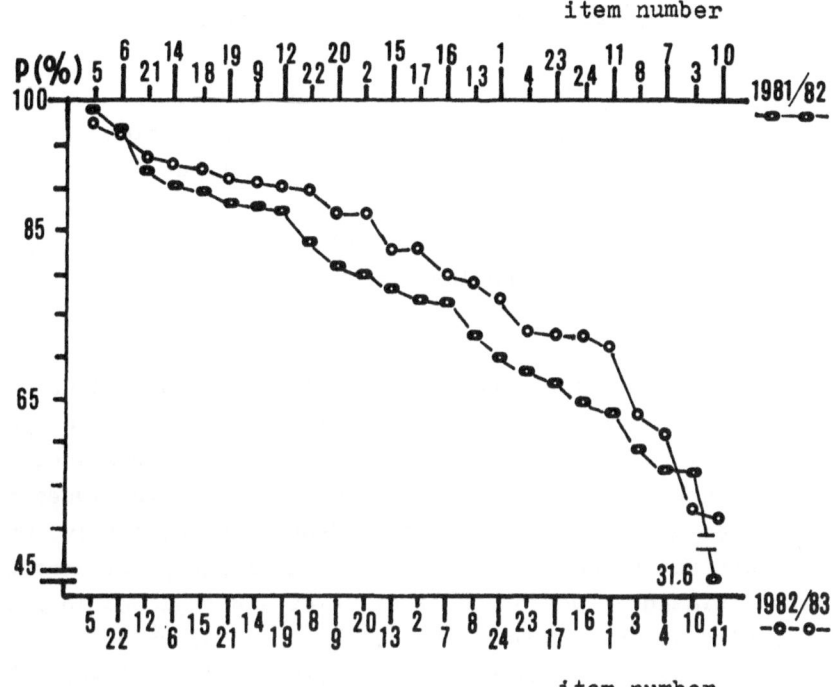

Fig.2: Plotting of items according to the decreasing value of the difficulty index for both samples of students

The evaluated difficulty of the total examination programme is relatively low. This fact reflects that most of students mastered the principles of statistical inductive reasoning. The obtained results of the examination programme well correspond to the lecturer's experience.

REFERENCES

(1) Frič I, Zámková V, Zvárová J (1982) New concept of the discipline of social medicine at the Medical Faculty,Čs.zdrav.30,11:465-468
(2) Proceedings of the Interregional conference on teaching statistics to medical undergraduates (1978), Karachi, Pakistan
(3) Zvárová J (1982) Statistical methods in social medicine, SPN,Prague
(4) Guilbert J (1977) Educational handbook for health personnel,WHO publication No 35, Geneva
(5) Zvárová J, Zámková V (1983) Experience with problem-oriented examination programmes in social medicine education, Acta Univ. Car.Medica 29:157-160

USE OF COMPUTERS IN CONTINUING EDUCATION

Professor Aleš Šatánek, M.D.
Chief, Dept. of Medical Education
Postgraduate Medical Institute
Ruská 85
100 05   PRAGUE 10
Czechoslovakia

Postgraduate medical and pharmaceutical education in Czechoslovakia
is divided into two time periods. During the first period physicians
and pharmacist specialize in various branches of medicine. This first
period of specialty training includes two stages concluded by a specialty exam of the first and second degree, respectively, while the
first part is obligatory for all physicians and pharmacists. The specialty training is performed at district and regional level. The second period of postgraduate medical and pharmaceutical education concerns continuing education of specialits of both 1st and 2nd degree.
Educational courses at the highest level are prepared by various departments of the Postgraduate Medical Institute in Prague. The annual
turnover in this institute totals over 5 000 participants. (1)

The Department of Medical Education is more than 20 years dealing
with modern educational technology with the use of programmed instruction and teaching machines. 10 years ago we started to implement microcomputer technology to postgraduate medical education. (2)

At that time we have constructed our own microcomputer systems based
on 8 bit microprocessors. We have used for the first time Motorola
microprocessor family 6 800 and later also Intel and Zilog devices in
various configurations. For presentation of programs in group instruction we have used slide projectors controlled by a microprocessor system. Later we have introduced multimedia systems. In group instruction
each participant has a feedback unit connected to a microcomputer.
For individual training we built another computer systems which were
connected with a monitor screen. In this time we construct an entirely new microcomputer system featuring color graphic capabilities specifically designed for exploitation of color video tapes. We use the

video records for introductory information of a problem that is presented to the participant. Simultaneously further information are retrieved from a floppy disc and distributed by a single microprocessor
system to several trainees which can solve one or several problems
independently.

Feedback is, of course, provided to all participants, scanned, controlled, and evaluated. At all our microcomputer systems Basic is
used for compilation of educational programs. We have very good experiences with this language. It is a comprehensive and simple language
that provides possibility to every author of an educational program
to assemble his own software. We require all our educational programs
to meet following criteria:

Reliability   The software system should be as reliable as the hardware upon it runs. It should be capable of detecting, diagnosing and
recovering from most major errors due to user mishandling.

Protection   The software should protect both itself and the users
from errors caused by users.

Predictability   The system should respond to user requests with both
respect to time and variations in command sequence.

Convenience   Educational software is offered to the user to make his
job easier and to relieve him of the burden of allocating and managing
various resources. It should therefore not make life difficult for him
and it should be designed with basic human engineering factors in mind.

Efficiency   The software should be efficient in allocating resources.
It should maximize the use of data resources by the users and should
itself not use large quantities of resources.

Extensibility   It should be possible to add new features to the system in an evolutionary manner.

Transparency   The user should be able to remain ignorant about the
things beneath the educational content. However, he should be permitted to learn as much about the system as desired.

The degree to which the above objectives are compromised depends upon
the particular methodology chosen by the software architecture designer.(3)

After several year's use of computer based education we gained desired experiences. The computer allows to move away from spectator

learning for each participent of the educational process. A computer
can make learning interactive even with larger groups of participants.
But still the computer can query all participants so that we can thoroughly determine not only what the trainee knows, but also his intellectual skills and attitudes. The curriculum models can be adapted to
different backgrounds without any conscious realization on the part of
trainees. This approach enables us to detect, identify, and fill in
missing backround material or methods. After presentation of new ideas
the program can check using internal quizzes to see if the participant
comprehends. If not, the presentation can be reviewed or new approaches to that material can be offered to him. Thus, learning with the
use of computers can become highly individualized, differing for each
participant in terms of learning materials and time.

Another consequence of interaction is that we can determine the level
of interest of the participants. While this is more difficult to do,
it is possible in an interactive environment. Material that is weak
in interest can be changed, following a different approach.

Because of interaction we have very powerful mechanism for improving
the material. We save participants´responses which give us very detailed views of what is happening with them moment by moment.

Although the computer allows this highly interactive approach, with
various benefits following, not all computer based learning material
is interactive. It is necessary to develop standards for judging the
quality of interactions.

Computers have opened the way to superior quality training previously
impossible. However, for successful and efficient utilization of computers in medical education is a mastery of educational science and
technology by the lecturer staff a conditio sine qua non.

The use of computers in medical education should be emphasized particularly in:
1. Educational diagnostics
2. Programmed instruction
3. Expert systems
4. Clinical simulations

5. Decision making
6. Educational multimedia
7. Evaluation of educational effectiveness
8. Daily evaluation

Although exaggerated claims have been made by its proponents, there
is little doubt that computer based instruction appears to be considerably more effective than most other methods.(4)
Obviously a given program will cater for a certain range of abilities
and preknowledge. If we accept that challenging programs can be written
for any level of ability then we can prescribe the optimum situation;
this will require trainees to be alloted programs not according to
some arbitrary structure but rather as a result of their own ability
and knowledge.(5)

The production of computer based educational materials requires a lot
of efforts, such as information acquisition on particular subject, definition of educational objectives, preparation of methods of evaluating these objectives, creation of software architecture for practical realization of that educational approach. It is therefore obvious,
that these efforts must pay back in multiple utilization of the compiled educational material. It would be very sad if this were prevented
by hardware incompatibility of the computers. For this reason it is
necessary to select a hardware standard. As the present situation displays, it is most probable that the hardware standard will be the IBM
PC with a 16 bit operating system.(6)
Several programs are demonstrated.

References:
1. Šatánek,A.: Programovaná výuka ve zdravotnictví,AVICENUM Praha,1972
2. Šatánek,A.: Modernizace výuky v lékařství, AVICENUM Praha,1983
3. Šatánek,A.Jr.: Některé možnosti uplatnění mikroprocesorů ve zdravotnictví, Československé zdravotnictví,č.11,s.481-485,1984
4. Šatánek,A.Jr.: Mikropočítače v akutní medicíně, Časopis lékařů čes-
   kých,č.4,s.102-103,1985
5. Šatánek,A.Jr.: Biochemické expertní systémy v akutní medicíně, Bio-
   chemia Clinica Bohemoslovaca,č.3,s.233-238,1984
6. Philip M.Wolfe, C.Patrick Koelling: BASIC Engineering and Scientific
   Programs for the IBM PC, Prentice Hall,London,1983

HEMATOLOGIC IDEOGRAPHIC ALPHABET AND ITS UTILIZATION FOR PERSONAL COMPUTER PROGRAM SUPPORTING THE INTERPRETATION OF BLOOD AND BONE MARROW MICROSCOPIC IMAGES

Andrzej Brodziak
5 th Department and Infirmary
of Silesian School of Medicine
ul. Żeromskiego 7, 41-902 Bytom, Poland

Graduate physician, apart from the theoretical knowledge should know some practical skills important for his own diagnosis of the most common diseases and their treatment. One of the most dificult practical skills is the classic, microscopic hematology.
Even the diagnosis of the typical images of smears of the bone marrow is possible only after a long experience and the training under the experienced hematologist.
These exercises should aim at three separate stages: /1/ to master the recognition of the particular cells, /2/ to have the ability to perceive the predominance or deficiency of some kinds of cells, it means to master the differentiation of several reactions of the bone marrow, /3/ to associate these types of marrow images with clinical data and with some results of laboratory tests. The third stage allows the diagnosis of the most typical haematologic diseases at least.
It is dificult to secure for any student the advices of an experienced hematologist for many hours of the exercises because they set a high value on their time as any highly educated specialist. Therefore it is dificult to master the three abilities mentioned above. We have decided to try to transfer, at least a part of this necessary training effort on a tool recently easily accesible i.e. a personal computer of a student or of a physician. We have elaborated for this aim a program in the BASIC language of Sinclair's - Spectrum computer. The theoretical assumptions of this program as well as, its present potentialities are presented below.

Alphabet of ideographic signs for the cells of blood and bone marrow

We propose to combine the learning of hematologic images, especially
during mentioned stages /1/ and, /2/ with the use of microscope as
well as with the use of a personal computer. At the same time we
propose for students and physicians to represent the details of the
microscopic image by a special set of signs. Each of these signs
coresponds with one of the discerned cells of blood and bone marrow.
The signs have the shape resembling "the appearence" of these cells.
The shapes are defined precisely enough to have a unique characteristic feature and a definite meaning.
Thus proposed exercises are based on the assumptions of ideographic
writings like, for instance, the contemporary Japonese alfabet "kanji". Below we quote some of "kanji" signs to visualize this analogy
So: man is 人 mountain 山 , eye 目 , river 巛 , one 一 , two 二 ,
three 三 , ten 十 , three 木 , women 女 , blood 血 . The proposed alphabet of hematologic ideographic signs is composed of 22 basic
signs and of 3 additional signs denoting: an unrecognized cell ⦸ ,
so called "naked unclassified nucleus of the cell ⊗ and a signs
which marks a pathological appearence of a cell ('). The signs are
presented in table 1. It ascribes the signs of our alphabet to the
known international names of the cells of blood and bone marrow.
Another literal designations of these cells are given there also to
allow quick naming of these cells, using a classic keyboard of
a personal computer.
It is possible however to forsee in a specialized version of a "he-
matological computer" the appropriate keys for all our 25 signs of
ideographic alphabet.
We have defined all our hematologic signs precisely by means of geometrical and topographical notions in another more extensive table.
Table 2 gives an excerpt of this spacious original table for some
signs only.

Present Possibilities of the program elaborated for Sinclair's Spectrum computer

Our program is composed of some parts having separate functions,
according to several phases of the training in the recognition of
hematologic images.

1/ First part teaches the alphabet. It presents signs and corespon-

Cells of blood and bone marrow

Erythreid:

E1	Pronormoblast
E2	Basophilic normoblast
E3	Polychromatophilic normoblast
E4	Ortochromatic normoblast
E5	Reticulocyte *
E6	Erytrocyte

Myeloid:

G1	Myeloblast
G2	Promyelocyte
G3	Neutrophilic myelocyte
G4	Neutrophilic metamyelocyte
G5	Neutrophilic granulocyte with band nucleus
G6	Neutrophilic granulocyte with segmented nucleus

S3	Eosinophilic myelocyte *
S4	Eosinophilic metamyelocyte *
S5	Eosinophilic granulocyte with band nucleus *
S6	Eosinophilic granulocyte with segmented nucleus

B3	Basophilic myelocyte *
B4	Basophilic metamyelocyte *
B5	Basophilic granulocyte with band nucleus *
B6	Basophilic granulocyte with segmented nucleus

Thrombopoetic:

T1	Megakaryoblast
T2	Megakaryocyte

Lymphatic:

L1	Lymphocyte (small cell)
L2	Lymphoblast *
L3	Lymphocyte (big cell)

Plasma cells:

P1	Plasmocyte

Monocytes:

M1	Monoblast *
M2	Promonocyte *
M3	Monocyte
M4	Macrophage *

Reticulum cells:

R1	Specific cell of reticulum
R2	Sinusoidal cell of reticulum
R3	Mastocyte

* Scarce. Separate symbol not introduced.

ding names of erytroid, myeloid and other developmental series of
cells. After it the program is accomplishing a check test of acquired
knowledge.

2/ Second part assists to train the recognition of type of bone marrow
reactions as "increased erythropoesis with a basophilic set-back",
"increased granulopoesis with shift to left", "hiatus leucemicus",
"plasma cell reaction", "lymphatic predominance". The program dis-
cerns 13 of such types of images now. The training is completed in
such a way that the program introduces to the screen of the monitor
different proportions of cells signs and asks about the type of the
reaction of bone marrow. These are evaluated after the answer.

3/ Third part could be treated as a tool for the continuation of training or as a tool helping to interpret the smear images. Here the
student can introduce to the screen the signs of cells which can be
seen under the microscope. He determines the kind of sign and its
position on the screen using an intuitively simple representation of
"parts" of the screen by analogously placed keys on the keyboard. The
program memorizes the tables of normal and other typical range of
percentage for any kind of cells. In this way it is possible to compare the collected data with memorized data and to generate the diagnostic measages which interprete the created image. If this part of
the program is used for a real data from the microscope it is necessary to introduce data from several "microscopic seeing fields" to enable the interpretation of 500 or 1000 cells. One of fields is presented in fig. 1.

Some data concerning the way of programing

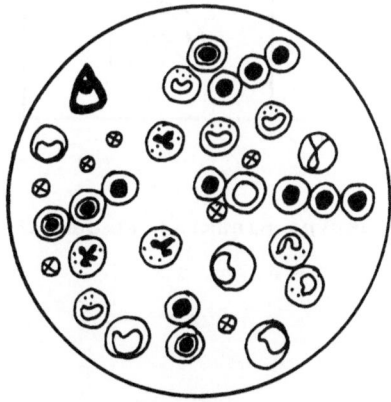

We searched for rather universal way
of the shape determination. Instead
of simple graphics only mathematical
notions like circle, elipse, sine-
wave have been used to program our
signs. It allows to present the same cell-sign in didiferent sizes
on the sreen using the same subroutine and changing parameters only.
The same subroutine is used to create images of different reactions of

the bone marrow. Even that condensation of all programing tasks leads to rather wide programs. All these three parts need a separate loading of the 48K memory of Sinclair's Spectrum. Our alphabet was defined initially for quick hand writing so colour is not necesary. However the majority of personal computers enables the presentations of our signs in colours. So we are preparing colour version of our program.

Name of the cell	Geometric and topographic characteristics of the sign	
E1 Pronormo-blast	Dimension of the sign /D/: big. Shape of the circumference of the sign /s.o./: round. Shape coresponding to the nucleus of the cell /s.n./ round, its inside /i.s.n./: non shaded.	
E2 Basophilic normoblast	D: less then E1 S.C.: round S.n.: round, i.s.n.: shaded	
E3 Polychromato-philic nor-moblast	D: less or eqal to E2 S.c.: round S.n.; round, i.s.n.: shaded In the border coresponding to the cytoplasma /b.c./ of the cell a thin ring	
G6 Neutrophilic metamyelocy-te	D: as G3 S.c.: oval In b.c. 3-4 spots, symbolizing the granulations	

Literature references:

Brodziak A.: Hematologia mnemotechnicznie. Skrypt Śląskiej Akademii Medycznej, Katowice, 1984.

LONG-TERM PLANNING MODEL FOR MEDICAL MANPOWER
TRAINING IN THE USSR

B.R. Loginov
All-Union N.A. Semashko Research Institute of Social
Hygiene and Public Health Administration, Ministry
of Health of the USSR, Moscow, Obukh str., 12, USSR

I. Introduction.

The parer deals with the description of methodology of long-term
planning of medical manpower training, physicians being taken as a
pattern. The methodology was developed at the Semashko Research
Institute and implemented at the Ministry of Health of the USSR.

The paper includes:
- description of model of dynamics manpower age structure in the
planned Health Care System;
  - convenient for calculation method of estimating model parameters;
  - description of method for searching optimal strategy in training
medical manpower to gain the objective specified for the whole planning period.

Usually the objective is determined as standard or any other
manpower requirement. The elaborated model has been computerized and
widely applied for Health Services planning in the USSR and for fore-
casting of medical manpower needs in the Czech Socialist Republic.

2. Description of the model.

The model represented here is quite similar to the population
model used at IIASA. The main difference is that the soviet model
makes it possible to plan the number of manpower by means of controlling output of graduates from Medical schools.

Mathematical model description can be formulated as follows:
$$\bar{x}(t) = P\,\bar{x}(t-1) + \vec{\rho}\,\omega(t-1) \qquad t = 1,\dots T$$
under known initial state, $\bar{x}(0)$, where $\bar{x}(t)$ is a column vector
whose elements represent the over one-year band distribution of manpower at time t, and $\omega(t)$ is total number of
graduates at time t taken for jobs within region Health Care Service
(below "output from training"), and $\vec{\rho}$ is column vector of age dis-

tribution of graduates, and P is a matrix in the following form:

$$P= \begin{Vmatrix} 0 & 0 & \cdots & 0 & 0 \\ p_1 & 0 & \cdots & 0 & 0 \\ 0 & p_2 & \cdots & 0 & 0 \\ \cdot & \cdot & \cdots & \cdot & \cdot \\ 0 & 0 & \cdots & p_{n-1} & 0 \end{Vmatrix}_{n \times n}$$

where 'n'is maximum length of service, and p_i is transition rate from one-year band, i , to the same band, i+1 .

Besides T means length of planning period being defined before.

We assume that transition rates involve such factors as wastage and migration. Therefore p can be more than unit.

In general P and $\tilde{p}$ change through time but in our case they are assumed to be constant over time.

To decrease the number of model parameters and to make the utilization of expert opinions easier a function, l(z), should be introduced instead of set p_i , i=1,2,...n-1 . The function is connected with p_i by ratio

$$p_i = \frac{l(i+1)}{l(i)} , \quad i=1,2,...n-1$$

If now we approximate l(z) by polynom of degree 'K'then the manpower model will have only 'k' parameters. Here the most important thing is that 'k' is much less than 'n' .

The essence function, l(z), is part of output from training having worked up to age 'z'. Typical curves l(z) for manpower problems are shown in Figure 1.

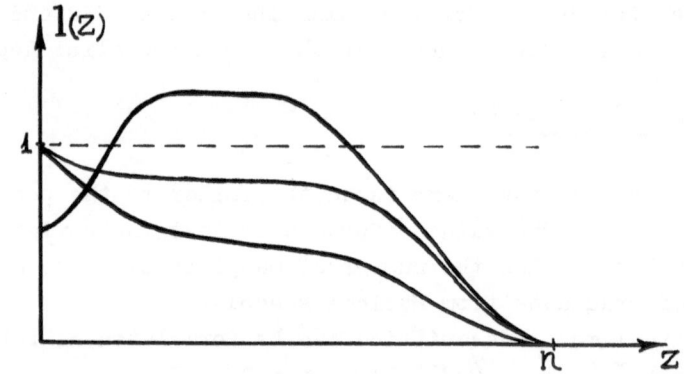

Fig.1

3.Estimation of model parameters.

To use the model for planning manpower of a particular region function, l(z) , should be determined. It seems known demography methods could be used for this purpose. But often we can't do it because input data are inadequate. A method is suggested to search for $l(z)$ under restricted input data conditions. It's advantage is that the whole accessible information including expert opinion is used in data processing. Calculation $l(z)$ is based on least-squares technique, that in our case can be expressed as follows.

Let us follow real transition of manpower in a region for 's' years. The interval will be called model instruction period. Let empirical data on $\widehat{\omega}(t)$ $t=1,2,\ldots$'s' within the given period and some information $\widehat{\beta}(t)$ $t=1,2,\ldots$'s', on age structure at time t be known.

It is significant that the content of $\widehat{\beta}(t)$ can be changed from time to time, still our estimation method remains applicable. For example as the last resort $\widehat{\beta}(1)$ is five-year bands structure at the very start of the instruction period and $\widehat{\beta}(t)$ $t=2,\ldots$'s' are total numbers without any distribution by age groups. Moreover 's' is within rather a wide interval raging from 5 to 30 years.

In general case empirical data consist of a few age manpower structures and total numbers at other times. Obviously the higher is the number of known age structures the higher degree of accuracy of the estimate, $l(z)$, should be obtained.

Model parameter $l(z)$ is chosen so as to minimize criterion Q
min $Q(\beta(t), \widehat{\beta}(t), \widehat{\omega}(t), t=1,2,\ldots s)$ where $\beta(t)$ is modelled value, defined by $\beta(t)=\Psi_t(\vec{x}(t))$ where Ψ_t is measuring operator, that changes with time.

As it was mentioned above $l(z)$ is searched for in terms of polynom $\quad l(z)=\sum_{i=0}^{r}\alpha_i z^i$ with $r+1$ parameters α_i .

The feature of the task is that Q has a lot of local optimums. In this case it's very important to decrease the feasible area of search for $l(z)$. In our procedure the feasible range is defined by the model user by writing down a set of inequalities

$$L^-(z_j) \leqslant l(z_j) \leqslant L^+(z_j), \quad j=1,2,\ldots r+1$$

The limitations are introduced into the criterion, Q , replacing the α_i by their expression obtained from the solution of the set of equations $\quad l(z_j)=\sum_{i=0}^{r}\alpha_i z_j^i =L^+(z_j)-\left[L^+(z_j)-L^-(z_j)\right]\sin^2\varphi_j$, $j=1,\ldots r+1$ where φ_j are new optimization parameters without any restrictions.

The method represented above has been applied to manpower models in all the republics of the USSR and the ČSR.

By means of the polynom l(z) of degree 3, data on the 10-year
length of instruction period including the only five-year bands age
structure of physicians at the start of the period as well as total
numbers of physicians at other years average percentage deviation between the modelled and empirical data on total physicians being in
the range of 0.01% - 1.5% have been obtained for all the republics of
the USSR.

4.Optimization planning method.

The method has been developed to define such output from training $\omega(t)$ t=1,2 ... T as to reach and keep the balance between the
planned value x(t)=($\bar{e}$, $\bar{x}(t)$)   and the target $\eta(t)$ (manpower needs)
for the shortest time within planning period T.

Optimization planning problem is shown in **Figure 2** and formulated
as follows:

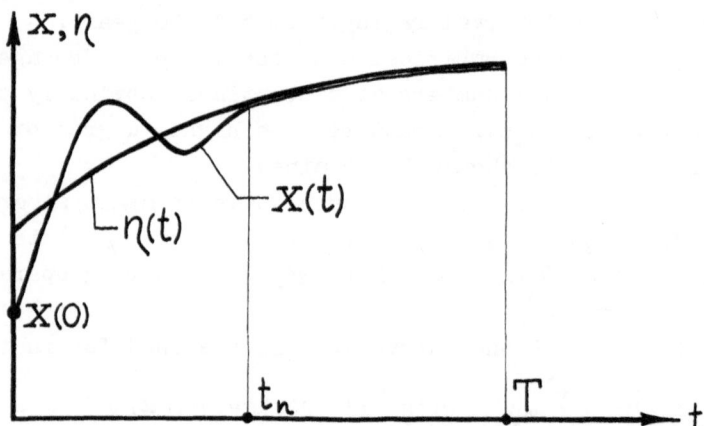

Fig.2

Let t_n be the time of reching target $\eta(t)$ and after t_n the
balance $x(t) = \eta(t)$ can be kept by means of feasible $\omega(t)$ t=1,2 ...T.
Then the strategy of output from training $\omega(t)$ is considered as optimal one if we have

$$\min_{\omega \in \Omega} t_n (\omega(t), \; t=1,2,...T)$$

where Ω is limitation on $\omega(t)$ usually represented in the form of

$$\gamma^+(t)\omega(t-1) \leq \omega(t) \leq \gamma^-(t)\omega(t-1)$$

where γ^+ and γ^- are high and low bounds on pace of $\omega(t)$ defined
by the planner. It is essential that $\gamma^+(t)$ and $\gamma^-(t)$ tend to the
unit.

To solve the optimal planning problem special method has been developed. It is based on the idea of dinamic programming.

To find the reliability solution of long term planning it is necessary to choose the proper length of planning period 'T'. The task is not easy because t_n depends on value T.

The dependence is shown in Figure 3.

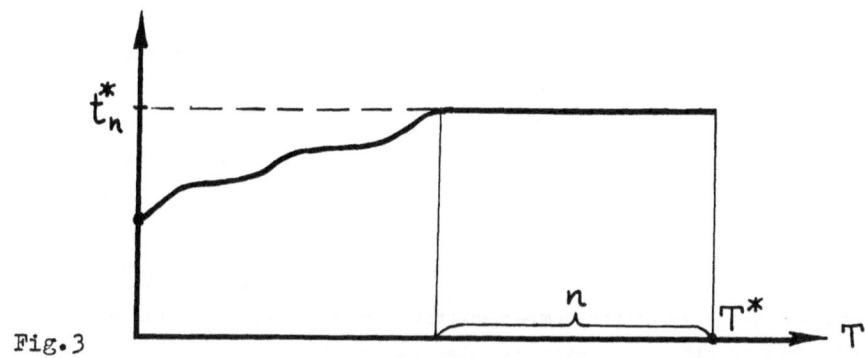

Fig.3

It would seem advisable to assume T* equal to or more than 2n, where 'n' is maximum length of service. To be more exact T* should be defined in the following way. Length of period T* should be increased until optimal t_n^* remains constant for 'n' recent years.

Foe reference careful calculation over one region, i.e. parameter estimation and optimal planning, takes about eight-ten hours of computer service including evaluation of results.

R E F E R E N C E

1. Pelling M. A multistate manpower projection model. Reprinted as IIASA Report WP-82-12.
2. Popov A.G. The problems of medical manpower. M.: Medicine, 1974.

THE IN-VIVO MEASUREMENT OF EXTRAVASCULAR LUNG WATER USING A MICRO-COMPUTER-BASED SYSTEM

M. J. Taylor & W. A. Corbett*

Departments of Computer Science and Surgery*

University of Liverpool

Liverpool L69 3BX UK.

Introduction   Respiratory failure is a frequent and well recognised complication in critically ill patients.   The abnormal respiratory function is often associated with an increase of lung water in the extra-vascular compartment (pulmonary oedema). The clinical hallmarks and characteristic chest X-ray changes of pulmonary oedema are usually found when the extra-vascular lung water has increased at least threefold and then not in every case (Staub 1974).

Special techniques have been tried in order to estimate changes in extra-vascular lung water but most give either semi-quantitive results over a limited range or are affected by factors other than extravascular lung water.   The use of a double indicator dilution technique with suitable markers has been shown to produce estimates of lung water that are both reliable and reproducible and which give the promise of a clinically useful tool (Severinghaus 1972).

Technique   Two indicators form the basis of this measurement technique. Firstly 10 ml. of ice-cold saline is used as a thermal water marker and 2.5 mg.of Indocyanine green, which binds rapidly to plasma proteins, is used as a blood marker. These indicators are injected simultaneously close to the right side of the heart into a major vein, the superior vena cava, and during their transit through the lungs the diffusion of the thermal water marker across the pulmonary capillary bed produces a difference in distribution when compared with the blood marker which remains within the vascular system.   The indicators then pass through the left side of the heart and are measured in the systemic circulation by a catheter inserted via the femoral artery.   The thermal water marker is detected by a thermistor on the outside of the femoral artery catheter and the blood marker by the withdrawal of blood by a constant speed pump to an external dichromatic green-dye densitometer system (Waters Instruments).

Hardware   Signals from the thermistor and the green dye densitometer are transferred to a 12 bit ADC in an Apple II microcomputer via special interface electronics that effectively isolate the patient from the mains supply (240v).

Software   The processing of data may be performed at the bedside or at a later stage by the retrieval of data from disk.   The processing of the indicator dilution curves follows the sequence.

      (1)   Analysis of baseline characteristics.   The first 6 seconds prior to injection of the indicators provide the information for baseline level, degree of

physiological noise and baseline drift.

(2) Analysis of curve form.   Each indicator curve is scanned in turn to identify the maximum positive deflection and the maximum negative deflection. This provides a simple evaluation of curve structure and can be used to reject poor quality curves of low amplitude or with excessive noise.

(3) Detailed curve analysis.   Based on the initial scan of the curve the integration is performed from the upswing to the 30% level on the downslope. Further integration by extrapolation of the monoexponential decay is achieved using simplelinear regression techniques using values from 70% to 30% of the downslope. Integration is complete when the extrapolated value reaches two standard deviations from the mean value of the baseline. In parallel with the integration the first moment of the curve, the mean transit time, is calculated. Cardiac output is computed by dividing the injected indicator by the area beneath the curve. The product of the mean transit time and the cardiac output for each indicator give a volume of distribution which is different for the thermal water marker and the blood marker. The difference in distribution between the two is in large part a measure of the extravascular lung water.

Though the software was written in basic for the Apple II facilities exist for data transfer to an IBM 4341 mainframe for both long term storage and use in developing improved curve fitting algorithms.

Results   The thermal/green dye system has been tested in a bench-top circuit which validates the estimate of flow made by the system, (r=0.99) over a wide range.   Experiments with sheep models of permeability and high pressure pulmonary oedema have shown a good correlation between the in vivo estimation of extra-vascular lung water and that obtained by the gravimetric method post-mortem in the animals (r=0.96).   The thermal/green dye technique has been applied to a study of patients following major aortic reconstructive surgery in which clinical progress has been assessed in relation to estimated values of extra-vascular lung water and all results to date are entirely in keeping with the clinical situation.

References

SEVERINGHAUS.   Thermal and conductivity dilution curves for rapid quantitations of pulmonary oedema.   Journal of Applied Physiology 32 : 770 : 1972.

STAUB.   State of the art review : "Pathogenesis of pulmonary oedema"
AM REV RESP DIS 109 : 358 : 1974

WATERS INSTRUMENTS Inc. Rochester, Minnesota, 55901, U.S.A.

A SYSTEM TO CONTROL BREATH BY BREATH THE CO_2 AND O_2 FRACTIONS IN END-EXPIRATORY GAS

E.W. Kruyt and Th.J.C. Faes
State University of Leiden
Department of Physiology
P O Box 9604, 2300 RC Leiden
The Netherlands

Introduction

At our laboratory we study the control of breathing in cat. To identify that part of the respiratory controller which has arterial blood gas tensions as input and ventilation as output we stimulate it with a forcing function in end-expiratory CO_2 or O_2 concentration and measure the ventilatory response during spontaneous breathing.

To stimulate the ventilatory control system we force either the arterial CO_2 or O_2 concentration sinusoidally or stepwise, while the non-forced gas concentration is kept constant. We also used step changes in end-expiratory CO_2 concentration followed by ramp functions to investigate the conditions under which with the "Read rebreating technique" [1] the steady state ventilatory sensitivity to CO_2 is obtained [2].

The partial pressures of CO_2 or O_2 in arterial blood can not be influenced directly, nor be measured fast enough. In healthy mammals however the end-expiratory gas concentration are a good index for the arterial blood gas pressure. Therefore we use a forcing function generator which controls the end-expiratory concentrations by driving the inspiratory gas concentrations (fig.1).

In the literature several systems have been described to maintain a constant arterial CO_2 tension in patients [3]. In those systems the patient is ventilated artificially, while the arterial CO_2 concentration is measured using e.g. electrodes with a time constant in the order of minutes. In contrast we are interested in processes with time constants in the order of seconds during spontaneous breathing. Robbins et al. [4] developed such a system to generate fast changes in the alveolar gas concentration in men. Our system has been tuned for cats and operates with a proportional type of valves. It computes prediction values in real time. Moreover special attention has been paid to synchronize the generated function with the breathing cycle of the animal. Because the end-expiratory gas concentrations can be measured only once a breath, the forcing function generator will be a sampled data controller. Moreover the changes in gas concentrations can only be administered and measured after some time delay which imposes constraints on the stability of the forcing function generator.

After stating the requirements, the different elements of the system will be analysed. Then we shall explain how we modelled the cat, and how we designed and realized the function generator. We close with a discussion of some results.

Requirements

The system must be able to generate a sinusoidal change, step change, ramp, or combination of step change and ramp in the end-expiratory CO_2 or O_2 concentration. All parameters of those functions must be adjustable on-line. Because one of the time constants to be estimated in the respiratory controller of the cat is smaller than 10 seconds, and the duration of one breath is roughly 3 seconds, the step change must be realized within one breathing cycle. As the absolute accuracy is of less importance, the non-forced gas concentration has to be kept constant within 1-2% to exclude the influence of changes of this gas concentration on the ventilation. To be able to study the variability in the estimated parameters, the forcing function has to be highly reproducible, both in delivered end-expiratory concentrations as in timing, viz. the respiratory phase, at which a step change is delivered. The system has to be fail-safe to prevent the delivery of fatal gas-concentrations in error conditions, and must react as good as possible to artefacts in the measured quantities (eg. after swallows) and to sudden changes in the ventilatory pattern of the cat (after sighs).

System analysis

In fig.1 a block diagram of the total system is presented. To be able to design the function generator we first analysed and modelled all components of the measurement system. In this section we will pay attention to the valves, tubing, gas analysers, and data aquisition system. In the next section the cat will be analysed and modelled.

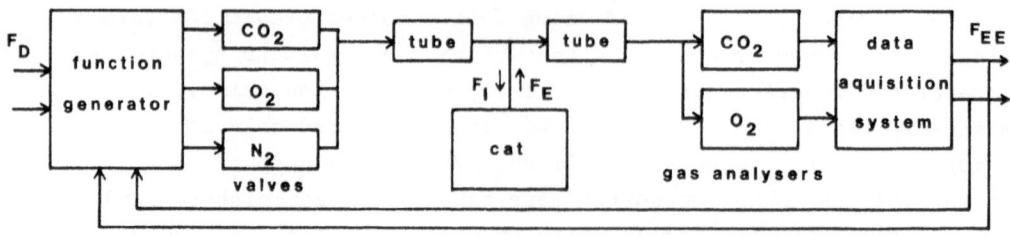

Fig. 1

We use mass flow controllers (MFC) (Advanced Semiconductor Materials AFC-260) as valves to dose the inspiratory gases. They deliver a mass flow which is in the steady state, within certain limits, linear dependent on the voltage applied. The description of the dynamic behaviour of the MFC's is complex because it depends on the size and direction of change of the input. We found the following transfer function to be suitable as mathematical description. The response of this transfer function to a step change is presented in fig.2.

$$H(s) = K \frac{\omega_o^2}{a} \cdot \frac{s + a}{s^2 + 2\beta s + \omega_o^2}$$

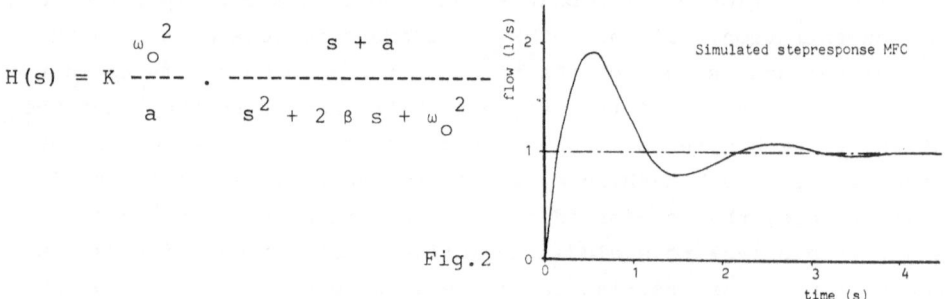

Fig.2

In which: $K = 0.14$ $1.V^{-1}.s^{-1}$; $\omega_o = 3.5$ $rad.s^{-1}$; $a = 1.68$ s^{-1}; $\beta = 0,4$ s^{-1}.

The tubing from the valves to the cat give raise to a delay of 0.3 s; that from the cat to the CO_2 and O_2 analysers of 0.4 and 0.7 s respectively.

The CO_2 gasconcentration is determined by a fast infrared meter (Gould Godart Mk2 Capnograph) and O_2 concentration by a fast oxygen cell (Jaeger O_2 test). Their dynamic behaviour can be described by a first order system with a time constant of 20 ms, which can be neglected. The gas analysers deliver a continuous analog output which is sampled and analysed by a data aquisition system [5] which extracts the end-expiratory

values from the converted and calibrated signals. Due to the peak value
detection and noise suppression algorithms, the end-expiratory values
are sent to the forcing function generator with a delay which depends
on the breathing frequency and on the shape of the CO_2 and O_2 signals.

Modelling the cat

The cat is modelled by three sets of difference equations, one set for
the lung, one for each body compartment and one for the respiratory
centre. The sets consist of one equation for CO_2 and one for O_2. To
describe the diffusion process in the lung we can use the mass balance
equation:

$$\frac{d}{dt} [V_L(t)F_A(t)] = \lambda \dot{Q}_b [C_{\bar{v}} (t-T_1)-C_a(t)] + \dot{V}_A(t)F_F$$

In which V_L is the mean lung volume; F_I is the fractional concentration
in t he inspired gas; F_A is the fractional concentration in the alveoli;
$C_{\bar{v}}$ is the mixed venous gas concentration; C_a is the arterial gas
concentration; $\dot{Q}_b$ is the blood flow through the lungs; T_1 is the
transport time of blood from the body compartment to the lungs; λ is a
coefficient depending on the units used; $\dot{V}_A$ is the alveolar
ventilation. During inspiration $F_F = F_I$, during expiration $F_F = F_A$. In
this model of the cat the lung acts as a sampler. During inspiration
the cat senses the inspiratory gas concentrations, during expiration
the cat delivers the expiratory gas concentrations from which we
determine the end-expiratory concentrations.

For the diffusion process between the blood and tissue a similar set
of equations can be used, for CO_2:

$$V_t \frac{d}{dt} [C_{\bar{v}}(t)] = \dot{Q}_b [C_a(t-T_2)-C_{\bar{v}}(t)] + \dot{V}CO_2$$

In which V_t is the tissue volume of the body compartment; T_2 is the
transport time from the lungs to the body compartment; $\dot{V}CO_2$ is the CO_2
production.

Concentrations can be converted to partial pressures using linearizat-
ions of the dissociation curves. The respiratory controller can be
modelled by equations for the peripheral and central chemoreceptors:

$$\tau_p \frac{d}{dt} \dot{V}_p + \dot{V}_p = [S_p + G_p \exp \{ -D \; PaO_2 (t-T_p) \}] \; PaCO_2 (t-T_p)$$

$$\tau_c \frac{d}{dt} \dot{V}_c + \dot{V}_c = S_c \cdot PaCO_2 (t-T_c) - G_c \exp \{ -DPaO_2 (t-T_c) \}$$

$$\dot{V}_E = \dot{V}_p + \dot{V}_c + \dot{V}_E^{\circ} \quad , \quad \dot{V}_A = \dot{V}_E - \dot{V}_D$$

In which τ_p is the time constant of the peripheral drive, τ_c of the central drive; G_p is the gain of the peripheral drive, G_v of the central drive; $\dot{V}_E$ is the ventilation; $\dot{V}_A$ is the alveolar ventilation; $\dot{V}_D$ is the dead space ventilation.

Design of the function generator

To design the controller of the function generator we used the above model to simulate the total system, using the PSI software tool for control system design [6].

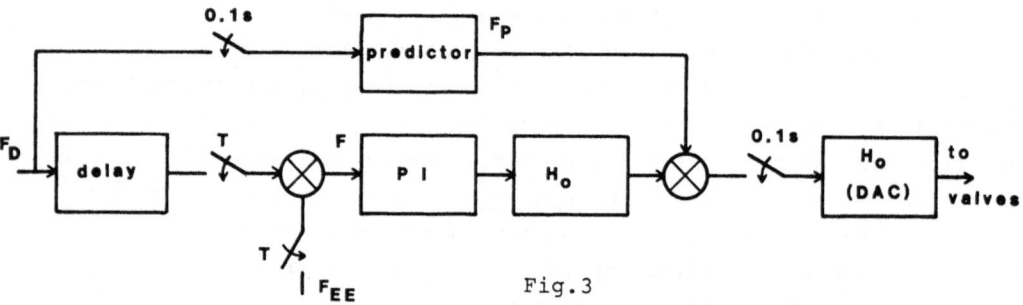

Fig.3

In fig.3 the block diagram of the controller of the function generator is presented for one of the gases. The parameters of the PI block were estimated using the Ziegler and Nichols criterium and optimized during the simulation with PSI.

To guarantee that the function generator starts with realistic values of the inspiratory gas concentrations, and change to new desired va-lues as fast as possible, the controller predicts the output from the desired value. Ideally the transfer function of the predictor should be the inverse of the transfer function of the cat. This inverse function however is not physically realizable. Moreover the parameters of the transfer function of the cat vary widely from one to cat. To overcome this problem we used an heuristic approach in which the predictor com-putes the steady state values and can supply a certain overshoot after

a step change during one or two breaths, followed by an exponential
decay. The height, duration and time constant of the overshoot are
supplied by the user and can be tuned after applying an initial learning step change.

To keep the non-forced gas concentration as constant as possible we
predict the inspiratory gas concentration for this gas from the estimated CO_2 consumption and the actual (measured) ventilation.

The delay, which is shown in the block diagram, cancels the delays of
the tubing and data aquisition system for the predictor. In this way
the measured end-expiratory gas concentrations are compared with their
corresponding desired values.

The controller algortithm as implemented can be written as:

$$F_I = F_p + H_p (\Delta F)_n + H_i \sum_{j=1}^{n-1} T_j (\Delta F)_j$$

$$(\Delta F)_n = (F_D)_n - (F_{EE})_n$$

Where F_I is the inspired fractional concentration to be generated; F_p
is the predicted inspiratory fraction; H_p is the proportional gain; H_i
is the integral gain; T_j is the duration of breath j; F_D is the desired end-expiratory fraction; F_{EE} is the end-expiratory fraction measured. The F_{ICO_2} and F_{IO_2} are converted to flows of CO_2, O_2, and N_2.

Realization

The function generator is programmed in Pascal and runs on a LSI 11
single board computer (SBC11/21) under the Minibos operating system
[7]. The end-expiratory gas concentrations are sent from the data aquisition computer (PDP11/23) via an asynchronous serial line protocol. Output
to the mass flow controllers is provided by 12 bit DA convertors. The
user interacts with the system by means of a video terminal.

Step changes in inspiratory gas concentrations have to occur at the
onset of an expiration to allow the valves to settle during the expiration and have the cat to inspire the new concentration. This has been
realized by scheduling the moment at which the function generator starts
a function. This moment is determined from the duration of the previous
breath, the time at which the last end-expiratory values was received,
and the known time delays in the system.

When the cat sighs or swallows the end-expiratory values are quite
different from those during normal breathing. The controller would
react immediately by adapting the inspiratory gas concentrations. To
avoid these transient deviations the tidal volume of every breath is
compared with the tidal volume of the preveous breath. Gas concentrations at outlier breaths are skipped. During transients in the desired
gas concentrations this procedure is not applied.

Discussion

The function generator is in use for almost a year and proves to be of
great value to identify the respiratory controller of the cat. After
some tuning of the parameters of the function generator fast and highly
reproducible functions are realized in the end-expiratory gas concentrations (fig.4). Note that in fig.4 the end-expiratory CO_2 values are the
highest values at each breath (exept at the transient), and the end-
expiratory O_2's are the lowest values.

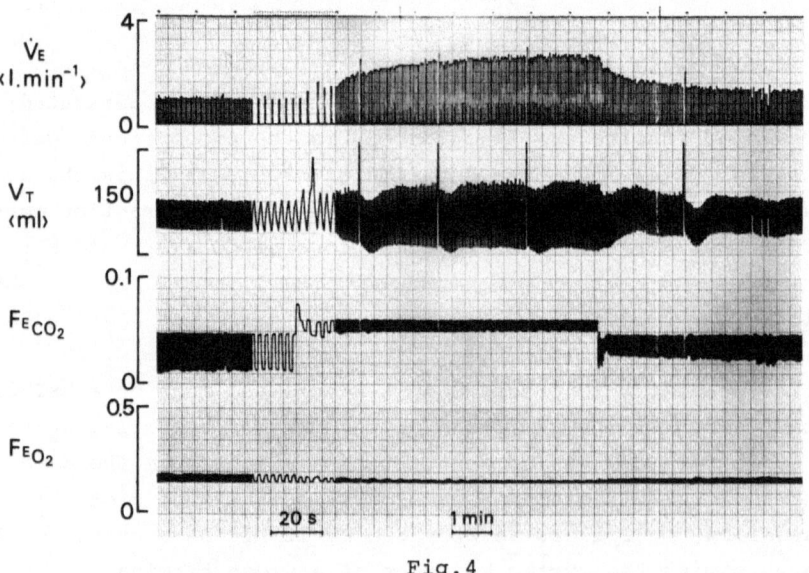

Fig.4

The system may also be suitable for clinical use to deliver a step
change in end-expiratory CO_2 concentration followed by a ramp to measure
the respiratory CO_2 sensitivity in patients. A pilot study for such an
application has been performed in cats 2 In the near future we plan
to improve the stability of the O_2 controller and to replace the manual
adjustment of the parameters of the predictor by an adaptive control
algorithm.

References

(1) Read D.J.C. and Leigh J., Blood-brain tissue realationships and ventilation during rebreathing, Journal of Applied Physiology, 1967, 23: 53-70.
(2) Schuitmaker J.J. et al, Determination of the steady-state ventilatory CO_2 sensitivity with a non-steady-state technique, In: Proceedings of the 19th annual congress of the SEPCR, The Hague 1985.
(3) Noshiro M., Design of a control system for maintaining a normal arterial pCO2 by arterial respiration, Medical & Biological Engineering & Computing, 1984, 22: 418-425.
(4) Robbins P.A., Swanson G.D., Micco A.J. and Schubert W.P., A prediction-correction scheme for forcing alveolar gases along certain time courses, J. Appl. Physiol.: Respirat. Environ. Exercise Physiol. 1982, 52(5): 1353-1357.
(5) Kruyt E.W., RESREG, A data aquisition and data processing system for studies of the ventilatory system, In: van Bemmel, Ball, Wigerz, ed., MEDINFO-83, North-Holland, Amsterdam 1983: 1285.
(6) van den Bosch P.P.J., Interactive system analysis and system design using simulation and optimalisation, In: IFAC-Proceedings Computer Aided Design of multivariable Technological Systems, Lafayette USA, 1982: 211-218.
(7) Boleij H.F. and Hortensius A., Miniboss: an operating system for preprocessors, Procedings of the Digital Equipment Corporation Users Society, 1976, 3(1): 333-336.

A COMMERCIALIZED PROGRAM ON APPLE-COMPUTER FOR A 24H CONTINUOUS INTRAESOPHAGEAL pH-MONITORING.

R. Lepoudre, Y. Vandenplas, L. Sacré-Smits, W. Sonck, S. Kuyk.

Departments of Paediatrics (Prof. H. Loeb), Nuclear Medicine (Prof. M. Jonckheer), Toxicology (Prof. A. Vercruysse), Academisch Ziekenhuis, V.U.B. and NFWO, Brussels, Belgium.

ABSTRACT

The miniaturisation of the investigation techniques and the automation thanks to the computer made it possible to do long lasting investigations on gastroesophageal reflux in newborns.
pH-Metry is a new investigation technique used in adults and children(1). We adapted this method to be used in newborns. We developed a program for Apple IIe computer. pH-data were stored in a Novo Memolog 600 system.
A 24-hour continuous pH-monitoring in the newborn is a non-agressive investigation technique in physiological circumstances, which adequately completes and/or replaces the traditional examinations on gastro-esophageal reflux. This method enables an objectivation of the favourable effect of therapeutic means, and is very interesting in the follow-up.

MATERIAL AND METHODS

The Novo Memolog^R 600 consists of a portable collection control unit, and an interface console, Novo Memolog RS-232 C Interface, which links the Novo Memolog 2A to our Apple IIe computer, making it possible to transfer the collected data for processing and printout. The pH-electrode is introduced transnasally. The location in the middle third of the esophagus is determined with the aid of a thorax X-ray. A flexible glass electrode (type MI-506; Microelectrodes Inc) with a maximal outer body diameter of 1.6 mm is used. The pH-range is between 1 and 13. The response time is between 5 and 15 seconds. The maximal noise level in vitro is 0.03 pH; the in vivo pH error is maximum 0.5 pH.

The Memolog-600 system collects the registered data until the memory is fully loaded, after which it switches itself off. The data recorded up to that time are retained in memory. The liquid crystal display shows in five decimal digits the number of registration. Sample frequency was fixed at 7.5 sec, but can vary from 0.02 sec to 480 sec. The memory capacity (if one channel is used) allows 12288 samplings. If a simultaneous intragastric and esophageal pH-monitoring is performed the memory capacity allows 6144 samplings for each channel. A real time control of the measured values is possible. The measured values are converted into true time values. The memolog has a marker for manually indications or events.

The pH input module amplifies the small voltage signals generated by the pH-electrode and converts then into the digital pulses which are required by the collection control unit.

The pH-module has a high input impedance. The sensor connection is a micro plug. The read-out of data stored in the memolog is performed using an Apple-IIe computer. With an RS-232C interface we can transmit data from the memolog to the Apple IIe. The transmission speed in which the memolog memory is transferred to the computer is called the bant rate (total bits transferred per second). We use a fast transmission of 4800. The output is formulated as follows:
- start byte (BTX ASCII02)
- information about whether one or two channels has been measured (ASCII 31 - ASCII 32)
- data
- if one channel has been used, the memory is transmitted in blocks of 4 bytes. If two channels have been used the memory is transmitted in blocks of 8 bytes.
- stop byte (EOT ASCII 04)

The software is delivered on a diskette. The hardware needed for applying the software is a personal computer Apple IIe. This computer consists of a system unit, a keyboard, a monitor and 2 disk drives.

Our Apple-IIe has a total central memory capacity of 128 Kbit and an asynchronic serial interface. The program is written in Basic and uses Assembler routines to read the data out of memory and write it on disk. It takes only one minute to read the 12288 data out of the memory. The memory is written on diskette under the patients name. The data are processed using a menu-form program. A choice leads to the execution of the service or function wanted. The data recorded by the Memolog are calculated and graphically processed to give the user a wide varity of easily accessible and understandable information about the measurements.

One curve gives an averaged picture of the distribution of the data: one point represents the mean of 50 points (6.25 min). Other curves of 250 points each, give a real representation of the data registered. 50 curves (each point representing the pH during a 7,5 sec interval) can be plotted. Selected parts of the curve can also be plotted separately.

We then calculate the number of data points with a pH under 4 and generate a histogram of the number and duration of the refluxes.

The mean pH and the standard deviation, calculated for each deliberately chosen period, and the moment and duration (in seconds) of the refluxes is calculated. The standard deviation of the mean pH, indicates the variability of the pH-moment and duration of the refluxes.

STUDY

In order to demonstrate the possible applications of the method we studied gastro-esophageal reflux in 30 babies with a risc for sudden infant death syndrome, before and under treatement with caffeine (table 1). Caffeine is classically administered to stimulate the respiration in these cases. In adults it diminishes lower oesophageal sphincter pressure (4).

As normal parameters in newborns were not available in the literature, we grouped the results obtained from 200 investigations in healthy neonates and used the mean as reference values.

Our results show that all pH-monitorings before therapy were in the normal range and that, in a highly significant way, as well the number of refluxes as the duration increased when the drug was administered.

CONCLUSIONS

We commercialized a program for the analysis of continuous esophageal pH-monitoring (Memolog 600 System) on an Apple IIe computer.
An example (secundary effects of caffeine treatment in newborns)
shows the general interest of this investigation technique,
especially its advantage in the follow-up of patients during treatment.

TABLE 1 : RESULTS OF pH-MONITORING ($m \pm$ SEM)

	Before caffeine	Caffeine treatment
Duration of pH < 4 (min)	8.9 $\pm$ 3.6	70.0 $\pm$ 23.4
Number of refluxes	5.3 $\pm$ 2.0	17.1 $\pm$ 3.4
Number of refluxes lasting longer than 5 min.	0.6 $\pm$ 0.5	5.9 $\pm$ 2.1
Duration of longest reflux (min)	2.8 $\pm$ 2.2	13.7 $\pm$ 5.2
Mean pH	5.68 $\pm$ 0.91	5.62 $\pm$ 1.34
Standard deviation of pH	0.59 $\pm$ 0.21	1.01 $\pm$ 0.43

REFERENCES

1. Jolley S.G., Johnson D.G., Herbst J.J., Pena A., Carnier R.
   An assessment of gastroesophageal reflux in children by extended pH monitoring of the distal esophagus. Surgery 1978;
   84(1): 16-24.
2. Vandenplas Y. , Lepoudre R., Sacré-Smits L. 17-Hour continuous intraesophageal pH-monitoring analysis on computer.
   Lecture Notes in Medical Information, 24, 290-295, 1984.

3. Vandenplas Y., Sacré-Smits L. Seventeen-hour continuous pH-monitoring in the newborn; evaluation of the influence of position in asymptomatic and symptomatic newborns. J. Ped. Gastroenterol. Nat. (in print).
4. Comen S., Bootti G.H. Gastric acid secretion and lower esophageal sphincter pressure in response to coffee and caffeine. N. Engl. J. Med. 1975; 293: 897-899.

ACKNOWLEDGMENT

The authors thank Mr. E. Coppens (NOVO-Industries, Belgium) for his willingness to contribute to the succes of this study and the commercialisation of the program.

REDUCTION OF RINGING IN ULTRASONIC ECHOGRAPHY
BY IMAGE DECONVOLUTION

Julio GONZALEZ Bernaldo de Quirós
Professor Dr.
Universidad Politécnica de Madrid, Spain.

The response of the system to a non infinitely narrow
transmitted pulse can be focused and an improved clinical image can be obtained using deconvolution techniques. Several deconvolution methods are described
to achieve image improvement in real time, using digital processing.

1.- INTRODUCTION.-

Piezoelectric transmitters produce an ultrasonic oscillation when they
are excited by a single pulse. This is due to a resonance effect.
Ideal transmitters should produce an infinitely narrow pulse to ob -
tain reflected signals that represent the limits of tissues such as
bones, blood, etc... However, the response of the object to a wider
signal is a complicated signal which does not represent exactly the
object.

The oscillation of the piezoelectric transmitter is called "ringing".
This may be damped to a certain extent, but not completly eliminated.
The response of the object to a wide signal is "convoluted" with that
signal, introducing the ringing of the transducer in the image as a
defocusing effect.

There are several methods of compensating convolution, they are called
"deconvolution". In this paper we will mention three methods of deconvolution which will recover the ideal system response. We think that
the third method is the best and we will give an example of a deconvolution filter for a particular case.

2.- THE CONVOLUTION INTEGRAL.-

Let h(t) represent the response of the object to a narrow transmitter pulse. h(t) is then the echo signal with an ideal transmitter pulse. The response of the system to the real transmitter, g(t), will be obtained by adding the response $h(t - t_1)$ to the infinitely narrow parts $f(t_1) dt_1$ from the begining of the transmitter pulse to the end of it at the time T. f(t) will be the signal produced by the piezo-electric transducer. The whole response, so obtained, is the convolution integral of $f(t_1)$ and h(t). We have:

$$g(t) = \int_0^T f(t_1) \ h(t - t_1) \ dt_1 = f(t) * h(t). \quad (* \text{ means convolution}).$$

where T is the with of the real transmitter pulse.

In the usual case of sampled systems, we proceed to sample all signals at time interval multiples of t. Let h(k), g(k) and f(k) be the values of the functions at the time k t. The convolution integral is now sustituted by the discrete time equation :

$$g(n) = \sum_{k=0}^{k=k_1-1} f(k) \ h(n - k)$$

where k_1 is the number of sampled pulses contained in the transmitter pulse, due to the ringing of the transducer.

In the case of ringing, it is particularly convenient to take t equal to the half period of the transmitted signal. In most ultrasonic systems the received signal is rectified, and a narrow object (or "target") will give us a signal such as the damped oscillation represented in figure 1. The echo of a narrow target represents exactly the transmitted signal. The ringing appears as a damped repetition of the target, after the real image, and disappears under the receiver thresold.

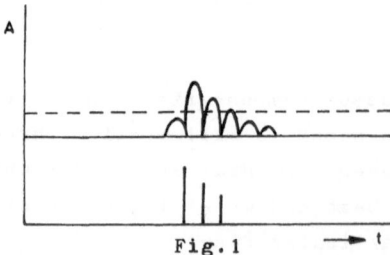

Fig. 1

3.- DECONVOLUTION METHODS.-

The problem of deconvolution is to calculate the function h(t) from the known function f(t) and the actual measured echo g(t), which is suppose to be the convolution of h(t) and f(t).

There are several methods to obtain deconvolution. The first method includes operational techniques. If we call G, F and H the Fourier transforms of g(t), f(t) and h(t), we have : G = F H. From this expression, we can easily calculate H by dividing G by F. The practical problem is to find quickly the Fourier transforms G and H, divide them and find the inverse Fourier transform of the quotient, all in real time.

The digital methods are based on writing the discrete convolution equation in the following form :

$$g(n) = \sum_{k=0}^{k=k_1-1} f(k) \, h(n - k) = f(0) \, h(n) + \sum_{k=1}^{k=k_1-1} f(k) \, h(n - k)$$

From the expression above, we can calculate f(0) h(n), which is the echo that we would have without ringing. We have :

$$f(0) \, h(n) = g(n) - \sum_{k=0}^{k=k_1-1} f(k) \, h(n - k)$$

This is a recursive equation. It is now easy to design a program to solve this equation in real time, using a microprocessor.

Instead of a program, we can use a recursive filter to solve the same equation. This filter is represented in figure 2 for the case of three ringing pulses.

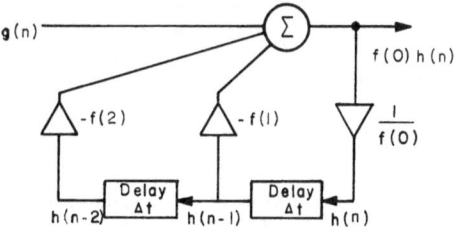

Fig. 2

4.- APPLICATION OF THE DECONVOLUTION FILTER.-

The deconvolution filter must be inserted after the digitizer, to obtain a filtered display. The complete system is represented in figure 3. In this figure, the system is used to obtain the image of a test block under water.

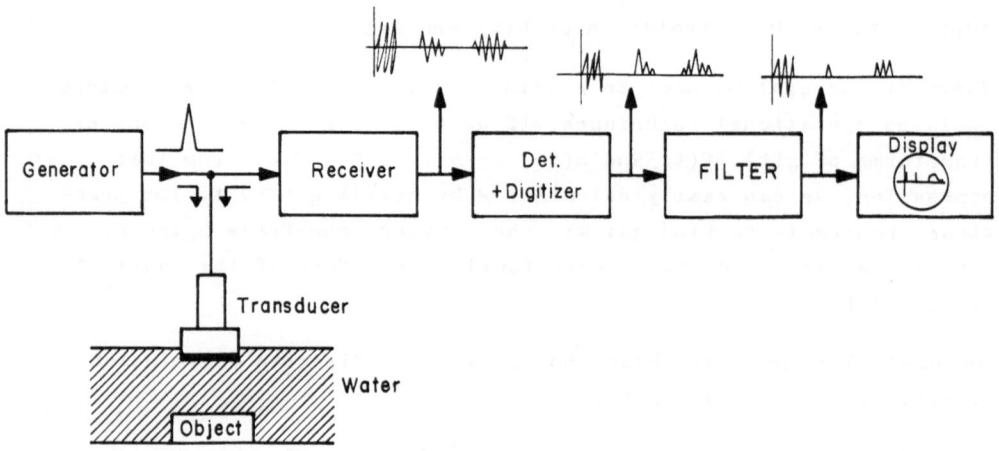

Fig. 3

Figure 4 shows the A- mode display before and after the deconvolution filter. The first pulse is the boundary between water and the test block, and the second bunch of pulses is the boundary between the test block and the table below.

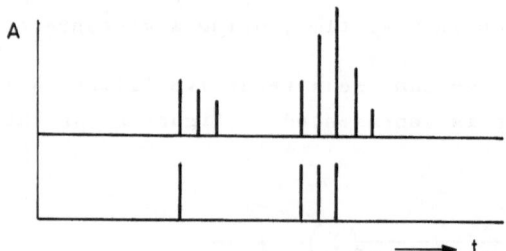

Fig. 4

REFERENCES.-

Herment and others, Algorithm for On Line Deconvolution of Echogra phic Signals, Acoustical Imaging 10 (Plenum Press, New York, 1.982).

J. González, Application of image deconvolution, Applications of Computers in Cardiology (North Holland, 1.983).

COMPUTER WAYS OF EXPLICITATION OF THE COMPRESSED ECG DATA.

Hilário Bastos Machado
Faculty of Medicine, University of Lisbon, Portugal

Advanced technology has always been applied to ECG equipment. However, classical electrocardiography has not followed the technical progress, since hardly any new information has been added during the past four decades. The main reason for this paradox may be the insistence of the using limb extremity leads, these are standing tradition, since Eintho ven used them in the beginning of the century. A salt water bath was needed. Nevertheless, his scientific work was based on the heart vector concept, this being defined in spherical coordinates (1). The limbs were used as an extension of the human torso. Many researchers tried to find different lead systems. The physical based Frank lead network reached a general agreement, and usage in vectorcardiography. Despite the aim for a better diagnostic performance, overall in myocardical in farction, vectorcardiograms (VCG) did not have the wide expansion of the ECG, because of the unpractical, unportable equipment that needed a shielded room and also, although the better explanation of the QRS, the usual VCG did not apply to the rhythm analysis.
Computerized Electrocardiography could be an opportunity to increase the ECG performance. However, some systems use the empiric 12 lead ECG (2) - and are out of progress of the vectoranalysis, used in the modern electrocardiology; others use the XYZ Frank ECG, performing a statistic analysis of the QRS after normalization (3) - and the cardiologist can not check routinelly the ECG contour analysis. Yet to achieve a better diagnosis, a bias was introduced by using the Bayes theorem, which must be only used for global decision about the patient's situation, the ECG being only a contributory test.
Dower developped a system (4) in which the Frank lead system is used, but the underlying philosophy is different: from compressed XYZ signals the central computer can display high-quality praphics, either familiar (derived 12-simultaneous lead ECG) or not, leaving a creative field for the cardiologist interested in developing new vectorana lysis displays - also, adding for instances some new ECG information.

THE PRE-PROCESSOR CART

The cart is a battery operated, microcomputer controlled, mobile unit
that performs the bed-side recordings and a series of operations prior
of sending digitized data via standard telephone lines to the central
minicomputer. It can also be used as a conventional electrocardiograph. The XYZ signals are: submitted to spherical or polar transforma -
tion; base-line clampped immediately before the QRS, to get reliable
angular measurements and a straightened base-line on the graphics; di
gitized at 1000Hz, getting both the high-quality graphics and the analysis at the level of the millisecond; compressed according to a digi
tal code, saving transmission time and computer file space; memorized
and sent in batches to the central minicomputer.

THE CENTRAL MINICOMPUTER

Here, the QRS identification is made on the spatial magnitude tracing
with high accuracy   , and the diagnostic and measurement programs
are performed. For each patient a complet set of measurements of ECG
events, intervals and angles are produced together with the patient's
identification, clinical data and computer diagnostic comments to aid
the cardiologist. The displays are drawn by electrostatic means in an
high-resolution printer-plotter. Every Frank ECG are kept in compressed form on magnetic files, for comparative or epidemiologic studies.
Data from more than 100 000 patients are now avaiable.

SOME DISPLAYS

It is obvious that all the clinical information existing in the vector analysis displays is already present in the Frank ECG, but not in
a well explained way. It is rewarding for the researchers to have an
explanation by QRS contour analysis, some new information, not yet
seen in the previous displays.
THE ECGD is the 12-simultaneous lead ECG synthesized from vectorcar -
diographic signals X Y Z, according to Dower's coeficients derived
from Frank data. Because of both the high sampling rate on digitation
and the straightening of the base-line, it generally has a better
look than the conventional ECG; and as each beat is derived from the
XYZ signals, the 12 leads are simultaneous.

In two independent computer studies of cases of MI, a system, programmed to read the conventional ECG was used, to read both the ECGD and
the conventional ECG from the same patients; the specificity was the
same and the sensitivity was increased in 10% for the ECGD. The figures were identical for both hte studies (5,6). So, even using the MI
classical diagnostic criteria, it seems that the ECGD represents a
real progress in clinical electrocardiography.

The ECGD is usually produced together with the measurement program data
and   computer comments, and is the familiar display routinelly requir
ed   and yielded by the system. In doubtfull cases, when there is not a
consistent MI diagnosis in all shown beats, a vectorcardiogram (VCG)
is drawn automatically, for the cardiologist checking.

THE THREE PLANAR LOOPS OF THE VCG are only shown in the cases reffered
above, giving a new increase to the system performance.

THE POLARCARDIOGRAM (4)   is formed by a set of graphics represented
in polar or spherical coordinates (spatial magnitude, latitude and
longitude) of the heart vectors, against a time scale. Along with the
better display of the measurements given by the development of the lo
ops, the spatial magnitude and the magnitude on the three orthogonal
planes are drawn in each degree, millisecond and 1/100 millivolt.This
fine analysis is only possible with the digitizing sample rate use .

The QRS waves identification is made in the spatial magnitude tracing,
and most of the simplified diagnostic program is based on the Polarcar
diogram. The Frank ECG is already drawn together. This display is not
usually edited.

THE SPHEROCARDIOGRAM is a new tridimensional vectoranalysis display, in
which the consecutive heart vectors are plotted on the planar projection of a sphere, according to Aitoff. It can be divided into octants,
corresponding to those of the classical vectorcardiography. In the cho
osen orientation (Fig 1), the equatorial plane corresponds to the fron
tal plane. The Spherocardiogram was described in 1978, and since then
some sparse refferences were made, mainly to show the versatility of
the system to display new vectoranalysis graphics . We perform
a sistematic study of normal (7) and abnormal cases (8), some stri-
cking visual diagnostic criteria or MI were being studied in a learning set and in a test set. Using only this simple criteria, not related to classical ECG - or vectorcardiographic usual criteria, the diagnostic performance of the Spherocardiogram was slightly superior to
that of the empiric ECG; however, this performance can be increased by
refinements of those criteria and with the implementation of others.
One interesting feature of the Spherocardiografic MI criteria is that

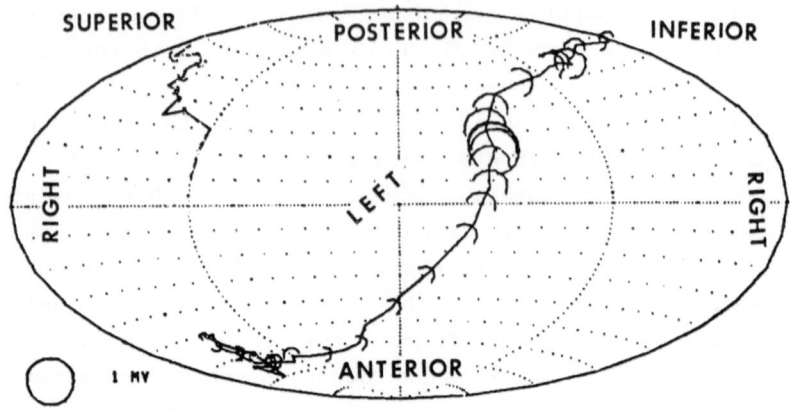

Fig. 1 - Normal Spherocardiogram. The latitude 0º, and the lon
gitude 0º and 90º divided the Aitoff plot into the correspondent octants of the classical vectorcardiography. The curve is
the direction of instantaneous vectors; the semi-circles repre
sents the spatial magnitude in each 2 mseg, its convenxity indicating its progression.

they are based on the relationship between the heart vectors direction curve and the equatorial plane (equivalent to the frontal plane,in
the shown orientation). So, the frontal plane was used to the diagnosis of both, anterior and inferior MI (Fig 2).

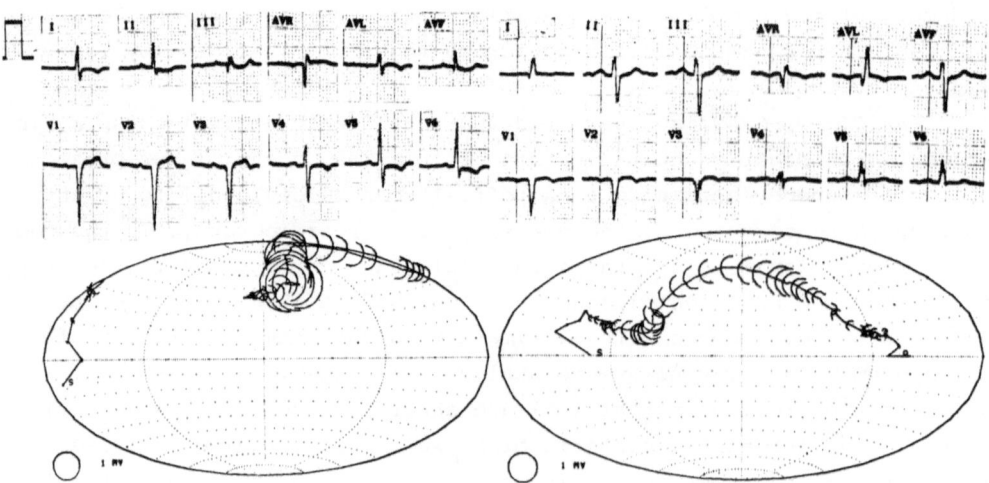

Fig. 2 - Upper part: The ECGDs mounted to comparative effects
         Bottom part: the Spherocardiogram of the same cases of
anterior myocardial infarction Note,the visual impressive differences in direction curves, in relationship to the equatorial
plane: easy reading, easy programming - in a single, rather than
12 graphics.

NEW INFORMATION DISPLAYED

There is some redundancy in the computer-derived displays from the
Frank vectorcardiographic signals. Redundancy also exists in the conventional ECG, one of the tests more often used in clinical pratice.
The computer can routinely simulate and edit the ECGD, which has sho
wn a performance 10% superior to the conventional ECG - this means
that some new information is added. Also, the ECGD is edited with mea
surements and vector analysis to aid the reading by the cardiologist.
The computer comments are based on displays that are not usually edited, but they are useful when the human reading does not agree with
them.

The Spherocardiogram added some unexpected new information to clinical
electro-vectorcardiology. Indeed, the frontal plane is not used to the
diagnosis of the anterior MI, both in the classical VCG or in the ECG.
In our study, all cases of anterior MI were diagnosed in relation to
it. The new information was contained in the Frank ECG - but was not
explicit. Its explanation seems to add, really some progress to the
modern electrocardiology, not necessary to be plotted, but to be used
as a tool in diagnostic software.

REFERENCES

1 - Burch GE and De Pasquale NP: A history of electrocardiography.Year
    Book Med Publ, Chicago, 1964

2 - Bonner RE, Crevase L. et al: A new computer program for analysis
    of the scalar electrocardiogram. Comp Biom Res. 5:629, 1972

3 - Pipberger HV, MCCanghan D et al: Clinical application of a second
    generation electrocardiographic computer program. Am J Cardiol 35:
    597, 1975

4 - Dower GE, Osborne J et al: A new system for ECG analysis oriented
    toward polarcardiography. In: Computers in Cardiology. IEEE Compu
    ter Society, Roterdam, 1977, 497

5 - Dower GE and Machado HB: X Y Z data interpreted by a 12-lead com-
    puter program using the derived electrocardiogram. J Electrocar-
    diol. 12: 249, 1979

6 - Bruce RA, Belanger L et al: Sensitivity for telemed diagnosis ...
    J Electrocardiol. 15: 157, 1982

7 - Machado HB and Silva MEP: Some findings on normal Spherocardio -
    gram ... In: Electrocardiology 81. Ed Antalóczy and Préda. HAS
    Budapest 1982, 343

8 - Machado HB, Silva MEP and Dower GE: QRS contour analysis ... In:
    The Applications of Computers in Cardiology: State of the Art ...
    Ed. Martin Quetglas et al. Elsevier Sc. Publ, IFIP - IMIA,1984,71.

A Computer-aided Physiological Teaching Software

of Circulating System

Qin Dulie   Han Daying
(Dept. of Mathematics)   (Dept. of Physiology)
Beijing Second Medical College
Beijing,People's Republic of China

1.Introduction

In these years digital computer's simulations of physiological systems are being popular gradually.MACMAN,MACPEE,MACDOPE,MACPUF are famous programs for physilogical teaching operated on mini-computers.Our program is operated on microcomputer.Its model was based on Starling law and Guyton relation and presented by Carl F.Rothe in 1978. This model may be used to assist in understanding the mechanizm of homeostasis and to simulate the effect resulted in by disturbances of cardiovascular system.

2.Model and dynamic system

The model is simplified one. Only one 'heart' is used and cardiac output is a linear function of filling volume. Only one vascular pathway is present and vasculature is lumped into only one artenal bed and one venous bed. Reflexes are neglected. We assumed that the product of heart rate and stroke volume is a constant. In real life,compensatory mechanisms tend to maintain the stroke volume with an increased rate.The mean presure of heart during diastole(filling) Ph is a constant. In fact there may be many segments and a pulsatile flow.A linear compliance is assumed. The volume is the volume causing the vasculature to be distended and does not include the volume present if the transmural pressure is zero.The venous pressure is the peripheral microvenous pressure and about the same as the mean circulatory filling pressure.The heart pressure Ph is the central venous pressure.A simplifying assumption is that the intrathoracic pressure is zero, so Ph is also the transmural filling pressure of heart. The 'heart' diastolic distensibility is assumed to be linear with no limit.

15 parameters are used in the model. They are as follows:

Fha: Flows from heart to arteries
Fav: Flows through the arterial beds
Fvh: Flows through the vanous beds
Pa: Arterial pressure
Pv: Venous pressure
Ph: Heart pressure(Central venous pressure)
Ca: Arterial complince
Cv: Venous compliance
Ch: Compliance of heart
Rav: Arterial-to-venous resistance
Rvh: Venous-to-heart resistance
Rha: Heart-to-arterial resistance(is assumed as 0)
Va: Arterial volume
Vv: Venous volume
Vh: Heart volume

According to Starling's law and Guyton's relations following equations may be set:

1. Fha = Kh*Vh   (Kh as 'contractility')
2. Fav = (Pa-pv)/Rav
3. Fvh = (Pv-Ph)/Rvh
4. Pa = Va/Ca
5. Pv = Vv/Cv
6. Ph = Vh/Ch
7. Va(t+Δt) = Va(t) + (Fha-Fav).Δt
8. Vv(t+Δt) = Vh(t) + (Fav-Fvh).Δt
9. Vh(t+Δt) = Vh(t) + (Fvh-Fha).Δt

The logic of equations7,8,9 is based on the differential equation for conservation of material.

3. Functions of the program

This program is heuristic and there are four operating modes:exercise mode,aneamia mode,hemorrhage mode and cardiac

failure mode.Its all operating stepsm includes displaying
schematic diagram of the model,answering questions of basic concepts,selecting a mode,displaying the table of nomal values of
parameters and curves of cardiac and systematic functions and
nomal operating point on screen,inputing necessary parameters'
changes,giving immediate values of iteration of parameters up to
reaching compensatory equivalence,displaying the table of values
after reaching equivalence and cardiac and sytematic curves at
set point,giving the table of control and reselecting a mode.The
operation of this program is flexible.

We take the aneamia as a example. For different degrees of
aneamia the changes of functions of cardiacvascular system may
be different.For slight aneamia the hematocrit value of erythro-
cyte and the viscosity of blood reduced, the lackness of oxygen
in organizations made blood vessels distend,the peripheral resis
tance and blood pressure reduce, all of this caused increasing
of contractility of myocardium reflexively. For serious aneamia
blood dilutes, the peripheral resistance is lower than slight
aneamia,however The lackness of oxygen in myocardium is obvious
and the contractility decreases. These may conceal reflexive
increasing of contractility of myocardium ,thus final effect is
that the contractility of myocardium decreases. At the begining
of the mode users may select slight aneamia or seious aneamia.
For the case of slight aneamia they will be required to enter
decreased value of arterial resistance and increased value of
contractility of myocardium.For the case of serious aneamia the
users will be required to enter decreased values of arterial resistance and myocardium's contractility respectively.

4. Acknowledgements

Authors wish to express their gratitude to professor Liu
Zengfu for his usual guidance. We also wish to expresss our gratitude to Dr. Khursh Ahmed for his generous offering of programs
of MACMAN,MACDOPE,MACPEE and MAACPUF and related literatures.

Reference

Rothe,Carl F. A computer model of the cardiovascular system for
effecteive learning, in Frontiers in the Teaching og Physiology:
Computer Literacy and Simulation, edited by Tidball, Chales S.
and M.C. Shelesnyak, Ammerican Physiological Society,pp 27-33,
1981.

THE MONITORING OF HEART RATE VARIABILITY IN THE ASSESSMENT OF DIABETIC AUTONOMIC
NEUROPATHY

J. H. Todd, W. J. Jeffcoate, M. Shenton, J. E. Evans and D. R. Tomlinson
Department of Medical Physics and Diabetic Clinic
City Hospital
Nottingham
United Kingdom

1. Introduction

Diabetic Autonomic Neuropathy (DAN) is a complication of chronic diabetes affecting
the autonomic nerves (1). In extreme cases the heart-rate cannot change in response
to even mild exertion such as standing up.

Several tests for DAN have been devised but the most common and the one we use is the
respiratory sinus arrhythmia test (2, 3). The change of heart-rate due to respiration
is monitored by measuring the difference between the highest heart rate on inspiration
and the lowest on expiration. In normal subjects the difference is >15 beats/min.
Subjects with a difference of <10 beats/min. are considered to be definitely abnormal.

The conventional method of assessing heart-rate variability is to mark events on an
electrocardiogram and then to measure R-R intervals after completion of the test.
This is time-consuming, providing only a numerical index and discarding any other
information which may be available within the recording. In our clinic we have evaluated a microcomputer system which provides on-line calculations and graphical display
of heart-rate with time.

2. Materials and Methods

The electrocardiogram was recorded using four limb leads. Simultaneous computer
monitoring used two additional leads attached to each arm. The R-wave was detected
using an isolated amplifier and used to generate a 40 msec duration pulse fed to the
analogue part of an Acorn BBC 'B' microcomputer. The heart-rate was continuously
displayed on a video monitor and the results of the test printed.

It was noticed that in some patients the amplitude of the R-wave decreased on inspiration and was not detected by the amplifier. Before commencing any test the operator
executed a programme which displayed the gating pulse derived from the R-wave and
adjusted the R-wave amplification.

The software was written by the authors and incorporated a screen dumping routine, GDUMP (D. A. Computers Ltd.), to print the graphical display.

The protocol for the test was:-

The patient was instructed to breathe deeply at six breaths per minute (5 inspiration, 5 expiration) for one minute. The manual recording was marked at the start of each period of inspiration and of expiration. The shortest and longest R-R intervals in each cycle were measured and the mean difference calculated for the one-minute period.

The computer programme displayed graphically the heart-rate, enabling the operator to ensure that the patient was relaxed and in a steady state before commencing the test. The heart-rate continued to be displayed during the test, providing the prompt to the patient to "breathe in" or "breathe out". The difference between minimum R-R interval and maximum R-R interval for each cycle and the mean difference for the one-minute duration of the test was displayed and printed.

The graphical display of the test can be printed (Fig. 1).

The operator can elect to display the histograms of R-R interval during inspiration and during expiration (Fig. 2).

Two groups of subjects were studied:-

i.   Normal non-diabetic - each of five subjects was tested on five consecutive days and on one day five tests of respiratory sinus arrhythmia were performed.

ii. Diabetics - Ten subjects with known DAN had three tests of respiratory sinus arrhythmia on different days.

3. Results

a. Validation of computer measurement of R-R interval

Computer measurements of R-R interval were correlated with manual measurement of the electrocardiogram for the normal subjects using the respiratory sinus arrhythmia test. There was very close correlation between the two methods ($p < 0.001$). It was concluded that the computer system was measuring the R-R interval as accurately as manual measurement. The range of heart-rates studied was 40 - 150 beats/min.

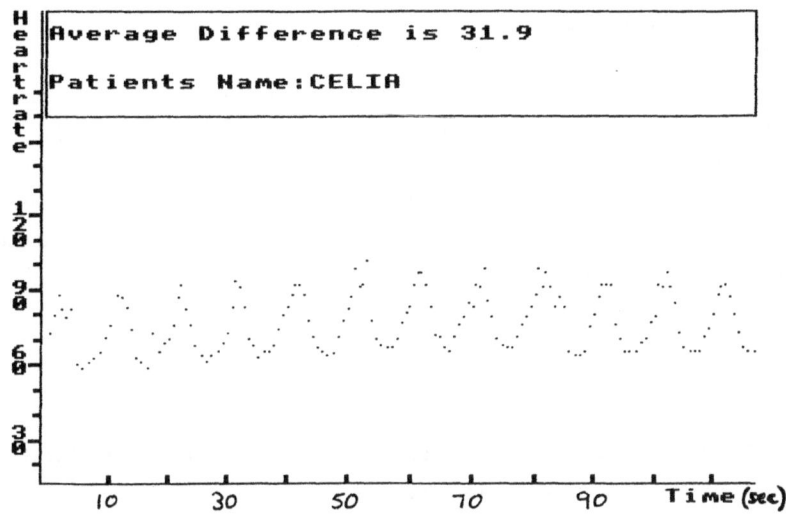

Figure 1. Normal respiratory sinus arrhythmia with deep breathing at 6 breaths per minute

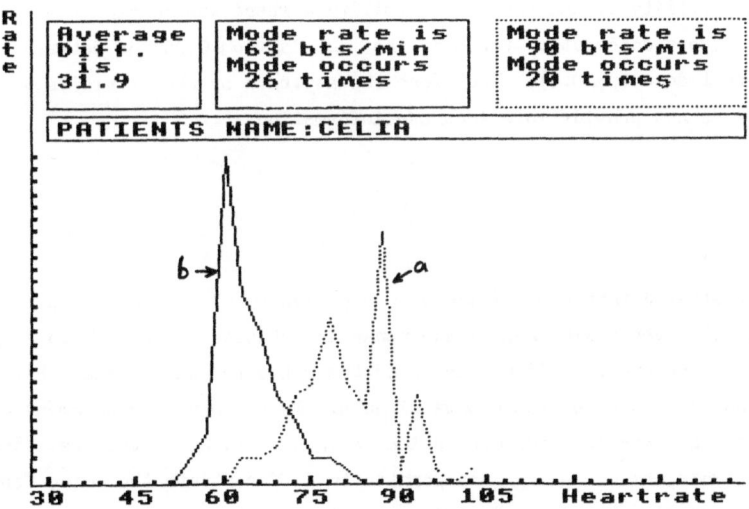

Figure 2. Histograms of the distribution of heart-rate during normal (a) deep inspiration and (b) expiration

b. <u>Respiratory Sinus Arrhythmia</u>

The computer calculations of heart-rate variability on deep respiration had good correlation with manual measurements for the normal subjects (p<0.001). However, there were instances when noise "spikes" were interpreted by the pulse generator as R-waves. During manual measurements these appeared on the E.C.G. tracing but were ignored by the operator. Consequently, differences of up to 50% between the two methods were occasionally observed.

c. <u>Clinical Results</u>

i. Normal subjects generally demonstrated a large heart-rate variability on deep breathing (range 11 - 44 beats/min).

ii. DAN subjects demonstrated a small heart-rate variability on deep breathing (range 2 - 14 beats/min). In both groups of subjects there were instances of substantial differences between computed and manually measured variability of up to 50%, particularly in the variability range of 10 - 20 beats/min.

iii. Reproducibility of heart-rate variability - There was no significant difference between consecutive tests on the same day (p>0.05) or between tests on different days (p>0.2). Therefore repeat tests or repeat visits to the clinic do not provide more accurate information.

4. <u>Discussion</u>

It has been demonstrated that a small microcomputer system can be used to accurately record R-R intervals over a wide heart-rate range in subjects who remain in a single postural position. However, rapid movements of the subjects causes noise which our software could not distinguish from R-wave signals. In the manual assessment of an electrocardiogram the operator uses discretion to ignore obvious artefacts. Enhancements to the software are now being incorporated to differentiate the noise "spike" from the true R-wave signal. The use of finger pulse monitors is also being investigated, which will remove the need to use an expensive E.C.G. amplifier and may also reduce the subject movement noise.

There is a considerable time saving by using the microcomputer for the respiratory sinus arrhythmia test which makes this test more acceptable in the clinic. Results are immediately available and our study has confirmed that subjects with known DAN have a very low heart-rate variability.

Software routines have also been written for the other commonly used tests for DAN, namely the postural change 30/15 ratio, the valsalva and the apnoeic face immersion tests (4, 5). Clinical trials of these tests will be undertaken.

The system described is to be routinely used in the diabetic clinic to test for DAN.

5. References

1. Hosking, D. J., Bennett, T., Hampton, J. R.:
   Diabetic autonomic neuropathy. Diabetes 27, 1043-54,(1978).

2. Wheeler, T., Watkins, P. J.:
   Cardiac denervation in diabetes. B.M.J., 584,(1973).

3. Bennett, T., Farquar, I., Hosking, D. J., Hampton, J. R.:
   Assessment of methods for estimating autonomic nervous control of the heart
   in patients with diabetes mellitus. Diabetes 27, 1167-74,(1978).

4. Mackay, J. D., Page, M. McB., Cambridge, J., Watkins, P. T.:
   Diabetic autonomic neuropathy - the diagnostic value of heart-rate monitoring.
   Diabetologia 18, 471-7, (1980).

5. Ewing, D. J., Campbell, I. W., Clarke, B. F.:
   The natural history of diabetic autonomic neuropathy. Quart. J. Med. 49,
   95-108, (1980).

A monitor for quality control in the routine of a department for obstetrics and gynecology *)

Thurmayr, R., Schöffel, J.: Institut für Med. Statistik und
                            Epidemiologie der TU München (IMSE)

  v. Hugo, R., Graeff, H.:   Frauenklinik, Klinikum re.d.Isar
                             der TU München

Summary

Monitors for quality control are being used in the Frauenklinik
der TUM to control the operative field, deliveries and bacteriology. Using Data from three previous years limits for measurements und frequencies were established, which transgressing
signals unusual findings. A patient oriented, daily used, was
set up, as well as a monthly and yearly monitor.
The control through the three monitors of the real happening was
able to show deficiencies in the data recording, in the obser
vance of instructions for the patient care and real problem
fields. In such cases retrospective or prospective studies in
form of thesis are performed to analyse the problem more thoroughly or to control the success of the measures.

1. Introduction

Quality improvement is a prerequisite for further development in
surgery. A hospital needs tools for a continuous survey of the
medical patient care (3,4). In the Frauenklinik des Klinikums
re.d.Isar of the Technical University of Munich were survey
tools implemented for three sections (perinatology, surgery,
bacteriology) so that a lot of patients of the clinic would be
recorded.
These monitors for quality control are implemented to point out
the facts of these 3 sections which are inconspicuous and then
obviously under control, respectively to create signals for
divergences which point out domains which may be out of control.

2. Data acquisition

Data acquisition for the quality control monitor in surgical
field is achieved with the computer aided writing of the physician's report. After the patient's discharge the physician fills
out a questionnaire including data about quality control and
some more data for the physician's report (2). The data is typed

---

*) Dedicated to Prof.Dr.H.-J.Lange (Head of IMSE) to his
   sixtyth birthday

in dialog in the computer by a data manager, a patient record is automatically printed out, and the data is stored for quality control. Due to the double use of the questionnaire, there is no additional work for the physician. The bacteriological data can be in fact obtained out of the bacteriological report for the Microbiological Institute to the clinics.

Perinatal data are acquired through a questionnaire which is being used for 170 hospitals in Bavaria (70%). These questionnaires are filled in by the physicians and are going to be used in the near future for the computer aided writing of the physician's report completed by additional information (6).

3. Set up of monitors

To set up monitors, frequencies of the variables for data material from 1981 - 83 were being used and stratified according to the diagnoses and operations. Criteria for quality control range from length of hospital stay to postoperative complications and increasing resistance of bacteria against antibiotica. Three monitors were set up:

- patient oriented monitor

This monitor is being used as soon as patient data are being entered. On one hand it checks the consistency of the data, for example the conformity of the diagnosis and of the operation and on the other hand points at unusual phenomenon in the data. Values of the variables which were not being found so far, were built in the monitor as unknown events. In the same way events which occured only up to 1% in the sample, were classified as seldom. In addition qualitative variables were sorted by their frequency and all events were included up to the sum frequency of 1, whereas for quantitative variables the upper and lower percentiles prevailed. In that way 152 questions could be defined for 25 features.

- monthly monitor

for the setup of the monthly monitor the monthly means of 30 variables from the surgical field were determined, in fact according to the operation and every variable was plotted with time on the abscissa (January '81 to December '83, fig. 1).

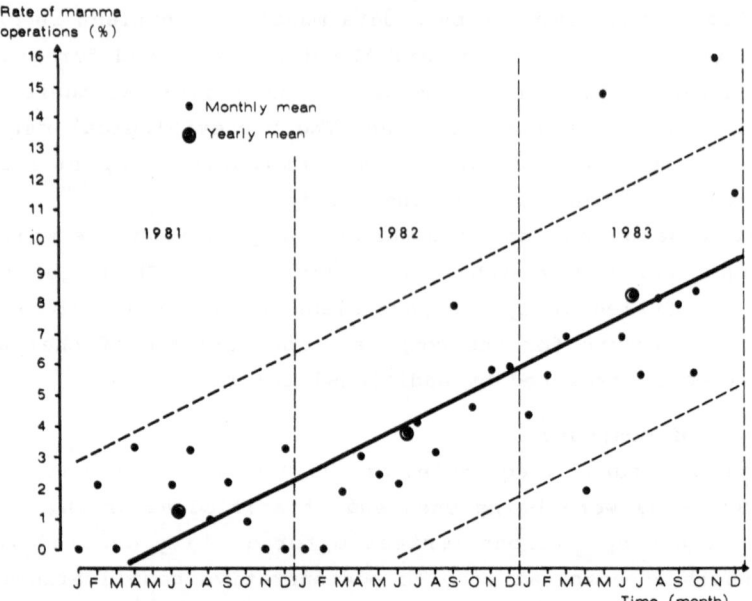

Fig. 1: Monthly quality control monitor rates of mamma
         operation 1981 - 1983

This plots include the annual means and the linear regression
line. In addition 2 lines were drawn in parallel that include
80% of all means, i.e. 33 of the 36, within and 3 outside of
these 2 lines, thus marking the central 80% percentile. Use of
the regression line for determination of the extreme values not
only considers the tolerance range but also the trend, since
more than half of the variables show a time related trend that
was statistically significant. For the monthly monitor the plots
for the variable are recorded on a monthly basis. Values that
are located outside the 80% percentile can be recognized at
first sight. In that way the monthly monitor indicates areas of
the medical care which need to be controlled.

- yearly monitor
At the request of the clinicians an annual statistic was compiled
featuring 14 tables and 7 histograms. This statistic is updated
annually.

4. Measures for quality control

In 1984 the patient oriented monitor gave 250 error messages for the 1460 operations. 50 of which were logical errors. 120 of the messages proved to be an input error and 80 were real unusual events. They are forwarded to the head of the department together with a copy of the physician's report for direct discussion with the physician involved.

1984 the monthly monitor indicated 50 unusual means for the surgical field that were analysed every 2 months in the clinic conference. Part of these unusual data is caused by the restoration of the surgical area during the 2.half of the year. The annual statistic is also being presented as the role issue during a clinic conference and confirms the trend of the data of the monthly monitor, e.g. the increase of breast intervention during the recent years.

These limited analyses demonstrated, for example, the difference between the specification bacteriuria in the questionnaire of the surgical field and the frequency of a bacteriuria according to the stored bacteriological results. As a consequence a separate definition of the germ count limits for midstream- and catheterurine were defined. For simular reasons the definition of infection related fewer had to be redefined as fewer of at least 38.5°C on two consecutive days.

For consequent solution of the problem specific studies were conducted for example in regard to the infection rate following Caesarian section. A previous prospectively conducted clinical study had shown that prophylactic antibiotics given to patients at risk resulted in a clearcut decrease of the rate of infection following Caesarian section in comparison to patients without prophylactic treatment (5). Based upon the results of the previous study the physician in chief ordered prophylactic measures for all patients at risk starting July 1, 1982. Reassessment of the consequences of this order - in the sense of the bi-Cycle concept (1) - showed - by the current study - , that during the first three months this order was followed in 69% of patients at risk and that the infection rate of these patient was 3.2% (fig.2).

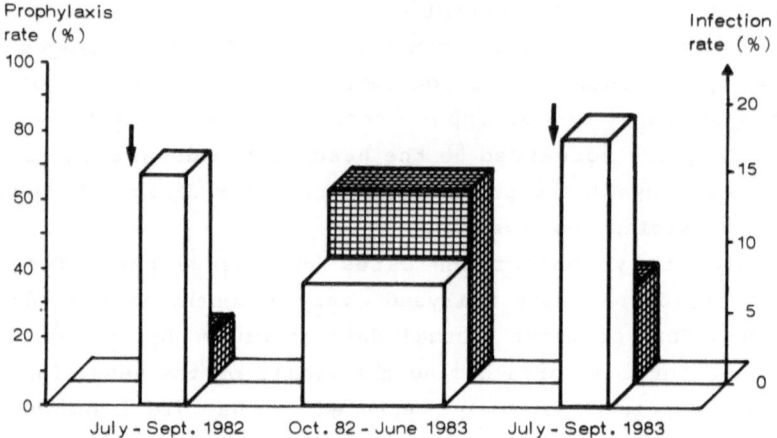

Fig. 2: Rate of antibiotic prophylaxis on 161 patients at risk
after written recommendation and infection rate

▱ Rate of antibiotic prophylaxis on patients at risk of infection
◼ Infection rate of patients at risk after sectio
▮ Occurence of a written recommendation to make prophylaxis

During the subsequent 9 months the adherence to the order decreased to 36% and the rate of infection increased to 14%.
Following a repeat, written order of the physician in chief in
July 1983 concerning the antibiotic prophylaxis the rate of
prophylactic treatment increased to 79% and the rate of infection decreased again to 6.9%. On one side the study showed the
performance gap that is to be controlled specifically in the
patient monitor as well as the efficiency of prophylactic antibiotic treatment in routine praxis by the reproduced reciprocal
action between prophylactic measures and infection.

5. Discussion

Linking data acquisition for quality control with computer
aided writing of the physician's report, the physician is not
charged with extra work. On the contrary, data are acquired
that can be used for the acquisition of data of medical performance as well as for basic documentation.

Control of the completeness of the quality control is without
problem since the surgical intervention as well as the deliveries are listed in consecutive numbers in the corresponding
journals. At the end of the year 130 questionnaires were missed,

most of the patients were transfered to an other department or
were only one day in the department.

To achieve complete data is by far more difficult since one depends upon the information of the physicians it is necessary
that physicians understand quality control not as a weapon
against themselves but as a help for their medical acting. The
setup of data acquisition and disclosure of unusual data using
the computer at the current state of the technology was without
problem. It will fulfill its objective only when every physician ready is his deviations from standards in diagnosticand
therapy to substantiate.

References

BROWN, C.R., FLEISHER, D.S.:
    The Bi-Cycle Concept-Relating continuing Education
    Directly to Care
    N.Engl.J.Med. 284 suppl. (1971) 88-97

LANGE, H.-J., THURMAYR, R., BECKERT, D.:
    Klinische Datenverarbeitung
    Beispiel: Klinikum rechts der Isar der Technischen
    Universität München
    Siemens Schriftenreihe 'data praxis' - 1984

SELBMANN, H.K., ÜBERLA, K.K.(Eds.):
    Quality Assessment of Medical Care.
    Bleicher-Verlag, Gerlingen, 1982, 206 S.

SELBMANN, H.K.:
    Qualitätssicherung ärztlichen Handelns
    Bleicher-Verlag, Gerlingen, 1984

WARNECKE, H.H., GRAEFF, H, SELBMANN, H.K., PREAC-MURSIC, V.,
ADAM, D., GLONING, K.Ph., JÄNICKE, F., ZANDER, J.:
    Perioperative Antibiotika-Kurzzeitprophylaxe bei
    Kaiserschnitt.
    Geburtshilfe Frauenheilkd 9, 654-661 (1982)

ZANDER, J., SELBMANN, H.K. (Hrsg.):
    Wege zu einer verbesserten Perinatalversorgung
    Deutscher Ärzte-Verlag 1982

COMPUTER ANALYSIS OF THE ANAESTHETIC ON-CALL SYSTEM IN A MATERNITY HOSPITAL

B Richards and A Lau
Department of Computation
University of Manchester Institute
   of Science and Technology
Manchester
England

J Kirby
St Mary's Maternity Hospital
Manchester
England

Introduction

There are two areas currently giving cause for concern within obstetric units in the United Kingdom. The first is the continuing concern over maternal mortality and the second is the problem of managing to adequately staff the anaesthetic service in times of severe financial pressure. This Study was carried out to discover whether the present service was adequate and if not to indicate how it should be improved.

A prototype for the present study can be found in the work of Jennings et al (1) and (2) and more latterly, in Dingwall, Richards and Miller (3), although these studies were concerned more with the area of general anaesthetics than with the specific area of obstetrics and gynaecology discussed in the present paper. These two studies looked at the work-load on the anaesthetics in a single hospital or small group of hospitals, whilst other studies and reports have looked at the situation throughout the nation. One thinks here of the Short Report (4) and the survey by Scott (5).

It is in the light of the above that the present Study was set up.

Structure of the Hospital System

The St Mary's Maternity Hospital is a large Teaching Hospital with some 260 beds devoted to obstetrics and gynaecology on the one hand, and to neonatal surgery and paediatrics on the other. There are between 4000 and 5000 live births annually. Anaesthetic cover is needed for the 24-hour epidural service offered in the Central Delivery Unit, for deliveries made under general anaesthetic (Caesarian Sections) and for Gynaecological cases. At present, some 30% to 35% of mothers receive an epidural during labour.

The anaesthetic cover for St Mary's is provided as an integral part of the work of the Anaesthetic Department within the Central Manchester Hospital complex. There are ten consultant sessions allocated specifically to the Central Delivery Unit and this is supported by full

24-hour cover provided by either a Senior Registrar or Registrar
However, during the day, the Registrar is almost exclusively confined
to the CDU. Outside this period, the on-call Registrar is responsible
for providing not only obstetric cover but also cover for emergency
gynaecological cases. The on-call Registrar is resident in the Hospital
but will generally not commence work outside CDU until he has been
assured of cover for CDU by a Senior Registrar. Gynaecological
emergencies occurring during the day are covered by the anaesthetist(s)
doing the routine operating lists in that Department.

```
              STUDY OF ANAESTHETIC SERVICE

Study No.  ┌─┬─┬─┐          Patient's Name
           └─┴─┴─┘          Patient's Hospital No.
                            Name of Anaesthetist

Date of request       ┌┬┬┬┬┐   Time of Request          ┌┬┬┐
Date of agreed start  ├┼┼┼┼┤   Time of Agreed start     ├┼┼┤
Date of arrival on scene├┼┼┼┼┤ Time of Arrival on scene ├┼┼┤
Date of actual start  ├┼┼┼┼┤   Time of Actual start     ├┼┼┤
Date of finish        └┴┴┴┴┘   Time of Finish           └┴┴┘

                            Duration (minutes)          ┌┬┬┐
                                                        └┴┴┘

Nature of work.....................................
Degree of urgency stated...........................
Degree of urgency as assessed by Anaesthetist......
If delay, how many minutes.........................
If delay, reason for delay in starting.............
Identity of person performing the task.............
If not Mat. Reg. what was he doing at this time?...
How many minutes before Mat. Reg. would have been available?...
If not Consultant, what was he doing at this time?.....
How many minutes before Consultant would have been available?..
Where was the person responding to the request?...
What was the activity of the person responding to the request?.


        ─────────────────────────────

If Gynae. emergency at 5.00 p.m. or at weekend...............
                                            1st    2nd    3rd
Identify of Anaesthetist requested to act as cover
Activity of Anaesthetist requested to act as cover
How many minutes until free to act as cover


        ─────────────────────────────

              FOR OFFICE USE ONLY

If Gynae. emergency between 9.00 a.m. and 5.00 p.m.............
Nature of work performed on CDU during this period

a) ┌┬┐    b) ┌┬┐    c) ┌┬┐    d) ┌┬┐
   └┴┘       └┴┘       └┴┘       └┴┘
```

Figure 1. An Incident Form

Methodology

The whole of the anaesthetic work-load for a four-week period (November/ December) was studied. All obstetric and gynaecological procedures were included in the study. The anaesthetist completed a pro-forma questionnaire for each procedure. These forms were then checked by one of the authors before being processed on a micro-computer. A copy of the pro-forma is shown in Figure 1.'

A few words of explanation related to the pro-forma are not inappropriate.

The Agreed Start is what it says, namely, the time agreed between the anaesthetist and the obstetric staff when the request is first made. The anaesthetist will then arrive on the scene hoping to allow the procedures to commence. Because of the frequent occasions when the procedure cannot start, the Arrival Time and the Actual Start Time are both recorded. The various reasons for the delay in starting are given in Table 1.

00	–	No delay
01	–	Theatre in use
02	–	Nursing staff not ready
03	–	Technicians not ready
04	–	Patient not arrived (i.e. Porters not ready)
05	–	Surgeons not arrived
06	–	Anaesthetist late-previous task took longer than expected
07	–	Anaesthetist late-requested to attend higher priority call
08	–	Anaesthetist requested delay to wait for cover to become available
09	–	Obstetricians undecided as to management of patient
10	–	Patient indecision

TABLE I Reason for delay in starting

The Degree of Urgency was assessed by using 5 levels of priority. These correspond to the classification used by the previous authors and are shown in Table II.

Priority		Definition
1	Immediate	Within 3 Minutes
2	Urgent	Within 15 Minutes
3	Emergency	Within 90 Minutes
4	Semi-emergency	When arranged
5	Cold/elective	When arranged

TABLE II Classification of Priorities

The anaesthetist responding to the emergency call could be in one of nine difference categories of place when the call comes in, some of

which include being in one of three other hospitals covered by the
Department of Anaesthetics, being elsewhere within the Maternity
Hospital, or in transit between sites.

Results

Tables of results were produced from the Commodore PET computer for each
individual week and for the whole of the four-week period. Activity
Charts were then derived by hand from the output.

The first parameter warranting attention must clearly be the degree of
priority and a table was produced showing the priority of the case as
determined by the anaesthetic staff on arrival and that stated by the
obstetric staff when the procedure was booked. (See Table III).

Priority	STATED		OBSERVED	
	CALLS	%	CALLS	%
1	3	1.53	3	1.53
2	17	8.67	13	6.63
3	103	52.55	105	53.57
4	50	25.51	51	26.02
5	23	11.73	24	12.24

TABLE III   Differences between Stated and Observed
Priorities

There is a good agreement between the 2 assignments, in fact there
was complete agreement in 191 out of 196 cases. The four cases where
discrepancy occurred were (a) a case in week 1 rated Priority 2 (P2)
by the obstetric staff and Priority 4 by the anaesthetist; (b) two
cases in week 2 rated P2 but found to be P3 when the anaesthetist
arrived; (c) one similar case of P2 to P3 in week 3 and (d) one case of
P3 to P5 in week 4.

The next procedure needing examination is the delay occurring in the
Priority 1 and Priority 2 cases. Here we have evaluated the time
period between the request being made and the anaesthetist arriving
ready to start the procedure. The time permitted for a Priority 1
case is 3 minutes and for a Priority 2 case it is 15 minutes. These
times are used by Jennings (1). In our Study, we found that 2 out of
3 Priority 1 calls were delayed (23%). These numbers are too small to
form an opinion as to statistical significance. Whilst any delay in
these categories is unacceptable, Jennings did admit that up to 5%
of Priority 1 cases might have to wait; and not more than 2.5% of P1
and P2 cases waiting more than 15 minutes could well be the best that

could be done with sensible staffing levels. The delays were 2 and
8 minutes for the two P1 cases and an average of 10 minutes for the P2
cases.

The incidence of the various priorities throughout the 24-hour day were
studied. Table IV shows the results. The three P1 cases were all
Caesarian Sections thought to be necessary because of Foetal Distress.
Of the 17 Priority 2 cases, nine were also for emergency Caesarian
Sections and a further 4 were for Epidural Analgesia.

Priority	08.00-17.00		17.00-14.00		00.00-08.00	
	No	%	No.	%	No.	%
1	1	0.5	2	1.0	0	0
2	8	4.1	6	3.1	3	1.5
3	51	26.0	27	13.8	25	12.8
4	40	20.4	8	4.1	2	1.0
5	18	9.2	5	2.6	0	0
Total	118	60.2	48	24.5	30	15.3

TABLE IV   Occurrence of Emergencies

This Table also shows the distribution of the work-load over the five
priority levels. We see that the lower priorities are very much
concentrated in the first period with a total of 78% (58) of the P4
and P5 cases in the period. It appears that all the emergencies
performed after 17.00 hours were anaesthetised by the on-call Registrar,
with the exception of one P3 case. The on-call Senior Registrar
performed that task.

One of the main reasons for the study was to examine the reasons for
the delays in the commencement of the anaesthetic procedures. Table V
shows the type of cases that incurred delays while Table VI shows the
reasons for the delay in starting a procedure.

Procedure	Number Performed	Number delayed	% delayed
Epidural LSCS	17	7	41.2
GA LSCS	41	22	52.5
Epidural analgesia	71	16	22.5
Shirodkar suture	3	1	33.3
Removal retained placenta	9	6	66.6
EVAC	38	20	52.6
Laparoscopy	4	0	0
Laparotomy	5	3	60.0
Drainage abscess	5	3	60.0

TABLE V   Types and Numbers of cases which incurred delays.

Reason	No. of delays	% of total number of procedures performed
Theatre in use	18	9.18
Lack of nursing staff cover	15	7.65
Lack of technicians cover	2	1.02
Lack of porters	5	2.55
Surgeons not ready	13	6.63
Anaes. not ready-last procedure over-ran	13	6.63
Anaes. not ready-asked to attend higher priority call	5	2.55
Anaes. not ready-waiting for cover before starting gynae. case	2	1.00
Patient reluctant to sign consent	1	0.51
Obstetric indecision as to immediate management of patient	4	2.04
	78	

TABLE VI The reasons for delay in starting a procedure

Discussion

There are several relevant conclusions which can be drawn from the study. One is that, by analysing the total duration of all the cases, it appears that the on-call Registrar is loaded for 14.35% of his time. Hence it is deemed that the cover is adequate. The staffing profile in the Maternity Hospital fulfills the requirement of the Short Report (4).

Examination of the reasons for the delay in starting the procedure show that the anaesthetist was responsible in only 20 out of 78 delays which occurred. Problems associated with the operating theatres were the biggest reason for non-anaesthetic delays. On 18 occasions, the theatre was already in use when the emergency occurred. In a further 15 cases, the theatre was empty but there were no theatre nurses available at that instant; the procedure had to wait until they became available.

In summary, it is held that the level of anaesthetic staffing in the hospital is adequate. Any short-fall should be covered by additional back-up service from the central department. There seems to be the start of a case for an additional theatre or better scheduling of the existing theatres.

References

1. Jennings, "A Study of Anaesthetic Emergency Work" BJA 41 70-75 1969.
2. Jennings, "Anaesthetic Emergency Services at Three Hospitals - a Decade of Change" BJA 54 267-277 1982
3. Dingwall, Richards and Miller "The On-call Service Offered by the Department of Anaesthesia, Manchester Royal Infirmary, BJA 55, 877-883, 1983.
4. "The Second Report from the Social Services Committee into Perinatal and Neonatal Mortality Session 1979-1980". Chairman Renee Short, (H.M.S.O.).
5. "A Survey of Anaesthetic Services to Obstetrics in the United Kingdom". The obstetric subspeciality committee of the Association of Anaesthetists in Great Britain and Ireland, chaired by D B Scott, 1977.

A COMPUTER BASED QUALITY ASSURANCE SYSTEM FOR ASSESSMENT OF ULTRASOUND MEASUREMENTS

B Richards[∅]   M Gowland[+]   P Laycock[∅]

[∅] University of Manchester   + Bolton General Hospital
   Institute of Science and Technology   Bolton
   Sackville Street   Lancashire
   Manchester   England
   England

1.   Introduction

This paper describes a study carried out with the objective of comparing
members of the ultrasound team, one with another, as regards the
reproducibility of measurements on the same patient. With any measurements involving human subjective judgement, there will be a variation
between the observations made by different observers using the same
machine to measure the same patient. In a "factory type" situation,
it would be acceptable to take many measurements on the same, inanimate,
specimen using a team of recorders. However, with patients it is not
considered desirable that more than two people from the team (of four
in our case) should scan the same patient. Hence, in order to compare
different members of the team against each other, it is necessary to
devise an "incomplete block" factorial experiment in which no patient
is scanned more than twice and every member of the team scans the
same number of patients.

Ultrasound is used in obstetrics for several purposes, some concerned
with the measurements of the growing foetus,[1] others with the search for
possible abnormalities of growth.[2][3] In the case of the former, the first
measurement, often made between 14 and 16 weeks is important as it is
used to establish the "base-line" against which latter measurements can
be compared. This "base-line" scan can give a fairly accurate statement
as to the elapsed period from conception to the time of the scan.[4]
Conversely, on the not too rare occasions when the date of conception
is supposedly known, it can very accurately establish a base-line
against which subsequent scans can be compared.

2.   The Incomplete Block Layout

Using statistical theory and by carrying out the subsequent matrix
analysis,[5][6] it is possible to arrive at an experimental protocol which
is susceptible to a simple implementation within the Ultrasound
Department. Figure 1 below shows the design.

One can then postulate that an individual measurement made on patient
j by operator i can be expressed in model form by the equation:-

$$x_{ij} = \mu + \alpha_i + \beta_j + \varepsilon_{ij} \qquad \ldots\ldots\ldots(1)$$

where $i = 1,\ldots 4$; and $j = 1, 2,\ldots 6$

ULTRASOUND ANALYSIS

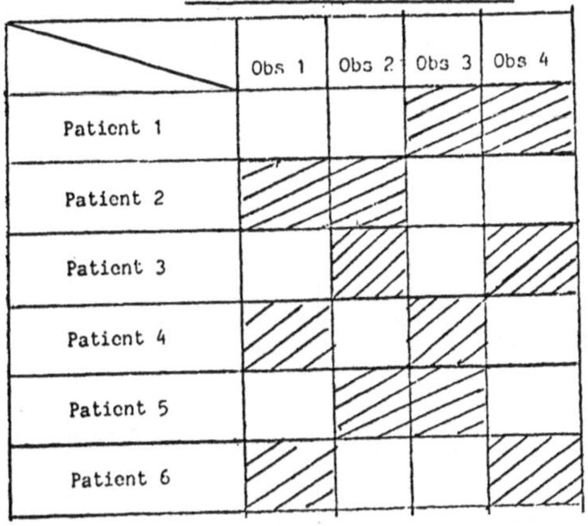

Figure 1 : The Incomplete Block Layout

One imposes the constraint that $\Sigma\alpha_1 = 0$ and $\Sigma\beta_j = 0$. This results in twelve equations in the nine unknowns, these latter being μ, α_1, α_2, α_3, and $\beta_1, \ldots \beta_5$.

In matrix form the system of twelve equations become

$$\underline{X}_{12 \times 1} = \underline{M}_{12 \times 9} \; \underline{C}_{9 \times 1} + \underline{E}_{12 \times 1} \qquad \ldots (2)$$

Here X is the vector of the twelve observations; M is the matrix of the coefficients; and C is the vector of the nine unknowns.

Solution of these least squares equations enables formulae to be found for μ, the α's and the β's.

The matrix solution is

$$\underline{C} = (\underline{M}^T \underline{M})^{-1} \; \underline{M}^T \underline{X} \qquad \ldots (3)$$

In this solution μ is the mean of all the observations but the formulae for the α's and β's are far from simple. One can also evaluate the variances of the α's and β's and these can then be used to test the various hypotheses as to uniformity amongst the operators. Further statistics can be computed, which are not shown in the Figures, in order to evaluate differences between any two specific observers.

3. Verification of the Model

In order to demonstrate the accuracy of the model, six theoretical patients were produced and four "observers" with known tendencies were used to "measure" these patients. The observations in the tableaux below, Figure 2, were obtained by derivations from exact values (shown) according to the operator involved.

The twelve observations were fed into a program running on a micro-

computer and estimates of the fitted parameters were obtained. From
Figure 3, it will be seen that the model fits the data exactly, since
there has been no biological variation on the part of any of these
"consistantly biased" observers.

	Obs 1	Obs 2	Obs 3	Obs 4	Exact Value
Patient 1	35.0	38.0			35
Patient 2			33.0	36.1	36
Patient 3	37.0		34.0		37
Patient 4		41.0		38.1	38
Patient 5	39.0			39.1	39
Patient 6		43.0	37.0		40

Observer No. 1 reads exactly

Observer No. 2 reads 3.0 units high

Observer No. 3 reads 3.0 units low

Observer No. 4 reads 0.1 units high

Figure 2   :   Test Data No. 1

PT	OBS1	FIT1	OBS2	FIT2
1	35.000	35.000	38.000	38.000
2	33.000	33.000	36.100	36.100
3	37.000	37.000	34.000	34.000
4	41.000	41.000	38.100	38.100
5	39.000	39.000	39.100	39.100
6	43.000	43.000	37.000	37.000

VALUE OF MEAN (MU) =   37.52500
VALUE OF ALPHA1   =   -0.02500
VALUE OF ALPHA2   =   2.97500
VALUE OF ALPHA3   =   -3.02500
VALUE OF ALPHA4   =   0.07500

VALUE OF SIGMA   =   0.00000
SIG OF MU   =
SIG OF ALPHA1   =
SIG OF ALPHA2   =
SIG OF ALPHA3   = $t_3(5\%) = 3.182$
SIG OF ALPHA4   =

Figure 3   :   Ultrasound Results Data 1

The fit was too perfect for us to adequately demonstrate the model. A
further set of Test Data were produced, Date 2 (Figure 4). This time
the fit wasn't "perfect" and it was possible to obtain, not only the
values for the parameters, shown in Figure 5, but also the Student's t
values for the departures from the mean of the various observers, i.e.

the significance of the $\alpha_1 \ldots \alpha_4$. Since $t_3(5\%) = 3.182$, we see that the α_2 is statistically significant, i.e. observer No. 2 is making unacceptable misreadings. (We <u>know</u> that the observer is consistantly reading 3 units too high).

	Obs 1	Obs 2	Obs 3	Obs 4	Exact Value
Patient 1	35.0	38.0	/////	/////	35
Patient 2	/////	/////	34.0	36.1	36
Patient 3	37.0	/////	35.0	/////	37
Patient 4	/////	39.0	/////	36.1	36
Patient 5	37.0	/////	/////	37.1	37
Patient 6	/////	36.0	34.0	/////	36

Observer No. 1 reads <u>Exact</u>

Observer No. 2 reads 3.0 units high

Observer No. 3 reads 2.0 units low

Observer No. 4 reads 0.1 unit high

Figure 4 : Test Data No. 2

4.   Use in the Field

The model was then used by the Ultrasound Team in one of the Local Hospitals. The observers all used the same scanner, namely an Hitachi EUB4, Real Time Linear Area Scanner with a 3.5 MHz transducer. Measurements, in millimetres, of the Biparietal Diameters (BPD) of the foetal skulls were made.

Figure 6 below shows the real observations and Figure 7 shows the result of the computer analysis. Happily this team are excellent scanners and there are no statistically significant deviators.

PT	OBS1	FIT1	OBS2	FIT2
1	35.000	35.375	38.000	37.625
2	34.000	34.375	36.100	35.725
3	37.000	36.625	35.000	35.375
4	39.00	38.625	36.100	36.475
5	37.000	37.000	37.100	37.100
6	36.000	36.750	34.000	33.250

```
VALUE OF MEAN (MU    =  36.19167
VALUE OF ALPHA1      = .-0.27500
VALUE OF ALPHA2      =   1.97500
VALUE OF ALPHA3      =  -1.52500
VALUE OF ALPHA4         -0.17500

VALUE OF SIGMA       =   0.86603
SIG OF MU            = 144.76667
SIG OF ALPHA1        =  -0.51854
SIG OF ALPHA2        =   3.72410     t (5%) = 3.182
SIG OF ALPHA3        =  -2.87557      3
SIG OF ALPHA4        =  -0.32998
```

Figure 5 : Ultrasound Results Data 2

From the various trials, the example shown in Figure 8 (Data 4) has been selected. This contains two patients who had foetuses in very obscure positions, so much so that it was almost impossible to measure accurately the BPD. The observations were starred (*) at the time of recording by the author, prior to any computer analysis. The subsequent analysis, Figure 9, shows that observer No. 1 who had the two difficult

ULTRASOUND ANALYSIS

Data 3

	Obs 1	Obs 2	Obs 3	Obs 4
Patient 1	28	22		
Patient 2			39	39
Patient 3	34		35	
Patient 4		32		32
Patient 5	37			36
Patient 6		33	35	

Figure 6 : Live Data, Data 3

PT	OBS1	FIT1	OBS2	FIT2
1	28.000	26.750	22.000	23.250
2	39.000	39.500	39.000	38.500
3	34.000	34.875	35.000	34.125
4	32.000	31.125	32.000	32.875
5	37.000	37.375	36.000	35.625
6	33.000	32.625	35.000	35.375

VALUE OF MEAN MU = 33.50000
VALUE OF ALPHA1 = 1.50000
VALUE OF ALPHA2 = -2.00000
VALUE OF ALPHA3 = 0.75000
VALUE OF ALPHA4 = -0.25000

VALUE OF SIGMA = 1.55456
SIG OF MU = 74.64953
SIG OF ALPHA1 = 1.57568
SIG OF ALPHA2 = -2.10090 $t_3(5\%) = 3.182$
SIG OF ALPHA3 = 0.78784
SIG OF ALPHA4 = -0.26261

Figure 7 : Ultrasound Results Data 3

ULTRASOUND ANALYSIS

Data 4

	Obs 1	Obs 2	Obs 3	Obs 4	
Patient 1	34	31			*
Patient 2			34	34	
Patient 3	35		31		*
Patient 4		23		22	
Patient 5	33			32	
Patient 6		39	39		

Figure 8 : Live Data. Data 4.

PT	OBS1	FIT1	OBS2	F1T2
1	34.000	33.750	31.000	31.250
2	34.000	33.750	34.000	34.250
3	35.000	34.500	31.000	31.500
4	23.000	22.500	22.000	22.500
5	33.000	33.750	32.000	31.250
6	39.000	39.250	39.000	38.750

VALUE OF MEAN (MU) = 32.25000
VALUE OF ALPHA1 = 2.00000
VALUE OF ALPHA2 = -0.50000
VALUE OF ALPHA3 = -1.00000
VALUE OF ALPHA4 = -0.50000

VALUE OF SIGMA = 0.91287
SIG OF MU =122.38015
SIG OF ALPHA1 = 3.57771
SIG OF ALPHA2 = -0.89443
SIG OF ALPHA3 = -1.78885 $t_3(5\%) = 3.182$
SIG OF ALPHA4 = -0.89443

Figure 9 : Ultrasound Results Data 4.

patients, had a significant deviation. Fortunately, the operator had taken part in previous tableaux and had been found to be consistantly accurate. In short, this example has been included to show the necessity of only allowing accurate data to go into the computer system. In routine practice, Data 4 would have been aborted and the trial re-commenced. Results from trials at several different hospitals are available and these have been able to select out occasional, less careful scanners.

5. Conclusions

This system is simple to use from the operator's point of view: it produces no great inconvenience to the patients (in fact, having had the procedure explained to them, many patients welcomed the study and thought that a hospital far-sighted enough to do this, and to be concerned about quality control, was one of the better ones), and the results can be available very quickly after the trial.

Clearly this system is not restricted to measurements of the BPD but can be used on any obstetrical ultrasound measurement: further it can be used in any ultrasound unit where very accurate measures are essential, e.g. measurements of the ventricle sizes in the neonate.

References

(1)   Deter, R.H., Harrist, R.B., Hadlock, F.P., Carpenter, R.J.,
       "The Use of Ultrasound in the Assessment of Fetal Growth:
       A Review", Journal of Clinical Ultrasound, Vol 9, pg. 481, 1981.

(2)   Campbell, S.
       "Early pre-natal diagnosis of neural-tube defects by Ultrasound"
       Clinical Obs.and Gyn. Vol. 20, pages 351-359, 1977.

(3)   Campbell, S.
       "Diagnosis of fetal abnormalities by Ultrasound", pg 431-465 in
       Genetic Disorders and the Fetus, Ed. by A Milnusky, 1980,
       New York, Plenum.

(4)   Hadlock, F.P., Deter, R.H., Harrist, R.B., Park, S.K.,
       "Fetal Biparietal Diameter : a critical re-evaluation of the
       relation to menstrual age by means of real-time ultrasound"
       Journal of Ultrasound in Medicine, Vol. 1, page 97, 1982.

(5)   Johnson, N.L., and Leone, F.C.,
       "Statistics and Experimental Design" Vol.II, Wiley, New York,
       1964.

(6)   Steel, R.G.D., and Torrie, J.H.,
       "Principles and Procedures of Statistics" 2nd Ed. McGraw-Hill,
       Kogakusha, Tokyo.

---o0o---

ATTITUDES TO A COMPUTER-BASED INFORMATION SYSTEM AND THE DECLINE OF PAPERWORK

Pirjo Hynninen
MN
Director of Nursing Services
The Health Centre of Varkaus
Finland

Attitudes towards computers held by physicians, nurses and ancillary personnel in five Finnish health centres and the impacts of the real-time computer-based information system Finstar on the working patterns of nursing and ancillary personnel were surveyed. The results of both studies are reported in this paper.

Attitudes to computer-based information systems in health care

A computerized information system will either decrease costs or improve productivety /3/. Whether or not the installation of an automated data processing system does produce desired impacts on productivity and costs depends on the extent to which users of the system are willing and capable of using it /3,8/.

Despite the apparent importance of understanding the process of personal adaptation to automated information technology only few studies of user adaptation have been conducted /3,4/. According to one of few reviews of reactions to the implementation of computerized systems in health care, resistance may emerge because of characteristics of the setting, the system itself and the people involved /3/.

Important personal characteristics appear to include attitudes towards automation; personality variables such as general acceptance of changes: age; education and occupational group /3/. Studies of attitudes towards computers have indicated that a favourable attitude increases with age and that men have far more positive attitudes than women /3,11,12/. Males' more positive attitude has been explained with the cultural stereotype of the woman as apt to be more easily threatened by technical devices /12/.

In the medical setting physicians and technical personnel have been found most positive towards computers, nurses and nursing students least positive and clerical staff in an intermediate position /3,5,12,14/. Ancillary personnel in various studies have exhibited lowest attitude scores /3,10,12/.

Educational level and length of the time working at the organization being computerized are positively correlated with attitudes towards computers /3,14/. At least some college education apparently fosters a more favourable opinion of computers, undoubtedly because that environment affords a greater opportunity to learn about computers and their application /14/.

In many studies it has been proved that bringing a staff into closer regular contact with computers, increased experience of automation and formal education have undoubtedly most contributed to the decrease of resistance of computerized systems /7,10,12/. The professional groups with none, one course and some computer experience achieved lower total attitude scores than did the extensive and daily users /7,10,13/. Educational programmes specially designed to provide information and understanding of computer techniques would be expected to influence attitudes towards computers in a positive direction /12/.

The decline of paperwork due to computer systems

Ranking of a computerized information system's benefits by its users showed that cost-benefit and the freeing of health care professionals from clerical duties were perceived as assets by more than 70 per cent of respondents /7/.

The reduction in clerical work of nurses was experienced so great improvement produced by an automated data processing system that nurses unanimously preferred the computer system to the manual /9/.

The cost of a computerized data processing system can be recovered in terms of saving of staff time or by the more effective use of resources /1,2,10/.

It has been estimated that 25 to 33 per cent of a hospital budget is spent in the acquisition and communication of information /2/.

Labour savings by a computer system may be even 95 per cent of the total cost savings, and nursing labour constitutes most of the labour savings /5/. Nurses have been found to spent up to 40 per cent of their time writing nursing records /6/. A study report states that before nurses used computers for their notetaking, charting time averaged 13 minutes per patient per shift and after the computerization only 6,3 minutes per patient per shift are required for this chore /15/.

Attitudes in five Finnish health centres

Attitudes towards the developing of information systems were surveyed in five Finnish health centres which were in different phases of installing the computer based information system. In the health centre of Varkaus a computer-based, real-time patient information system (Finstar) had been used for two years; in the health centre of Joensuu the Finstar-system had recently been installed. In the health centre of Espoo the installation of the Finstar-system was going on. A computer based information system for statistical functions had been used for years in the health centre of Raisio. The fifth health centre, Mikkeli "had not got touched" by a computer.

Attitudes towards electronic data processing were surveyed using a questionnaire, which included 10 variables of participants and 39 statements about the impacts of computer. The participants expressed their opinions on the Likert-scale. In the survey there were 715 respondents of which 81 physicians, 69 dentists, 112 public health nurses, 49 staff nurses, 326 assistant nurses, 78 orderlies and clerical persons. The real-time computer system Finstar was developed in the health centre of Varkaus and the staff strongly participated in the developing process. The change was not quick because the developing of the Finstar-system took three years and the staff had plenty of time and opportunities to get familiar with the computer system.

The distribution of attitudes showes that greatest resistance was manifested by the youngest (< 25 years) and the eldiest (> 55 years) groups, while the middleaged group (35-44) was the most positive in their attitudes (table 1).

Table 1. Distribution of attitudes by age groups (%)

	Age groups					
	< 25 (N=50)	25-34 (N=302)	35-44 (N=202)	45-54 (N=109)	> 55 (N=26)	Mean (N=689)
Positive	34	44	47	36	27	43
Neutral	16	17	18	18	11	17
Negative	50	39	35	46	62	40

Although in the literature there has been presented the statement that women are more disposed than men to resist changes /3/ there were no differences between sexes in this study (table 2).

Table 2. Distribution of attitudes by sexes (%)

Sexes		
	Women (N=643)	Men (N=70)	Mean (N=713)
Positive	42	43	42
Neutral	18	17	18
Negative	40	40	40

According to the results of previous studies the favourability to computers is related with the level of education, physicians being most positive in their attitudes /3,13/. In this study staff nurses presented the greatest amount of positive attitudes while the group of orderlies and clerical personnel with perhaps least education showed the greatest amount of negative attitudes. Dentists were more positive than physicians, who were most negative after the group of orderlies and clerical personnel (table 3).

Table 3. Distribution of attitudes by professional groups (%)

Professional groups						
	Physicians (N=81)	Dentists (N=69)	Public health nurses (N=112)	Staff nurses (N=49)	Assistant nurses (N=326)	Clerical orderlies (N=78)
Positive	37	51	44	55	43	24
Neutral	21	25	18	23	14	21
Negative	42	24	38	22	43	55

Only 27 per cent of the respondents had got education concerning computer techniques, but they were far more positive than those without (table 4).

Table 4. Distribution of attitudes versus education about computer techniques (%)

The amount of education about computer techniques		
	Without (N=523)	Little (N=182)	Plenty (N=11)
Positive	38	54	64
Neutral	18	16	0
Negative	44	30	36

The certain amount of favourability to computers can be seen in the attitudes of those who have got experience about working with computers. Of all participants 26 per cent had either little or plenty of computer experience and their attitudes were more positive than those without any computer experience (table 5).

Table 5. Distribution of attitudes versus computer experience (%)

The scale of the computer experience			
	Without (N=526)	Little (N=88)	Plenty (N=98)
Positive	38	42	66
Neutral	17	25	12
Negative	45	33	22

The positivism of attitudes was greatest in Varkaus where the personnel had had most time to get used to a computer. The greatest negativism was expressed in Mikkeli, where the staff had not had anything to do with a computer (table 6).

Table 6. Distribution of attitudes by the health centres (%)

Health centres					
	Varkaus (N=116)	Joensuu (N=172)	Espoo (N=230)	Raisio (N=64)	Mikkeli (N=137)
Positive	60	37	47	34	29
Neutral	16	21	15	11	23
Negative	24	42	38	55	48

The decline of paperwork

One of the most essential objectives of the Finstar-system was to decrease the time spent by nurses in data processing and to release them for more time to examine, care and councel patients for which their education has prepared them.

The division of the working time of the staff in the open health care in the health centre of Varkaus was surveyed before the installation of the Finstar-system in 1980 and in 1983 when the Finstar-system had been in routine use for two years. The purpose of the follow-up research was to determine the impacts of the computerized real-time patient record system on the work of the staff. Special emphasis was directed to the distribution of data processing tasks and the actual nursing care in the work of nurses. The survey of the nurses' working day and its comparison in various points of time will show, if the Finstar-system has been able to reach one of its objectives: to decrease the amount of time spent by nurses in data processing.

Although the whole staff except physicians and dentists took part in the research this paper illustrates only the results of the research concerning the nurses. The nurses belong to different groups according to their education. The groups and the years of nursing education or training within parenthesis are following: nurses (2.5), public health nurses (3.5), laboratory nurses (2.5), radiographers (2.5), practical nurses (1.5) and dental nurses (1.0).

The working day data was collected on premade form using a self-recording system. The tasks were classified in eight areas and included altogether 20 partial factors.

In the year 1980 altogether 61 nurses took part in the survey and in the year 1983 there were 80. There were 411 follow-up forms in the survey of 1980 and 502 for the year 1983.

The amount of time spent in data processing by a nurse was on the average 30 % (142 min) 1980 and 28 % (124 min) 1983 in a day. The amount of time spent in nursing care was, on an average 37 % (165 min) in 1980 and 40 % (177 min) in 1983 per day. The greatest amount of time spent by a nurse group in data processing was 218 minutes in 1980 while the mean of all nurse groups was 142 minutes in a shift per nurse. The change in the time spent in data processing varied among the nurse groups from an increase of 15 minutes to the decrease of 77 minutes the mean being the decrease of 18 minutes, which meant savings of three nurses' work per day in the health centre of Varkaus.

A very important nurse group, public health nurses, spent 25 minutes less time in data processing in 1983 than in 1980. While 23 public health nurses were participants in the surveys in both years (1980 and 1983), the savings in paper work changed to half an hour long patient visit mean 20 visits more per day and 4.800 visits per year in the health centre of Varkaus. A public health nurse used 25 minutes per day more in nursing care in 1983 than in 1980 and so she used the 25 minutes saved from data processing for nursing care. The mean of the increase of the time spent by a nurse in nursing care was 12 minutes. The greatest increase in the time spent in nursing care (57 min) per day was seen in the dental nurse's work.

The practical nurses assisting physicians in polyclinics spent the most of all nurse groups time in data processing (218 min per day) before the installation of the Finstar-system. Contrary to the objectives of the Finstar-system a practical nurse spent 15 minutes more time in data processing in 1983 than before.

Conclusion

Contrary to the results of previous surveys neither were the males in this study more positive than women in their attitudes towards computers nor was the favourability of the most educated staff group (physicians) greatest. Formal education on computer techniques and direct continuous exposure to the operations of the computer have also in this study been proved to influence attitudes in a positive direction.

Although the general objective to save time spent by nurses in clerical tasks was partly achieved by the Finstar-system a more remarkable change was expected than realized in 1983. Lack of formal education on computer technology and unwillingness to change working routines claimed to be characteristic of nursing personnel may be reasons of insufficient changes in nurses' working patterns.

References

1. Barker Marilyn, The Era of the Computer and Its Impact on Nursing, Supervisor Nurse, August (1971).

2. Carpenter Catherine R., Computer Use in Nursing Management, The Journal of Nursing Administration 13,11 (1983), 17-21.

3. Counte Michael A., Kjerulff Kristen H., Salloway Jeffrey C., Campbell Brune C, Implementation of a Medical Information System: Evaluation of Adaptation, Health Care Management Review 8 Part 3, (1983): 25-33.

4. Drachman R.H., Zukerman A.E., Becker M.H., Computers and Ambulatory Health Care, In Advances in Pediatrics 20, edited by I. Schulman, Chicago: Year Book Medical, (1973), 119-27.

5. Gall John E., et. al, Demonstration and Evaluation of a Total Hospital Information System, El Camino Hospital, Mountain View, California, National Center for Health Services Research, Rockville, December 1975, V.S. Department of Commerce, National Technical Service.

6. Kiley Marylou et. al, Computerized Nursing Information Systems, Nursing Management 7,14 (1983):26-29.

7. Klonoff Harry, Campbell Clark, Measuring Staff Attitudes toward Computerization, Hospital & Community Psychiatry 12,26 (1975), 823-25.

8. Lundeberg Mats, Goldkuhl Göran, Nilsson Anders, A Systematic Approach to Information Systems Development-I Introduction, Information Systems 4, (1979).

9. Mather B., Sherwood, Nursing Staff Attitudes, The Australian Nursing Journal 1,3 (1979): 20-22.

10. Melhorn J. Mark, Legler Warren K., Clark Gary M., Current Attitudes of Medical Personnel toward Computers, Computers and Biomedical Research 12, (1979): 327-334.

11. Miner John B., The Management Process. Theory, Research and Practice, New York 1973.

12. Reznikoff Marvin, Holland Charles H., Stroebel Charles F., Attitudes toward Computers among Employees of a Psychiatric Hospital, Mental Hygiene 5,1 (1967): 419-425.

13. Singer Joseph, Sacks Henry S., Lucente Frank, Chalmers Thomas C., Phycician Attitudes toward Applications of Computer Data Base Systems, JAMA 12, 249 (1983): 1610-14.

14. Startsman Terry S., Robinson Robert E., The Attitudes of Medical and Paramedical Personnel toward Computers, Computers and Biomedical Research 5 (1972): 218-227.

15. Viers Valdyne M., Introducing Nurses to Computer, Nursing Management 7,14 (1983): 24-25.

TRAINING NURSES TO USE COMPUTER SYSTEMS.

M.J. BARBER, Senior Systems Analyst,
West Midlands Regional Health Authority,
Birmingham, UK.

N.C. BAKER, Senior Nurse, In-Service Training,
North Staffordshire Hospital Centre,
Stoke-on-Trent, UK.

SUMMARY.

During the last three years Computer Systems have been installed in hospitals across the West Midlands region of the United Kingdom. In seven of these hospitals, computer video terminals (VT's) have been put onto wards and nurses have been trained to use them. This paper describes the methods the authors adopted to train the nursing staff so as to disrupt the day-to-day working of the hospital as little as possible, and in a way which would fit in with their existing professional duties and working hours.

INTRODUCTION.

In 1974 a computer system was installed at the North Staffordshire Hospital Centre (NSHC) to facilitate the admission, discharge and identification of patients (1) in a very large hospital complex (population served 460,000). Nursing staff in hospitals have to supply a considerable amount of administrative information as part of their professional responsibilities and at the NSHC this information was collected for the eight years up to 1982, via a computer system using a network of ward based datapens (which read bar coded labels) and teleprinters sited away from wards - each serving a number of ward areas. This system was experimental at first but eventually proved to be useful and effective, and in 1981 a decision was made to replace it by more modern equipment and extend it to other hospitals. The replacement of this equipment by a network of VT's and the extension of the system to other hospitals in North Staffordshire (2), made it necessary to train 1300 qualified nurses to use the whole range of computer transactions (3), and during 1984 the implementation of these computer systems in other hospitals in the West Midlands (4), has required the training of a further 600 nurses in two other hospitals.

STRATEGY.

A Working Party was set up by the senior Nursing Management in conjunction with the hospital Computer Department, consisting of two Ward Sisters, two In-Service training officers and a member of the computer staff. After much discussion the working party agreed on a set of aims and objectives i.e.

> The overall aim was to ensure that all nurses would be competent in the use of the video terminals and be well motivated in order to maintain 24 hour use of the system, and to ensure continuity and up-to-the-minute information.

The objectives were that each trained nurse would be able :-

(i)   to operate the video terminal on a day-to-day basis,

(ii)   to use the computer transactions to keep the hospital bedstate up-to-date,

(iii)   to make use of the information stored in the computer for queries e.g. Policies, Procedures, Drug Interactions etc.,

(iv)   to correct errors and re-record correct information.

The working party then set about producing a training package to achieve these aims and objectives.

DEVELOPMENT OF THE TRAINING PACKAGE.

INTRODUCTION.

The main considerations as the working party saw them were :

(i)   The design of the Computer System.

(ii)   Nurses attitudes to technology not actively beneficial to patients.

(iii)   Nurses professional responsibility for confidentiality and maintenance of patient records.

(iv)   Nurses flexible working hours.

(i)   The Design of the Computer System.

Any training package obviously has to take into account what the subject matter to be trained for is. The new computer system had been designed by an iterative process with computer development staff producing a series of computer video terminal screen formats, letting a group of nursing officers and sisters view them and try them out, and then, according to their reactions, the screen formats or the complete approach was changed till something acceptable to both sides was reached.

This produced a system which was workable for nurses within a general philosophy that all instructions or information a nurse might need while using the computer would be displayed by the V.T. This philosophy required that any computer user could request a 'menu' of available computer transactions as illustrated below:-

Transaction available to this terminal

```
1    IN      -   To accept a patient on your ward
2    OUT     -   To transfer or discharge a patient
3    INF     -   To input and view general information
4    RAP     -   Referral appointment for an inpatient
5    FAP     -   Follow up appointment for an inpatient
6    QU      -   Shows/Amends/Cancels outpatient appointments
7    QL      -   Shows a list of patients on your ward
8    QW      -   Shows patients present hospital/ward
9    QC      -   Shows patients present Consultant
10   QD      -   Shows patients registration details
11   QDIS    -   Shows summary of discharges/transfers
12   CANCEL  -   Cancels last action on a patient
13   CHCONS  -   To change a patients consultant
14   BEDSTATE -  To view current ward bedstate
15   FREEBED -   To view current hospital bedstate
16   WDLEAVE -   To record a patients ward leave
17   COL     -   To view messages sent to your terminal
```

Enter required number / e(X)it / (N)ext page '   '

The computer user selects the transaction required, then that transaction guides the user as to what replies are needed, and what to do next. The computer system thus produced was then used in some training exercises for a period of four months, after which time any difficulties experienced by those using it for training were taken into account and changes made to improve the system. On reflection we feel that this method of developing the computer system contributed a great deal to the simplicity of training, ease of implementation and, eventually, to its final success.

(ii)   Nurses Attitudes to Technology.

As a caring profession, nurses can be very suspicious of machinery but will gradually accept it if it can be shown that this machinery is activly helping to support the patients life or augmenting the quality of life in some way - e.g. Heart Monitors, Life support machines, haemodialysis etc. but a computer based information system does not fall into this category because it does not directly 'help' the patient in any way - nurses may feel it only helps the administrators and other staff.

(iii)   Nurses Professional Responsibility for
         Confidentiality and Maintenance of Patient Records.

The third very important factor to bear in mind is that nurses are bound by a professional code of confidentiality of patients information and records. We then ask them to use a system where this very information would be taken away from ward security and recorded on magnetic media in the 'Computer Department'. Therefore it was essential, very early on, to ensure from management, and stress to the nurses, that only basic identification details would be kept on computer and that no medical or private details would ever be divulged or added now or later.

Organisation of Training.

Before training started the question of responsibility for
the use of the computer had to be clarified. It is no use
training nurses how to use computer equipment if they feel it
is not part of their nursing duties. The Chief Nursing
Officer instructed all her staff that use of the computer is
an extension of patient documentation and thus part of a
nurses professional responsibilities. Those who instruct
staff were asked to emphasise this to all being
trained, so that it was clear to all nurses that the
training was necessary and useful, and not just a
polite exercise to keep hospital staff informed of recent
development in hospital technology.

(iv)   Nurses Flexible Working Hours.

The care of patients in a hospital is a 24 hour,
seven-day-a-week service. Any system of training for nursing
staff must be devised bearing their unusual shift patterns in
mind. The trainers must be willing to undertake the training
any time, day or night, to suit the needs of the nursing
service.

The Training Package.

It was decided to utilise the way the computer transactions had been
designed as mentioned above to make teaching a nurse to use the
computer terminal more like teaching a nurse any other skill on a
ward. This involved treating the VT operation as a "learning set",
so that training would move from simple to complex gradually to build
confidence. Time had to be allocated for practice so that the
required skill could be developed. As all staff take varying times
to become confident the training package would consist of a series of
self paced exercises related directly to their everyday working
environment with extra sessions made available to meet possible
additional needs. Any training should only give a minimum of
background information before practice starts and the training
exercises should be meaningful, that is, adapted to the circumstances
nurses are familiar with: the identity of the wards, type of patient
and consultant consistent with the wards, patients and consultants of
the hospital where they work.

Having experimented with various ideas a final package was agreed
and produced, consisting of three overhead projection (OHP)
transparencies, three practice sheets of typical ward activities, a
realistic data base simulating the real hospital situation on which
to practice and a booklet summarising the transactions and codes
required for reference. The essence of the OHP transparencies were:

    1.   Read what is on the screen.
    2.   Type in the reply asked for.
    3.   Press the "SEND" button on the VT.

The three practice sheets, each more difficult than the preceding
sheet were devised to include all transactions which nurses would be
required to use.

These were:

Practice Sheet 1.

Introductory exercises starting with the more easy to use computer transactions.

(Designed to take less than the 1½ hours allocated to allow for a short 10 minute introduction).

Practice Sheet 2.

At least one example of every computer transaction with some of the easier ones duplicated. (This usually took nurses the full 1½ hours).

Practice Sheet 3.

Several examples of each of the less common transaction with some of the simple ones previously learnt - for reinforcement.

This was more easily assimilated than sheet 2 because of the previous lessons, practices and familiarity and hopefully left nurses feeling that they had mastered the computer and felt competent to use the 'live' system.

Time required for Training.

We tried out the training package on a small group of nursing staff - allowing 4½ hours of training time in 3 x 1½ hour sessions away from the work situation in the computer training room. We found this to be successful and deduced that each member of staff would need a similar amount of time with some maybe requiring more to become competent. We also ensured that there was a suitable time gap between the installation of the VT's on the wards and the day the system went live to allow the training to reach all potential users. Training sessions were held mornings, afternoon, evenings and at night time to reach all staff during their hours of work.

Training Method.

A "Cascade" method of training was decided upon, that is, to train a core of nursing officers who would train the ward sisters responsible to them. The ward sister would then train the staff on their ward (qualified nurses) with the knowledge that the original working party were available for advice and help if necessary.

However, in North Staffordshire, this method did not work so well in practice, because, for reasons beyond their control, such as sickness, busy wards, holidays etc., the core trainers did not have time to fulfil this role and ultimately the bulk of the training was done by members of the working party with help from individual nursing officers who showed aptitude for training this particular skill. It did work better in the other hospitals in the West Midlands, partly because adequate time was made available and partly because the system adopted by the West Midlands Regional Health Authority was a simplified version of the original software.

CONCLUSION.

Having deployed this method of training with the reservations expressed above, it proved to be very successful judging by the fact that the system ran very smoothly from day one! In restrospect we realise, and indeed our own experience bears this out, that a small group of trainers responsible for training all staff was the most effective means of achieving our objectives. It was also an ideal means of keeping records of attendance at training. We were very pleased to discover during the training period that our fears about negative attitudes to computers on the part of nurses did not manifest themselves and in fact the nurses were most co-operative and interested in being involved in modern developments.

REFERENCES.

1.   Beech, P, Carmichael, M.R., Friend, J.H., Goddard, M.A., Mountford, G., Richardson, M.D., Sewell, W., The Inpatient System. Computers in Health Care. 1975, 69-106, Staffordshire Area Health Authority.

2.   Gossington, D.M. Amending and extending an existing Patient Administration System. The Impact of Computers in Nursing, Eds. Scholes, M. Bryant, Y, and Barber, B., 1983, 406-410, North-Holland, Amsterdam.

3.   Barber, M.J. and Smith, R.J. An Information System for Nursing use. Proc. Man/Machines Systems, 1982, 234-237, Institute of Electrical Engineers, London.

4.   Sargent, S. The Implementation of P.A.S. by the West Midlands R.H.A. Current perspectives in health computing. Ed. Barbara Kostrewski, 1984, 23-31, Cambridge University Press.

THE DEVELOPMENT OF A TECHNOLOGICAL
SUPPORTED NURSING COMMUNICATION SYSTEM

Dr. R. Trill
Forststr. 53, D 1000 Berlin 41

1 Preliminary note

The scope of the following representation is to explain some fundamental
ideas, which are important developing a technological supported Nursing
Communication System (NCS). Represented principles base on empirical
inquiries carried out in hospitals of Berlin in 1983 and 1984. A parallel
is likely to be drawn for the overall situation in hospitals of the Federal Republic of Germany.

2 The importance of communication processes in hospitals

Hospitals are very complex social organizations. In times of increasing
environmental complexity and competition between hospitals, also rising
costs and the necessity of keeping up with medical progress, the handling of informations (quality and quantity are both relevant dimensions)
is a basic function. Especially in the medical domain extremely high demands are set up regarding informations (particularly contents of information, operational area and representation). Wrong or inaccurate informations can bring irreparable damages for the patient. The problem of
information-management is able to be solved by supporting man by communication technologies (communication means transport of informations).
It will be the most essential task to support interpersonal communication
(most relevant in hospitals) by man-machine communication. The most successful method to build a communication system like this is the interdisciplinary systems approach(7).

The ward has to be seen as the central place of hospital activities.
Therefore the following explanations will concentrate to thinkings about
this subsystem.

3 The importance of communication processes on the ward

Communication processes on the ward play a substantial role. They are
important for

- relations between the ward and other subsystems of the hospital (e.g.
  diagnostic and therapeutic departments, administration, pharmacy,
  supporting services);

- relations among medical staff (nurse, physician - not mentioning communication difficulties due to status);

- relations between medical staff and patient (to this point the knowledges of medical sociology should be integrated in analyses).

The sequence mentioned above shows also the decreasing possibility of support by technologies.

In two empirical studies the author quantified the importance of communication processes on the ward. The aim of these studies was, first to collect informations about a subsystem, which is not explored very often and second to get a foundation for conceptional thinkings. One study took place in a large hospital with about 1200 beds and "Gruppenpflege" and the study for comparison in a hospital with about 530 beds and "Funktionspflege" ("Gruppenpflege" and "Funktionspflege " are two opposite systems for share care duties among nurses). In both studies the same method has been used (multimoment-frequency technique as an element of the work studies)(6).

Remarkable findings are written below (in the view of nursing personnel):

Of all nursing duties are (column I = results of study I; column II = results of study II; all statements in percentages)

	I	II
- pure communication activities	39.9	37.0
- combination of communication with practical work	37.1	30.7
- pure practical work	14.1	18.7
- absence	8.9	13.5 .

Another interesting finding (from study I; in percentages of all communication activities) shows the relevance of the communication partners of the nursing personnel:

- nurses did communicate with nurses	about	46 %
- nurses did communicate with patients	about	24 %
- nurses did communicate with physicians	about	8 %
- nurses did communicate with others	about	22 %.

It is important to mention, that there is no standard, especially for the communication with patients, to value these percentages. Two element of communication are not considered in both studies - the quality and the result of transported informations (there are three levels of possible errors: the technical, the semantic and the influential level)(4).

Study I shows also that verbal communication predominates (about 63 % verbal communication; about 37 % written communication). A special fact

which has to be pointed out here is that more than 50 % of the total
written communication happened between nurses. It was first of all the
documentation of practised nursing care. In contrast to study I the ward
visited for study II did not use a standardized nursing care documentation system. Therefore the percentage of written communication was much
lower (about 10 %).

4 Nursing care documentation as an essential work of nursing personnel

In contrast to the verbal meaning of "nursing care documentation" (documentation of pure basic and special nursing procedures), documentation
of medical procedures by the physician (in chart, formulars, anamnesis
and others) are kept. The latter documentation is mainly a comprehensive
medical documentation written by physicians. The documentation of nursing
procedures (setting of nursing care goals, nursing care plans, nursing
procedures) is relatively unstructured or even there is no documentation
of this kind(1).

While today the integration of medical and administrative data in a computer-based nursing care documentation system should not be problematic
(there are many realizations of computer networks in hospitals) the documentation of the professional nursing procedures still need comprehensive
preparation(3).

All ideas and solutions for the ward has to secure the improvement of
patient care, that means first of all to accept the significance of interpersonal communication.

Some objectives of an effective nursing care documentation will explain
its high relevance (for patients and nurses):

- guarantee of nursing care continuity (e.g. changing of shifts, absence
  of nurses);

- guarantee and improvement of nursing care quality;

- foundation for a (realistic) personnel-management;

- foundation for juridical security of nursing staff(5);

- possibility to collect new and actual informations for nursing research
  projects.

Considering the present state of development four levels of nursing care
documentation systems are classified as follows:

- level I   : no nursing care documentation;

- level II   : nonuniform nursing care documentation;

- level III : standardized and conventinal systems for nursing care do-

cumentation (german producers offer only a little number
of systems);

- level IV   : technological supported nursing care documentation system.

The author tried by inquiring all Berlin hospitals to prove the status
quo in relation of the levels mentioned before. Returning quotas of 64 %
from the responding hospitals in relation of 82 % regarding their numbers
of hospital beds give a quite reliable evidence, not taking into account
level I and IV (because no hospital can afford a non-documentation of
nursing care and on the other hand no hospital has achieved level IV
yet):

  25 % of the hospitals have a standardized, conventional nursing care
      documentation system (these hospitals only represent 19 % of
      the number of beds);

  28 % of the hospitals plan to realize such a system;

  47 % of the hospitals do not have such a system yet.

The following results show the relation between ownership of hospitals
and applications of nursing care documentation systems of level III:

common hospitals   14 %;

hospitals owned by churches
or other organizations   30 %;

private hospitals   20 %.

The results should be surprising, because of the considerable advantages
for patients and nurses. It has to be seen that every loss of information means a risk for the patient and a psychological load for the nurses.
On the other hand such a system opens the possibility to control the individual work load and the possibility to control the realization of
nursing goals. Another fear of some nurses base on the idea that a formalized system could "produce" unpersonal care.

Mostly the first step to develop a standardized nursing care documentation system was done by the nursing management. Some initiatives could
not come to a good end, because of objections by physicians.

5 Nursing care documentation by an EDP-system - a future task?
The questionmark points out the opportune and necessary doubts here. An
inquiry of hospital software producers in the FRG in autumn 1984 showed
that only one of the responding producers had such a modul in his offer
of programs.

In principle (and this was confirmed during many discussions between nursing personnel and the author) the engagement of an EDP-system is possible. Hardware is not the problem. The organization of this particular EDP-system into the daily routine of the ward will demand a lot of ideas and efforts(2).

Now, some conditions should be mentioned, which have to be taken into consideration as minimum demands developing a nursing care documentation system (maybe as a modul of a wide-spreaded HIS):

- the users (nurses) should be integrated in the development of _their_ system;

- nursing care has to be standardized intensively (this is no contradiction to individual or wholistic nursing care);

- before the implementation an extensive training has to be carried out (more than just the ordinary handling);

- the dialog has to be arranged comfortable and flexible (paying attention that the workload is not aggravated, that usually data entering has to be interrupted and that the nurses have access at any time retrieving certain informations-e.g. catering or menuplans);

- terminal(s) and printer(s) have to be placed close to the actual working area, but preferably at a place which can be locked (it is not possible to give a standard for the number of hardware components);

- the (essential) interpersonal communication with the patient has not to be limited (!);

- a personal control of work performance should not be done by non-nursing personnel.

In spring and summer 1985 moduls of a nursing care documentation system will be developed, talking into consideration the factors mentioned above.

References
(1)A.Bechtler/E.Köhler:Einführung der Pflegedokumentation,in:Deutsche Krankenpflegezeitschrift No.5/1984,p.285-288

(2)F.Dittrich:Computer in der Krankenpflege,in:Deutsche Krankenpflegezeitschrift No.1/1985,p.3-5

(3)D.E.Gagnon:Use of Automation in improving nursing efficiency and operations,in:World Hospitals Vol XIX No.4/1983,p.23-25

(4)R.D.Garrett: Hospitals-a Systems Approach,Philadelphia 1973

(5)M.Stoppel: Juristische Aspekte der Pflegedokumentation,in: Deutsche Krankenpflegezeitschrift No.4/1983,p.192-194

(6)S.Thiel/R.Trill:Kommunikationssystem des Pflegebereichs-Ergebnis einer empirischen Untersuchung,in:das Krankenhaus No.2/1984,p.61-65

(7)R.Trill:Design of a communication system for an efficient hospital, in:W.vanEimeren/R.Engelbrecht/Ch.D.Flagle:System Science in Health Care,Berlin/Heidelberg/New York/Tokyo 1984,p.747-750

COMPUTERS AND NURSE EDUCATION

R. A. Hoy

39 Congreve Road

Eltham, London SE9 1LW

United Kingdom

The micro-computer's ability to store, manipulate and process information makes it an extremely useful adjunct to the learning process, a point that was realised relatively quickly by educationalists within the general field, and by central government who allocated funds to prepare youngsters for the electronic age. Nursing, however, did not appreciate the full potential of computer assisted learning for, I would suggest, two reasons:-

Nurse education and training within the United Kingdom has been, in the past, and still is, very rigidly controlled, and is geared to an examination system to such an extent that the system controls education and training. There is a lack of computer literacy and expertise amongst nurse educators and nurses generally. This is changing and there is now a movement away from the traditional approach to teaching nurses, but the philosophy that student nurses are adults and therefore nurse teachers should respond to their needs, their past experiences and their objectives is some way away, as this presupposes a self paced and competency learning program, tailormade for computer assisted learning.

The potential that computers have for nurse education in the first instance lies in the ways that students can interact with the computer. This they can do in three ways:-

(i)   In drill and practice sessions designed to supplement regular teaching.

(ii) As a tutorial tool aiding the understanding of concepts and skills based on those concepts. The great advantage here is that the computer fulfills the role of a very patient tutor and does not get bored or upset with a series of incorrect answers and responses.

(iii) Through simulation or dialogue. This will enable the learner to experiment with and react to a given situation and then to review the outcomes of that intervention. This as a method will, I would suggest, move nurse education nearer to reality as students can initially become involved with a hypothetical patient, through a computer program, and can identify nursing problems, can test solutions and discover the results of the interventions without endangering real patients. Thus the learner can practise and monitor skills before being exposed to patients. This is an important concept in nurse education as any failure to learn could have life threatening consequences.

"Students can initially become involved with a hypothetical patient through a

computer program. They can identify nursing problems, test solutions and discover the results of their interventions without endangering real patients."
(de Tamway 1970)

Although the term 'computer assisted learning' is in common practice, the learner, in
reality, reacts with the program. If the program is designed as a self teaching program
allowing the student to move to more advanced work, or even to back track into a remedial mode, a give and take system can be identified which is learner controlled. Such
a system is a movement away from the traditional stance taken by nurse educators in the
United Kingdom which is based upon the supposition that all learners learn at the same
rate and in the same way. This has been disproved by work carried out in Banbury in
Oxfordshire where like groups of students were educated using two methods - the traditional method and mixed ability grouping. The latter allowed the students to explore
problems in their own way. The results showed that academically, as measured by examination results, there was no difference in achievement but that the mixed ability group
enjoyed their experience and were more committed to on-going education on leaving
school than were the 'traditional' group. There is a lesson here for nurses as nurses,
in the U.K., have not in the past been committed to on-going professional education.
Could it be that the training experience offered was stullifying?

As well as being a danger it is, I think, a stage that must be taken in the development
of computer assisted learning. I refer to rote learning. There is in any learning
situation, and nursing is no exception, a degree of rote learning that must be undertaken. The danger is use of the computer for this exclusively which will in effect
relegate the computer to the level of the old teaching machines that were all the vogue
a few years ago. I would argue that text books are cheaper than computers and that
there are enough of them about to allow the student to choose that which they prefer.
Having said that, there is a place for rote learning by computer which can give the
tutor more free time for the very important human interaction so essential in any
learning situation. It may be a criticism of nurse teachers in the United Kingdom
that they do not have a lot of practical credence. Could this be that we spend too
much of our time rote teaching that which could be learned privately? Would not the
planned use of the computer give nurse teachers more time for clinical practice and
research? Would this not make us better teachers and more effective teachers?

Before computer assisted learning can be used to its full potential two conditions
must be obtained:-

The collection of data on individual students. This will allow for some predictions
to be made and conditions to be allowed for when determining the types of interactions
that could occur when designing teaching programs and feedback sequences within those
programs.

Bundy in 1967 said:-

"The storage in the computer of all the relevant data related to a given student will
allow the development of a learning program that can select the appropriate learning
sequence that best matches the student. As the student works through the program
and responds actively to the material presented, the computer learns more about the
student and therefore will be able to modify and improve upon its feedback."

The identification of learning problems. Tutorial teaching via a computer program will
allow the tutor to obtain a print out of a given student's progress. This will enable
the identification of students with learning difficulties who require remedial teaching. This will also allow on-going curriculum evaluation determining whether the
course objectives are realistic or whether content or method should be changed. The
logical next step from this is the use of the computer in the management of learning,
which will allow curriculum parts to be converted into strategies for learning and
teaching.

The big question is:- Is this reality? I think it is but the concept pre-supposes
variations in curriculum time, curriculum content and teaching method, as these are all
interdependent, in order to meet the student nurses needs. It should not be forgotten
that the philosophy of nurse education will also change. This will effect the working
situation. At the moment trained staff have certain expectations of learners based
upon the training program in force within the hospital and training school concerned.
These, at present, do not vary a great deal from hospital to hospital, such is the
central control upon the curriculum, but in the future there must be considerable
change in expectation of skill and knowledge from student to student. Thus, will student nurses no longer be able to form the major part of the ward work force? The
financial implications of such a change will be considerable.

What then are the advantages of computer assisted learning?
(i)   As stated above, computer assisted learning lends itself favourably to the inde-
       pendent study approach to learning.
(ii)   Computer assisted learning can facilitate the development of a more creative
       and more flexible approach to problem solving within the learner. To my mind
       this is one of the greatest benefits that can be bestowed upon the teaching of
       student nurses, given the diversity of problems, physical and psychological,
       that the trained nurse deals with throughout the working day.
(iii) The computer is able to test, check, grade and keep records of the learning
       process. This means that tutorial time can be used more effectively. This is
       rather important as, at this time, there is a shortage of nurse tutors nationally
       which is having a somewhat detrimental effect to nurse training programs.
(iv)   The computer can be a good motivator as it will provide immediate feedback during
       the learning process. Should that feedback be negative, then this remains a

private interaction between the computer and the student. Thus it can be stated that the computer will allow more efficient learning. There is, in the United Kingdom, a high wastage rate amongst student nurses especially during the first year of training. Could it be that we as nurse educators are not meeting the educational, intellectual and professional needs of these students? If this is so, then perhaps the use of computers with good programs may reduce this loss of manpower and, indeed, money.

(v)   The computer allows a multi sensory approach to learning.

(vi)   The computer is consistently patient, fair and tolerant.

There are however a number of disadvantages that need to be discussed:-

(i)   The first of these is the cost factor. When considering cost, sight must not be lost of the cost of time. It has been said that it takes about 100 hours of programming time to produce 1 hour of effective teaching, but as expertise is gained this time can be reduced. The hardware costs are reducing all the time, but what is needed is research to show the number of machines required for student nurses that would allow effective teaching to take place. This takes us into the world of content control. If as stated above there is the very great investment in time required in order to produce good programs, there is the danger of leaving the production of such programs to the soft ware firms. They are, incidentally, becoming increasingly aware of the commercial potential of good software within schools of nursing. The danger that we are facing is to allow these firms to produce programs and then to use them in schools of nursing, building learning experiences around the programs. If this is to be allowed to happen, I would argue that this is the same as abdicating to these firms important decisions about nurse education which should remain within the hands of nurse educators. This presupposes that a partnership could exist between the expert programmers and the expert nurse educators. Without such a partnership, programs developed will become just another bit of course material, possibly meeting the needs of the programmers rather than the students.

(ii)   Tutorial Staff. The reason that I have placed tutorial staff under the heading of disadvantages is twofold:-

(a)   that teachers of nursing in the U.K. do not have clinical credence.

(b)   hitherto they have been dispensers of knowledge.

Thus, two questions are posed:-

Could tutors feel threatened when their role changes as change it must when computer assisted learning becomes reality and will they attempt to relegate the computer to a rote learning role, thus protecting their perceived role?

If the use of computers is taken up fully by schools of nursing, will this not give the tutors more time to teach the practical aspect of nursing where it is practised, that is in the ward and departments?

The answer to these questions lies partly in the training of tutors which must reflect these changes.

(iii)　Isolationism.　Schools of nursing within the United Kingdom are recognised as being independent units, a system that has led to the schools of nursing doing their own thing independently of others reinventing the wheel as it were.

(iv)　Theories of learning.　I place this under the heading of a disadvantage because some research is needed to determine how computer assisted learning does influence the speed, quality, retention and transfer of learning.　It can be argued that by grafting computers into a traditional system it will reduce their effectiveness as teaching aids.

(v)　The educational process.　Bloom, Nordaus and Hastings have suggested the following factors that should be considered when determining an educational program:-

Identify the overall goal

Devise a general plan

Analyse:　The learner's needs

　　　　　The teaching process

　　　　　Specific outcomes

Devise a detailed plan

Prepare the instructional materials

Implement and evaluate the programme.

Before this regime can be implemented the question must be asked, who are the learners and where are they to be found?

In the past learning has been the exclusive prerogative of those training to enter the nursing profession, little cognisance being taken of the need for learning after qualification.　Happily this trend is being reversed and nowadays the emphasis is on the concept that in the pursuit of knowledge all are learners.　For the purposes of the rest of this paper therefore when referring to learners we will be referring to all nurses, no matter where they be found.　Thus, the question is posed, will nurses be able to determine their own on-going learning needs.　Possibly in the past nurses have not been able to do this to any great degree and I would argue that this has been to the detriment of the nursing profession and its relationship with other health care professionals.　Given the flexibility of the computer the possibility of continuing education for all nurses becomes very real and very practical.　One big argument in the nursing profession is related, as I have already hinted, around the best place for learning to take place.　I don't think that many people would object to the answer to that question being, wherever care needs to be given.　The computer is ideal for this. Given its flexibility, and given its portability, but provided nurses are able to determine their own learning needs, it becomes possible to have learning programs devised to suit individual wards, departments or indeed types of patients, so that nurses will be able to key into training programs whenever they feel that it is necessary or whenever a problem arises.　Thus learning can become fully integrated with reality.　In order to achieve this more research is needed.　It does however bring

nurses of all grades into the area of programming for the computer. Such an approach
will mean that the learning process can continue long after qualification no matter
which branch of the nursing profession that the nurse decides to take but that that
learning experience can be meaningful to the nurse and can enhance the practical care
that needs to be given to the patient. Thus, the service to the patient will be
improved.

Although differing groups of nurses will have differing learning needs and a great
amount of intragroup variance, they will have one need in common, if they are to benefit from the use of computers, and that is computer literacy. Nurses practising in
the wards will need for example to be able to operate a terminal on their unit, department or ward, as will nurse managers, but the latter will need a higher level of literacy so that they will be able to operate programs that will make predictions for the
future given a set of circumstances. This means that the teaching of computer literacy
should start in the classroom during the nurse's period of preparation that is needed
in order to enter the profession. Can I at this point criticise the profession again.
Youngsters leaving school and entering schools of nursing are used to computers and
expect to find them within a school of nursing. The fact that they don't find them,
the fact that teaching methods may be outmoded could in some way account for the high
wastage rate amongst learner nurses already mentioned.

Computer technology will play an essential part in the education of nurses in the
future, but the central focus must be upon the minds of the nurses and not on the
machine.

"The role I give to the computer is that of a carrier of cultural germs or seeds whose
   intellectual products will not need technical support once they take root in an
   actively growing mind." (Papert 1982)

References

Papert S.   1982   Mindstorms. Children, Computers and Powerful Ideas.
                                      The Harvest Press.

Scholes M. (Ed.)   1982   The Impact of Computers on Nursing.
                                      North Holland Press.

Kotrewski B. (Ed.)   1984   Current Perspectives in Health Computing.
                                      Cambridge University Press.

Bundy R.F.   1967   Computer Assisted Instruction. Now is for the future.
                                      Audio Visual Instruction. Vol. 12, pg. 344-348.

Bloom B.
Nordaus G.   1980   Evaluation to Improve Learning.
Hastings T.   McGraw Hill, New York.

COMPUTER DEVELOPMENT AND THE NURSE AS THE ADULT LEARNER

Mrs. U. Jolly, SRN., SCM., RCNT., RNT., Dip.N(Lond),
FPA(Cert, Oncol(Cert), B.Ed(Hons), M.Ed.
Senior Nurse,
Research and Development,
Preston Health Authority, Lancashire.

1.   Introduction

Continuing Nurse Education is an attempt to assist the learners in the process of fulfilling their own potential or fully-functioning persons in their chosen roles. In a
context of continually growing knowledge of technology one cannot even by unlimited
extension of time in initial learning, kit-out nurses with sufficient knowledge, attitudes and skills to last them forever. One can, however, make learning an experience
from which the nurse can learn how to learn, and catch the desire to do so, leading
to a life-long education.

The opportunity to incorporate a system of information technology into the nurses professional work was the task of the writer as co-ordinator in a large Health District.
The discussion which follows incorporates an overview of education and training on
computers in nursing. Adult learning theory, and the writer's experience of the implementation of a system together with an evaluation and discussion. The chief assumption of the writer is that although the realisation of the adult potential has become
the sign of our times, we do not take account of this potential and enrich opportunities available to them.

2.   Computers in Nursing: An Overview of Education and Training.

In order to achieve the World Health Organisation objective "Health for All By The
Year 2000", the nursing profession need to utilise fully the new advancements in science
and technology. This was emphasized by Dame Catherine Hall in her opening address at
the Impact of Computers in 1982 (1).

If the Health Service is to benefit from the use of computing systems, personnel need
education in relation to knowledge, attitudes and skills. Nurses would then participate knowledgeably and confidently with their colleagues. The Health Service has indeed a deep interest in the introduction of new technology, but sadly the users do not
appear to have an adequate and systematic education and training. Barber believes that
computers are fast becoming a big influence on Nursing. He states that "Nursing Informatics must be pushed higher up in the professional consciousness of Nurses". (2).
In the past, nurses were unable to communicate the needs of nursing to the computer
programmers, and designers of machines. Berg believes that nurses have been brought
to implement systems without a grasp of its long-term implications. (3) In the

education of nursing students in computer technology Ronald has recognized issues such as differing cultures, and diverse settings. (4) But there appears to be no mention of the adult learner who is presently required to use a system with responsibility. Zielstorff indicates that the main focus in any hospital orientation programme is on how to use the equipment and the specific programme. (5) According to M.A. Sweeney very few nurses seem to be neutral towards computers. They usually elicit a strong positive or negative tendency. He claims that affective responses influence the cognitive and psychomotor domains. He has stressed that "Hands on" routine of exercises need to be planned by the instructor and the technical knowledge must be simple. (6). Startsman and Robinson's findings illustrate that the overall attitudes of Nurse Educators were positive. At least in relation to computer efficiency, and the importance in Society. The attitudes were least positive with respect to the willingness to use and accept the use of computers. It appears there were no significant differences in attitude based on the nursing programme, age or instruction time. (7). Virts in his concern for introducing a hospital-wide information system says that it is imperative to create an environment of acceptance, participation, direction, control, co-ordination realistic expectations, and a hospital/vendor relations. (8).

3. Adult Learning Theory.

Curriculum planners and adult learning theory suggest that adult education programmes are most effective when they are learner centred. The facilitator need to promote learning in a climate of mutual respect. The role of the nurse educator is intended therefore, to achieve this objective in an educational enterprise.

Adults influence the learning situation, therefore, it is the learning situation that one ought to be concerned. A learning situation is conceived with the identification of what is to be learned. Appropriate strategies for learning which involve the active conscious participation of the learner also have to be worked out. One then moves into the realm of teaching concerned as a system of planning, setting objectives, standards and devising methods which will help the adult to realise the goals set for him or which he sets for himself. Exactly how the objectives are identified is a complex issue. The writer is influenced by the views of Eisner (1969) that objectives are expressive and provides both the teacher and the learner with an invitation to explore, defer or focus on issues. It is evocative rather than prescriptive. (9). Both the adult educator and the adult learner are often concerned about trends in learning during adulthood. Adults tend to under-estimate their learning ability by over-emphasizing their early school experience and under-emphasizing their recent informal experiences. Knox (1977) (20) /0 indicates that in practice, adults perform substantially below their capacity. In 1963 Birron claims that social background, health and educational experiences are more effective in predicting learning ability than age. His work illustrated that certain intellectual skills concerned with cognitive and other significant learning processes are maintained well into the sixties and beyond by those who use it. (11) Bromley's work

illustrates the fact that the older adult experiences an increasing registration deficit. Their errors entail forgetting rather than mistakes. (12). Welford highlights
the view that much of the decline in educational performance by adults, reflect a
speed deficit rather than a decline in power. Thus reducing speed and emphasizing
accuracy. 13). Knowles (1978) rates the resource of highest value in adult education as the learners experience. (14). This view was illustrated by Carl Rogers
(1972) in that adult learning was self-initiated, pervasive, evaluated by the learner
geared to a quality of personal involvement and the essence was meaning. (15). Bruner
(1967) believes that adults are self-directing, and the adult education needs to engage in the process of mutual inquiry with them rather than transmit knowledge and
then evaluate the learner's conformity. He claims that adults become more autonomous
if they are permitted to think their way through to a new understanding. Personality
patterns established in childhood prevail in adulthood was highlighted by Zahn (1969)
(30). She indicates that those adults with strong feelings of powerlessness will fail
to learn and control relevant information. This review at least to some extent could
make the adult education aware of a positive approach to new technology and coping with
adjustment.

The System Development and Evaluation.

4:1 Terms of Reference:
The writer was appointed as co-ordinator by a large Health Authority to implement a
specific computer system for collecting, storing and using nursing information. The
time allocated for the system to be in readiness for operating 'live' was four months.

4:2 The General Objectives:
(a) To provide initial information of the system to all senior and middle managers.
(b) To provide information to members of staff organisations.
(c) To assist middle managers in the completion of personnel input documents of their
    staff.
(d) To ensure that all potential users were given 'hands-on' instruction/practice on
    the use of the visual display unit and printer.
(e) To ensure continued update opportunities.
(f) To ensure that the implementation of the system is phased in with ease.

4:3 Methodology:
The design was divided into three distinct phases. In the **first phase** the writer was
engaged in a process of open-minded familiarisation with the exploration of the specific
computer system. In the **second phase** the writer focused the inquiries as issues began
to emerge from the initial consultations which required sustained and systematic study.
In the **third phase** the writer clarified and interpretated issues during individual
training/learning sessions.

4:4 Schedule of Work:
The Schedule commenced with the computer system's Information Package being sent to all
middle managers. This was followed by scheduled discussion on a person to person con-

tact with a mean time of 1½ hours each. This decision was taken by the writer in order to assist individual needs as illustrated by Zahn, Knowles, Brüner and Tough. The objective of this decision was to introduce the concepts of the System, discuss and answer questions, allay anxiety in both day and night staff. 2,740 personnel input documents were given to the middle managers with written instructions on how to complete. These were checked and collated by the writer within three months. The completed information was processed by a Data processing bureau and 'keyed-in' to the System by a central team of officers within the next month. The Health Authority installed 8 visual display units and printers and 8 modems at different locations within the District.

4:5 Description of the Sample:

The sample for this study was 45 Nursing Officers, which included 30 female and 15 male. The age distribution of the nursing officers was 25-53 years. Those who worked on night duty were 6. Explicit individual differences ranged from mixed experiences, breaks of service and long experience in one area. The types of units that the sample worked were **General, Mental Illness, Midwifery and Community,** which included **District Nursing and Health Visiting.** 7 of the Sample had a knowledge of typewriting, 6 had piano playing skills, 2 played the organ, 5 experimented with Home Computers. To the writer's knowledge, not one individual had more than one keyboard skill.

4:6 Design:

All members of the sample were initially informed by the Senior Nurse Managers that commitment to the project was a requirement of their job. To understand how professional practice could be enhanced by the acceptance and use of computers was stressed by them. It is believed that this information had been received by the Sample with mixed feelings. The writer sent out a fact sheet of the computer system to all nurses. The Sample had no choice but participate with the new system. A carefully planned instruction sheet was prepared for the Sample. This included a log-in/off procedure, options, retrieval procedure, and use of the printer. Individual information on the principles and concept of the new System, keyboard skills and the application of the System in their own unit were of high priority in their learning sessions. All 45 members of the sample presented themselves for their learning. 20 sessions took place during the mornings, 23 sessions in the afternoons and 2 on night duty. The mean time for each session was 2½ hours, but this included an introductory period to make the individuals at ease, and a cup of tea/coffee according to the person's wishes, or when the writer identified a physiological or psychological limit. The 15 male nursing officers received their learning session at their work location due to difficulties of transport.

5. Evaluation

5:1 The Affective Domain : During and after the initial meeting of the writer with the Sample, the implementation of an automated system was generally perceived by them as threatening, and unrealistic in terms of their expectations. 30 respondents had neutral attitudes towards the new system. In 3 respondents it had evoked strong positive feelings and 12 displayed strong negative attitudes. At the end of their scheduled 'hands-on' learning session, however, 13 of the 30 respondents who were neutral had a positive attitude towards computers. They were most positive in their willingness to accept it and use it. In the 3 respondents who had strong positive attitudes, their interest in computer efficiency had grown. Of the 12 who displayed strong negative attitudes, 9 remained so; with their feelings most negative towards their willingness to use the computer, and their attitudes least negative towards it. The 3 whose attitudes had changed, were neutral towards the whole concept of computerisation.

5:2 Cognitive Domain: A needs-assessment survey would have been of great assistance at the commencement of this project. But this was not possible. However, the writer assessed the respondent's knowledge of computers qualitatively. It appeared that 36 had no theoretical or practical knowledge of computers generally. It was difficult to acquire the degree of knowledge of the rest. Therefore in planning and teaching it was difficult for the writer to cater for individual differences, such as varying the depth of content with the needs of the respondent yet maintaining a fruitful experience. Observation during the sessions indicated that all respondents had difficulties in concentration for long periods.

5:3 Psychomotor Domain: Throughout the instruction period the writer observed that all respondents were intense on accuracy at the cost of time. At the end of each initial 'hands-on' instruction period the writer assessed the overt behaviour of the application of principles: **(a)** logging-on to the system accurately; **(b)** logging-off the system accurately. The length of time taken to do so was not taken into account in this instance. It appeared that those respondents who were equipped with another keyboard skill were in the category 'good'. The writer believes that with these learners a transfer of learning may have taken place. It was interesting to note that those who were graded 'not good enough' were also the same individuals who had negative attitudes towards computers. The 3 respondents who were graded 'Excellent' were in the group who changed their neutral to positive attitudes after the learning schedule. Of the 20 who were graded 'good' 18 had their learning session in the morning, which may indicate a suitable temporal setting.

6. Discussion : Hospital organisations have been quick to make decisions on implementation at the cost of the individual in the organisation. Training of nurses at present is specific to a computer system as applied to the organisation. Trainers are selected not for their ability but to 'get the job done'. Inadequate preparation of the nursing staff affects the new innovation. The adult learners are unable to pace themselves to the new learning due to its urgency in operation of the system. Responsible investigators need to survey the opinions of individuals prior to initiation of computer activities. If discreetly presented this would arouse interest and perpetuate a feeling of genuine concern for the individual's opinion.

1. **HALL Catherine (Dame) 1983:** Perspectives in Nursing in Impact of Computers on Nursing - An International Review: Scholes. M., Bryant Y., Barber B. (Eds) ElSevier Science Publishers, B.V., North - Holland P.10.

2. **BARBER 1983 :** ibid - Computers Need Nursing. P.24.

3. **BERG C.M. 1983 :** ibid - The Importance of Nurses' Input For The Selection of Computerised Systems. P.42.

4. **RONALD J.S., 1983 :** ibid - Educating Nursing Students About Computers. P.248.

5. **ZIELSTORFF R.D. 1976 :** Orienting Personnel to Automated Systems. Journal of Nursing Administration. March-April pp. 14-16.

6. **SWEENEY M.A. 1983:** Computers and Nurse Education: Change and Challengers in The Impact of Computers on Nursing. Op.cit.

7. **STARTSMAN T.S., ROBINSON R.E. 1972:** The Attitudes of Medical and Paramedical

8. **VIRTS S.S. 1977 :** Introducing the hospital wide information systems to hospital and medical staffs. Medinfo 77. Shires/Wolfs (Eds) North - Holland Publishing Co.

9. **EISNER E.W., 1969 :** Instructional and Expressive Educational Objectives: Their formulation and use in Curriculum. AERA Monograph Series on Curriculum Evaluation. Rand McNally, Chicago.

10. **KNOX A.B., 1977 :** Adult Development. San Francisco. Jossey Bass.

11. **BIRREN J.E., 1963 :** Adult Capacities to learn in Kuhlen R.G. Ed. Psychological Backgrounds of Adult Education. C.S.L.E.A., Chicago.

12. **BROMLEY D.B., 1966:** Psychology of Ageing. Harmondsworth. Penguin.

13. **WELFORD A.T., 1975 :** Ageing and Human Skill: Oxford University Press.

14. **KNOWLES M., 1978 :** The Adult Learner - The Neglected Species. Gulf Publishing Co. Houston, Texas.

15. **ROGERS C.R., 1972 :** Freedom to Learn - Merrill. Columbus.

16. **BRUNER J.S., 1966 :**

17. **ZAHN J., 1969 :** Some Adult Attitudes Affecting Learning ; Powerlessness, Conflicting Needs and Role Transition. Adult Education: Vol. XIX. No.2 pp 91-97 Winter.

EXPERIENCE IN USING A COMPUTED-AIDED LEARNING PACKAGE IN A SCHOOL OF NURSING.

B Richards and A Campbell
Department of Computation
University of Manchester Institute
   of Science and Technology
Manchester M60 1QD
England

J Minshull
School of Nursing
South Manchester Health Authority
Manchester
England

Introduction

In the field of education, students have been familiar with learning
through reading books and listening to lectures. New on the scene is
learning through the video program. The advantages of the latter over
the long-standing book is that animation and film-inserts can be used
to impart information to the student. The advantage of the lecture
versus private study is that the lecturer, if he is so minded, can
pause in his lecture and ask questions of the class. In this way, both
the teacher and the pupil/student can discover whether the student has
absorbed what he has just been taught. With the computer, the occasion
arises to provide the opportunity for the student to interact with the
source of knowledge, or with the questioner; a thing he cannot do with
the television or the textbook. With computer-aided learning, one can
impart information to the student, quiz him or her, on the extent to
which that knowledge has been understood, and explain where he is going
wrong when he does not get the right answers.

The topic of this paper goes under many related but different, terms.
Thus we find Computer-Aided-Learning (CAL), Computer-Aided-Instruction
(CAI), Computer-Based-Education (CBE), and so on. What concerns us here
is Computer-Aided-Examinations in which the computer is used to examine
the student, to measure their performance by awarding a mark, and to
indicate where the student has gone wrong when incorrect answers are
given. With the computer, one can interact with the student on an
individual basis, giving him a personalised tutorial.

CAE In Nurse Education

Computers have been used in various spheres of education, ranging from
primary schools (nine and ten year olds), through to University students.
The task in hand in a School of Nurse Education is the same as in any
other area of education: if computers can help elsewhere they should
be able to help in nursing as well. The potential of the computer in
education has long been recognised, see for instance Tawney (1979) and
Rusby (1979), (1983). In nursing, progress has been made in the U.S.A.

with activities in progress since the late 1960's. The U.S.A. scene has
been admirably reviewed by Tymchyshyn (1983) and updated (1984). One
reason for the take-off of CAL in America has been the provision of
the PLATO system by Control Data Corporation.

The Present CAE Package

The package being described herein runs on a BBC-Micro-Computer equipped
with twin-disc drives and a printer. The package is truly CAE as
distinct from a computerised form of Multiple Choice Questions (MCQ)
in that not only does it test the student's state of knowledge but it
ensures that it comes up to par by the end of the test.

The System, the Manchester Computer-Aided-Learning in a School of Nursing
(MCALSN) provides a complete System for the whole School and records the
marks obtained by every student, on every course, after sitting each
Module.

The Modules

After every period of teaching, usually a two-week block, the students
can sit a Module of questions based on the knowledge they are supposed
to have acquited. A Module consists of ten questions. Each question
poses a ward situation and then asks the student to put into the
correct order, three of six possible, courses of action for the nurse
to take to respond to the situation described. Thus the student is
presented with a list of six possible actions all of which are usually
relevant to the situation. They must be put in chronological sequence.
The example given below will make this clear.

SCENE

Mrs Clare, a patient with severe anaemia is receiving
a blood transfusion as part of her treatment. During
your routine observations of her temperature, pulse
and blood pressure, you note a pyrexia and that the
patient is breathless.

The student has then to list her first three actions, in priority
order, chosen from the following list:-

A.   Report to the Senior Nurse.
B.   Reassure Mrs Clare
C.   Stop the transfusion
D.   Administer prescribed oxygen
E.   Tepid sponge the patient
F.   Change the infusion to normal saline.

If the student selects an answer not in the first three, the computer
will.respond, indicating this fact and giving the student an explanation
as to why his chosen answer is not correct. Thus, in our chosen
question, answer (E) is incorrect and the computer responds with:-

>   E.   Tepid sponge : Incorrect
>   This must not be carried out unless instructed to
>   do so by the Senior Nurse. Inappropriate tepid
>   sponging can lead to rigors and shock.

When the student finally gets the correct three actions, and in the
correct sequence, he or she is told why these three actions are
important and why each has that place in the sequence.

The student then completes the other <u>nine</u> tests in that Module. The
computer then tells him the total marks acquired, out of one hundred,
and then stores this total in the computer's memory, on a floppy disc
in fact. The computer is then left in a quiescent state awaiting the
next student nurse.

At the end of the period prescribed for students to take the test, the
Tutor can ask the computer to print out a list of students, showing
the date on which they sat the test and the total marks obtained..

The Students' View of the System

The student nurse approaches the computer and finds it in a quiescent
state displaying the MCALSN Logo. The student answers the questions
one by one. We note that the student cannot proceed to the next
question until the correct answer has been obtained, even though the
student may not collect any marks on that question if he has too many
guesses. If the candidate does not do too well, he may see a screen
similar to that displayed below:-

```
YOUR SCORED 40 MARKS OUT OF 100 ON
MODULE 8 WHICH IS BELOW AVERAGE.

YOUR MARK INDICATES THAT YOU ARE HAVING
DIFFICULTY WITH THE SUBJECT - PLEASE
CONSULT YOUR TUTOR FOR ASSISTANCE.

TO REMOVE YOUR MARK FROM THE SCREEN
PRESS <RETURN>
```

Results

The System has been used by several groups of trainee nurses. The reactions of the students are given below. A questionnaire was produced and issued to each student nurse after she had taken a test. A test normally takes about 15 to 20 minutes, depending on whether the student gets the answers right on the first attempt or not. One would expect a strong negative correlation between the marks obtained and the time taken.

On the questionnaire, the students were asked if they found the Computer System easy to operate. (They were only asked to press three letters followed by RETURN). Almost all the students found the System easy to use, even when they had not seen or used the System previously. This bodes well for the success of the experiment.

The students were then asked what they thought the benefits to Tutors would be if they, the students, were tested regularly by the System. The students thought that bringing the System into regular use would (a) Give the Tutors more free time whilst the learners get on with the test; (b) Let the Tutor know of your mistakes in private rather than before the whole class; (c) Help identify those students in need of extra attention; (d) Require less paperwork being done by the Tutors; (e) Provide a more accurate method of marking the students' work. These, and similar comments, suggest that the students see some benefit for the Tutors by the students sitting the computer tests.

The questionnaire then attempted to obtain the views of the Students regarding the benefits to them of the Computer System. Some recognised that being tested and marked so soon after the lecture course brought home to them how little they really had absorbed. The students also welcomed the style of the questions, since they, the students, recognised the need to get their priorities right, to get their actions into the right order. Another point recognised by the students was that, when seated before the computer, they had to make reasonably quick decisions - as in a ward situation, whereas the students were aware that when writing essays, they had much more time to think about things.

In contrast, one nurse said she welcomed the opportunity to play with the computer but felt that the course material would not help in her future nursing career.

In another section of the questionnaire, the students were invited to add their comments. One student thought that "the computer was very impersonal" and this was later explained to mean that the computer did not particularly care for her or her problems.

The view of the Senior Tutor to the exercise was that there was not an awareness on the part of the teachers of the need to help the students to put their actions in order of priority.

Conclusion

The Computer System clearly works and works well. There are several modules now in use and these can be made available for use elsewhere.

The System can be operated by non-experts and proves to be very resilient.

Finally, a new dimension has been introduced into the School of Nursing, one which is evidently here to stay. Clearly, CAE has a proven role to play in Nurse Education.

References

1.   RUSBY, N.J.   (1979)   "An Introduction to Education Computing"
                                 Croom-Helm.

2.   RUSBY, N.J.   (1983)   "Computer-Based-Learning - State of the
                                 Art Report", Program Infotech.

3.   TAWNEY, D.A. (1979)   "Learning Through Computers", Macmillan
                                 Press.

4.   TYMCHYSHYN, P.(1983)   "Nursing Education in the Computer Age
                                 in Retrospect and Prospect", in The
                                 Impact of Computers in Nursing,
                                 300-306, North Holland.

5.   TYMCHYSHYN, P.(1984)   "Computer Proliferation : An Experience
                                 to Share", in Medical Informatics
                                 Europe, 1984, Springer-Verlag.

THE RATIONALIZATION OF

EDUCATIONAL SOFTWARE RESOURCES

IN THE U K

Graham Wright

Nurse Tutor

Open Software Library

Education Centre

Warrington District General Hospital

Lovely Lane

WARRINGTON, England

History frequently points the way to the future. An appreciation of potential difficulties prior to implementing educational innovations can be afforded by scrutinising the nursing literature. Townsend holds that such an examination would provide some points for computer based learning (1)

The current interest in learning programs utilising computer technology has been likened to the popularisation of programmed learning and teaching machines such as the Bristol tutor, the demise of which seemed singularly related to a lack of valid cost effective software.

In addition a volatile market already exists in the U.K., as witnessed by the collapse earlier this year of Acorn Computers, despite the patronage of the prestigious B.B.C. educational programme. The educational implications of micro-computers in schools are now well established, and these in turn have caused a flurry of articles to appear in the nursing press, extolling the virtue of Computer Aided Learning (C.A.L) in nurse education.

Many authors (2,3,4) argue forcefully the appropriateness of selecting suitable software, before purchasing computer hardware. There remains, however, a dearth of educational software in spite of the large volume of published work regarding this area of computer use (5).

The principal generation of learning materials heralds from two distinctly different encampments: the commerce-based and the enthusiast. Many publishing companies have for years produced textbooks on a predominantly commercial basis. The plethora of low quality material is a reflection of the economic pressures which these companies face. Fortunately for the nursing profession notable authors emerge, seemingly at random intervals to justify the efforts of their patrons, who have in the past tended to foster quasi-medical rather than nursing texts. It is not surprising that computer software has parallel and interrelated developments with the written word. In the major geographical growth areas of computer use the emergence of commercially based and programmer developed C.A.L. appears to be following the same pattern.

In the U.S.A. commercial interest has been minimal because only a very limited number of major publishers have wanted to become involved in distributing educational software in the early stage of development (6). This has been tempered by the costs and related budgetary concerns, which are often determined on the basis of the traditional book publishing model (7). This in turn has allowed many small entrepreneurs to fill the demand with low quality material. This fractured cottage industry is dominated by enterprising programmers no educators (8). The situation has produced a lack of consistency in the overall quality of available programs.

This lack of direction, absence of assessment criteria and user ignorance has prompted an educational computer consortium director in the U.S.A. to comment "There is so much trash out in terms of software that it's very difficult for the teacher to buy intelligently" (9). Caputo called on educators in the U.S.A. to form a strong, educational network to take firm control of all areas of educational computing development (10).

Rushby (11) realised that finance may be perceived as a stumbling block to the integration and acceptance of C.A.L and in this light suggested that co-operative projects might be established to share materials and expertise. These philosophies have been upheld in a number of ventures in the United Kingdom. The Network of Users of Microcomputers in Nurse Education (N.U.M.I.N.E) formed in 1982 continues to encourage the exchange of information and ideas (12). Other groups involved in similar efforts include the Scottish Computer Liaison Group formed also in 1982, at the instigation of the Chief Nursing Officers (13), and the Nursing Specialist Group of the British Computer Society (B.C.S), which was formed in 1982 following the International Medical Informatics Association (I.M.I.A) Working Conference on the Impact of Computers in Nursing held in September, 1982 (14).

Early in 1981 the author realised that dissemination of information alone would not enhance the exchange of software amongst nurse educators (15). It was thus in 1984 that the concept of a voluntary software distribution network became a reality, under the title Open Software Libary (O.S.L) David McKendrick, a senior nurse and fellow member of the Warrington Computer Club (W.C.C) together with the author enlisted the help of colleagues from the W.C.C., Manchester Polytechnic, and other Schools of Nursing to collect, evaluate, register and distribute low cost software to nurse in the U.K. The first catalogue of material was published

in April of that year and has been reprinted at two monthly intervals to include
new material. In the past year the mailing list has been extended to include all
members of N.U.M.I.N.E and the B.C.S. Nursing Specialist Group, through both
organisations' newsletters. Although primarily an educational network the library
also includes programs which aid research (16)

As stated earlier one of the factors which has a great influence on the production
of educational software is monetary reward. Open Software being cognisant of this
facet of author motivation offers competative royalty rates. It is hoped however
that software writers are not pursuing C.A.L development for purely personal gain,
for they would certainly find more remunerative endeavours.

Authors who submit programs to O.S.L are asked to present flow charts and listings
of their material along with the user documentation and program, so that an initial
assessment can be speedily processed. Assessment is conducted on three broad areas
application, content and program structure by a nursing expert in the topic and
an experienced programmer from either the W.C.C or Manchester Polytechnic. Many
of these expert nurses are tutors from Schools of Nursing throughout the U.K who
have volunteered to evaluate learning material mostly using their own home computers.
If a program is rejected a full analysis of the problems encountered by the
evaluators is returned to the author, so that modifications can be made to make
the software comply with O.S.L standards. This can be via the authors or Open
Software's volunteers.

Four existing tools for program evaluation have been identified, CONDUIT (17) and
MicroSIFT (18) from the U.S.A and from the U.K. Protocols from both the Open
University (19) and the National Computer Centre (20). Although helpful none of
these Protocols is all embracing and the author is of the opinion that a specific
model for assessment is required to allow national standards of assessment to be
meaningful. The future of C.A.L requires nurses to learn from the past and direct
the authoring, assessment, distribution and evaluation of learning material. These
are similar logical skills to those which nurses use so well in patient care planning.
It is not necessary to be a computer programmer, designer or expert to be an
effective and realistic user of computers in education. Cobin (21) noted that
"the opportunity to influence the way computers are used in nurse education will
not come again", is fortunately still true, for the moment.

1. Townsend I. The Second Coming (Resurrection or Reservation?), Scholes M. Bryant
Y, Barber B, (eds), The Impact of Computers on Nursing, 1983, Elsevier Science
Publishers B.V. (North-Holland). ,:334

2. Mace S, Major book publishers are getting into the software business, Info World
4 (May 10,1982) 13-19. (Info World, 375 Cochituate Road, Box 880, Framingham, MA
01701, :13.

3. Townsend I, Norman S. Seven steps to success NUMINE Newsletter 1983

4. Rankin J, Koch B. Choosing a swift idiot. Senior Nurse 1 (36) December 5,1984, :21-22.

5. Wright G. Which Micro? Senior Nurse 1 (32) November 7, 1984, :10-12

6. Grobe S.J. Protocols for software selection, development and evaluation for nurse education. Scholes M, Bryant Y, Barber B, (eds), The impact of Computers on Nursing, 1983, Elsevier Science Publishers B.V. (North-Holland),:310

7. Steffin S.A. The educator and the software publisher: a critical relationship T.H.E Journal 9 (March 1982) 63-64. (Technological Horizons in Education, P.O. Box 992, Acton, Ma 01720),:63.

8. E.P.I.E. Report, Microcomputer Courseware-Microprocessor Games, 98-99m. Educational Products Information Exchange, Box 620, Stony Brook, NY 11790, 1981 ,:4.

9. Mirin S, Making the Most of the Microcomputer in Nursing Education, Scholes M, Bryan Y, Barber B, (eds), The Impact of Computers on Nursing, 1983, Elsevier Science Publishers B.V. ,:298.

10 Caputo, P. The Computer Industry and Education; The Issue of Responsibility, 1 (1): 1,6,7, September/October, 1980.

11 Rushby N.J. Selected Readings in Computer based Learning : AETT Occasional Papers Publication, No 5 London: Kogan Page, 1981.

12 Townsend I. A forum for educational computer users. Nurse Education Today 2 (6) 1984,:100-102.

13 Thompson B, Computer assisted learning in Scotland. Nurse Education Today 2(6) 1984, :102-104.

14 Editorial B.C.S. N.S.G. Newsletter 1(1) 1984

15 Wright G. Open Software Nurse Education Today 3(6) 1984,:138-139.

16 McKendrick D. Community Psychiatric Nursing data, Community Psychiatric Nurses Journal 4 (2) 1984,:5-11

17 Peters H.J. and Johnson J.W.. Author's Guide: design, development, style, packaging,review. (CONDUIT Co.P.O Box 388, Iowa City, Iowa 52244, 1981)

18 MicroSIFT: Evaluator's guide for microcomputer-based instructional materials. International Council for Computers in Education, Department of Computer and Information Science (University of Oregon, Eugene, OR 97403).

19 Open University Study Pack, Micros in Schools, 1984, The Open University, Centre for Continuing Education, P.O. Box 188, Milton Keynes, MK3 6HW.

20 Rothwell J (ed) National Computer Centre, Computer Based Training Library, Authoring Systems, Module 2, October, 1983, The National Computer Centre, Oxford Road, Manchester.,:125-129.

21 Cobin J. Combining computers with caring. Nursin Times Lecture 79, 1983,: 24-26.

Inger Sannes
Institute of Informatics
University of Oslo

WILL COMPUTER TECHNOLOGY LEAD TO MORE AND BETTER NURSING?
MAY NURSES DIRECT THIS DEVELOPMENT?

Professionals may influence and direct the development of their
own profession on condition that they know the technology that
is introduced. The "Florence-project" at Institute of
Informatics, University of Oslo, started July 1. 1984. The aim
of the project is to develop and disseminate knowledge about
how computer technology may be used as a tool in "proper
nursing".
The project is also aiming at giving computer scientists some
information on how they may develop tools in cooperation with
the professional groups using the technology, so that
technology may be adjusted locally by the professionals. The
project is organized and financed through the Scandinavian
research program SYDPOL (SYstem Development environment and
Profession Oriented Languages). The project group at Institute
of Informatics consists of 4 computer scientists, 1 social
anthropologist, and 1 nurse. Professor Kristen Nygaard is
responsible for the project.
Today many nurses are in contact with edp at work, but this is
often a technique having been introduced without their
participation.

THE WAY EDP IS USED IS IMPORTANT.

The users' experiences (positive and negative) depend on the
way edp has been introduced as well as on the technique itself.
Edp (or any other technique) that has been "forced upon" nurses
has often
- created opposition and
- created bad systems.
The opposition has often resulted in not very successful pilot
projects, where it is difficult to draw any conclusions of the
value of the edp-technique itself. The lack of user
participation has often resulted in systems not fit for the
users in their daily work. On the other hand, nurses whose
main concern is "proper nursing" should participate in
the development of systems to be used in nursing. There is an
evident **risk** that nurses whose main concern is edp (or
who are more concerned with technology than with nursing), are
those who develop systems for nursing.

WHAT IS "PROPER" NURSING?
When I have emphasized the importance of nurses being concerned
with "proper" nursing engaging in the way edp should
be used in their profession, I owe to say something about what
I consider to be proper nursing.

"The collaboration" between the one who receives and the one who gives care is probably the most important factor in nursing. I maintain, that "proper nursing" occurs when the collaboration is in such a way
1) that it stimulates good health,
2) that people being cut off from normal life because of chronical diseases, handicaps etc. experience life as good and meaningful,
3) that people being in acute or life threatening situations may experience confidence and calmness,
4) that dying people experience peace.
All persons providing such care "provide nursing" even if they are not trained nurses.
However, nurses have
a) a responsibility for **practising such care,** and they have
b) a responsibility for **developing and spreading knowledge** of which factors in this collaboration provide such results.
Proper nursing necessarily implies a consideration of the quantitative factors. It is the nurses' responsibility that all who need nursing are given care.
If proper nursing is provided to only a few, while the queue of those who need it increases, quality should be considered on the basis of the entirety. The application of edp should be considered on the basis of this.

WHO SHOULD DIRECT THE DEVELOPMENT WHEN COMPUTER TECHNOLOGY IS APPLIED IN NURSES' WORK SITUATION?
When edp-systems are introduced in nursing, certain work processes and aspects of these are emphasized. It is important to notice the risk that these aspects will awake so much interest and attention, that the most important qualities of nursing, those not suited for technology, are underestimated. Concerning employees in libraries, this dilemma is discussed in the LOFIB-report (Learning Oriented Tests in Libraries), no. 19/83, Work Research Institutes, Oslo:
It feels natural to draw parallels to nurses' work conditions. The way computer technology will be applied will vary according to nurses' attitudes of their job/profession, and the already existing work processes. **I therefore find it urgent to stress the importance of engagement, i.e. that nurses being concerned with providing proper patient service, caring and nursing, and who estimate the possibilities and constraints of technology in relation to this, are engaged in directing this development.**

DEFENSIVE OR OFFENSIVE WAYS OF RELATING TO TECHNOLOGY
The report "Sjukvårdsarbet och datorn" (Hospital Work and Edp) (ADIS RAPPORT 1983-10-05) discusses the problems met by health service when adjusting to computer technology instead of adjusting the technology to health service. "It is e.g. talked about computerizing health service instead of developing tools for health service by means of computer technology." (Author's translation.)
One of the reasons is, that technology is met defensively. One relates to more or less fixed information systems (as already mentioned), transferred from other occupations. Computer technology is introduced because "it has come to stay" and one may experience, that after all, there is no need for it in the work situation.

Professor Charles Stabel at the Norwegian School of Management claims in his doctorate paper from MIT, Boston, that there are different needs for computer technology solutions in professional and bureaucratic organizations respectively. In professional organizations, there is more demand for systems supporting the employees in taking better and quicker decisions (decision-helping systems, expert systems).
In bureaucratic organizations, computer technology will replace routine decisions and the manpower needed for such decisions. The initiatives and the decisions concerning the purchase of edp equipment are often taken at another level of the organization than the actual level where the equipment will be used (the bureaucratic level of the health organization).
In the Florence-project we have just finished phase I (September 1984 - March 1985). Through theoretical and practical education, the nurses at Voksentoppen have achieved an extensive basis for evalutating possibilities and constraints of computer technology. By seminars, excursions and tests of programs they have partly participated in developing, the period har led to interest, engagement and exciting ideas on how edp may be used as a tool for more and better nursing and treatment.
We have now just started phase II, continuing through 1985. As a result from phase I, the personnel at Voksentoppen are now more fit to choose computer technological solutions which may be supportive in the work taking place at hospitals.
Simultaneously, and in cooperation with the Florence-project, corresponding development work is going on at the medical front. Nursing and medical treatment are very close. The use of computer technology as support for nurses in their work should therefore be seen from a perspective taking the entire treatment service vis-a-vis the patient into consideration.

The aim of the Florence-project is not primarily to develop software programs for nursing and treatment, but rather to develop knowledge about factors of importance regarding nurses' possibilities to lead and be responsible for the development of their own profession at the introduction of computer technology. We pay special attention to three main areas:

1. HOW CAN COMPUTER TECHNOLOGY BE USED IN ORDER TO DOCUMENT NEEDS FOR NURSING - AND TO DOCUMENT WHAT NURSES DO.

a) Documentation of the patients' needs for nursing and care.
There is now a large input of resources and engagement in order to find simple, reliable measures to document patients' needs for nursing and care. In Scandianvia and the rest of Europe ideas to such registrations have been taken from different American systems.
Well-known is the "Rush-system" for patient classification, developed at the "Rush-Presbyterian St. Luke's Medical Center" in Chicago.
Since 1979 a more simple instrument has been in use at the catholic university hospital in Leuven, Belgium. Here, a system developed at San Joaquin Hospital, Stockton, California is used. It takes app. 10 minutes to register 30 patients.
The instrument gives only a rough estimation of the patient's need for care, but does however, illustrate the ward sufficiently enough to use it as a **basis for personnel planning.**
Only the need for and not the effect by nursing and treatment is registered.
It is possible, that simple registration systems, like the one used at Leuven university, provide just as good data as the Rush-system. The Rush-system may lead people to believe it is good just because it makes use of many categories (32, versus 9 in Leuven).

It may be valuable that the weaknesses are obvious, because it
creates improved consciousness concerning what is registered.
The above mentioned examples also indicate some dangers
computer technology may lead us into, because it is easier to
register large amounts of data than picking the essentials.
Demands to documentation of nursing- and treating- activities
should not necessarily be seen as negative. The demand stems
from a wish for fair distribution of resources, and is
therefore a positive challenge.
The instruments used for such registrations should not necessarily
be equal. A demand for common instruments may just as well lead
to a situation where some groups turn out badly, and therefore
become objects of injustice.

b) **Documentation and improvement of the nursing in practice.
     "Quality - assurance".**
In order to become "good nurses" it is important that we are
critical to the work we perform; if it serves the patient the
right way. Such a realization in the work situation may be put
forward when nurses make use of tools for constant evaluation
of quantity and quality of the efforts.
Granting institutions will gradually demand documentation also
concerning the quality of nursing and treatment. Demands for
such documentation by means of computer technology may easily
be misused, and lead to a feeling of control and supervision.
It should be presupposed that nurses are able to be responsible
for and have a certain knowledge of their work. Development of
knowledge and development in work do not happen through control
and supervision, but through a personnel policy where nurses are
believed in and made demands on.
The instruments applied should satisfy such demands, and should
be applied in such a way that this happens.
The demands do not only concern objectivity. The application
itself should stimulate more and better nursing.

c) **Enquiries**
The best source of information concerning how nursing and
treatment work, is the patient herself and her relatives.
Nursing is primarily offering correct treatment and improved
life quality during illness. Enquiries may give important
feed-back on how this offer is experienced, and whether the
patient has received the help and comfort he/she felt a need
for.
My experiences from using this instrument at Voksentoppen
show, that it gives insight and knowledge to the personnel
performing the work. It gives important information on what
should be adjusted concerning nursing- and treatment and the
organization of this. Here, edp may contribute to improvements.
Manual processing of enquiries is time- and resource-consuming.
Computer technology provides faster, cheaper and more secure
processing of large amounts of data with many variables.

2. **COMMUNICATION AND INFORMATION TRANSMISSION.**
   **HOW ARE QUALITIES LIKE SERVICE, COMFORT AND TIME FOR THE
   PATIENT INFLUENCED WHEN EDP IS INTRODUCED IN ORDER TO
   ORGANIZE WORK PROCESSES INVOLVING SEVERAL PROFESSIONAL
   GROUPS?**
Computer technology may influence the collaboration between the
one who gives and the one who receives care. This concerns both
the time nurses spend together with the patient, and the
quality of this contact. Too much attention may be directed
towards technology, as e.g. "monitoring screens" in intensive
care units may be examples to.

The time nurses spend on communication with and information transmission to other groups in the treatment team and institutions outside the treatment unit varies in different work situations. When computer technology is introduced in order to make communication and information transmission more effective, one should be conscious of such relations. Computer technology alone is often not sufficient. The way nursing is organized and cooperation within organizations are equally important factors to consider.

If many of the channels nurses use for information exchange are replaced with electronics, the basis for social network and hence cooperation may change. When new problems and challenges arise, it is difficult to assume that people who rarely see or talk to each other will cross routines and guidelines in order to help each other or solve new tasks.

"Intuition" and non-measurable observations are often important signals of a patient needing special attention, both medically and concerning nursing.

Computers cannot replace inter-personal contact, creativity and closeness to the patient, but may become important tools for nurses in order to spend more time on such qualities.

3. HOW CAN COMPUTER TECHNOLOGY BE USED IN RESEARCH, DEVELOPMENT WORK AND EDUCATION?

Computer technology is well fit for storing and treating large amounts of data, and thereby for the part of research- and development work concerning this.

In order to be meaningful, nursing research needs close collaboration between reality and theory. Paradoxically enough, research removes nurses from practical nursing, one of the factors being that treatment of data is time-consuming and comprehensive.

Through technology it is possible to combine work and research to a larger extent than earlier.

Language-use in nursing.

Computer technology limits and demands categorization of language. Research demands conceptualizations and clarifications. If nurses shall be able to make use of research results, language use and presentation should be similar to the language and concepts nurses are used to.

Computer technology and research demands a standardization of the documentation of the nursing process. Such a standardization may, if used correctly, make nurses conscious of their work and professional development. There is, though, a certain danger, that our richness of expresssions may be impoverished if exaggerated.

EXPERT SYSTEMS - SYSTEMS FOR WORKERS

Expert systems for nursing - medicine and other professions are today in use and are also being developed. These systems are being developed by an "expert group". The problem here is, that it may lead to an unfortunate professional development for the users. If responsibility for professional development is centralized, it may lead to a professional passivity among the workers. When developing new edp-technology one should be concerned with such relations. Thus it is important to develop edp-technology providing professional development in daily work. Professor Kristen Nygaard has in debates concerning knowledge based systems strongly maintained, that the responsibility for the use of such systems should be with the user. Consequently, the user has to both understand and keep control over the technology, and the knowledge base being used.

May Computer Technology Improve the Education Possibilities for Nurses?

Nurses' work- and duty-situation makes it nearly impossible to carry through good offers of education at the work place. There are now (especially in the United States) a lot of education programs on the market, meant for nurses in an education- or training situation. The periodical "Computers in Nursing" provides a list of such programs annually.

In an enquiery, leaders for different nursing schools in the United States (referred to in the book "Using Computers in Nursing"), assume, that computer assisted learning will occupy a considerable position both in educational situations and at the work place in 1-3 years.

Conclusion.

There should be paid special attention to several aspects if nurses are going to direct the development towards more and improved nursing, when computer technology is introdused in their work situation.

Little knowledge of what nursing is among those who make the decisions may lead to disastrous consequences for the treatment offered to the patients, and for the nurses' work situation.

Nurses, on their part, cannot expect their knowledge to be taken into consideration if not expressed. We have a special responsibility, not only to practice proper nursing, but also to disseminate knowledge concerning what leads to proper nursing and why this is important.

References.

1.The Research Program SYDPOL (SYstem Development environment
and Profession Oriented Languages)
NORDFORSK
Stockholm 1983

2.Omsorg som yrke eller omsorg om yrke
Hans Berglind og Ulla Petterson
Sekreteriatet for framtidsstudier
Box 7502
103 92 Stockholm
Stockholm, 1980

3.LOFIB Læringsorienterte forsøk i bibliotek
Tamar Berman
Arbeidsforskningsinstituttene
AI Dok 19/83
Oslo, 1983

4.Sjukvårdsarbete och datorn
Automatiseringar og Datoriseringar i Sjukvården
Rapport 1983-10-05
Stockholm, 1983

5.W.Sermus and H.Dierickx
Introducing an automated patient classification.
System for personell management in nursing.
in Medical Informatics Europe 84
Edited by F.H.Roger, I.L.Willems, R.O'Moore and B.Barber s.722

6.Sygeplejersken, nr.14 og nr.15, 1984

7.Sykepleien, nr.10 1984

8.EDB håndbok for sygeplejersker
Dansk sygeplejeråd
København 1979

9.Computers in nursing, 1984
J.B.-Lippincott Company

10.Using computers in nursing
Marion J.Ball and Karthryn J.Hannah
Reston publishing Company, Inc.
Reston, Virginia 1984

COMPUTERIZED NURSING CARE PLANS

H.B.J. Nieman
BAZIS, Leiden University Hospital
Leiden, the Netherlands

Summary

In order to organize and control patient care, nurses spend a great deal of time in recording and processing data.
Contents and volume of the nursing registration have been analyzed, in a surgical and a medical unit. Figures are presented on the administrative workload of nurses.
A further increase of the clerical effort is discussed, as well as the characteristics of nursing data.
A computer system has been developed, providing nursing care plans that should solve some problems related to paperwork and communication in the nursing unit.
The objectives of the project are described, as well as the concept and main functions of the system. Structure and contents of both standard and individual care plans are discussed. Attention is given to the limitations and benefits of the computerized care plan system.

Introduction

The BAZIS integrated Hospital Information System is being applied in over 20 hospitals in the Netherlands with together 11,500 beds. At Leiden University Hospital users communicate via terminals with a database that contains administrative and financial as well as medical data of 700,000 patients.
The real time system is available for 24 hours per day, seven days a week. The further development and support is organized in a cooperative structure [1].
The nursing applications, embedded in the HIS, provide functions in the field of nursing management, education, research and practice, for example :
- admission, transfer and discharge information
- student nurse and staff scheduling
- computer assisted instruction
- drug distribution and medication registration
- ordering of meals based on diet-date
- patient care classification
- personnel information
- online reporting of lab.test results, pathology reports, etc.
- online retrieval of nursing instructions and patient data.
At the moment, nurses use the inquiry functions of the HIS rather than the facilities for storage and processing of data.
The stage has not yet been reached that the HIS provides extensive support to the daily dataprocessing activities in the nursing unit, especially with regard to patient care. In order to explore the feasibility of computerization in this area, pilot-projects are being set up [2].
This paper reports on the development of a pilot system to support patient care and treatment, provided by nurses.

Volume of nursing administration

At the outset of the project the patient oriented administration of nursing units was analyzed. The results for a surgical ward of 34 beds can be summarized as follows :

Data	Number of forms	Registered by nurses	Data recorded per patient (%)
assessement, nursing/MD orders	5	3	16
reporting, charting data	6	4	37
worksheets	4	4	8
meals and medication forms	7	5	12
orders to ancillary depts.	18	9	25
miscellaneous	3	2	2
	43	27	100 %

In order to organize and control care and treatment of patients, over 40 different documents are used in the nursing unit; about 60 % is filled out by nurses.
Up to 100 data per patient are written on these forms, every day. The registration of one item on different documents is included in this figure.
The administrative nursing effort is focused on initiating and maintaining the patient file (Kardex) and patient's chart (50 % of the daily registration workload). On the chart, as a source of information at the bedside, 30 different items are recorded relating to the patient's condition, vital signs, treatment, medication, etc.
The communication with the service departments takes about 25 % of the administrative nursing effort.
Per patient approx. 7 forms are sent daily to other departments, e.g. laboratries, radiology and pharmacy.

These figures demonstrate the huge clerical effort, as performed by nurses in order to organize and document patient care.
The administrative workload will probably continue to increase, because :
- A patient is surrounded by a growing number of care providers, ranging from doctors and nurses to dietitians, clinical pharmacists and social workers.
  All these specialists need current and accurate patient data to make sure that the patient is given appropriate care and treatment.
  An increasing number of services are provided by specialized departments e.g. lab, physical therapy and radiology. Usually, nurses coordinate and provide the dataflow to these departments.
- Fast developments in medical science and technology and new trends in the nursing profession itself, cause an increase of the amount of data to be recorded.
- Due to budget constraints and the corresponding efforts to keep the quality of patient care at the desired level, hospital management needs more information.
  From the total expenses of the hospital, personnel costs take 70 %. Nursing personnel are about 45 % of all employees in an university hospital.
  So, data on nursing activities relative to patient care are important.
  Moreover, governmental organizations and third parties need information to direct their efforts to reduce the costs of health care. Finally, nursing management need data to promote and support activities in the field of nursing education, research and quality assurance.

Characteristics of nursing data

By analyzing the patient files we found some characteristics of nursing data which should be addressed when designing a nursing information system, [3] :
- Data change frequently, especially data that reflect the patient's condition and data, used in documenting basic nursing care.
- Information is needed on various locations and levels at the same time; this requires copying and re-arranging of data already recorded.
- Many abbreviations are used and there is a lack of standard terminology, to describe the patients progress and to record nursing observations and orders. Terms may differ by clinical speciality and nurse.
- Uniform patient files (Kardex) are introduced hospital wide, which might not meet the requirements of a specific nursing unit.
- Many nursing data are inter-related.
  For example : diagnosis oriented protocols are used that include information on intravenous therapy, medication, lab. tests and observations.
  By referring to these protocols the administrative effort might be reduced. However, present procedures and the structure of the patient file require the protocol data to be split-up and seperately recorded in different sections of the file.
- Patient files have become rather voluminous and inaccessible. However, to find out the patients progress and the results of the therapy, many care items have to be interpreted in relation with other data.
  To prepare the care to be given and to evaluate the care provided, data from various sections of the patient file have to be collected.
  Data are available in one fixed format only.
  Manual re-arranging and processing of data, stored in patient files is a time consuming activity.
- Many nursing data processing activities are repititious.
  For example : The admission of a patient and the pre-operative preparation, generate a series of routine administrative actions. The physicans order "next week lab. test X for patient Y, every day", may result in 7 requisition forms, labels, annotations in the patient file and 7 lines on the specimen pick-up list.

A computer system might solve some problems related to nursing administration and communication [4]. Especially, a great deal of the manual dataprocessing with respect to inter-related and repititious activities as well as the efforts to re-arrange data, may be eliminated.

Objectives

The care plan pilot-system is aiming at :
. A reduction of the administrative workload; freeing nurses from some paperwork so that more time will be available for direct patient care.
. Providing support to the communication on the nursing unit; especially with respect to shift changes, therefore enhancing continuity of care.
. Providing support to the further introduction of individualized patient care, based on the 'nursing process', which might lead to a qualitative improvement of care.

The 'nursing process' is a new approach in the delivery of care, in the Netherlands: Nursing practice is moving from task-based towards patient ortiented procedures. Whereas in the past a nurse performed certain tasks for all patients of the ward, at present a nurse provides the complete care for a limited number of patients.
This new way of nursing allows for following the 4 steps of the nursing process :
1. Assessment of the patients needs and problems

2. Set goals and plan the care to be given.
3. Provide care, tailored to the needs of an individual patient.
4. Evaluate the results achieved.
However, when performed with the traditional paper-and-pencil tools, the nursing process-approach requires a considerable, additional clerical effort.
Moreover, to apply this method succesfully nurses may have to change their attitude, skills and knowledge to some extent [5].
Guidelines are required on how to identify patient problems, to set goals and to evaluate the results of nursing actions.
The projectteam, with nurses of 7 hospitals and dataprocessing experts, decided that the computer system might serve as an agent for change. It should provide a tool to support the implementation of the nursing process.

The care plan system

In 10 meetings of the projectteam the functional specifications of the system were drawn up. The software development was done in 1984 and took 1 manyear. At this moment the system functions are being tested; in spring '85 the care plan application will be implemented on a limited number of nursing units, in 4 hospitals.
The care plan system-concept is shown below :

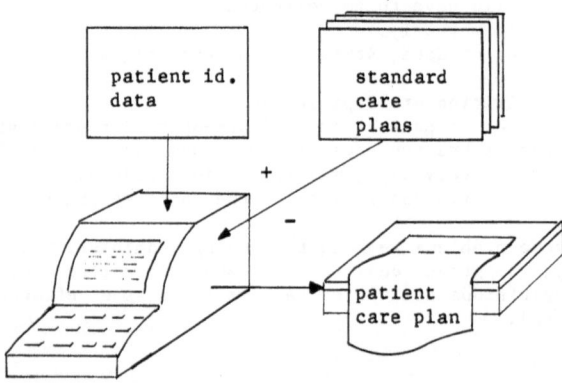

Nursing staff develops standard care plans, containing guidelines for care, based on e.g. a diagnosis, admission indication or operative treatment together with the sex and age of a patient.
These standard care plans are fed into the computer and stored in ward-based libraries.
An online function of the system allows for developing a patient care plan that shows the care to be given to an individual patient in 24 hours.
The planning process includes the following steps :
. Identify the patient on a screen, that displays all beds and patients within the nursing unit.
. Select the appropriate care plan(s) from an index, listed on the screen.
. Optional : review the information on previous plans for this patient.
. Select (problems) and modify data; add specific information.
. Print the patients care plan.

This approach implies that nurses find out to what extent the usual nursing care activities, are adequate for a particular patient.
By identifying patient problems and recording special items, as compared to the

standard approach, an individualized care plan can be produced [6].

The system provides some special features :
. Guidelines
  With an inquiry function, overall-information (admission period, duration of the operation) on each standard care plan can be accessed.
  Any item displayed on a screen will be further explained after typing a "?".
  The system is menu-driven, as to the main functions, and the options available are displayed on each screen.
  These facilities should reduce the instruction effort.
  It is expected that nurses will become familiair with the system's functions within a few hours.
. Reporting.
  In a free-text mode, vital signs, observations and specific M.D orders may be added to the patient's care plan.
  Items on standard care plans may be 'flagged'; as a consequence the reporting program generates questions that have to be answered i.g. just prior to a shift change. The data reported can be included in the patients care plans for the next days (optional).
. Long term storage of relevant data.
  All information on care plans can be retrieved online during the admission of the patient.
  A complete report may be printed in the nursing unit.
  When a patient is discharged, nurses identify the information to be kept in the computer. Other data will be deleted.
  So, information is available to authorized users, in case of another admission or follow-up treatment by the outpatients department.
. Questionnaires.
  With a special function, questionnaires can be defined to record data from, e.g the admission interview. Selecting such a 'computer-document' results in a series of questions on the terminal screen.
  Each answer may be identified to be printed on all care plans for that patient.
  Thus, all relevant information (allergies, protheses, patients habits) is available to each shift.

Structure and contents of care plans

In patient care plans the following data-sections are presented:
. patient identification (name, admission date, room/bed etc.)
. relevant information, collected in the admission interview.
. nursing goals (discharge criteria).
. reporting results (observations, vital signs)
. information derived from the selected standard care plan(s).

The care plan related information usually covers a certain phase in the hospitalization of the patient. For example : separate sub-care plans are designed for pre- and post operative patients.
Moreover, care items can be set on a specific day or period of time, e.g : "remove stitches on the 4th. post-operative day". That order will be displayed or printed on the indicated day only, i.e. some orders are cancelled automatically.
Thus, a patient care plan doesn't contain redundant and outdated information; it shows a set of current data, selected from standard sub-plans, that relates to 24 hours of nursing care.

The computer system allows for (combinations of) 3 different approaches in the careplan design :
1. Seperate care items may be grouped into broad categories, such as : mobility, dressings, hygiene and medications, tests, MD-orders that occur most frequently

in the nursing unit.
2. Checklists that include series of inter-related nursing activities with respect to a certain treatment/situation; for example : pre-op. care instructions.
3. Potential problems, information on nursing activities to solve these problems and expected outcomes that indicate the progress that has been made in the resolution of the problems.

To prepare for the implementation of the system a working-group of nurses, employed in various hospitals, was formed.
These nurses develop standard care plans and discuss the experiences obtained.
In future this group might coordinate the development efforts as well as the exchange of standard care plans between the participating hospitals.
The working group prefers the problem oriented approach, because it might provide major support to the further introduction of the nursing process.

Concluding remarks

In a joint effort of nurses and dataprocessing experts, a computer application has been developed that assists nurses in the production of care plans for individual patients.
The system provides legible and current information for assessment, planning, practice and evaluation of patient care. It might promote the use of standard terminology in nursing. The system supports the communication of care requirements, across shift changes.
A reduction of the administrative workload of nurses will be achieved. Data are registered only once; copying, with a chance for errors, is eliminated.
Some sections of the manually produced patient file will be replaced by computer output.
Relevant data remain stored in the database.
Care information is available online to authorized users on many locations in the hospital. The information can be accessed easily and fast.

The pilot system doesn't yet include facilities for :
. Extensive processing of data, for example : functions to select and present patient chart information, to produce task-oriented worksheets and to calculate the nursing care workload from care plan data.
. Automated transmission of data from the nursing unit to ancillary departments, for example : orders for lab. tests, drug supply and radiology appointments.

The project is considered to be an experimental development with a limited scope.
It should provide a tool for testing the feasibility of the care plan approach.
Thus, the basic functions of the pilot system were designed and implemented first, allowing nurses for the exploration of a new way of care delivery.
With the know-how and experiences obtained, further developments can then be discussed.

References

[1] Bakker, A.R., Organization of a cooperation for further development and implementation of an integrated Hospital Information System. Proceedings Medical Informatics Europe 1982, Ed. R.R. O'Moore et al., Springer-Verlag, Berlin, 1982, pp. 14-20.
[2] Nieman, H.B.J., de Stigter, W.C., Pilot projects on computer applications in the nursing practice. Proceedings Medical Informatics Europe 1984,

Ed. F.H. Roger et al., Springer-Verlag, Berlin, 1984, pp. 705-710.

[3] Grijpdonck, M., Automatisering van verpleegkundige informatie en communicatie :
een bijdrage tot de kwaliteit van de verpleegkundige zorg ?.
Acta Hospitalia, Ed. Blanpain et al, Leuven, 1983, pp. 45-56.

[4] Bakker, A.R., Mol, J.L., Hospital Information Systems.
Effective Health Care, Vol. 1, no. 4, 1983, Ed. F. Grémy, A.S. Mason and F.F.H.
Ruthen, Elsevier Science Publishers b.v., Amsterdam, 1983, pp. 215-222.

[5] Hughes, S.J., Developing a patient care planning system for automation.
Nursing Information Systems, Ed. M.R. Grier, H.H. Werley, Springer-Verlag, New
York, 1981, pp. 143-148.

[6] Mayers, M.G., A systematic approach to the nursing care plan.
Appleton – Century – Crofts, New York, 1978.

CONTINUITY OF NURSING CARE IN PRIMARY CARE IN FINLAND

ANNELI HALTTUNEN

HEAD NURSE
THE HEALTH CENTRE OF VARKAUS

The backround of the study

   Quality assessment of health services has been an important area in health care
research over the decades. The demands of efficiency and cost containment have guided
guality assessment in a prodominantly direction (Vuori, 1970). Only recently the
perspective of guality assessment has been broadened. Quality assurance has become an
intresting topic also in nursing research.

But there are certain problems in primary health care which make it difficult to assess the guality of care. It is generally diffucult to define the beginning and end
point of a treatment period or even a definite diagnosis. The documentation of information is not consistent. It is difficult to control the compliance of the patients
(Christoffel et Loeventhal, 1977).

The quality of health care can be defined by several means. American Public Health
Association (APHA) has defined the elements of "good medical care", used by e.g. Vuori.
There are: accessibility, quality, continuity and efficiency (Vuori, 1970, Vuori, 1982).

WHO has specified the three basic elements for the quality of care in a scientific-
technical sense: adequacy, efficiency and scientific-technical quality. According to
the APHA, when measuring the continuity of care, one should estimate the individuality,
and the degree of centralization and coordination of care.

Hennen considers the continuity of care one of the most important elements of primary
care. He considers accessibility, coordination and comprehensiveness, to be the basic
components (Hennen, 1975).

The continuity of care should be measured by the provider, geographical location and
timing of the contacts (Kekki, 1982).

Göran Ejlertsson has developed a continuity index which can be used to measure e.g.
the continuity of care in terms of a provider in a given period of time (Ejlertsson,
1978).

The purpose of this study is to measure the continuity of nursing care in ambulatory
health care and to estimate its quality.

The following questions have been selected:

1.   What is the level of continuity of nursing care in the Health Centre of Varkaus?

2.   Are there differences in the continuity of care between the provider groups
     (physicians, nurses, assistant nurses)?

3.   What are the shortages in documentation of patient data in terms of quality
     assessment?

4.   What are the possibilities to measure the quality of the nursing care?

Material and methods

The study is conducted in the Health Centre of Varkaus, which is responsible for the the primary health care of 33.000 inhabitants.

For the study all home care visits during the years 1983-1984 will be analysed. The total number of visits by all professional groups is about 27 600.

The continuity of care by providers is measured in this study using the continuity index developed by Göran Ejlertsson.

Information system

In the Health Centre of Varkaus a comprehensive computer based information-system, Finstar, was used routinely during the years 1983-1984 (Hosia et al., 1985). Information of all contacts between the providers and patients was stored in the computer memory and can be retrieved either individually or collectively. A traditional patient record has been replaced by an interactive computer system.

However, in the home care department of the health centre, encounter forms are still needed, because there are no portable terminals in use. A summary of every home visit has been entered in the computer which enables the follow-up of the home care using the Finstar system. Also all other primary care contacts of these patients can be accessed through the computer system.

In the Finstar system there is a subsystem for management and reporting which is used to select the patients and contacts relevant to this study. The basic data including the diagnoses, procedures, treatments etc. can be tabulated. A special program to calcutale the indices of the care have been added to the system.

Results

First results (May 1985) indicate that the continuity index in nurse and assistant nurse group is quite good.

The base of the continuity index is, how many providers (in this study e.g. in the nurse group) one patient meets during one year (Ejlertsson, 1978). The index number varies from 0 to 100. If the number is zero there is no continuity at all. If the number is hundred there is the perfect continuity of care (same provider during every contact).

In the nurse group the continuity index varies in years 1983-1985 between 77 and 73. In the assistant nurse group the same numbers vary between 77 and 88. There is no information about studies of the same kind to compare these figures in nursing research. However, the continuity index in general practitioners´ work in Finland was in a rural health centre only 41,8 (Kekki, 1982).

The final results will be presented at the conference. Also the possibilities to apply the presented method in other health centres will be discussed. The method is planned to use in other Finstar-health centres; in accordance to measure the quality of nursing care.

Table 1. The continuity index in different patient age groups in home care department
1983 in Varkaus Health Centre.

| PROVIDER | PATIENT AGE GROUPS | | | ON |
	< 65	65-75	76 <	AVERAGE
NURSE	63 (N=26)	81 (N=81)	77 (N=202)	77 (N=309)
ASSISTANT NURSE	93 (N=9)	82 (N=37)	73 (N=85)	77 (N=131)

Table 2. The continuity index in different patient age groups in home care department
1984 in Varkaus Health Centre.

| PROVIDER | PATIENT AGE GROUPS | | | ON |
	< 65	65-75	76 <	AVERAGE
NURSE	67 (N=27)	72 (N=67)	74 (N=171)	73 (N=265)
ASSISTANT NURSE	86 (N=18)	94 (N=36)	83 (N=66)	88 (N=120)

REFERENCES

Christoffel, T & Leewenthal, M (1977). Evaluating the quality of ambulatory health
care; a review of emerging methods. Medical care, 15:877-987.

Ejlertsson G (1978). Assessment of patient-doctor continuity in primary care. World
Conference of Family Medicine, Montreaux.

Hennen B (1975).Continuity of care in family practice. Journal Family Practice
2: (371-372).

Hosia, et al. (1985). Finstar-development, dissemination and maintenance of a Costar-
based information system in primary care in Finland.

Kekki P (1982). Potilashoidon jatkuvuus ja koordinaatio terveyskeskuksessa, Suomen
Lääkärilehti 24.

Vuori H (1970). Terveydenhuollon ja sairaalahoidon mittaaminen, Sairaalaliiton tut-
kimusosaston julkaisuja F:2.

Vuori H (1982). Quality assurance of Health Services, Public Health in Europe n:o 16,
WHO, Copenhagen.

World Health Organization (1967). The effeciency of medical care, Report of a symposium Copenhagen 1966.

THE THERAPEUTIC INTERVENTION SCORING SYSTEM (T I S S) COMPUTERIZED IN A CORONARY CARE UNIT

S. de Graaf, P.P. Kint and C. Schellekens

C.C.U. Thoraxcentre
University Hospital Rotterdam
The Netherlands

1. Introduction

The nursing staff of a Coronary Care Unit (CCU) are not only concerned with the day to day data on individual patients, they also need to know longer term characteristics of the case group they care for. Both bedside and administrative staff want to know such things as the average age of the patients admitted to the unit, the average stay in the unit, the workload at any time, the mortality rate and much more. Such information is not only time-consuming and tedious to collect but the analyses of the results are normally only available at a much later date and are seldom easiliy accessible to the bedside nurse. In addition, using personnel without critical care training to collect and evaluate the data does not often improve the reliability of results. We now feel that we have found a solution to a number of these problems which puts a very powerful tool in the hands of bedside and administrative staff alike. Both can now obtain immediate answers to many of the questions about our unit which have previously too often remained unanswered due to lack of relevant information.

The basis of our scheme is the implementation within the Coronary Care Unit of the Therapeutic Intervention Scoring System (TISS) developed by D.J. Cullen, using the central computer system available in the unit. The nursing staff themselves handle data collection and data entry, combining keyboard and mark-sense card input, and the data after validation is used to build a local database geared to the needs of the nurses. They also request their own analyses.

2. The Therapeutic Intervention Scoring System

TISS was developed by D.J. Cullen et al. at the Massachusetts General Hospital in Boston. Since its introduction in 1974, it has become a widely accepted method for classifying critical care patients. The system applies to 76 medical and nursing interventions, each of which is assigned a score from 1 to 4 depending on severity. For instance, an intubation procedure scores 4 points while ECG-monitoring scores 1 point. The sum of all points resulting from the interventions for a patient on a specific day is called the TISS. Using the TISS, patients can be classified into four classes:

Class 4 >40   points   Class 3 20-30 points
Class 2 10-19 points   Class 1 <10   points

Nurse to patients ratios can be assigned using this classification. Class 4 patients require a 1:1 ratio and additional help may be needed on occasion. A class 3 patient who requires intensive nursing but who is relatively stable can be paired with a class 2 patient and be managed by one critical care nurse. Four class 2 patients can usually be adequately cared for by one critical care nurse. Class 1 patients do not require intensive care, except for those admitted with a suspected myocardial infarction.

3. Data collection and data entry

We have designed forms for data collection. These forms are in two parts. The left hand part is used to record administrative data (patient registration, admission and discharge diagnosis, origin and destination) while the right hand part forms the mark-sense card. TISS items are marked in this section, which can be detached for entry into the computer. Each card can contain data on a single patient for up to twelve days' stay in the unit (one day per column), two continuation cards are allowed for long stays.

The administrative data are entered on the card at admission and discharge. The TISS items are filled out during the night shift around 1 a.m. New flowsheets are being made then and the nurse can easily check whether a TISS item was performed for the patient in the previous 24 hours. Collection time is therefore minimal, perhaps only one or two minutes extra. The final TISS points are collected when the patient is discharged from the unit.

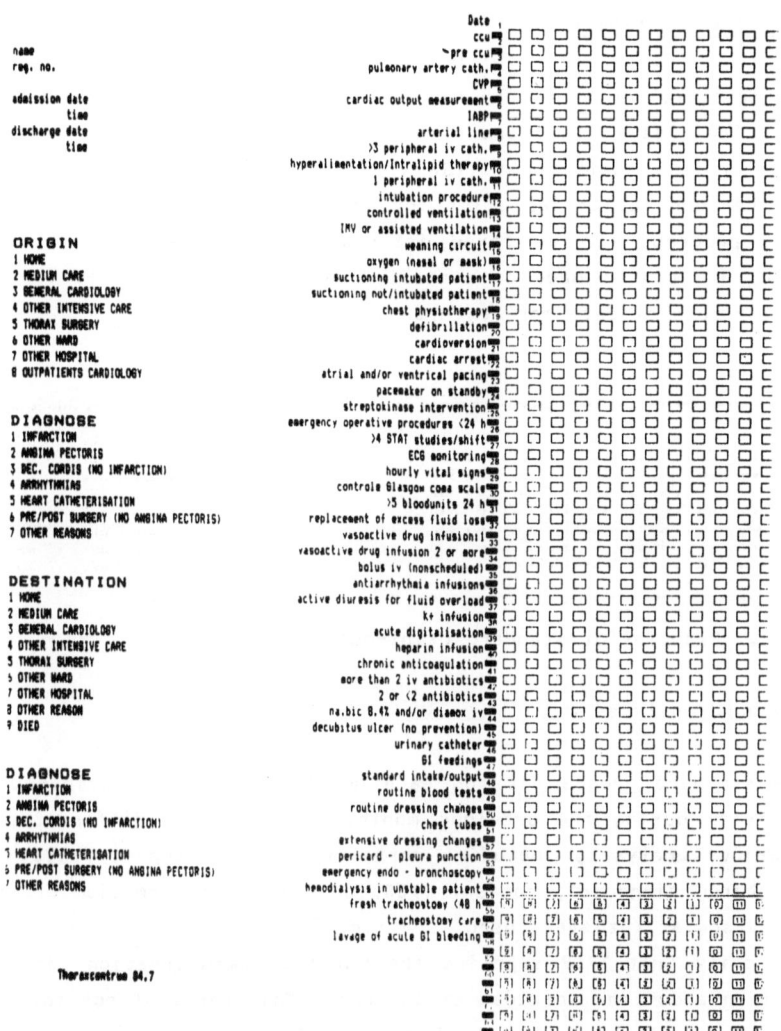

Figure 1. Mark sense card

The data are usually input immediately after the patient's departure. However this can be done later if time is short. The administrative data are input manually and the mark sense card is read using an optical mark reader attached to the terminal. Data is validated immediately and the nurse can correct errors and confirm unlikely items on the spot. The data are then stored directly in the database.

4. Use of the database

The database contains both registration and administrative data together with the 'raw' TISS items and derived data, such as patient age, length of stay, daily TISS, daily unit TISS (the total for the unit) and other parameters. Various facilities exist for analysing the data. Some of these are standard programs run at fixed intervals, others are run on demand. In addition, use can be made of central Thoraxcentre facilities for analysing particular sets of data for research studies.

REVIEW NR:10 ADMISSION TIME><WEEKDAYS <<CCU>> FROM 011184-301184 = 30 DAYS

89 CCU patients = 100%

	MON	TUE	WED	THU	FRI	SAT	SUN	TOT
0 ---- 4 hr	1.1%	2.2%	1.1%	0.0%	1.1%	5.6%	2.2%	13.5%
4 ---- 8 hr	0.0%	1.1%	0.0%	1.1%	1.1%	0.0%	2.2%	5.6%
8 -- 12 hr	2.2%	2.2%	4.5%	3.4%	4.5%	3.4%	3.4%	23.6%
12 -- 16 hr	4.5%	4.5%	3.4%	4.5%	4.5%	4.5%	1.1%	27.0%
16 -- 20 hr	4.5%	4.5%	1.1%	4.5%	1.1%	1.1%	3.4%	20.2%
20 -- 24 hr	0.3%	1.1%	2.2%	1.1%	2.2%	1.1%	2.2%	10.1%
Total average	12.4%	15.7%	12.4%	14.6%	14.6%	15.7%	14.6%	100.0%

REVIEW NR:22 TISS UNIT/SCORE><WEEKDAYS FROM 011184-301184 = 30 DAYS

	CCU	pre CCU	TOTAL
Monday	154.5	14.5	169.0
Tuesday	174.3	24.0	198.3
Wednesday	163.8	27.0	190.8
Thursday	129.6	22.4	152.0
Friday	124.8	20.0	144.8
Saturday	136.0	9.5	145.5
Sunday	123.3	10.0	133.3
Total	142.6	18.4	161.0

Figure 2. Examples of standard print-outs

4.1 Standard analyses

The standard program is run each month. It provides print-outs of the CCU activity during the previous month. There are 25 different print-outs with various analyses, including mortality rate, occupancy rate, admission and discharge diagnoses, patient TISS, unit TISS, information or the number of intravascular catheters used (see fig. 2).

The daily unit TISS supplies the nursing administration with important information about the workload of the unit. This makes it possible to employ more nurses at times with a higher unit TISS and so create a more stable workload for the unit.

The print-outs of mortality rates, diagnoses and interventions give the nursing staff useful insight into the patient population. They also make it easier to see whether any parameters change with time.

4.2 Individual information program

This program allows all nurses to create temporary sub-groups in the database and to analyse data from these sub-groups. For instance: questions like, "Is there a relationship between age and resuscitation procedures?"

or "Is it true that on friday afternoons a majority of our patients are referred from other hospitals?" could not be answered. Before we had this program there were a lot of speculations about the answers. At the moment we can directly check these questions on the ward which we feel is a great improvement over the previous situation.

Conclusion

The system at present in use was initiated in 1984 and contains nearly 1000 patient records (January 1985). While it makes use of the facilities already available in the unit for other functions (the computer handling most Thoraxcentre database needs, the optical mark sense reader and printer used for automated discharge letters and the terminals used for various purposes), the system itself was entirely developed by and for the nursing staff. It includes an extensive training program to help the inexperienced user, as well as elaborate cross-checking and validation.

The system has already become an important tool for both nursing administrator and bedside nurse in our unit. It provides us with a great deal of easily accessible, reliable information about our unit, our patients and our care for them. The possibilities of the system are still being explored. We do not yet know where they will end.

Finally, we are not only providing data for our own unit, we are helping to check the accuracy and completeness of the central Thoraxcentre database and hence the reliability of the computer-held patient records.

Literature

Coebergh, J., Pluyter, E.S.P.: Intensive care in het ziekenhuis. Tijdschrift voor ziekenverpleging 1982;15:490.

Cullen, D.J. et al: Therapeutic Intervention Scoring System: a method for quantitative comparison of patient care. Crit. care med. 1974;2:57.

Keen, R., Cullen, D.J.: Therapeutic interventions scoring system: update: 1983. Crit. care med. 1983;11:1.

Schwartz, S., Cullen, D.J.: How many intensive care beds does your hospital need? Crit. care med. 1981;9:625.

UTILIZATION OF A COMPUTERIZED REAL-TIME DATASYSTEM IN CHILDREN'S CLINIC OF HELSINKI
UNIVERSITY CENTRAL HOSPITAL

Ritva Tiikkainen, Assistant director of Nursing & Elina Lohva, Special nurse &
Marjut Nummela, Special nurse
Children's Clinic
Helsinki University Central Hospital (HUCH)
Stenbäckinkatu 11, 00290 Helsinki

Introduction

In Children's Clinic of the Helsinki University Central Hospital (as well as in the
whole HUCH) has the content of nursing, its documentation and nursing dependency
classifications been developed. After the start of the development of the computerized real-time datasystem for the patient administration in the outpatient departement of Children's Clinic in 1982, has the proportion of nursing staff been notable
in the development. The development has been done as project work with the ADP-office
and Children's Clinic and it is still continuing. The nursing dependency classification and the classifications of the external causes of the children's accidents,
which are included in the system, are developed by the nursing staff (Lohva 1982,
Tiikkainen 1982). Both classifications have been researched, the obtained results
have been evaluated and developed further. In this lecture will the computerized datasystem of the patient administration of the Children's Clinic of HUCH be represented
for the part of its content. Furthermore the system of classification of the nursing
dependency in the outpatient department of the Children's Clinic will be represented
and evaluated. The computerized datasystem of the patient administration in the out-
patient department and the opinions of the nursing staff before and after the introduction of ADP and has after one years use been evaluated. The results of this study
will be represented.

Outpatient department of the Children's Clinic

In the Finnish healthcaresystem the examination and care of children's diseases is
divided to health centre-, hospitalcenter-, centralhospital- and university-central-
hospital levels. The outpatient department of the Children's Clinic of HUCH operates
on all of these levels, though most of the patients need the level of demanding special care. The yearly number of outpatient visits varies from 34 000 to 36 000, which
means in the working days 150-170 visits, from which 25-30 are emergency cases. There
are 25 pediatrical and surgical subspecial consultations.

Computerized datasystem of the patient administration in the outpatient department of the Children's Clinic

Since autumn 1983 a computerized real-time datasystem for patient administration in the outpatient department of the Children's Clinic has been introduced step by step. The development of this system was made as a projectwork for the computing-section of HUCH and Children's Clinic. The users have also defined the data-content.

The system has been carried out by a PDP 11/44 computer installed in the computer-centrale of HUCH. For the use of the system 24 terminals were installed in the outpatient department and in two wards nursing dayhospitalpatients. The system involves following functions:

- dealing with dispatches
- programmes of the consultations
- appointments
- workinglists of the outpatient department and stick-on labels of patients
- registration
- admission of the wardpatients
- input of the visitdata
- display of the visitdata
- control of the patientpayments
- reports and statistics
- transfer of statistical data

In addition to the patientregister of the outpatient department the following supporting registers have been developed:

- population register, population under 17 years in the capital district
- commune register
- post office register
- institution register involving in addition to the names of the health-care organizations also the address-data of children-stations for consultation and school-health care in the district of HUCH and the address-data of educational institutions in the whole country
- titles for the reason of the visit, diagnose, treatments, nursing dependency classification
- accident-data system

The system also involves the background-data of the outpatients from the written nursing care plan.

Nursing dependency classification in the outpatient department of the Children's Clinic

The nursing dependency classification was developed in HUCH in 1977-1979 primarily for the bedwards (Tolvanen 1982). Since then this classification was developed to be suitable to measure the nursing care of the outpatients. In the outpatient department the patients nursing dependency has been measured continuously since the beginning of 1982.

The current system

The outpatient nursing dependency classification is aimed to measure the patient's direct nursing care, basic and special care and the time used for the nursing care. It is indicative of the nature and amount of nursing. Data on nursing dependency is based on assessment by the nurse. The assessment is based on professional knowledge and skills and has been written on the nursing care plan for the individual patient.

The basic care means nursing care given by nursing staff to help the patient on the area of the basic needs to manage his individual health care. If the patient because of his illness or another reason is not independent, the nursing staff helps him by necessary actions. They are by the dependency classification tasks which requires either much or little nursing staff resources. Basic care is described with four categorys and their symbols are the letters M, A, T and J.

The special care is nursing care caused by the patient's illness. It involves treatments ordered by the phycisian to be fulfilled by the nursing staff and nursing care which the nursing staff estimates to perform according to their competence. The special care is also described with four categorys, labelled 1, 2, 3 and 4. The amount of the special care increases from 1 to 4.
Both basic and special care take the patient's physical, emotional and social needs into considerence.

The time of the patient's care used by the nursing staff will be separately patient-relatedly measured in minutes and hours. Time spent for the nursing care of the patient is described with four categorys, labelled: 5 = under 15 minutes, 6 = 15 to 30 minutes, 7 = 31 to 60 minutes and 8 = over 61 minutes. They will be documented as real nursing time.
A category of nursing dependency involves always a criterion for both basic and special care and for the time spent for the nursing care, for example M 2/5, T 4/6, A 3/8 etc. Choise of the nursing dependency is directed by timefactors and factors of the nursing content.

The evaluation of the usefullness of the real-time data system

The opinions of the nursing staff were surveyed by two questionaires, from which the one was made before changing to the ADP system – during the manual data system – and the other after the new system has been used about one year in autumn 1984 (Nummela 1984). The nursing dependency classification has been evaluated by comparing the data of nursing dependency of the patient with the time reserwed in the consultations and in the emergency-rooms in March of 1982, 1983 and 1984.

In the research from March 1982 (Lohva 1982) the nursing dependency of children-sur-gical and pediatric outpatients was explained. At that time the aim was even to eval-uate the suitability of the newly introduced classification of nursing dependency and its developmental needs for measuring the nursing care of the outpatients in Child-ren's Clinic. On this grounds the nursing dependency classification was developed in such a way, that the time criteria used for the nursing care was separated from the criteria of direct nursing care, basic and special care. In 1982 and in the beginning of 1983 the nursing dependency data of every outpatient was collected on its own sta-tistical form from which the data was retroactively feeded twice a month into ADP in the Statistic office. In autumn 1983 the outpatient department of Children's Clinic gradually changed over to a realtime-ADP-system and at the beginning of 1984 the whole patient administration system had changed into a realtime-ADP-system. In March 1984 could all patient-related visitingdata have been fed into ADP from a terminal immediately after the visit by the persons of all professional groups. By comparing the materials before and after the realtime-ADP-system can the benefits and disad-vantages of ADP be evaluated from the point of view of the measurement of the nursing care.

Results

It has been investigated twice what the nursing staff thinks about the new datasys-tem and how they use it. In the spring 1983 (before using this system) and in the autumn 1984 (the new system has been used about one year). At both times the infor-mation has been gathered with questionaires. At the first time the object was the nursing staff of the outpatient department. The answered questionnaires were about 92 % (N = 36). At the second time in addition to this staff there were also some persons from other units. The answered guestionnaires were about 90 % (N = 46). The majority had positive attitudes to the system at both times, but the opinions were more positive at the second time (75 %/90 %; nurses 90 % and special nurses 100 %). No one would return to the practice before real-time data system in the patient ad-ministration.

As central results are represented: the main benefit was, that the appointment of the patients had changed quicker, more flexible and easier than before (mentioned by 30-50 %). 70-90 % of nurses mentioned that the service of customers in the out-patient department therefore had become better, because of the earlier data of the patient was easier to get with the new system. The customers could be better informed through letters (in Finnish and Swedish) anouncing the time reserved and giving ad-vices for the visit in the outpatient department or bedwards.

In the planning-phase of the ADP-system it was of great importance for the flexible function and trustworthy of the data, that it will be recorded where it is produced. Many different employers were participating in the dataprocessing during the patients visit in the outpatient department.

The personal-data is recorded by the clerk in the admission, the visit-data produced during every consultation - for example actions by the phycisian or the nurse, the accident-data, the medical diagnose and at least the nursing dependency scale and the names of the phycisian and the nurse participating in the care of the patient - are recorded by the nurse who is responsible for this consultation. Because there are too few terminals in the outpatient department it is necessary to use the forms for the visit-data. The majority (60 %) found the fulfilling easy. The data conserning the patients care is also documented in the written nursing care plan and the medical data in the medical record, both manually fulfilled. Recording the visit-data found 64 % from the persons, who answered, easy; about 70 % of them made the recording just after the consultation. They worked in the office (39 %) or where they found a free terminal (42 %). The visit-data should after their opinions primarily be recorded by the nurses (38 %), the clercks (27 %), children's nurses (23 %) and the phycisians (3 %). 9 % had the opinion, that everybody should record for his own part.

Inquiring, which other units besides the outpatient department should be involved in the ADP-system, were following units mentioned: the laboratory (18 mentions), the bedwards (14 mentions) and the action units (11 mentions). As the worst deprivations of the present system were mentioned the functional problems, too few terminals and some problems with the software and hardware. The greatest benefit mentioned was the easy using of the system (25 mentions). From the point of view of the nursing care it's notable that about 90 % of the nurses found the reports and statistics they got from the system usefull. They also mentioned many fields where the benefits were to be seen, for example planning the function, the assessment, planning, follow-up, evaluating the patients care and the development of the own profession. About 40 % of the persons answered have not noticed that they would have got more time to serve the customers and care the patients. In the first questionnaire about 33 % had wished that they would get more time to serve the customers and to nurse the patients.

The evaluation of the nursing dependency classification was made by comparing how in March 1982, 1983 and 1984 cared childrens-surgical and pediatric patients were situated in the different categories of the nursing dependency classification. In 1982 and 1983 the data was recorded into the system from the statistical form in the statistical office of HUCH. In 1984 the nurses recorded the data into the system in the outpatient department just after the consultations. In 1983 the content of the nursing (the symbols M-J and 1-4) was separated from the time criteria. The nursing dependency of the patients has been realized more steady in the different categories in 1983 and 1984 than 1982, when the same measure included the time criteria.

The nursing dependency classification in its present form may be suitable as one indicator to describe the nursing in the outpatient department. Different kind of statistics and reports produced by ADP will be used in planning the nursing resources and in allocating them in the unit internally. The nursing staff has positive attitudes to the ADP-system and wants to use and develope it further to serve the nursing.

References:

Hokkanen, E et al., Kirjallinen hoitosuunnitelma potilaan hoidon apuväline (Written nursing care plan helping in the patient's care), Sairaalaliitto 2/1980

Käsikirja kirjallista hoitosuunnitelmaa varten (Manual for written nursing care plan) HYKS 1977

Lohva, E, HYKSin polikliininen hoitoisuusluokitus (Outpatient department nursing dependency classification in HUCH), opinnäytetutkielma 1982

Roper, N, Current thought and practice in the assessment of patient/client needs for nursing care and methods/tools to plan for meeting the needs, WHO medium term programme in nursing/midwifery in Europe, Copenhagen 1977

Somers, J, Information systems: the process of development, Journal of Nursing Administration, January 1979

Study group on NIS: Computerized Nursing Information Systems: An urgent need, Research in Nursing and Health, Vol.6, 1983

Tiikkainen, R, Lasten tapaturmien rekisteröintijärjestelmän kehittäminen Auroran sairaalan lastenpoliklinikalla (Development of the children's accident registration system at the outpatient department of Aurora hospital), Kuopion korkeakoulu 1982

Tolvanen, S, Hoitoisuusluokitus hoitotyön prosessimenetelmän sovellutuksena (Nursing dependency classification as an application of nursing process), HYKS tutkimusjulkaisuja 1/1982

DECISION SUPPORT IN CLINICAL MEDICINE

A Critical Look at Some Critical Issues

by

F. T. de Dombal MA MD FRCS

Reader in Clinical Information Science
University of Leeds,
LEEDS,
England.

INTRODUCTION

The use of computers to provide decision support in clinical medicine is increasing rapidly. In contrast with only a few years ago, there appears now to be only two remaining schools of thought[1]. The first predicts widespread use of decision support systems when the crop of computer literate school children enter medicine. This is the pessimistic school! The second school holds that technology will insinuate its way into medical decision-making well before the close of the present decade. The latter groups cite as examples, the systems in the United Kingdom and the Unites States which are currently becoming available on a widespread basis.

It becomes relevant therefore at the present time to examine decision-support for clinical doctors; but to do so in a critical way, looking hard at the crucial issues involved. Such is the purpose of the present paper.

1. WHY DECISION SUPPORT?

Traditionally doctors are the source of much wisdom and indeed it is impossible to emerge from any study of the clinical diagnostic process without a profound respect for the ability of the experienced doctor to take life and death decisions under conditions of great uncertainty. Unfortunately, however when one turns to the study of inexperienced doctors, a very different picture emerges which gives no grounds whatsoever for complacency.

Acute abdominal pain, for example, is a common problem often dealt with on an emergency basis by inexperienced doctors. Recent national studies (in the U.K. and elsewhere) confirm that there is a less than 50% chance that the first hospital doctor to see a patient with this common problem will make the correct diagnosis[2]. Negative laparotomy rates range up to 60% in some countries and some centres[3], whilst the proportion of appendices which perforate before removal is almost as high in some hospitals[4]. It has even been claimed that around half of all deaths associated with acute appendicitis are preventable[5].

Given these disquieting facts which in no way support the "cosy" notion

that doctors are doing a grand job!, some kind of decision support seems
logical.   This is not a diatribe against the hard-pressed doctor, but
a sober appreciation of observed fact.

2.   WHY DO WE NEED IT NOW?

Current health care technology is in something of a shambles and we need
urgently to increase the effectiveness of its use.   For in the U.K. (as
elsewhere in Europe) we have a massive and compelling dilemma:-

(i)   The population is getting older and iller (rather than less
        ill as the founding fathers in the N.H.S. envisaged).

(ii)   Technology is becoming more expensive (as CT scans replace
        plain X Rays)

(iii)   Public expectations increase (not least as a result of the
        stunningly successful public education programmes on television).

These factors combine to make nonsense of even the most rational resource
allocation.   In this day and age it _is_ possible to spend more and get
less, and it _is_ possible to "inflation proof" allocations and still face
closures.   In the U.K. alone it has been estimated that we need to save
one billion pounds per annum merely to stand still and unless rapid and
effective action is taken then (to use current political polemic), the
N.H.S. is not safe with anybody.

The sheer scale of this problem implies that doctors performance levels
must be changed (since any other solution constitutes mere tinkering with
the problem).   Moreover, if these substantial changes are to be made then
it is logical to start at the point of medical decision, for if one can
support and alter methods of effectiveness with which doctors make decisions
then maximal impact may be expected both upon resource utilisation and
patient care.

3.   WHAT DECISION SUPPORT?

A number of proposals have been put forward for supporting clinical decisions

by some form of automated system.   Areas of controversy have emerged
and it may be helpful to look critically at some of them.

1.   Role of the Computer.

A variety of roles have been suggested for the computer.   These are listed
in Table 1.   By and large there is some resistance amongst the medical
profession to the use of a computer as a surrogate consultant and also towards
audit of their (traditionally somewhat mystical) practice.   More favourable
reaction has been elicited by the introduction of systems partly aimed at
educating inexperienced staff and partly used as "just another test", so
that the net effect is to aid the inexperienced doctor rather than replace
the experienced doctor.   Perhaps most favourable, acceptable and powerful
of all is the influence of the computer as a stimulus of good clinical
practice.

2.   Expert vs Probabilist Systems.

Much argument has been expended on this controversy.   The artificial
intelligence fraternity have strongly argued a case for decision support
systems to behave like an expert, dealing with large areas of clinical
medicine and offering a "consultative opinion".   In contrast, the
"probabilist" school of thought has argued quite forcefully that doctors
are familiar enough with numbers emerging from the laboratory, and that
a computer which merely produces a numbered probability certainly is not
only acceptable but preferable.   Currently this controversy is unresolved
partly as a result of the current lack of any acceptable comparative trial
between an "expert" and a "probabilist" system.

3.   Source of Data.

In contrast, it seems increasingly obvious that the controversy over the
source of data is fading.   The school of thought which proposed the adoption
of "expert thoughts" seems to be on the wane;   having been replaced by a
school of thought which proposes - as a basis for the computer's prediction -
data from a representative real-life source of similar patients.

4.   ARE SUPPORTED DECISIONS BETTER?

The U.K. has probably ammassed a greater experience of computer-aided

decision support in medicine- performed real time and involving real
patients - than anywhere else in the world.   The Leeds group's studies
alone have involved over 50,000 cases[6].

Actually there is now quite good evidence from a series of studies over
the past 15 years that in some fields of medicine the sensible use of
decision support packages can alter clinical performance quite rapidly.
The Leeds studies of acute abdominal pain constitute one good example
of this.

Preliminary studies in three U.K. hospitals[7,8,9] showed that the
diagnostic accuracy of junior clinicians could be raised from 50% to 65-70%
and the number of unnecessary operations reduced by about half.   Preliminary
data from a further national trial involving 17,000 patients attending
eight hospitals indicate the same trends.   Significantly, the three original
hospitals are still using the system and present results indicate comparable
findings even after ten years use[10].

The resources freed in these studies amounted to only around 10% of those used.
Nevertheless the nominal savings for the various hospitals concerned have
exceeded one million pounds per annum (and it should be remembered that the
acute abdomen accounts for only 1% of hospital admissions and the hospitals
involved serve only 2-3% of the U.K. population).   Clearly it is facile
to stick noughts on the back of the one million pound's worth of resources
saved.   The data however, do support the concept that relatively small
changes in doctors performance can be brought about relatively painlessly
and yet have profound effect upon resource utilisation and patient care.

5.   FOXGLOVES OR DIGOXIN?

It becomes relevant to question the modality of this improvement;   and
some possible means are suggested in Table 2.   First,   it is undoubtly
true that the use of a "stupid" computer system, which demands precise data
in a pre-agreed format is actually highly advantageous - for it forces the
doctor both into a disciplined mode of data gathering and to use a pre-
agreed and therefore common medical terminology.   Second, undoubtedly the
feedback which the doctor receives is effective in giving the doctor from
time to time some extra information to think about, and also in an educational

sense so that mistakes are not repeated. Finally, undoubtedly there is
an element of "big brother" about such systems, though their proponents
would prefer to refer to this latter element as a stimulus to good clinical
practice.

We are thus in a position to some extent of Witheycombe studying the foxglove.
We know that an improvement takes place but it is far from clear which of
the above modalities predominates - even if it is clear that no one modality
is singularly responsible. Thus to some extent we are administering
foxglove extract rather than a major dose of its active principal but this
is no reason for not administering the extract!

6.   HOW MUCH CAN WE SUPPORT?

Previous paragraphs have referred to the acute abdomen.   Various other areas
have been studied intensively, principally acute chest pain[11], jaundice[12],
dyspepsia[13,14], inflammatory bowel disease[15] and upper gastro-intestinal
bleeding[16].

As a result of these studies it seems reasonable to suspect that maybe
10-20% of medicine is supportable in the way described and with the results
listed.

7.   WHAT DO WE NEED?

The amount of research needed to bring this about is formidable.   For a
given area of medicine problems have to be defined with care, as do the
questions to be asked of each patient and even the disease categories.
Data collation must take place from a large series of cases to form the
computer's databank about a problem.   Wide and careful testing of the
resultant system must precede any use in routine clinical care.

From this it is apparent that both computer scientists and clinicians need
to provide their expertise and their experience in the short and medium
term future on a fairly large scale - to ensure the development is
co-ordinated, sensibly used and assists rather than replaces the caring

concerned clinician.   There is also considerable need for action both at
national and international level, for the problems faced are international,
and the solutions proposed should not be piecemeal.   Indeed, unless there
is international coordination to such effect (such as that of the World
Organisation of Gastro-enterology[17,18], there is a real danger of fragmentation
and dissipation of effort.

In terms of solving the problems posed by the explosion of medical
technology, re-education of doctors and decision support - backed by
emphasis upon cost containment and involving the sensible use of computers -
is thus the only alternative to compulsion or chaos.

TABLE 1.

Suggest Modalities of Computer's Role

Role	System	Reference
Consultant	MYCIN,	(19)
	INTERNIST	(20)
Audit	BANGOUR	(9)
Special Test	LEEDS	(2)
Education	LEEDS	(2)

- -

Stimulus to good practice	ALL	

TABLE 2.

Possible Modalities Responsible for Improvement in Decision-Making.

	Modality.	Derived from
1.	Disciplined data collection	Proformata
2.	Common terminology	Prior discussion
3.	Feedback (instant)	Computer
4.	Feedback (delayed)(educational)	Computer
5.	Audit	Subs. analysis.

REFERENCES

1. Editorial: Why can't a doctor be more like a computer?. Economist (1984) December 1 issue, p101

2. de Dombal F.T. Computers and the surgeon: A matter of decision. In: Nyhus LM (ed). Surgery Annual (1979a) New York: Appleton-Century Crofts, p33.

3. Lichtner S and Pflantz M. Appendicectomy in the Federal Republic of Germany. Medical Care (1971), 9: p311

4. de Dombal F.T. Picking the best test in acute abdominal pain. J Roy Coll Physns London (1979b), 13 (4) p203

5. Pledger HG and Buchan R. Morbidity and mortality from the acute abdomen. Br Med J (1969) 4,p466.

6. de Dombal FT. Computer-aided diagnosis of acute abdominal pain. The British experience. Rev. Epidem. et Sante Publ. (1984) 32, p50

7. de Dombal FT, Leaper DJ, Staniland JR, Horrocks JC and McCann AP. Computer-aided diagnosis of acute abdominal pain. Br Med J (1972), 2, p9

8. McAdam WAF. Computer-aided diagnosis of acute abdominal pain in a District General Hospital. Report to the Department of Health and Social Security of the U.K. (1978).

9. Gunn AA. The diagnosis of acute abdominal pain. J Roy Coll Surg Ed. (1976) 21, p170

10. de Dombal FT. Clinical decision-making and the computer: consultant, expert or just another test? Br J Health Care Computing (1984), 1, 1, p7

11. de Dombal FT. Evaluation of decision-making by humans and computers in acute abdominal and acute chest pain. In: Beneken JEW, Lavelle SM (eds). Objective Medical Decision-Making. IEE 1983. Springer Verlag, Berlin, p42.

12. Knill-Jones RP, Stein RB, Girmes PH et al. Use of sequential bayesian model in diagnosis of jaundice by computer. Br Med J (1973), 3, p530

13. Clamp Susan E and Wenham Janet S. Interviewing by paramedics with computer analysis: Gastro-intestinal Cancer. In: Rozen P and de Dombal FT (eds). Frontiers of Gastrointestinal Research. Computer Aids in Gastroenterology. S. Karger AG, Basel, Switzerland (1984), p186.

14. Davenport PM, Morgan AG, Darnborough A, de Dombal FT. Can preliminary screening of dyspeptic patients allow more effectiveuse of investigational techniques. Br Med J (1985), 290, p217

15. Myren J, Bouchier IAD, Watkinson G, Softley A, Clamp S.E. de Dombal FT. The O.M.G.E. Multinational Inflammatory Bowel Disease Survey 1976-1982. In: Studies Co-ordinated by the Research Committee of the World Organisation of Gastroenterology. Scand J Gastroent (1984), 19, Suppl 95, p1

16. Morgan AG and Clamp SE. O.M.G.E. International Upper Gastro-intestinal Bleeding Survey 1978-1982. Scand J Gastroent (1984), 19, Suppl. 95, p41

17. Bouchier IAD and de Dombal FT. Studies co-ordinated by the Research Committee of the World Organisation of Gastro-enterology. Scand J Gastroent. (1979), 14, Suppl. 56.

18. Bouchier IAD and de Dombal FT. Studies co-ordinated by the Research Committee of the World Organisation of Gastro-enterology. Scand J Gastroent. (1984), 19, Supp. 95.

19. Shortliffe EH. Computer-based medical consultations. MYCIN. New York: Elsevier, (1976)

20 Miller RA, Pople HE Jr, Myers JD. INTERNIST-I, an experimental computer-based biagnostic consultant for general internal medicine. N Eng J Med (1982), 307, p468

A CP/M BASED MICROCOMPUTER FOR OFF-LINE PROCESSING OF NUCLEAR MEDICINE IMAGES AND
TIME/ACTIVITY CURVES

D. Pearson and J. H. Todd,
Medical Physics Department,
City Hospital,
Hucknall Road,
Nottingham.
NG5 1PB.
United Kingdom.

Introduction

With the increasing use of computing to manipulate images and time/activity curves
in nuclear medicine it is becoming more important to have a programmable image processing computer available. Many of the manipulations are simple and do not require
vast amounts of memory or computing power. The aim of this work was to provide a
small, relatively cheap microcomputer that would process time/activity curves and
images which had been transferred by RS232 interface from non programmable gamma camera
computers.

Hardware

Any Z80 based machine with 64k of memory and a programmable serial port running the
CP/M operating system is suitable. Our minimum hardware configuration was an SMI
single board computer with a Z80B processor running at 6MHz, 64kbytes of fast, dynamic
memory, integral colour VDU with 160 x 96 resolution graphics, dual $5\frac{1}{4}$ inch floppy
disc drives, monitor and keyboard. An additional feature which was used to speed
processing times was a 256k silicon disc. Other additions were a printer and video
display system to display 256 x 256 images to eight levels of grey.

Memory Usage

Locations up to 100H are used as workspace and pointers by CP/M. CP/M starts at BC000H
and the intervening space is used as the transient programme and stack. F000H upwards
is used for disc support routines, leaving over 6kbytes of memory free between D61FH
and EFFFH. This is memory that will not be corrupted by chaining from one programme
to another and so was chosen to store images and curve data.

Operation

Serial data was transferred at 9600 baud using software handshaking taking 5s for a
64 x 64 pixel image. There is no requirement for high quality image display as processed images can be transferred back to the gamma cameras for display and output to
hard copy. A suite of curve analysis and image processing programmes have been written
in compiled BASIC with machine code subroutines. Image processing operations as complex as 128 x 128 pixel frame arithmetic are possible. Programmes are loaded onto
the silicon disc automatically on startup for fast access from one programme to the
next.

The cost of the basic system is around £1700.

INFORMATION SYSTEM OF THE CLINICAL CHEMISTRY
AND HEMATOLOGY LABORATORIES
IN THE UNIVERSITY CENTRAL HOSPITAL OF TURKU

Anne Kaitila   Liisa Nordman   Leila Simula

There is an information system for the clinical chemistry and hematology laboratories at University Central Hospital of Turku. The
system contains actions from test reguest to sending of results.
Statistics are also collected. The quality control is not yet taken
with the system.

The wards fill up the requests beforehand and send them to the laboratory, where they are fed into the files. The labels for the test
tubes are printed out before the sampling. The labels have an indentification number, which connects the patient and the samples. After
the sampling the laboratorytechnician confirms the samples taken and
rejects the samples not obtained. The samples are analyzed according
to the working sheet produced by the computer. After the analyses
have been done the results are added on the working sheets manually
or automatically, accepted and stored to the patient file.

The results of urgent tests are sent as rapid results either directly
to the printer in a ward or they are printed in the ADP department
or in the laboratory and sent to the wards immediately.

The daily reports are produced twice a day, the first one contains
results of the day and in the other are listed in addition all the
requests nor yet analyzed.

A cumulative report is produced daily. It is summary of the analyses
and results of a certain patient during the present treatment period.

The system was taken into use in 1982 first for feeding in the
requests and production of labels. In the year 1984 daily reports
and rapid results have been produced to the wards. The system will
have greater coverage after the wards and out-patient departments
are connected with more terminals.

The system is running on PDP 11/44 MUMPS stand-alone system, which
is connected with the patient record system in the central
computer (VAX 11/750).

EEG SLEEP PATTERN RECOGNITION BY CLUSTER ANALYSIS

P.Grass and H.Fruhstorfer
Institute of Physiology
D-3550 Marburg / FRG

The sleep EEG is a highly individual signal containing an abundance of different patterns; atypical EEG patterns may additionally appear under the influence of psychopharmaca, stress, pain and other stimuli. Therefore a dynamical classification scheme, free of a priori assumptions of universally valid sleep states, is indicated for sleep analysis permitting also the detection of unknown patterns. The main features of the EEG are the power and coherence spectra; they form a timevariing vector that moves through the feature space during night. A principal component transformation is performed in order to reduce the dimension of the vector space and to minimize the correlations between the variables. The grouping process of the transformed data is iterative; for an increasing number of groups a nonhierarchical cluster analysis in combination with discriminant analysis is performed to evaluate the amount of really separable clusters. The sleep states are defined by the location in the feature space, the covariance matrices, the realisation and transition probabilities. Once the individual sleep states are defined they are used as a basis set for the classification of data from further nights of the same subject. The allocation of a vector to a known sleep state is determined by the smallest Mahalanobis distance on condition that the constraints of homogeneity are not violated. Otherwise the vector is marked as a potential element of a new, hitherto unknown group which has to be set up if more similar vectors occur. Thus, the capability of this classification algorithm is not restricted to the sleep states of the basis set, but it is able to detect new patterns. Additionally it is possible to define EEG states in advance by the declaration of the cluster centers and covariance matrices of patterns which are of special interest. Until now this method has been employed in two studies on the effects of daytime stress on night sleep; altogether 94 sleep EEGs of 19 subjects were analysed and classified. The automatic EEG analyser has proved to be a practicable and sensitive tool in sleep research. As it is adapted optimally to the individual EEG of a subject, it is able to detect even small differences to the normal course of sleep.

THE MICROCOMPUTER AIDED ARCHIVISATION OF DIAGNOSTICAL – THERA-
PEUTIC PROCEDURES IN THE CASES OF EROSION OF UTERUS CERVIX –
CYTO-INFO SYSTEM

K.Gwóźdź, L.Wolański
ZETO – Computing Center
50-069 Wrocław, Poland

I. INTRODUCTION: Uterus collum erosions, regarded as a precancer
state, make a phenomenon which is close to an epidemic.
The rate of all mature women who are afflicted with uterus
collum erosions is approximately 30%. As the problem has become
momentous recently, an all-country network of out-patient cyto-
oncological consulting units has come into existence. Besides
their major diagnostic – therapeutic functions the units keep
also record of multiple and detailed medical data which in their
traditional form are very difficult to handle and process.
II. OBJECTIVES: It has been the aim of the authors to develop
a microcomputer technique based system dedicated to recording
the course of diagnostic and therapeutic uterus collum treatment
procedures. The CYTO-INFO system is intended to automatically
process the data gathered in the system data base of the system.
Selective processing will enable to catch new trends and correlations as for as the biological parameters under examination are
concerned. The system will help also to handle patients traffic.
III. ASSUMPTIONS: The CYTO-INFO is a mono-modular, monothematic,
multifunctional microcomputer system which is intended to record
medical data concerning uterus collum diagnosis and treatment.
The data are stored on floppy disks.
IV. METHODOLOGY: – defining the role of a microcomputer in the
operation model of an exemplary uterus collum erosions consulting unit – establishing the role of a microcomputer in the organizational structure: eriosions consulting unit – ginecological
hospital ward, histopathological laboratory, – computer hardware
specification.
V. SUMMARY: The major objective of the CYTO-INFO microcomputer
system is to optimalize the diagnostic and therapeutic procedures of uterus collum erosion treatment /lowering the complications rate, shortening the diagnostic cycle, reducing the
number of cases requiring hospitalization/.

A COMPUTERIZATION PROPOSAL OF THE REGISTRATION OF ROUTINE ULTRASONOCEPHALOMETRIC EXAMINATION OF THE FETUS.

K.Gwóźdź, L.Wolański
ZETO-Computing center
50-069 Wrocław, Poland

As cephalometric ultrasonography of the population of the fetuses provides a great amount of numeric information, the traditional methods of handling the data have become more and more timeconsuming and therefore less efficient. In general, our procedures of input, storing, processing and output of medical data on fetus development make possible, among others, a better evaluation of fetus's mass which is a decisive parameter in respect to the post-natal care of a neonate, and allows to determine the probability of fetus's pre- or post-delivery lethality. The computer input data are to be found on the form entitled "CEPHALOGRAPHIC EXAMINATION of FETUS by ULTRASONOMETRY" which is made up of three parts. Part I: DEMOGRAPHIC and Anamnestic Data. This part appears only once. Part II: Fetometric Data. This part appears at each examination. Part III: Neonate's Data. This part appears only once. There are three modes of operating the system: Automatic: The ultrasonograph operates on-line with a CPU. The Demographic and Anamnestic Data are keyed into the memory and visualized on the screen. The Fetometric Data from the ultrasonograph are automatically entered into the computer. The Neonate's Data are entered by a nurse or a physician. Semiautomatic: the ultrasonograph operates off-line. The computer or terminal, i.e. the VDU, keyboard and printer are located are located near the ultrasonograph. All data are entered manually by a nurse or a physician and visualized on the screen for verification. Manual: The ultrasonographic laboratory operates in isolation form the computer system. The measurement results are filled into appropriate source documents which are physically transferred to the system input station and entered manually. The layout of the source documents please find enclosed.

PROTOCOLS DESIGN IN MEDICAL ORIENTATED LOCAL AREA NETWORKS

Milan Šárek
Technical University
Brno, Czechoslovakia

A local area network is distinguished from other types of data networks in that communication is usually confined to a moderate geographic area such as a single office building, a hospital or a campus and can depend on a physical communications channel of moderate to high datarate which has a consistently low error rate.

The ISO open systems interconnection reference model (OSI RM) is a way of designing communications and networks. The OSI RM defines seven layers of communications protocols, with specific functions isolated at each level. The OSI RM layers are: application (the identification of users , selection of services), presentation (the conversion of data from standard to application dependent format), session (the connection establish and maintain), transport (making a reliable end to end connection across an imperfect network - repeat the message, sequence checking), network (the routing of information from node to node), data link (information flow and error control on the physical path), physical (defines the electrical and mechanical characteristics of the network).

The current activity of the Intitute of Electrical and Electronics Engineers (IEEE - project 802) and the European Computer Manufacturers Association (ECMA - standards 80,81,82 and TR/14) is focused on specifying the data link and physical layers, partly on the network layer. The data link layer is broken into two sublayers: logical link control and media access control. The media access control sublayer is depended on the type of access method to a communication medium. The standards prefer following methods: CSMA/CD (carrier sense, multiple access with collision detect), token ring and token bus. The network layer is divided into sublayers: global network (interconnection between LANs using bridges, interface to public networks via gateways) and network services.

Many articles is concerned on the physical and data link layers. This attention should result in the availability of standard components that a variety of manufacturers can use. The higher layers are out of scope.

A higher layers discussion is based on a comparison of the Network Systems (Advanced Computer Communications), Digital Network Architecture - phase II (Digital Equipment Corporation) and OSI RM.

Network Systems		OSI RM	Digital Network Architecture
Clearinghouse		application	Data Access Protocol
Courier		presentation	Network Service Protocol
		session	
Internet Transp. Protocol	Sequenced Packet Protocol	transport	
	Internet Datagram Protocol	network	Transport Layer
Ethernet		data link	Digital Data Communication Message Protocol
		physical	

SEVENTEEN YEAR EXPERIENCE OF A COMPUTERIZED MICROBIOLOGY LABORATORY INFORMATION SYSTEM

P.Grönroos
University Central Hospital of Tampere
33520 Tampere
Finland

At the beginning of 1970, a modest computer based hospital information system (HIS) was built in the University Central Hospital of Tampere (UCHT). The 1340-bed hospital has about 40000 inpatients and 150000 outpatients a year. Basic information on every patient, including the outpatients, was recorded in the HIS. The including discharge data on every patient. This information provided the central core of a regional data base developed later for all inpatients in the different hospitals in this region of 420000 inhabitants. For all the inpatients a laboratory test request and results reporting system was developed using pre-identified port-a-punch cards. There were different cards for clinical chemistry, hematology, physiology and one card for bacteriological tests.

The system produced a ward summary on all tests done during the past few hours and in the evening a cumulative report on every patient. The latest cumulative report became a sheet in an otherwise manually kept but strictly structured unit medical record of the patient. The system is now working online, using a parallel cluster system VAX 750 with three machines. The system has many subsystems of which the microbiology system is described in some detail here. There is a definite need for interpretative reporting in clinical pathology and especially in microbiology. The tremendous capabilities of modern hardware should be used to create a real information system for the benefit of the clinician. This of course requires a flow of information in both directions, from physician to laboratory and back. We can no longer rely on one single and simple request form. The data needed by the laboratory to perform different tests in microbiology are diverse and require several request forms. The data from these forms are recorded in the computer. When the time comes for the physician to collate the final results he has at his disposal all the information mentioned above as well as the patients "treatment diagnosis", and can furnish the results with statements on the test results. In the evening a cumulative report for every patient with new laboratory test results (clinical chemistry, hematology, microbiology and some parts of physiology) is printed out, including earlier results from the same treatment period ("patient-related cumulative report") that is kept in the unit medical record.

A COMPUTERIZED LONG-TERM FOLLOW-UP OF ANTIBIOTIC SENSITIVITY PATTERN FOR A HOSPITAL REGION

Paul Grönroos M.D.
Central University Hospital of Tampere
33520 Tampere
Finland

A laboratory test request and reporting system has been in use in the Central University Hospital of Tampere (1238 beds) since 1969 as the initial stage of a hospital information system. The system has been operative throughout this time also for microbiology.
The sensitivity determination has been done all these years by the so-called PDM method of the Biodisk company. The method has a specially designed medium that is quality controlled in the factory against the standardized antibiotic containing 6 mm paper discs sold by the firm. After strictly controlled incubation times etc. the diameter of the inhibition zone for each antibiotic is measured by a caliper and the results recorded in the computer data file. Biodisk provides the users with regression lines for every single antibiotic that gives the relationship of the inhibition zone (mm) to the corresponding MIC values for the bacteria. The regression lines are kept in the computer and permit the calculation of the MIC- values when needed. Usually, however, the results are converted for the benefit of the clinician into SIR groups. The individual results may be collected into a file for multiresistant bacteria. The regression lines mentioned are changed from time to time for long-term storage, however, the data files will keep only the millimetre of the zone diameters. This makes it possible to follow over the course of time the changes that take place in the sensitivity patterns of the different antibiotics.

REGISTRATION OF HOSPITAL INFECTIONS

Paul Grönroos, M.D.
Central University Hospital of Tampere
Department of Microbiology
33520 Tampere, Finland

The Hospital League of Finland definition for a hospital infection is: An infection acquired during hospitalisation, i.e. it was not observable or incipient at the time of the patient's admission (unless it is regarded as a sequel of an earlier hospital stay). A nosocomial infection often appears after discharge from hospital. Hospital infection refers in practice to an infection established in the patient after his/her third day of treatment. In the University Central Hospital of Tampere (1238 beds) hospital infections have been recorded since 1964. A three level approach has been used.

1) In the wards a special form is kept with space for the registration of 3-6 patients. The form contains basic data on the patient and their infection (s). Patient ID (the official Finnish ID number specific for each individual), name, date of infection, type of infection and for surgical patients the so called operation wound classes. Various statistics has been produced since 1964. During 1985 this system will go on-line.

2) The hospital has been using a computerized laboratory test request and report system since 1968. The system generates a cumulative report on all laboratory data for every patient. The above-mentioned definition of a hospital infection has been programmed into the computer. 3) The laboratory system has operated in an on-line mode since 1979. The physician who is responsible for the final test report and uses the computer for comments on the results may at this juncture decide to store the information on that patient in a special data file.

Method no 1 seems to keep the interest in reporting hospital infections alive. This is important for sustaining preventive measures by the staff at a high level. The method is rather insensitive for disclosing impending hospital infections. The planned extension of the method will most probably be useful.

Method no 2 is fast and detects many cases. Too many, in fact, to be coped with effectively. Some of these are not hospital infections by any definition.

Method no 3 has been found to be sensitive and useful for purposeful supervision of hospital infections.

PLANNING OF A SURGERY DEPARTMENT ON THE BASIS OF SURGERY AND
ANESTHESY STATISTICS

T. Niinimäki
Oulu University Central Hospital, Department of Surgery, Oulu, Finland

Surgery departments usually have some kind of statistical system in
their routine use. The contents include basic data concerning the
amount of the production, also specifying medical details. This is
generally done by a codal list of the procedures. These statistics are
needed for the management of the department. These data are also
necessary in planning, especially if the need for a change-over is
great. The number of staff needed, number of theatres and the costs of
materials are the most important facts necessary.

The question we desired to answer was: Is it possible to estimate the
staff and the time needed for each procedure in exact reliable calculations for the future making it possible by the aid of simple statistics containing only the names and the number of the procedures ?

We collected the theatre times and number of staff in every single
operation from the patients' entry to time of dismissal. This data was
compared with the data, which concerned the same matters but were
produced artificially by long-time statistics, estimation and an
arbitrative procedure. The whole list of operations was under close
inspection. Also the number of staff and material costs were inspected.

The result was that the mean times, materials necessary and the
personnel needed were near equal and therefore approved. This estimat-
ive process also gave a sufficient accurate basis for planning. Most
groups were uniform in a 5 per cent limit, whilst those within a
10 per cent limit can probably be developed to the same accuracy.

In this poster we show the models and the results of this calculation.

STATISTICAL DATA PROCESSING BY MICROCOMPUTER

István Ratkó
Computer and Automation Institute
Hungarian Academy of Sciences
Budapest, Victor Hugo u. 18-22 , H-1132

Physicians, biologists and other - non mathematician - experts often use various mathematical processes. It seems, however, that they not always apply procedures best suitable for the examined problems, sometimes even resort to methods not applicable to the problem. What to do then? A possibility: the user sits up to the computer, feeds the data set into the microcomputer and by keeping answering the questions of the microcomputer, the microcomputer selects the statistical procedures to be followed on the basis of the obtained answers.

We note that simultaneously with the data input the program controlling the data input executes also the following: 1) Checking the data whether a) the given data fall within the given limits b) is there incompatibility among the values of any data pair or data trio 2) The microcomputer monitors the data fed in and notes at the end of the data input that which of the data can be considered discrete and which continuous. It turns even out after the end of the data input that there are special distributions (normal, Poisson, exponential, binomial etc.) or not among the particular variables.

The structure of the algorithm selecting the statistical method can be illustrated by a directed graph G.

A purpose of the questions is to decide on the following: a) Which data take part in the statistical processing? The codes of which data are to be converted?

b) The data have a nominal, ordinal, interval or quotient scale. This is, as a matter of fact, relevant to the selection of the best method. c) Search for relation; average, deviation, comparison; distribution comparison; the completion of other tasks is the aim to be attained.

All other information (independence of the samples; one sample, two samples, k-samples; whether there is a special distribution, number of the elements of the sample etc.) will be obtained on the basis of the data set and the answers given to the questions.

A MICROCOMPUTER-BASED CLINICAL LABORATORY SUBSYSTEM

I. Bordás and A. Jávor

Documentation and Information Centre

County Hospital, Szekszárd, Hungary

We have been occupied since 1977 in development of computer-based laboratory information system. We consider this work as one of the fundamental parts of hospital information system. Of late years we have begun to create a complete hospital information system on microcomputer network with the help of developmental and operating experience we have got by a previous centralized information system model. The clinical laboratory subsystem is one of the fundamental parts in this new system too.

The most important functions in our system:

- To collect and to distribute the test requests,
- To collect and to control the test results,
- Automatic Quality Control,
- Daily and cumulative reports,
- Archive data storage,
- Statistics, and
- Subsequent data processing.

The system - as forms a part of hospital information system - collaborates with other subsystems e.g. Patient Administration System, Clinical Support System. The connection among subsystems is realized via Local Area Microcomputer Network (MMT-HNS). The direct connection reduces the input data and administrative work, it increases the precision of informations and makes easier the complex data processing.

The system can work in autonomous mode (without network connection) too. It is flexible and modular completable. We are convinced by many years collected experience, that a system is far better, more effectual which is possessed of modern external connections, than that "autonomous" system which is in communication with hospital departments old mode.

MEDUCATION, A TEACHING PROGRAM TO RECOGNIZE SYMPTOMS AND
SIGNS EMPLOYING A GENERAL MEDICAL DATA BASE.

P.L.M. Kerkhof, J.J.A. Schreuder, J. Helder, J.Y. Kresh and K. Gill.
Medwise Working Group, P.O. Box 1621, 3600 BP Maarssen, Netherlands, and Jefferson
Medical College, Philadelphia, PA. 19107, U.S.A.

SUMMARY
On the basis of a general medical data base (MEDWISE) we developed a program which
aids the student and evaluates his performance, when studying characteristics (e.g.
symptoms and signs) of various diseases. Drawbacks of the present version of the
program are the succinct expressions rather than conversation type of phrases to
describe the attributes. Advantages include the fact that the teacher is not necessarily involved, and that the user has easy access to detailed information in connection with the disorder analyzed.

INTRODUCTION
Computer assisted learning enables the student to acquire and evaluate information
without the instructor's constraints in terms of time and fatigue, whereas the
teacher's work investment is limited to the preparation of single lessons. The latter
task, however, often appears to be circumstantial, because one has to anticipate on a
wide spectrum of turns of thought from the side of potential users.
Therefore, many programs are usually designed such that the student has merely to
make selections from a fixed list of alternatives generated by the machine, and preferably not by himself. To further reduce time investment for the instructor, we developed a general program that produces an endless stream of teaching material to
train recognition of features of any disease selected.

DESIGN
We are developing a general medical data base MEDWISE (1), which includes information
on symptoms & signs, therapy, complications, prognosis and laboratory investigations.
Ultimately, the system will cover all diseases listed according to the ICD-9-CM code.
Besides all applications as a documentation system, this data base can also be utilized as a teaching aid. To reach this goal, we developed a program (MEDUCATION)
that combines the features of a preselected disease, with a variety of characteristics which are not relevant for this particular disorder. Consequently, the multiple
choice list produced contains pertinent as well as irrelevant items, all presented
as short key words (e.g. nausea / hypertension / preclinical marker). Since the dummy
alternatives are randomly collected from adjacent ICD-disorders, the presentation of
the case can be infinitely repeated, without the need to consult the teacher.
Thusfar, we applied this method to the field of recognizing symptoms and signs, hematology and laboratory analysis data related to individual diseases. However, the
same procedures can be employed to verify correctness of complications, therapy,
prognosis etc. The program runs on an Apple II microcomputer with dual disk drive.

APPLICATION
The student may enter the name of any disease he wants to study, and determine the
number of alternatives to choose from. The length of this list can be longer (maximum is 100 items), as the student gets more familiar with the characteristics of
the disorder selected, thus enhancing the level of difficulty. From the survey then
presented on the screen, he should determine all correct answers. After the efforts,
all selections realized are displayed again, and it is indicated which alternatives
are considered correct, along with the score reached. Next, the exercise can be repeated with a fresh list, while the program generates new alternatives for the same
disease. At a certain stage, the user may desire to receive all correct answers, and
a full survey will be presented containing all text from the data base and not just
the single key words. Finally, the student may wish to incorporate aspects of the
data base itself, and request further information on incidence, therapy, prevention
or prognosis. In this manner all aspects of a particular disease can be integrated
during the learning process. As mentioned before, the flexibility of the program
implies some loss of elegance regarding the formulation of the individual case.

REFERENCE:
P.L.M. Kerkhof et al. Automedica 5 (1984) 333-341

THERESA: A COMPUTERIZED MEDICAL INFORMATION SYSTEM
Grady Memorial Hospital, Atlanta, Georgia, U.S.A.

Mattie L. Ridley, Director
Medical Records Department
Grady Memorial Hdspital
Atlanta, Georgia 30335

There is a wealth of information which can be systematically explored through a computerized medical information system. Such a system, called THERESA, is being developed at Grady Memorial Hospital by Medical Systems Development Corporation. THERESA is a true Management Information System (MIS) for the practice of medicine. Through interactive access to the wealth of clinical experiences reflected in patient records at Grady (over one million encounters with 350,000 patients annually) capabilities for patient care, clinical research, teaching, cost containment, and administrative control and planning will be greatly enhanced.

For computerization to be practical, medical information needs to be entered from a selection of pertinent documents from the patient's record. THERESA therefore will include: Diagnosis-Problem Lists, Drug Profiles, X-ray reports, Laboratory reports, Discharge summaries, Clinic visit key data, Pathology biopsy reports, EKG reports, Surgical operations, Autopsy reports.

Also, there are other practical uses for the THERESA System:
1. A record tracking and locator system
2. A system for diagnostic coding and indexing on-line
3. A physicians' index on-line
4. A computerized abstract system on-line from which medical statistics and reports can be generated.

As a record tracking system, using bar-codes and light pens, records can be tracked and reports can be generated as to the timeliness of providing the record, the timeliness of the return of the records, the identity of the users of the records, etc.

With coding and indexing on-line, data would be available immediately for the financial office for billing purposes. Also, information would be current and available for research studies and teaching.

Physician profiles could be generated and the physicians index information would be available for review and management.

A medical record abstract system would provide current medical statistics for review of service allocation and staffing.

Finally, the abbreviated medical record would be available for use in lieu of the complete medical record--capable of being used at several locations at the same time--saving time and providing data in emergency situations when the hard-copy record might be in use elsewhere.

NOSOCOMIAL INFECTIONS IN NEWBORN INTENSIVE CARE UNITS.

W.B.Kędzia
University School of Medicine
Department of Pharmaceutical Microbiology
Sieroca 10
61-771 Poznań, Poland

The study was performed in the Institute of Microbiology and Infectious Diseases and in the Neonatal Intensive Care Units /NICU´s/ of the Institute of Obstetrics and Gynaecology in Poznań.Admission to the NICU´s was reserved for critically ill neonates and for underweight infants. The samples were collected from inanimate objects, from hospital personnel and newborns. All bacterial strains were isolated, identified and typing by serological,pyocine and bacteriophage methods. Serious hospital infections in newborn babies were caused by K.pneumoniae, P.aeruginosa, E.coli and S.aureus. There were only sporadically Enterobacter,streptococci group A and B, Flavobacteria and S.marcescens infections.Three outbreaks of epidemics have been observed. Two of them were caused by P.aeruginosa and one epidemic by K. pneumoniae. Hospital strains have shown typically bacteriophage or pyocine pattern and have also been isolated in hospital environment, from skin of hands of the personnel and from the equipment. 59 newborns suffered from pneumonia, sepsis and meningitis and 78 suffered minor infections. The K.pneumoniae outbreak was caused by the strain multiply-resistant to antibiotics. The epidemic strain was resistant to chloramphenicol, ampicillin,cephalotin, gentamycin, kanamycin and tobramycin. One of the epidemic strains of P.aeruginosa was resistant to aminoglycoside antibiotics but the second epidemic strain of Pseudomonas was sensitive to aminoglycoside antibiotics. Sources of infection of the epidemic strains were a mother with infection of the delivery tract and a baby with intrauterine infection. Environmental cultures have been found in reservoirs such as : sinks, toilets, standing water, suction apparatus, nebulizing humidifiers, mops, gastrointestinal tract. The most important way of transmission of the hospital infections were hands of the personnel and sometimes the hospital equipment.Factors influencing nosocomial infections rates in newborns are : underweight,low immunological respons, malformations, diabetes and anoxaemia. For surveillance and control of infection we recommend handwashing and antiseptic of the hands skin before passing from one patient to another one. We consider this the basic point in preventing nosocomial infections. The guideline has also contained methods of cleaning, disinfection and sterilization of the hospital equipment to protect transmission of infections. Care must also be taken with wet sources as well as tap water and distilled water as these might be the reservoirs of microorganisms, especially gram-negative rods. The adoption of these recommendations by the Neonatal Intensive Care Units resulted in a decrease of the rate of infections from 19 to 8 per cent of all admitted patients. The Working Group at the Hospital Center worked out worksheets for surveillance of infections. Such information can also be adopted for a transfer to punch cards or computer tape.

DESCRIPTOR - A SOFTWARE TOOL FOR CONSTRUCTION OF FLEXIBLE DATA BASE

M.Dvořák and O.Gotfrýd
Research Institute of Traumatology
Ponávka 6, 66250 BRNO, Czechoslovakia

Surgical (traumatological) information system CIS-1.T developed in 1984 in our institute is working under an operating system DSM-11. In that system and programming language DSM the information is stored on the disc in a tree structure. That fact may be used for structurizing the data base to "files" - each file being a subtree for each patient. Each patient file consists of data records being again subtree of the patient file. Every record consists of data items that, from the user's point of view, are elementary types of information.

The authors of CIS-1.T have developed a special descriptive structure. It is called "descriptor"and it describes the internal structure of information record (IR). In the system there exist about 80 different types of IRs, i.e. the same amount of descriptor's types. The descriptor contains list of items of which corresponding IR consists, their names, types and other necessary auxiliary information. Every IR of particular type contains only values of defined items and number of version of corresponding descriptor. If a change in the structure of IR occurs from any reason, a new version of descriptor is created supposing the old version remains in the structure as an auxiliary substructure for decoding the IRs created earlier. The flexibility of medical data base allows to write a universal input/output programme suitable for great deal of user programmes.

The described method of processing the IRs has been used in last two years in design of four different clinical information systems in Czechoslovakia. These systems work on traumatologic, internal, neurologic and ophthalmic clinics. The systems working on different clinics may contain nearly equal programme modules. Their different field of professional activity is described by different information contained in the descriptors. Modification of an information system having the described features is easy even if the application software should be applied on the clinic of different type. This organization also allows easy changes in IRs' structure when required.

pDMS a Data Management System in Health Care Application

K. Kovács
Computer and Automation Institute
Hungarian Academy of Sciences
Budapest, P.O. Box 63. H-1502

This poster presents an application of pDMS in an integrated hospital
information system [2]. The first medical utilization of this software tool was a drug register [1].
pDMS is a Personal Data Management System. It can be installed on any
Z80 microcomputer having 64 kB memory and CP/M operating system. It is
designed to create, modify and report on any number of data base systems, each consisting of main (data) and auxiliary (data) files.
A DBS is ordered by VSAM structures. A VSAM structure itself forms a
separate file. It is defined by specifying which field is the key field.
The records are ordered by their keys. Any number of VSAM structures
can form a part of the DBS.
The role of auxiliary files is to provide additonal information about
the records of the main files. This approach has the advantage that
repetitive information can be put in the auxiliary files where it can
easily be edited and changed. The relations between the data of the
main and auxiliary files are managed also with help of VSAM structures.
There are six field types used: string, integer, real, date, binary
integer and logical. The data input is carefully controlled. All not-
string types are stored in compressed format, reducing space requirements by 50 percent. The system has a number of utilities not usually
implemented on microcomputers: it makes a journal of data processing,
providing the opportunity to restore the consistency of data base in
case of any injure, it uses the printer through a spooler, allowing
user accesses in the same time, etc.

References

1. Bakonyi P. et al., A Microcomputer-Network Based Decision Support
   System for Health-Care Organizations, Preprints, IFAC 9th World
   Congress, Budapest, Vol. XI, eds. J. Gertler L. Keviczky, pp.85-92,
   1984.
2. Kerékfy P. et al., An Approach to the Microcomputer-Network System
   in the Hungarian National Institute of Cardiology, (manuscript for
   MIE 85).

AUTOMATION OF THE INDIVIDUAL MENUCHOICE BY PATIENTS IN HOSPITAL IN RELATION TO MINIMIZING PRODUCTION COST

R.S.J. Rikken

St. Radboud Hospital, Dept. of Medical Information Processing
Geert Grooteplein Zuid 10, PO Box 9101
6500 HB Nijmegen, The Netherlands.
Telephone: 080-517065/513979. Telex: 48232 ACZHS NL.

An automated individual menu-choice system has been operational at the St. Radboud Hospital from the beginning of 1984. The system permits all in-patients and guests to compose meals of their own choice.

Daily all patients choose their meal. The computer composes a menu with options for the individual patient on a daily basis and including only food, suitable for the patient. All the individual choices are collected and worked up by the computer, making derivation for the patient diet. As close as possible to the mealtime all changes in diets and menus are worked up.
About two hours before the distribution of the food, the system makes a working list for the central kitchen.
For each patient a coded meal order card is made for preparing and serving out the individual meals in the kitchen and distribution to the nursing stations.
The system is table-driven, with a minimum of maintenance and a maximum of flexibility to changes in menus, diets, patient transfers and patient discharges
The users of the system are: wards, kitchen, transportation service and dietary.

The realisation of the objectives according to reduction of food over-production is a continuous process. The next points are important:
- the choice should be made as close as possible to the mealtime.
- detailed information about the daily choices per ward.
- statistical information about patient's choices in relation to their diets.
- discovery of special trends in the supplied components.
- consolidated management information.

The reduction of the over-production of food (900 meals, 3 times a day) will be about 150 litres a day, in Dutch Guilders ƒ 300.000,-, against an exploitation cost of ƒ 100.000,- a year for the total system.

A DRUG-REQUISITION AND DRUG-INFORMATION SYSTEM USING AN IBM-PERSONAL COMPUTER-XT

Poul Walløe , Hospital Pharmacist
Skive Sygehus
DK-7800 Skive, Denmark

Erik Kirkeby, EDP-Manager
County Hospital Administration
Skottenborg 26
DK-8800 Viborg , Denmark

Over the past two or three years personal computers - Pcs - have gained much ground wherever on-line connection to large data processing centres was unnecessary or inexpedient.

A new EDP-system for the requisition of drugs is described. The system, which has been in use in the medical depots of 3 Danish hospitals in the county of Viborg since October 1984, is based on an IBM-PC-XT. Medical depots are hospital departments which mainly buy their supplies from local, privately owned pharmacies, but the system could also, if slightly changed, be used in hospital pharmacies.

The system is based on 4 main files: The EDP master drug-file of the Association of Danish Chemists, a file containing the names and addresses of suppliers of drugs (pharmacies and wholesalers), a file of the consumers of drugs (wards, clinics and other departments), and a file of the drugs recommended for each individual consumer (standard list of drugs).

Drugs are purchased and dispensed by means of cards with BAR-codes printed by the system-printer.

The system is extremely well suited for controlling the consumption of drugs and the expenditure involved, at both ward and hospital level. The system also supplies the drug committee of the hospital with valuable documentation material.

The retrieving of any information requested and the changing of file data is quick and simple.

If one or more of the about 15 search criteria are used the master drug-file of the system could easily function as a general drug-information system.

Multi-level quality control procedures in a clinical database management system (CLINIC/3000).

N. Issakides, Y.N. La, M.A. de Rotrou and R. Gomeni
Laboratoires d'Etudes et de Recherches Synthelabo (L.E.R.S.)
Department of Clinical Research,
58 rue de la Glacière, 75013 Paris France

1. Introduction.

The objective of a clinical trial is to evaluate drug efficacy and safety in a selected population of patients in order to detect all kind of errors and source of bias during clinical data management. Quality control procedures should cover every area of data processing : data collection, data entry, data editing and data modification. DDL/3000 language (1) allows to create a database structure reflecting the case report form. All information and relationship between the different sections of a case report form are recorded on a STUDY-DICTONARY which is used by all quality control procedures.

2. Data entry.

A double data entry system records data on a temporary database. The data entered on separate occasions are compared and a code replaces the mismatching data. Each medical record is logged on an AUDIT file.

3. Data editing.

In CLINIC/3000 system, data editing takes place when data are in the temporary database or when data are entered into the master database. According to the study dictionary, detection of outliers and protocol violation check can then be performed using univariate and multivariate tests.

4. Data integrity.

Reports are generated in order to display the different kind of errors found during test procedures. Records with unsolved problems cannot be transferred into the master database. All modifications on the master database are logged in a special file which saves old and new values of the modified items.

5. Conclusion.

High quality of data is performed by supplying a set of automatic tools which can guarantee, given an appropriate analysis, that results are reliable and interpretable.

REFERENCES

1 - N. Issakides, M.A. de Rotrou and R. Gomeni : CLINIC/3000 a clinical trial management system. Lecture notes in Medical Informatics, MIE84, Springer Verlag, New York, 406-411, 1984.
2 - G. Averkin and B.M. Beaver : Quality assurance in clinical data management, D. Inf., 67-69, 1984

DEL/3000 : Local and remote data entry language for a clinical database management system (CLINIC/3000).

Y.N. La, M.A. de Rotrou, N. Issakides and R. Gomeni
Laboratoires d'Etudes et de Recherches Synthelabo (L.E.R.S.)
Department of Clinical Research
58, rue de la Glacière - 75013 Paris, France.

DEL/3000 is an interactive language designed for CLINIC/3000 (clinical database management system). It allows to enter clinical data either locally or from a remote site in order to reduce the timelag between data collection and data availability on a mainframe.

For each clinical trial, an independent structure is created :

- a STUDY DICTIONARY to record the information and the relationship between different sections of a case report form,
- a TEMPORARY DATABASE (TDB) where data are initially entered
- a MASTER DATABASE (MDB) in which data are transferred from TDB after validation.

Local data entry :

In order to ensure a high quality of clinical data, a double blind entry is performed on each datum and a track of every transaction is recorded on a special file : the AUDIT file

To ensure data consistency, no blank item value is accepted. Each item should be affected by an alphanumeric value or an error code (missing, not pertinent or unreadable).

1) **Temporary database (TDB):**

  a) First entry : data are entered in the TDB but cannot be printed or transferred to the master database
  b) Second entry : data are re-entered and compared with the first ones. In case of mismatching, no confirmation is asked and doubtful data are replaced by a code.
  After the second entry, reports are generated and submitted to clinical monitors for review.

2) **Master database (MDB)** : Data can finally be transferred to the master database when all errors are rectified.

Remote data entry :

DEL3000 allows to collect clinical trial data by remote entry directly from the investigator's office. Data entered via the remote data entry sub-system have to be validated on the central site before being included in the master database. Two different types of remote data entry are supported according to the available hardware : terminal (and additional equipments) and micro-computer.

GAIA – GASTROENTEROLOGICAL ARTIFICIAL INTELLIGENCE APPLICATION

Simon L., Aszalós J. and Jávor A.

Dept. of Gastroenterology and Computer Center, Tolna
County Hospital, Szekszárd, and SZÁMALK, Budapest
Hungary

During the last few years several attempts have been made to
introduce the idea of computer-assistence for the medical decision making.

In our gastroenterological information system clinical support
subsystems and a risk-specific surveillance subsystem are already in routine use. In the near future several microcomputer-based "expert"-systems are planned to extend this structure.

As the first model of such sub-systems an expert system for
the differential-diagnosis of jaundice has been developed.

GAIA: essential features

GAIA deals with two classes of problems, the "data oriented"
and the "goal oriented" ones. In the first case the problem is
to detect the possible causes of the observed symptoms /diag-
nostic problem/, in the second one the system tries to interpret the symptoms on the base of a specific hypothesis /inter-
pretation problem/. In both cases the task of planning the relevant and possibly most economical diagnostic procedure can
arise /configuration problem/. GAIA can be used as a Question-
Answer system related to the diagnostic knowledge stored in the
knowledge base.

The knowledge in GAIA is organized according to two different
structuring schemata. The first presents knowledge independent
of the problems to be solved: general knowledge. The situational
knowledge, on the other hand – structures knowledge according
to the requirements of the problem situations. To avoid redundancy only general knowledge is stored permanently in the system.
All these informations are stored and represented as PROLOG
clauses, sentences and rules, and MiniPROLOG for the used MOD-81
64 Kbyte microcomputer, as well.

The differntial-diagnostic possibilities are published by the
system in a decreasing order of probability.

COMPUTER BASED INFORMATION SYSTEM ON PROTECTIVE GLOVES AND BARRIER CREAMS FOR OCCUPA-
TIONAL USE

G. Mellström and A. Boman
National Board of Occupational
Safety and Health
Research Department
S-171 84 Solna
Sweden

A database has been developed containing test data on protective effects of safety
gloves and protective creams against chemicals. Permeation data for gloves, clinical
data and other experimental data for gloves and protective creams are collected and
after dermatological assessment put into different files in the database. The main
purpose of this database is to give up-to-date and relevant information to those who
have to choose and recommend suitable gloves or other skin protection to workers handling or working with hazardous chemicals. The databse consists of 5 files. Each file
contains data on glove materials and protective creams found in literature or provided
by retail seller or manufacturers. The files are a) Product and retail seller file,
consisting of names and description of products and adresses to retail sellers. b)
Chemical resistance file, consisting of data from technical material testing found in
literature ·   c) Medical report file, consisting or results from clinical and
other experimental investigations and side effects of gloves and protective creams reported in the literature ·   d) Reference file, consisting of all references from
which data to the other files have been extracted. The information from the database
is presented to the users in form of printed documents which can be regularly up-dated ·

To day test results published in the literature are not always comparable because many
different investigation methods are used. In order to make it possible to compare test
results from various manufacturers, or test laboratories, still more work has to be
done to create internationally accepted standard or reference methods (in vitro and in
vivo) and internationally accepted rules for presentation of the test data. This would
make it easier to evaluate the protective effect against chemicals of protective glove
materials and protective creams.

Key-words: Database, protective effect, protective creams, rubber gloves, plastic
gloves, hazardous chemicals, test result.

AN INTERACTIVE SYSTEM FOR THE SURVEILLANCE OF INFECTOUS DISEASES IN ITALY.

Susanna Conti, Laboratory of Epidemiology and Biostatistics, Istituto Superiore della Sanità, V. Regina Elena 299, Rome, ITALY.

In Italy 21 infectous diseases were identified as the most important for public health. Since 1982 the 21 Italian Regions have been weekly sending data about these diseases to the National Health Institute.

The informatic system to handle these informations is implemented on an IBM Model 4341; its operative system, "VM", provides the feasibility to run interactively with Virtual Machines; so a virtual machine has been dedicated to the system of Surveillance. To enter the system it is sufficient to type the word "SURVEYOR" on the keyboard: then the Menu of the system appears on the screen, and you can ask for one of the following facilities: INPUT, REPORT ON A PERIOD and INTERACTIVE ANALYSIS.

The INPUT of data uses a Panel, which has some interesting features, such as: the cursor moves directly to the fields which are to be filled, avoiding trivial but dangerous errors; the system checks the formal validity of data; the zeros which appear on the screen are real zeros, so you have to type on the keyboard only non-trivial data. The procedure stores data on the File dedicated to the current year. When you ask for the REPORT ON A PERIOD, you have only to supply the date (/s) which identifies the period to analyze; the system then prints a Table containing, for each Region and for each disease, the number of cases and the rates X 100,000 referred to the general population.

The facility for INTERACTIVE ANALYSIS allows to obtain absolute numbers and rates, choosing in the panel any combinations of the three grouping categories: Time (only 1 or more weeks), Place (only 1 or more Regions) and Disease (only 1 or more diseases).

The programs are written in Fortran and the procedures are written in IBM-EXEC Language.

Advanced BASIC Programming Software Package
for Teaching

Qin Dulie

Dept. of Mathematics

Beijing Second Medical College

Beijing,People's Republic of China

Our advanced BASIC programming software includes 130 sample programs for teaching programming. Its contents are as follows:

1. Converting program of number system.
2. Limiting characteristic of Fibonacci series.
3. Techniques of processing strings.
4. Various sorting methods of strings.
5. Techniques of cursor control on screen.
6. Techniques of arrangementing data terms on screen.
7. Methods of preventing incorrect input of data.
8. Graphics on screen.
9. Word processing prgramming.
10. CAI programming.
11. 'INKEY$' simulation of INPUT statement.
12. Leisure programming.
13. Coding and encoding of compressed information.
14. Practicing of using complicated software packages.
15. Disk images of data files.
16. Use of POKE statement.
17. Some programs of scientific calculation.

Our teaching practice indicated that this package is effective in fostering the ability to develop application programs.

THE USE OF INFORMATION SYSTEMS IN DUTCH GENERAL HOSPITALS

A.J.G. van Rijen

Advisory Board for Automation in Health Care
P.O. Box 439, 2260 AK Leidschendam
The Netherlands

In the second half of 1984 a survey on the use of information systems in general hospitals was held. No less than 97% of the hospitals participated in the survey. The purpose of the survey was double: to provide Dutch hospitals with information on available information (sub)systems and to gain a deeper understanding in existing gaps in the supply of information systems. The resulting overall-view allows a connection between historical developments and the status quo in this field and at the other hand identifiable general trends in automation.

To illustrate the developments in hospital automation the development of the relative frequency of some subsystems is shown:

	1974	1979	1984
I Functions concerning the treatment of patients diagnoses and therapy:			
Clinical laboratory	2	6	35
Radiology	0	2	18
Pharmacy	0	2	15
Operating-room	0	2	9
Microbiologic laboratory	0	2	9
Pathology/anatomy	0	2	7
Nursing department	0	0	2
II Planningsfunctions:			
Bed control/census	2	16	74
Inpatient pre-admission	0	4	38
Outpatient appointments	0	1	19
Duty roster	0	2	8
Maintenance planning	0	1	6
III Support-functions:			
Billing/Accounting	6	27	84
Patientregistration	5	24	78
Treatment administration	5	24	76
Inventory/Stock control	3	15	56
Personnel administration	0	5	25
Purchase order management	0	1	15
Food supply/kitchen/Dietary	0	1	11
IV Functions concerning general medical management and hospital management:			
Hospital management statistics	3	10	46
Inpatient management information	0	6	35
Outpatient management information	0	2	14

The results of the survey indicate trends in hospital automation:
- within a couple of years all Dutch hospitals will have automated their support-functions (III);
- within a couple of years more than 50% of all hospitals will have one or more clinical subsystems for diagnoses and therapy (I) at their disposal;
- the existing concepts on hospital information systems will be developped to hospital information networks containing a variety of hardware facilities including a strong increase of the integration of personal computers;
- subsystems providing facilities for separate hospital departments and medical-technical systems (CT-scanners, Coronory Care Units, respiratory-functions, EEG-systems etc.) will be integrated in hospital computer networks.

CLASSES OF UTILIZATION OF DATA BASE MANAGEMENT SYSTEMS IN A HOSPITAL INFORMATION SYSTEM

Dieter Schreiter

Institut für Medizinische Informationsverarbeitung
Medizinische Akademie "Carl Gustav Carus" Dresden
GDR - 8019 Dresden, Fetscherstraße 74

For about three years we successfully use the data base management system MIMER developed by the Uppsala Data Center (UDAC) and the MIMER Information Systems AB, Uppsala. Besides other favourable properties MIMER has an extremely good portability and gets along also with limited technological resources.

In hospitals rarely large-scale computers are available, therefore often the question arises, whether and for which purposes data base management systems may be used, though.

During the atilization of the DBMS on the computers with limited resources, some universally valid findings could be abtained.

The systematization resulted in the following categories:

A. Kind of data base tables

    A1   "Constant" tables (e.g. catalogues)

    A2   "Static" tables (typical are INSERT functions)

    A3   "Dynamic" tables (complete application of the INSERT-, UPDATE- und DELETE-functions)

B. Modes of application of the data base tables

    B1   Query on gathered information/search (GET ... WHERE "group" - batch oriented)

    B2   Query on individual information (GET ... WHERE "ident" - real-time oriented)

The following table contains a code I to VI referring to the degree of difficulty and the requirements of the ressources in relation to the kind and mode of application of the data base tables.

	A1	A2	A3
B1	I	III	V
B2	II	IV	VI

M-STEFI

A MICROCOMPUTER NETWORK-BASED CLINICAL SUPPORT SYSTEM

D. Leposa, Gy.Turchányi, L.Péterbencze, S.Pintér, A.Jávor
Tolna County Hospital
Documentation and Information Centre
H-7loo Szekszárd, Hungary

Since l98l more than 4.000 patient per year have been dealt with
STEFI(based on standardized features and information of medicine),
wich is a comprehensive in - and outpatient interactive medical
record system in standalone hardware environment. Analysing the
experiences, the advanteges and drawbacks of STEFI operation have
been planned the M-STEFI system. Its hardware environment is a two-
level bus topology local area network, in wich the higher level
is the hospital bus, the lower one is the working office subnetwork,
wich contains a file server and some (max.8.) working stations.
M-STEFI has a user friendly, fast and convenient interaction between medical doctors and computer system via a menu technique (u-
sing memory disk and a self study process to reduce access time
to the menu-description file). Important is the code independent
from the menu-descpiption file, so the M-STEFI system is capable
to include any code system (SNOMED,WHO-ICT or auy special code).
Its modularity and flexibility are resulted from the data independence, the portability from PASCAL implementation. The extension of menu-description file concept makes possible the parame-
terised description of relatively simple algebraic or logic algo-
rythms and warnings, wich can be altered without modification of
the program.
M-STEFI's standardized data are encoded but the retrieved data
are free-text like. This highly structured data are suitable for
real-time processing in standalone or in connected environment via
the LAN and can be stored in a database. Our future plan is to
create the logical and physical connection between M-STEFI and our
pilot expert system.

THE ADAPTATION OF THE ADVANCED HOSPITAL INFORMATION SYSTEM HELP INTO THE ENVIRONMENT OF A GERMAN UNIVERSITY HOSPITAL

J. Dudeck[1] and P. Clayton[2]

[1]Institute for Medical Informatics, University of Giessen
Heinrich-Buff-Ring 44, D - 6300 Giessen

[2]Dept. of Biophysics, University of Utah, Salt Lake City (guest professor at [1])

HELP is an advanced hospital information system, developed at the Latter-Day-Saints-Hospital in Salt Lake City. It is the first system which includes a data driven medical decision support system in the communication process within the hospital.

Experiences with expert systems in medicine have shown, that the physician is not prepared to type in a large amount of data during the diagnostic process. It can be assumed, that expert systems will be accepted in the clinical environment only, if they are data driven and if they can provide the decision arrived at automatically. In HELP this approval has been chosen.

We are about to transfer and adapt HELP to the environment of a German university hospital. In particular the drug information part is investigated. The acceptance and the consequences concerning the physician's prescription behaviour are observed.
First results will be presented.

AN INFORMATION SYSTEM FOR COMMUNICABLE DISEASE SURVEILLANCE

by S.Mariotti,D.Greco,A.Verdecchia.
Laboratorio di Epidemiologia e Biostatistica,
Istituto Superiore di Sanita', Rome, Italy.

All European countries have a national notification system for communicable diseases. Most countries have developed today also a parallel surveillance network, which has been added to the official notification system, with the aim of improving speed and efficiency and avoiding burocracy. A periodical bulletin is usually published monthly, spread around each country to provide reference information for quick intervention purposes, and also sent to European central office. The WHO Collaborative Centre for Health and Disease surveillance (WHOHDS) was established in March 1983 at the Italian National Institute of Health in Rome, with the aim of providing a quick reference source of data on communicable diseases in the European region. Up to date national reports have been received from 28 out of the 35 European countries on some 37 different diseases. Disease frequencies are received from different countries for different time intervals, ranging from one week to one month and then converted to monthly equivalent frequencies. A computer system for easy input of data, statistical analysis and graphical presentation of data on Communicable Diseases was designed and implemented in the Centre. Data entry facilities are provided on an IBM 4341 computer system, and a data base is organized for simple and flexible data maintenance, using a general purpose inquiry language (IBM's APLDI). The inquiry facility can be used also by persons with no programming background. Two simple interface programs have been developed to provide routinely simple statistical analysis on one side and graphical presentations on the other side, simplifying the use of pre-existent statistical and graphical packages like BMDP and IBM's GDDM available at the installation site. A report is issued every six month on behalf of WHO, which presents time and geographical trends for various diseases.

QUALITY CONTROL IN CLINICAL PHYSIOLOGY LABORATORY

Sirkka Aunola and Vesa Kuusela
Rehabilitation Research Centre of the Social Insurance Institution
Peltolantie 3, SF-20720 Turku, Finland

Introduction

The development and specification of the interpretation of the physiological measurements has given rise to an increased use of some measures as diagnostic or screening instruments. This has brought up a requirement of higher standards. The recent development of the measurement equipment as well as the standardization of protocols present a solid basis for quality control procedures. Additionally, the advanced information systems make the data collection and analysis fairly easy.

However, there are many problems in the quality control in a physiological laboratory because there are several independent components causing variation in the measurements (e.g. Löllgen 1984). Some of the problems may be solved in case the components are identifiable and the data set is large enough.

Quality control system

The data collection is based on a standardized form in which most of the potential sources of variation are recorded (personnell, instruments, circumstances, protocols, co-operation, medication etc.). The data are stored in a cumulative data base. Preliminary checks are undertaken by a series of logical conditions between the measures.

The quality control analysis is done quarterly by standard statistical programs (BMDP, Dixon 1981). The focus is on the potential development of a trend. Additionally, the variation of the levels and variations of the results between nurses is monitored.

Results and discussion

Some results will be presented. Although experiences are still limited the system has already proved useful. For instance, in spirometric measurements there doesn't seem to be a significant trend nor seasonal variation (or any other kind of cyclic periodical variation). On the other hand, there seems to be a slight variation in the measurement levels between nurses.

References

Dixon WJ, ed. BMDP statistical software. Berkeley: University of California Press, 1981.
Löllgen H. Quality control and test criteria in ergometry. In: Löllgen H, Mellerowicz H, eds. Progress in ergometry: Quality control and test criteria. Berlin: Springer-Verlag, 1984:11-19.

EVALUATION OF THE PREDICTIVE VALUE OF NEUROLOGICAL CLINICAL SYMPTOMS AMONGST LOW-BIRTH-WEIGHT INFANTS FROM 3 TO 18 MONTHS OLD.

* J.B. GOUYON, ** N. DEBBAS, ** L. DUSSERRE, ** F. A. ALLAERT, * M. ALISON,
* J. L. NIVELON.
* Hôpital d'Enfants de Dijon (Pr M. ALISON - Pr J.L. NIVELON)
** Service d'Informatique Médicale (Pr DUSSERRE)

Boulevard Maréchal de Lattre de Tassigny 21034 DIJON CEDEX - FRANCE

Neuro-developmental outcome of very Low-Birth-Weight (<1500 g) infants has been widely described through highly specialized assessment scales. Nevertheless, these scales are difficult to use in the daily practice of general practitioners amongst the larger population of Low-Birth-Weight infants (<2500 g).

So we undertook a prospective neurological survey of L.B.W. infants including conventional items easily collected by general practitioners. The goals of the study were :
  1 - An appraisal of frequency of abnormal items to 3, 6, 9, 15-18 months of corrected chronological ages.
  2 - To pull out of 47 items the more reliable symptoms for early detection of neurological impairment.

The methodology of this study has been previously described (1). Neurological assessments were established by paediatricians and general practitioners. Data was available for 252, 203, 167, 86 infants respectively at 3,6, 9, 15-18 months of corrected chronological age. The more frequency abnormal items were :
  - 3 months : lack of any interest for adapted toys showed to the infant (15.3 %) ; infant does not watch his hand (11.6 %) and does not turn his head towards noises (11.6 %) On the whole, behavioral and tone abnormalities were respectively observed in 28.2 % and 19.5 % of the newborns.
  - 9 months : 10.3 % infants do not hold a sitting position and 23 % cannot stand up with support. Tone abnormalities : 13.8 %.
  - 15-18 months : 10.3 % cannot walk without help ; 21.1 % cannot pile up cubes.

CONCLUSION :

Some abnormal items are often significantly associated with others neurological abnormalities and have to be looked for with priority. The follow up to the study would permit us to precisely determine those which have the best predictive value for the ulterior neurological development of L.B.W. infants tonus.

REFERENCE :

1 - Gouyon JB, Allaert FA, Brichon P, Debbas N, Traore E, Dusserre L, Nivelon JL, Alison M. Psychomotric development of Low-Birth-Weight infants. Methods and preliminary results. In Third International Conference on System Science in health Care, Munich. Ed Van Eimeren W, Engelbrech R and Flagle ChD. Springer-Verlag Berlin Heidelberg New-York Tokyo. July 16-20 1984, 581-583.

DISCUSSION ON THE EXPERT CONSULTING PROGRAM OF THE GYNECOLOGICAL
DEPARTMENT OF TRADITIONAL CHINESE MEDICINE

Shi Cheng[1] and Liu Zhou-you[2]

[1]Gui Zhou Province Institute of Traditional Chinese Medicine,
Gui Yang Gui Zhou P.R.C.
[2]Gui Yang Medical College

This paper discusses the expert consulting program of the gynecological department of T.C.M. The consulting contents include treatment and diagnosis for menstruation and leukorrhea. The expert consulting program is written according to the clinical experience of Professor Liu Zhou-you in BASIC language. In this paper we simply introduce how to devise a mathematical model of T.C.M. The clinical information is collected using a symptom code. There are two output forms, one in Chinese and one in English (Latin). The output contents include the general rules of treatment, the medical formula, Chinese herbal medicine, acupuncture and moxibustion, order etc.

The program is composed of five files:1)Hello 2)English display (drage) 3)Chinese display (drage) 4) English display (acupuncture and moxibustion) 5) Chinese display (acupuncture and moxibustion).
The Chinese display needs a Chinese character generator.

In the mathematical model we choose the method of weight sum of small range, to decide the diagnosis. The weight and the lowest threshold are experimental value. For example the whole diagnostic scope in in menstruation is divided into ten parts:

1)Dysmenorrhea	2)Metrorrhogia
3)Hypermenorrhea	4)Hypomenorrhea
5)Advanced menstruation	6)Late menstruation
7)Irregular menstruation period	8)Amenia
9)Vicarious menstruation	10)Metroptosic

In every small range we can gain a maximum Pj.
Pj by the following expression:

$$P(Dj) = \sum Aibji \text{---(1)}$$

Where P(Dj) = the value of the possibility for the diagnosis of
Ai   = clinical symptom related to no i. The symptoms appear then $Ai=1$, if the symptoms disappear the $Ai=\theta$
Bji   = weight (the doctor's experience)

The program of the gynecological department of Traditional Chinese Medicine was welcomed by patients during three-year trial period.

AUTOMATICALLY CODED MEDICAL DATA FORMS

M. Madjarić and V. Lovrek

Clinical Hospital Centre, CZI, Šalata 2

41000 Zagreb, Yugoslavia

The majority of problems encountered in medical informatics, especially with respect to various modes of data entry, arises from specific nature of medical data. First of all, this applies to their scope, that is to number of attributes assignable to a patient. At the same time the number of pertinent data, that is of attributes providing relevant information is as a rule relatively small. In practice, this means that medical forms should provide a large number of questions, 80 to 90% of which will be answered negatively of will not be answered at all. And this is precisely the main problem attending the use of forms for medical data. Namely, the entire form must be entered into the computer regardless of the degree of completeness or the number of existing data. Since attributes are determined by their position on the form, the operator entering the data must seek the filled-in fields by counting or skipping empty fields, which is not only time consuming but also the source of a significant error rate.

In order to overcome this problem, the applicability of OSAK forms was investigated. OSAK is Croatian contraction standing for "automatically coded forms". The peculiarity of these forms is the provision of separate codes for all fields. Consequently, only filled-in fields neeed to be entered into the computer. The resultant saving in time and effort is by no means irrelevant: data entry by means of OSAK forms appears to be 3 do 5 times faster than entry from classical forms!

According to the experiances gained so far, the applicability of OSAK forms within the scope of medical informatics is manifold. First of all, mention should be made of their use in clinical departmental systems (CDS) for entering extracts from or entire medical records of in- and outpatients. Completing smaller forms of about one hundered attributes is a matter of several minutes, the more comprehensive documents requiring up to 10 minutes. Data entry likewise depends on the size of the form and the number of data supplied but it seldom takes more than 5 minutes to enter the longest documents (those containing over 700 attributes).

Medical research is another field of application of OSAK forms. Valuable experiance has been gained in occupational medicine where several dozen of different documents have been designed to meet the needs of different specialities, target groups and exposition factors.

OSAK forms have also been succesfully used in clinical research and in accounting applications in hospital institutions.

SCIENTIFIC-INFORMATION SECURING, PLANNING AND TAKING OF A

DECISION IN HUMAN MEMORY MODELLING

Simeon Jordanov MRCHEV
ul."Jordan Mishev" 21A , 8600 Jambol , BULGARIA

Procedure of the subsystem "Scientific-Information Supply".

⇓

Procedure of the subsystem "Planning of the Scientific Research".

⇓

Making the lists of:
- estimation factors;
- the experts, connected
  with the factors.

⇓

Making the matrix:
!!factor--estimation!!

⇓

Making the file of the experts answers: M x N ,
M - factors , N - experts.

⇓

Is the expert answer verbal ? —1→ The program "Text", estimating by fuzzy sets.

↓ 0

⇓

Are the experts signs freely graded ? —1→ Calculating the agreement coefficient at free grading of the signs (factors)

↓ 0

⇓

Calculating the agreement coefficient at classic grading of signs ⇒ Calculating the work-load coefficients of the experts and a choice of 10 experts with maximum coefficient

⇒

Printing the model of the system human memory i.e. the final order of the estimations.

∧

Determining the standartized average values of the factors.

∧

Calculating the weight of each expert (higher estimation accuracy).

∧

Determining the final order and number of the experts and estimations.

∧

Making the regression relation betwee the experts.

∧

Calculating the standardized dispersion value for each expert.

∧

A check for presence of hysteresis. Error estimation.

ECG DATA MANAGEMENT AND ANALYSIS IN THE
MONICA SURVEY AUGSBURG (WHO PROJECT)

S. Perz, S.J. Pöppl, J. Stieber

GSF-Medis-Institut

D-8042 München-Neuherberg, FRG

The electrocardiogram (ECG) is used for population studies, where a repeatable, valid and quantitative method is required for classification of ECG findings related to disease. Useful classification depends on standardized methods of data acquisition and data analysis.

Multinational monitoring of trends and determinants in cardiovascular disease (MONICA Project)

The main objective of the WHO Monica Project is to measure risk factor changes and incidence in cardiovascular disease at the same time in defined communities in different countries. In addition to the obligatory measurement of cardiovascular risk factors the WHO recommended also the recording of the resting ECG for surveys in the Monica project.

Monica survey Augsburg

The study area of the Monica Project Augsburg contains a population of about 530.000 people. To determine defined risk factor changes in age- and sex-subgroups 5312 men and women of the study area aged 25-64 were randomly selected.

Computerized ECG analysis

Within the survey 1984/1985 the resting ECG (twelve conventional leads) is taken using stand-alone ECG acquisition and analysis systems. Computerized ECG analysis is applied to improve data acquisition and reproducibility of both, ECG measurements and classification. The digitized ECG data and the results of the automatic ECG analysis, available within 1 1/2 minutes, are stored on floppy disk. For further statistical analysis codes are available with respect to the diagnostic statements. These results are also stored in a data base at the Medis computer center. Statistical analysis of the ECG data is performed including data of the other sections of the screening procedure (physical examination, interview, self-administered questionnaire, nutrition record.

Monitoring for the Health of Individuals Working in Industry and its Relationship to Their Environment

Knapp M.S., Knapp P.A., Webster C., Pearson K.

Varied problems, posed by a wide range of working environments and the range of established and potential hazards, sets problems when creating a computer-based monitoring system based on stereotyped formulated screens and on programmes that are difficult to change. Computer systems that provide the user with a range of options when introducing computing, and with the ability to rapidly change as the working environment changes, if new hazards are identified or when the law or government regulations change, are now available.

The needs of a range of industries were determined by a postal survey, and were then considered by this development team, which has had 6 years of experience of using a reconfigurable system, the CDS System, in different clinical situations. The development team worked with occupational hygenists, and staff with experience in several aspects of occupational medicine. The needs of this range of industries, with a range of occupational hazards, could mostly be met. The replacement of the paper record, with a computerised record, is a practical solution for many industrial situations, giving a high probability of improved surveillance and of environmental exposures being correctly identified and so limited, with a reduction in the morbidity and potentially in the mortality of staff. Computing can incorporate on-line monitoring using interactive computer graphics and statistical methods which automatically identify change points and, should either the environment or the health of workers change, permit the earlier detection of an occupational hazard.

The satisfactory resolution of some health monitoring incorporates three dimensional methods of graphic presentation which are now available.

Unit of Medical Information Technology, Obstetrics and Gynaecology, Queens Medical Centre., University of Nottingham and MedStat Ltd., Nottingham, U.K.

A KALMAN FILTER TECHNIQUE, GENERALIZED FROM RENAL TRANS-PLANTATION TO OTHER CLINICAL PROBLEMS

Knapp MS, Gordon K, Smith AFM and Pownall R.
Unit of Medical Information Technology
Department of Obstetrics and Gynaecology and the Department of
Mathematics, University of Nottingham.

Patients with Kidney disorders can be monitored prospectively using a computer program incorporating an adaptation of the multiprocess Kalman filter. This method was succesfully used to detect rejection in transplanted kidneys (British Medical Journal 1983. $\underline{286}$, 1695-1699). In order to develop the method for a range of other clinical monitoring, modifications and extensions to that methodology were needed. The method can now consider series with data provided at unequally spaced intervals, common in clinical work as there is often less frequent sampling when "risk" is considered to be low, and there are also "missing" values as a result of logistic or organisational problems. The method now also has the ability to consider other conventional time series models, other than the linear growth model previously reported, including quadratic, cubic growth and simple auto-regressive-moving average models.

A more varied selection of sudden changes can be monitored, many of which are more realistic in the biological situation, e.g. the effect of a drug given at a single time-point may cause a measurement to progressively diminsh or to increase. The new models enable one to detect the onset of an influence of the drug, they are also capable of distinguishing between several types of effect, such as a change in level or a change in direction of trend. The computer programmes written to utilise these procedures allow for user-induced interventions, whether additive or subtractive, such as dialysis-induced level changes common in the renal transplant situations. Many other features may be built in e.g. periodic waveforms. The models can be extended to handle several time-series at once for detection of more complex types of changes, helping to distinguish between transients that are errors of artefacts, and those that have a medical or biological significance.

A number of analyses of time-series, collected in a variety of clinical specialties, illustrate the range of the potential uses of the method now it has been modified.

Reference: Kidney International, Vol. 24 (1983), pp. 474-486. Mathematical and statistical aids to evaluate data from renal patients.

ON-LINE COMPUTING SYSTEM FOR THE DATA PROCESSING

OF CARDIOVASCULAR AND PULMONARY DYNAMICS

Valery M. Zaiko, Iosif M. Starobin, Alexander N. Sharikov
Department of Biomedical Informatics and Engineering,
Institute of Transplantology and Artificial Organs,
2/3 Pekhotnay Street, P.O. 123436, Moscow, U.S.S.R.

On line computing system is designed for the data processing and
identification of parametes of cardiovascular and pulmonary dynamics
and also for controlling the state of an organism during functional
investigations, cardiosurgery operations, transplantation of organs
and tissues and implantation of artificial organs.

The computing system consists of an "Electronic-60" Soviet microcomputer with peripheral input/output units and a "Salute" medical recording poligraph connected with a microcomputer by an analog-to-digital
converter. The system performs on-line analysis of the data to provide
immediate results which are displayed on a video monitor.

Aortal and venous pressure curves are recorded during cardiosurgery
operations and aortal, left ventricular and left atrium pressure curves and EKG are recorded during functional investigations of cardiovascular diseases with cardiac catherization.

Based on input information, the system also provides two types of data monitoring and identification. The first type is a calculation of
the main central hemodynamics parameters and the second type is a calculation of a large number of hemodynamic parameters intended for
diagnosis of some cardiosurgery deseases as well as for some research
areas.

The pulmonary computerized system is used for on-line estimation of
lung characteristics in the intensive care and cardiosurgery departments. Pulmonary parameter monitoring allows continous estimation of
the lung conditions during or after surgery. It is also possible to
use the system for functional lung investigation of patient with
other deseases.

MUMPS/FILE MANAGER/SNOMED-BASED COMPUTER PROGRAM FOR SURGICAL PATHOLOGIC SERVICES

K. Lauslahti, R. Karikoski-Leo and R. Aine
University Central Hospital of Tampere
Department of Pathology
Finland

The described data management system for surgical pathology services is located in the 1200-bed University Central Hospital of Tampere, Finland. The department of pathology serves over 37000 patients with 18000 tissue biopsies and 22000 cytological samples annually. Nearly 700 autopsies are performed per year. The system operates on a DEC PDP 11/23 computer and is programmed in MUMPS and File manager systems. The equipment consists of 2+2 disk bases (RL-02) with 10,4 megabytes each. All the data concerning patients, their hospital units, pathologists, special laboratory procedures (e.q. immunofluorescence studies, frozen section examinations, tissue frozen and stored), diagnoses and their comments are entered in on-line storage. All diagnostic data are coded via SNOMED. The data entry and retrieval are interactive through videoterminals.

The system has greatly increased the ease, speed and accuracy of responses to inquiries about the specimens. When needed the pathologist can get a printed list of previous specimens and their diagnoses concerning an individual patient under study. This information is receivable by identification of the patient or by the specimen number. Filesearching system is very flexible. It is possible to specify wanted retrieval groups of cases according to their SNOMED-codes (or by utilizing the hierarchial structure of SNOMED) or by a set of any combinations of variables used in the entry.

This data management system is used to (1) follow and (2) retrieve previous data of individual patients (for e.q. clinical meeting purposes), (3) searching spesific pathologic diagnoses for scientific work or education. (4) billing, and (5) monitoring the departmental activities.

"LARGE SCALE CONSUMERS" IN PATHOLOGY

R. Aine, R. Karikoski-Leo and K. Lauslahti
University Central Hospital of Tampere
Department of Pathology
Finland

The surgical pathologic and cytologic data of Tampere University
Central Hospital, Finland, were analyzed for evidence of variations
in the utilization of pathologic resources by the patients. The data
management system in this hospital with 1200 beds operates on a DEC
PDP 11/23 computer running on MUMPS and File manager systems. The
total number of patients in the files was 51139 and they had 91443
specimens of various types. 50 (0,01 %) patients with 15 or more
specimens were found. Median age of these was 67 yers (range 17-87)
and there was a predominance of men with a ratio of 2,4:1. These 50
patients had 942 specimens (0,01 %). The great majority of patients
were investigated for suspected lung disease. The majority of specimens were cytologic (73 %) and most of all sputum samples (33 %).
There were 244 (26 %) tissue biopsies. The final diagnosis was
revealed to be cancer in 26 (52 %) patients which included 12 lung
cancers, 3 urinary bladder cancers and 3 malignant lymphomas. We
conclude that the contribution of the pathologist may be essential
in diagnosing these patients with a large amount of specimens. Mis-
cellaneous clinical follow-up methods also increase the number of
specimens sent to the pathologist.

References:

Bohrod MG. What is a pathologic diagnosis? A prelude to computer
diagnosis.   Pathol Annu 1971; 6:197-208.

INDEX

Lecture Notes in Medical Informatics

Vol. 23: Selected Topics in Image Science. Edited by O. Nalcioglu and Z.-H. Cho. IX, 308 pages. 1984.

Vol. 24: Medical Informatics Europe 1984. Proceedings, 1984. Edited by F.H. Roger, J.L. Willems, R. O'Moore and B. Barber. XXVII, 778 pages. 1984.

Vol. 25: Medical Informatics Europe 1985. Edited by F.H. Roger, P. Grönroos, R. Tervo-Pellikka and R. O'Moore. XVII, 823 pages. 1985.

Lecture Notes in Medical Informatics